GLOSSARY OF BIOTECHNOLOGY AND NANOBIOTECHNOLOGY TERMS

FOURTH EDITION

GLOSSARY OF BIOTECHNOLOGY AND NANOBIOTECHNOLOGY TERMS

FOURTH EDITION

KIMBALL NILL

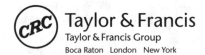

Taylor & Francis
Taylor & Francis Group
Boca Raton London New York

A CRC title, part of the Taylor & Francis imprint, a member of the
Taylor & Francis Group, the academic division of T&F Informa plc.

Published in 2006 by
CRC Press
Taylor & Francis Group
6000 Broken Sound Parkway NW, Suite 300
Boca Raton, FL 33487-2742

International Standard Book Number-10: 0-8493-6609-7 (Hardcover)
International Standard Book Number-13: 978-0-8493-6609-3 (Hardcover)
Library of Congress Card Number 2005051082

Library of Congress Cataloging-in-Publication Data

Nill, Kimball R.
  Glossary of biotechnology and nanobiotechnology terms / Kimball R. Nill.-- 4th ed.
    p. cm.
  ISBN 0-8493-6609-7 (alk. paper)
  1. Biotechnology--Dictionaries. I. Title.

TP248.16.F54 2005
660.6'03--dc22   2005051082

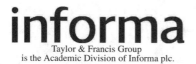

Taylor & Francis Group
is the Academic Division of Informa plc.

Visit the Taylor & Francis Web site at
http://www.taylorandfrancis.com

and the CRC Press Web site at
http://www.crcpress.com

Dedication

To my wife, Janet J. Nill

Preface

I began writing this book as a hobby, more than a decade ago, when it became obvious to me that the various specialists working in the then-emerging field of biotechnology (e.g., geneticists, chemists, molecular biologists, intellectual property attorneys, marketers, etc.) were often having difficulty simply understanding the terms utilized by their colleagues in their respective fields.

Subsequently, a number of organizations with various motivations have stated their concerns about agricultural biotechnology. In my experience, the level of concern inevitably diminishes when such people understand the terms used to discuss a given topic.

Therefore, when similar organizations recently began to assert safety concerns about the now-emerging field of nanotechnology, I added to this book those of the "nanotech" terms that are relevant to biotechnology.

I have attempted to write definitions in this book employing words that would enable the reader to conceptualize the idea embodied in the term, without the necessity of holding advanced degrees in biochemistry or molecular biology. In order to accomplish this, however, I had to make certain compromises between scientific rigor and definitions based on analogy, with the inherent possibility of oversimplification.

I offer this work in good faith, and in the hope that it will assist individuals who seek to gain some understanding of the terminology as it is currently used. However, the reader should be aware that the fields of biotechnology and bionanotechnology are rapidly expanding and evolving: New terms are entering the nomenclature at a rapid pace. In fact, the meaning(s) of some of the newest terms will undoubtedly be expanded or contracted as the technologies further develop. Although I have endeavored to be as accurate as possible, this work is meant to provide a general introduction rather than to be absolute and legally definitive.

Kimball R. Nill
Technical Issues Director
American Soybean Association
St. Louis, Missouri

About the Author

Kimball Nill is Technical Issues Director of the American Soybean Association's International Marketing Division, and is responsible for detecting emerging technology-related issues that could impact U.S. soybean exports and proactively dealing with those threats and opportunities.

Mr. Nill holds a bachelor's degree in chemistry from North Dakota State University and a master's degree in business administration from the Wharton Business School at the University of Pennsylvania. He has authored numerous papers and articles on various aspects of the marketing of agricultural biotechnology products for U.S. and European journals and other publications.

Prior to joining the ASA in 1996, Mr. Nill was International Marketing Manager for Moorman's Inc., an Illinois-based manufacturer of soy-based livestock nutrition products. Before that, he spent five years in positions supporting in-house venture capital and biotechnology research activities in a major biotechnology company.

Mr. Nill grew up on a farm in North Dakota. He is a member of the American Chemical Society, the Licensing Executives Society, and the American Association for the Advancement of Science.

A-DNA A particular right-handed helical form of DNA (possessing 11 base pairs per turn), which is the form that DNA molecules exist in when they are partially dehydrated. A-form DNA is found in fibers at 75% relative humidity and requires the presence of sodium, potassium, or cesium as the counterion. Instead of lying flat, the bases are tilted with respect to the helical axis, and there are more base pairs per turn. The A-form is biologically interesting because it is probably very close to the conformation adopted by DNA–RNA hybrids or by RNA–RNA double-stranded regions. The reason is that the presence of the 2^2 hydroxyl group prevents RNA from lying in the B-form.
See also B-DNA, DNA–RNA HYBRID, DEOXYRIBONUCLEIC ACID (DNA), BASE PAIR (bp)

A_w See WATER ACTIVITY (A_w)

aAI-1 See ALPHA AMYLASE INHIBITOR-1

***ab initio* Gene Prediction** (*ab initio* = "from the beginning")
The prediction of a gene's (exon) structure via algorithms (e.g., in a bioinformatics computer), based on the protein coded for by the gene.
See also GENE, PROTEIN, EXON, ALGORITHM (IN BIOINFORMATICS), SEQUENCE (OF A DNA MOLECULE), SEQUENCE (OF A PROTEIN MOLECULE)

ABC See ASSOCIATION OF BIOTECHNOLOGY COMPANIES (ABC)

ABC Transport Proteins See ABC TRANSPORTERS

ABC Transporters Refers to a class of **membrane transporter proteins** that "transfer" the following across cell membranes:

- Sugar molecules (used by cells as "fuel")
- Inorganic ions (needed to catalyze certain cellular processes)
- Polypeptides (i.e., protein molecules)
- Certain anticancer drugs (thereby making it harder to halt certain cancer tumors via use of pharmaceuticals)
- Certain antibiotics (thereby conferring **antibiotic resistance** on some pathogenic bacteria)

ABC transporter molecules are embedded in the plasma membrane (i.e., surface "skin") of cells.
See also CELL, PLASMA MEMBRANE, PROTEIN, CATALYST, ION, POLYPEPTIDE (PROTEIN), CANCER, CHEMOTHERAPY, ANTIBIOTIC RESISTANCE

Abiogenesis Spontaneous generation.
See also BIOGENESIS

Abiotic Absence of living organisms.
See also ABIOTIC STRESSES

Abiotic Stresses The stress caused (e.g., to crop plants) by nonliving, environmental factors such as cold, drought, flooding, salinity, ozone, toxic-to-that-organism metals (e.g., aluminum, for plants), and ultraviolet-B light.
See also CITRATE SYNTHASE (CSB) GENE

Abrin A toxin derived from the seed of the rosary pea.
See also RICIN, PHYTOCHEMICALS, TOXIN

Abscisic Acid A phytohormone (plant hormone) utilized to control the following:

- The size of **stomatal pores** — i.e., the openings in leaves through which plants exchange oxygen and carbon dioxide (and, inadvertently, water) with the atmosphere
- Abscission (e.g., shedding of flowers, fruit, etc.)
- Dormancy

See also PLANT HORMONE, GPA1

Absolute Configuration The configuration of four different substituent groups around an asymmetric carbon atom, in relation to D- and L-glyceraldehyde.

See also DEXTROROTARY (D) ISOMER, LEVOROTARY (L) ISOMER

Absorbance (A) A measure of the amount of light absorbed by a substance suspended in a matrix. The matrix may be gaseous, liquid, or solid in nature. Most biologically active compounds (e.g., proteins) absorb light in the ultraviolet (UV) or visible light portion of the spectrum. Absorbance is used to quantitate (measure) the concentration of the substance in question (e.g., a substance dissolved in a liquid).

See also OPTICAL DENSITY (OD), SPECTROPHOTOMETER

Absorption From the Latin *ab* = "away" and *sorbere* = "to suck into."

The taking up of nutrients, water, etc., by assimilation (e.g., transport of the products of digestion from the intestinal tract across the cell membranes from the gut and into the blood).

See also ADME TESTS, DIGESTION (WITHIN ORGANISMS)

Abzymes Catalytic antibodies that are synthetic constructs. They either stabilize the transition state of a chemical reaction or bind to a specific substrate, thereby increasing the reaction rate of the reaction.

See also CATALYTIC ANTIBODY, TRANSITION STATE, SUBSTRATE (CHEMICAL)

Ac-CoA Abbreviation for **acetyl-coenzyme A**. Ac-CoA is a chemical that is synthesized in cell mitochondria by combining the thiol (molecular group) of coenzyme A with an **acetyl group** (i.e., from breakdown or digestion of fats, carbohydrates, or proteins).

See also COENZYME, COENZYME A, FATS, ACETYLCHOLINE, LUCONEOGENESIS, ACETYL-CoA CARBOXYLASE, CHOLINESTERASE, CELL, MITOCHONDRIA, FATS, PROTEIN

Ac-P Acetylphosphate.

ACC Abbreviation/acronym for the compound 1-aminocyclopropane-1-carboxylic acid, which is produced from *S*-adenosylmethionine (SAM) in the fruit of certain plants. When the "sam-k" gene is inserted into the genome of these plants, the level of SAM is greatly reduced in their fruit, which inhibits (slows) ripening or softening of the fruit via a reduction or slowdown in the production of ethylene (the hormone that causes fruit to ripen or soften).

See also ACC SYNTHASE, ETHYLENE, SAM-K GENE, GENETIC ENGINEERING, GENOME, PLANT HORMONE

ACC Synthase Aminocyclopropane carboxylic acid synthase/deaminase; it is one of the most critical enzymes in the metabolic pathway and creates the hormone ethylene inside fruit. Because ethylene causes certain fruits (e.g., tomatoes) to ripen (soften), it is possible to significantly delay the softening (i.e., spoilage) process by controlling the creation of ACC synthase via manipulation of the ACC synthase gene.

See also ACC, METABOLISM, ENZYME, METABOLITE, INTERMEDIARY METABOLISM, PATHWAY, PLANT HORMONE, POLYGALACTURONASE (PG), ETHYLENE, SAM-K GENE

ACCase See ACETYL-CoA CARBOXYLASE

Acceptor Control The regulation of the rate of respiration by the availability of ADP as phosphate acceptor.

See also RESPIRATION, ADENOSINE DIPHOSPHATE (ADP)

Acceptor Junction Site The junction between the right 3 end of an intron and the left 5 end of an exon.

See also INTRON, EXON

Accession (germplasm) The addition of germplasm deposits to existing germplasm storage banks.

See also AMERICAN TYPE CULTURE COLLECTION (ATCC), GERMPLASM

Accession (sequence data) The addition (e.g., to a major public database) of the sequence data for a newly determined gene or protein molecule.

See also GENE, PROTEIN, SEQUENCE (OF A DNA MOLECULE), SEQUENCE (OF A PROTEIN MOLECULE), ALGORITHM (IN BIOINFORMATICS)

Acclimatization The biological process whereby an organism adapts to a new environment. For example, the body of a mountain climber who has spent a significant time high up on Mount Everest (e.g., 20,000 ft above sea level) produces twice as many red blood cells (to transport oxygen) than at sea level.

Often, this adaptation actually occurs at a molecular level. One example is when natural microorganisms adapt so that they feed on and degrade toxic chemical wastes; or change from using one sugar as a fuel source to another.
See also SUGAR MOLECULES, CATABO-LISM, RED BLOOD CELLS, COLD HARD-ENING, PHARMACOENVIROGENETICS

ACE Angiotensin-converting enzyme. It is an enzyme that is crucial (within the human vascular system) for catalyzing the formation of angiotensin, a hormone that causes narrowing/restriction of blood vessels; this increases the body's blood pressure as the blood is "squeezed" through these narrowed blood vessels.
The action of ACE can be inhibited by the pharmaceuticals known as ACE inhibitors. Research indicates that consumption of whey protein can also result in inhibition of ACE.
See also ENZYME, HORMONE, ACE INHIB-ITORS

ACE Inhibitors A "family" of chemically similar pharmaceuticals utilized to lower blood pressure in humans by blocking the formation of a hormone (angiotensin) that narrows/restricts blood vessels.
See also ACE

Acetobacter aceti A bacterium that can "spoil" alcohol-containing beverages by turning the ethanol into vinegar (acetic acid). Discovered by Louis Pasteur during the 1800s.
See also BACTERIA

Acetolactate Synthase See ALS

Acetyl Carnitine One of the metabolites of mitochondria, it is a substrate (i.e., substance that is acted upon) for acylcarnitine transferase (which converts the acetyl carnitine to carnitine).
Research indicates that consumption of acetyl carnitine helps to increase the levels of acetylcholine and nerve growth factor (NGF) in the brain.
See also METABOLITE, MITOCHONDRIA, ACYLCARNITINE TRANSFERASE, SUB-STRATE (CHEMICAL), CARNITINE, ACE-TYLCHOLINE, NERVE GROWTH FAC-TOR (NGF)

Acetyl-Coenzyme A See Ac-CoA

Acetyl-CoA Acetyl-coenzyme A.
See Ac-CoA

Acetyl-CoA Carboxylase An enzyme that catalyzes the chemical reaction (i.e., conversion of Ac-CoA to malonyl CoA via carboxylation), which is the first step in the series of chemical reactions through which some plants "manufacture" oils (e.g., soybean oil, canola oil, etc.).
See also ENZYME, FATS, SOYBEAN OIL, CANOLA

Acetylation See HISTONES, POSTTRANS-LATIONAL MODIFICATION OF PROTEIN

Acetylcholine A neurotransmitter (i.e., one of several relatively small, diffusible molecules utilized by the human body to "transmit" nerve impulses) that is synthesized (i.e., manufactured) near the ends of axons (i.e., one type of neuron). That synthesis is accomplished by the "transfer" of an acetyl group (portion of molecule) from Ac-CoA to a choline molecule (that is available in the body via consumption of soybean lecithin or certain other foods) in a chemical reaction catalyzed by cholinesterase.
Research indicates that consumption of a chemical compound known as **Huperzine A**, which is extracted from the Chinese club moss (*Huperzia serrata*), inhibits the enzyme that breaks down acetylcholine molecules within the human body.
Increased amounts of acetylcholine in the (human) brain has been shown to reduce the symptoms of Alzheimer's disease.
See also NEUROTRANSMITTER, NEURON, CHOLINE, Ac-CoA, LECITHIN, ALZHEI-MER'S DISEASE, THYMUS, ENZYME, CHOLINESTERASE, ENDOTHELIAL NITRIC OXIDE SYNTHASE (eNOS)

Acetylcholinesterase An enzyme that hydrolyzes (i.e., cuts into smaller pieces) molecules of the neurotransmitter acetylcholine after they have accomplished "transmission" of a nerve impulse. The hydrolysis serves to prepare the neurons (cells of the body's nervous system) for the transmission of new nerve impulses.
See also ENZYME, HYDROLYSIS, NEU-ROTRANSMITTER, ACETYLCHOLINE, NEURON

Acid A substance that contains hydrogen atoms in its molecular structure, with a pH in the range from 0 to 6, which can react with a base to form a salt. Acids normally taste sour

and feel slippery. For example, food product manufacturers often add citric acid, malic acid, fumaric acid, and itaconic acid in order to impart a "sharp" taste to food products.
See also BASE, CITRIC ACID, FUMARIC ACID ($C_4H_4O_4$)

Acidic Fibroblast Growth Factor (AFGF) See FIBROBLAST GROWTH FACTOR (FGF)

Acidosis A metabolic condition in which the capacity of the body to buffer changes in pH is diminished. Hence, acidosis is accompanied by decreased blood pH (i.e., the blood becomes more acidic than is normal).

ACP (Acyl Carrier Protein) A protein that binds acyl intermediates during the formation of long-chain fatty acids. ACP is important in that it is involved in every step of fatty acid synthesis.
See also FATTY ACID, ACYL-CoA, FATS

Acquired Immune Deficiency Syndrome (AIDS) A disease in which a specific virus attacks and kills macrophages and helper T cells (thus causing collapse of the entire immune system). Once the immune system has been inactivated, other diseases that under normal circumstances would have been overcome by the body, become fatal.
See also HUMAN IMMUNODEFICIENCY VIRUS TYPE 1 (HIV-1), HUMAN IMMUNODEFICIENCY VIRUS TYPE 2 (HIV-2), HELPER T CELLS (T4 CELLS), MACROPHAGE, TUMOR NECROSIS FACTOR (TNF)

Acquired Mutation A genetic change (i.e., mutation in DNA) that occurs within a somatic cell (i.e., cell **not** involved in the organism's reproduction), the mutation is, therefore, not passed down to subsequent generations.
See also SOMATIC CELLS, MUTATION, SOMATIC VARIANTS, CELL, ORGANISM, DEOXYRIBONUCLEIC ACID (DNA)

Acrylamide Gel See POLYACRYLAMIDE GELS

ACTH (Adrenocorticotropic Hormone [Corticotropin]) A polypeptide secreted by the anterior lobe of the pituitary gland. This is an example of a protein hormone.
See also POLYPEPTIDE (PROTEIN), ENDOCRINE GLANDS, ENDOCRINE HORMONES

Actin A contractile (i.e., periodically contracting) protein that is present within — or as part of the exterior — of eucaryotic cells. Via its contractions, actin is involved in the following actions of eucaryote cells:

- Movement (e.g., when it "pulls" the cell to a new position) within the body, much like a towrope. The "towrope" utilized is a long narrow structure extending from the exterior of cell, and is called a **filopodia**; it is composed of actin surrounded by a layer of the cell's plasma membrane.
- Separation of nuclear DNA during meiosis (dividing in two; a reproductive step in the life of a cell).

Actin analogues present in bacterial cells include **ParM, which separates DNA plasmids during meiosis, and MreB, which are located just beneath the outer membrane and determine cell shape in rod-shaped bacteria**.
See also CELL, PROTEIN, EUCARYOTE, DEOXYRIBONUCLEIC ACID (DNA), NUCLEAR DNA, MEIOSIS, CYTOSKELETON, ANALOGUE, BACTERIA, PLASMA MEMBRANE, MOTOR PROTEINS, CELL MOTILITY, *LISTERIA MONOCYTOGENES*, CHEMOTAXIS, MreB, ParM

Activation Energy The amount of energy (calories) required to bring all the molecules in one mole of a reacting substance to the transition state. More simply, it may also be viewed as the energy required to bring reacting molecules to a certain energy state from which point the reaction proceeds spontaneously.
See also TRANSITION STATE (IN A CHEMICAL REACTION), MOLE, FREE ENERGY

Activator (of enzyme) A small molecule that stimulates (increases) an enzyme's catalytic activity when it binds to an allosteric site.
See also ENZYME, EFFECTOR, ALLOSTERIC SITE, CATALYST

Activator (of gene) A protein molecule that increases the expression of a given gene by binding to transcription control sites (e.g., within that gene or in an adjacent intron).

See also PROTEIN, GENE, EXPRESSIVITY, TRANSCRIPTION ACTIVATORS, SIGNAL TRANSDUCERS AND ACTIVATORS OF TRANSCRIPTION (STATs), TRANSCRIPTION FACTORS, INTRON

Active Site The region of an enzyme surface that binds the substrate molecule and transforms the substrate molecule into the new (chemical) product (entity). This site is usually located not on a protruding portion of the enzyme but, rather, in a cleft or depression. This establishes a controlled environment in which the chemical reaction may occur.

See also CATALYTIC SITE, AGONISTS, PHARMACOPHORE, SUBSTRATE (CHEMICAL), ENZYME, ANTAGONISTS

Active Transport Cell-mediated, energy-requiring translocation of a molecule across a membrane in the direction of increasing concentration (i.e., opposite of the natural tendency). This is done via special membrane-bound proteins (i.e., protein molecules embedded in the cell's plasma membrane).

See also OSMOTIC PRESSURE, CELL, PROTEIN, PLASMA MEMBRANE, ION CHANNELS, G-PROTEINS, MEMBRANE TRANSPORT

Activity Coefficient The factor by which the concentration of a solute must be multiplied to give its true thermodynamic activity.

Activity-Based Screening See HIGH-THROUGHPUT SCREENING (HTS)

Acuron™ Gene A gene, trademarked by Syngenta AG, that can be inserted into plants via genetic engineering techniques. When this gene is inserted into the genome (DNA) of a plant, it confers tolerance to those herbicides whose active ingredient is a protoporphyrinogen oxidase inhibitor (therefore, such herbicides are known as PPO INHIBITORS).

See also HERBICIDE-TOLERANT CROP, GENE, GENETIC ENGINEERING, GENOME, DEOXYRIBONUCLEIC ACID (DNA)

Acute Transfection Short-term infection of cells with DNA.

Acyl-CoA Acyl derivatives of coenzyme A (acyl-S-CoA).

See also CARNITINE, COENZYME A, TRYPSIN INHIBITORS

Acylcarnitine Transferase An enzyme that converts the mitochondrial metabolite **acetyl carnitine** into carnitine.

See also ENZYME, ACETYL CARNITINE, CARNITINE

AD An acronym utilized to refer to the group of diseases known collectively as **autoimmune disorders.** These include diseases such as multiple sclerosis, lupus, rheumatoid arthritis, etc.

See also AUTOIMMUNE DISEASE, MULTIPLE SCLEROSIS, LUPUS

Adalimumab A monoclonal antibody approved by the U.S. Food and Drug Administration (FDA) in 2003 for use as a pharmaceutical treatment to inhibit the structural damage (to body joints) in the autoimmune disease rheumatoid arthritis.

Adalimumab specifically blocks tumor necrosis factor-α.

See also RHEUMATOID ARTHRITIS, AUTOIMMUNE DISEASE, FOOD AND DRUG ADMINISTRATION (FDA), MONOCLONAL ANTIBODIES (MAb), TUMOR NECROSIS FACTOR (TNF), PHAGE DISPLAY

Adaptation Refers to the "adjustment" of a **population** of organisms to a changed environment.

For example, when the Industrial Revolution caused large amounts of black soot to be deposited on the white bark of certain trees in England during the 19th century, it resulted in adaptation (via selective breeding) of the **population of a particular indigenous moth (*Biston betularia*), which consisted of a mixture of all-white and all-black members**. Because the soot blackened the formerly white bark of the trees that these moths rested on, predatory birds were able to easily catch and eat the all-white members of the moth population. Thus, there were fewer of the all-white moths present in the breeding population and a greater preponderance of all-black members.

During the 20th century, antipollution efforts in England resulted in a cessation of the release of airborne soot, so that the tree bark regained its original white color. Because the predatory birds were now able to more easily catch and eat the all-black members of the moth population, there were fewer of the all-black moths

A

present in the breeding population and a greater preponderance of all-white members.
See also ORGANISM

Adaptive Enzymes See INDUCIBLE ENZYMES

ADBF See AZUROPHIL-DERIVED BACTE-RICIDAL FACTOR (ADBF)

Additive Genes Genes that interact but do not show dominance (in the case of alleles) or epistasis (if they are not alleles).

A single additive gene does not "show up" in the phenotype, but a **collective group** of additive genes can result in a trait that is evident in the phenotype.
See also GENE, ALLELE, DOMINANT ALLELE, EPISTASIS, PHENOTYPE, TRAIT, ADDITIVE VARIANCE

Additive Variance Refers to the amount or percentage of an organism's genetic variance that results from a single given **additive gene**.
See also GENE, GENETICS, ADDITIVE GENES

Adenine A purine base, 6-aminopurine that occurs in ribonucleic acid (RNA) as well as in deoxyribonucleic acid (DNA) and is a component of adenosine diphosphate (ADP) and adenosine triphosphate (ATP). Adenine pairs with thymine in DNA and with uracil in RNA.
See also BASE (NUCLEOTIDE), BASE PAIR (bp), RIBONUCLEIC ACID (RNA), DEOXYRIBONUCLEIC ACID (DNA)

Adenosine Refers to the **nucleoside** (i.e., hybrid-with-ribose or -deoxyribose) **form** of adenine.
See also ADENINE, NUCLEOSIDE

Adenosine Diphosphate (ADP) A ribonucleoside 5-diphosphate serving as phosphate-group acceptor in the cell energy cycle.
See also CATABOLISM, ADENOSINE TRIPHOSPHATE (ATP), ADENOSINE MONOPHOSPHATE (AMP)

Adenosine Monophosphate (AMP) A ribonucleoside 5-monophosphate that is formed by hydrolysis of ATP or ADP.
See also HYDROLYSIS, ADENOSINE DIPHOSPHATE (ADP), ADENOSINE TRIPHOSPHATE (ATP)

Adenosine Triphosphate (ATP) The major carrier of chemical energy in the cells of all living things. It is ribonucleoside 5-triphosphate, functioning as a phosphate-group donor in the energy cycle of the cell. ATP contains three phosphate/oxygen molecules linked together. When a phosphate–phosphate bond in ATP is broken (hydrolyzed), energy that the cell can use to carry out its functions is produced. Thus, ATP serves as the universal medium of biological energy storage and exchange in living cells.
See also ATPase, ATP SYNTHETASE, HYDROLYSIS, CYCLIC PHOTOPHOS-PHORYLATION, BIOLUMINESCENCE, ATP SYNTHASE, ADENOSINE MONO-PHOSPHATE (AMP), UBIQUINONE

Adenovirus A type of virus that can infect humans. Like all viruses, it can reproduce only inside living cells (of host organisms). The adenovirus causes a protein (metabolite) to be made that disables the p53 gene. Because the p53 gene then cannot perform its usual function (i.e., prevention of uncontrolled cell growth caused by virus/DNA damage), the adenovirus "takes over" and causes the cell to make numerous copies of itself until the cell dies (thus, releasing the virus copies into the body of the host organism to cause further infection).
See also VIRUS, RETROVIRUSES, GENE DELIVERY, GENE THERAPY, CELL, PROTEIN, p53 GENE, DEOXYRIBONUCLEIC ACID (DNA)

Adenylate Cyclase The enzyme (within cells) that catalyzes the synthesis (i.e., "manufacture") of cyclic AMP.
See also CYCLIC AMP

Adequate Intake (AI) See CHOLINE

Adhesion Molecule From the Latin *adhaerere, meaning* "to stick to."

The term **adhesion molecule** refers to a glycoprotein molecular "chain" that protrudes from the surface membrane of certain cells and causes cells (possessing "matching" adhesion molecules) to adhere to each other. For example, in 1952, Aaron Moscona observed that (**harvesting enzyme-separated**) chicken embryo cells did not remain separated but, instead, coalesced again into an (embryo) aggregate. In 1955, Philip Townes and Johannes Holtfreter showed that "like" amphibian (e.g., frog) neuron cells will rejoin after being physically separated (e.g., with a knife blade), but "unlike" cells remain segregated (apart).

Adhesion molecules also play a crucial role in guiding monocytes to sites of infection (i.e., pathogens) because adhesion molecules in the walls of blood vessels (after activation caused by pathogen invasion of adjacent tissue) adhere to like adhesion molecules in the membranes of monocytes in the blood. The monocytes pass through the blood vessel walls, become macrophages, and fight the infection (thus, triggering tissue inflammation, etc.).

See also MONOCYTES, MACROPHAGE, POLYPEPTIDE (PROTEIN), CELL, PATHOGEN, CD4 PROTEIN, CD44 PROTEIN, GP120 PROTEIN, VAGINOSIS, HARVESTING ENZYMES, HARVESTING, SIGNAL TRANSDUCTION, SELECTINS, LECTINS, GLYCOPROTEINS, SUGAR MOLECULES, LEUKOCYTES, LYMPHOCYTES, NEUTROPHILS, ENDOTHELIUM, ENDOTHELIAL CELLS, P-SELECTIN, ELAM-1, INTEGRINS, CYTOKINES

Adhesion Protein See ADHESION MOLECULE, ENDOTHELIAL CELLS

Adipocytes Specialized cells within an organism's lymphatic system that store the triacylglycerols (sometimes also called "triglycerides") after the digestion of these fats and later release fatty acids and glycerol into the bloodstream (e.g., when needed by the organism).

See also CELL, TRIGLYCERIDES, FATTY ACID, DIGESTION (WITHIN ORGANISM), FATS

Adipocytokines See ADIPOKINES

Adipokines Refers to hormones that are synthesized by adipose cells, and that act to help the body regulate its metabolism, homeostasis, etc.

See also HORMONE, CELL, ADIPOSE, METABOLISM, HOMEOSTASIS, VISFATIN, LEPTIN, TUMOR NECROSIS FACTOR-α RESISTIN, ADIPONECTIN, INTERLEUKIN-6

Adiponectin An adipokine that activates AMP-activated protein kinase (AMPK) and modulates signaling pathways controlled by NFκB.

See also ADIPOKINES, AMP, PROTEIN, KINASES, SIGNALING, PATHWAY, NFκB

Adipose The term is utilized to refer to the **"energy storage" tissues** within some animals, consisting of fat molecules. Adipose

tissue tends to increase in animals' bodies if they consume more energy-dense food than needed for their level of energy expenditure (e.g., via exercise).

In humans older than 40, an increase in the body's amount of adipose tissue is correlated with an increased risk of premature death (e.g., from coronary heart disease).

Adipose tissue cells secrete a large number of compounds that impact the human body in a number of ways. For example:

- Leptin — a protein hormone signal to the brain that the body has "enough" energy stores and that also stimulates the body to consume calories faster.
- Visfatin — a protein that has some of the same effects as insulin (e.g., stimulates glucose uptake by the body, which lowers blood sugar levels, etc.).
- Tumor Necrosis Factor-α (TNF-α) — a cytokine protein that initiates the changes (inflammation) in vascular tissues that result in monocytes adhering to the internal walls of blood vessels, thereby becoming a macrophage and resulting in the formation of a plaque deposit. Additionally and separately, TNF-α can also cause some tissues to become insulin resistant.
- Angiotensin — a precursor molecule, which can become **angiotensin II** in the body. The hormone angiotensin II causes arteries to constrict (which can result in high blood pressure), promotes macrophage accumulation in plaque deposits on blood vessel walls, and enhances the metabolism of nitric oxide into free radical molecules.
- Adiponectin — a molecule that acts to inhibit both the development of insulin resistance in tissues and inflammation.

See also FATS, CORONARY HEART DISEASE (CHD), LEPTIN, LECITHIN, CHOLINE, VISFATIN, INSULIN, CYTOKINES,

MONOCYTES, ADHESION MOLECULE, MACROPHAGE, PLAQUE, METABO-LISM, NITRIC OXIDE, FREE RADICAL

Adipose Triglyceride Lipase See LIPASE

Adjuvant (to a herbicide) Any compound that enhances the effectiveness (i.e., weed-killing ability) of a given herbicide. For example, adjuvants such as surfactants can be mixed (prior to application to weeds) with herbicide (in water) in order to hasten transport of the herbicide's active ingredient into the weed plant. This is necessary because the herbicide must move from an aqueous (water) environment into one comprised of lipids/lipophilic molecules (i.e., the weed's cuticle or "skin") before it can accomplish its task.

See also SURFACTANT, LIPIDS, LIPO-PHILIC

Adjuvant (to a pharmaceutical) Any compound that enhances the desired response of the body to that pharmaceutical. For example, adjuvants such as certain polysaccharides or surface-modified diamond nanoparticles can be injected along with (vaccine) antigen in order to increase the immune response (e.g., production of antibodies) to a given antigen.

Another example is that consumption of grapefruit juice by humans will increase the impact of certain pharmaceuticals. These pharmaceuticals include some sedatives, antihypertensives, the antihistamine terfenadine, and the immunosuppressant cyclosporine. The adjuvant effect of grapefruit juice is thought to be caused via inhibition of the enzyme cytochrome P450 3A4, which catalyzes the reactions involved in the metabolism (breakdown) of these pharmaceuticals.

Yet another example is that consumption of the pharmaceutical known as clopidogrel (U.S. commercial name is Plavix) by people immediately following a mild heart attack — along with aspirin — greatly reduces the risk of death, strokes, and (new, additional) heart attacks vs. taking aspirin alone after a mild heart attack.

See also CELLULAR IMMUNE RESPONSE, HUMORAL IMMUNITY, POLYSACCHA-RIDES, NANOTECHNOLOGY, ANTIGEN, ANTIBODY, ENZYME, METABOLISM, HISTAMINE, CYCLOSPORINE, CYTO-CHROME P450 3A4

ADME Acronym for absorption, distribution (within the body), metabolism, and elimination of pharmaceuticals.

See also ADME TESTS, *IN SILICO* SCREEN-ING

ADME Tests Refers to the absorption, distribution (within the body), metabolism, and elimination tests historically required by the U.S. Food and Drug Administration (FDA) for approval of new pharmaceuticals or some new food ingredients.

Today, companies (e.g., pharmaceutical companies) perform such tests at earlier stages in their screening and assessments of new compounds, so that they can halt work on any compounds that are shown to be problematic. To assess the **absorption** of a new pharmaceutical (candidate compound), scientists can test its permeability through an artificial membrane (e.g., hexadecane), its permeability through artificial lipid membranes, and its transport through a single layer of Caco-2 cells (in a cell culture vessel). Because such cultured Caco-2 cells act very much like human intestinal mucosa cells, these tests provide a good prediction of the pharmaceutical's active transport, passive transport, and also its receptor-mediated efflux. **Distribution**, which is related to bioavailability, is closely associated with a compound's solubility (in body fluids) and its ability to be "bound" by plasma proteins. Thus, distribution (e.g., of a pharmaceutical compound) is assessed via a test to determine plasma protein binding (PPB). **Metabolism** can sometimes lead to toxicity. For example, in people whose bodies cannot degrade pyrimidines, the (pyrimidine) metabolites of the anticancer drug 5-fluorouracil can build up to lethal levels.

See also FOOD AND DRUG ADMINISTRA-TION (FDA), ABSORPTION, CACO-2, PLASMA, CELL CULTURE, RECEPTORS, ACTIVE TRANSPORT, PASSIVE TRANS-PORT, MEMBRANE TRANSPORT, PRO-TEIN, METABOLISM, INTERMEDIARY METABOLISM, METABOLITE, PHARMA-COKINETICS, PHARMACOGENOMICS, CODEX ALIMENTARIUS COMMISSION, ADME, ADMET, HAPLOTYPE, ADME/Tox, *IN SILICO SCREENING*

ADME/Tox Refers to tests of the absorption, distribution (within the body), metabolism, elimination, and toxicity of a given compound (e.g., a pharmaceutical candidate).

To assess the **absorption** of a new pharmaceutical (candidate compound), scientists can test its permeability through an artificial membrane (e.g., hexadecane), its permeability through artificial lipid membranes, and/or its transport through a single layer of Caco-2 cells (in a cell culture vessel). Because such cultured Caco-2 cells act very much like human intestinal mucosa cells, such **Caco-2 tests** provide a good prediction of a pharmaceutical's active transport, passive transport, and also its receptor-mediated efflux.

Distribution, which is related to bioavailability, is closely associated with a compound's solubility (in body fluids) and its ability to be "bound" by plasma proteins. Thus, distribution (e.g., of pharmaceutical compound) is assessed via a test to determine plasma protein binding (PPB).

Metabolism can sometimes lead to toxicity. For example, in people whose bodies cannot degrade pyrimidines, the (pyrimidine) metabolites of the anticancer drug 5-fluorouracil can build up to lethal levels.

Toxicity can be assessed, for example, via cell-based microarrays, which reveal a compound's quantitative impact on specific cells' integrity and cellular functions (with regard to toxicity).

See also ADME TESTS, ABSORPTION, CACO-2, PLASMA, CELL, CELL CULTURE, RECEPTORS, ACTIVE TRANSPORT, MEMBRANE TRANSPORT, PROTEIN, PASSIVE TRANSPORT, MICROARRAY (TESTING), METABOLISM, METABOLITE, HAPLOTYPE, CELL ARRAY, LIVE CELL ARRAY, TOXICOGENOMICS, *IN SILICO* SCREENING

ADMET Acronym for absorption, distribution (within the body), metabolism, elimination, and toxicity of pharmaceuticals.

See also ADME TESTS, *IN SILICO* TESTING, ADME/Tox

Adoptive Cellular Therapy The increase in immune response that is achieved by selectively removing certain immune system cells from a patient's body, multiplying them *in vitro* to greatly increase their number, and then reinserting these (more numerous) immune system cells into the same body.

See also CELLULAR IMMUNE RESPONSE, CELL CULTURE, *IN VITRO*, GENE DELIVERY, GENE THERAPY, *EX VIVO* (THERAPY)

Adoptive Immunization The transfer of an immune state from one animal to another by means of lymphocyte transfusions.

See also LYMPHOCYTE

ADP See ADENOSINE DIPHOSPHATE (ADP)

Adult Stem Cell Historically, this term referred to a stem cell that is derived (or extracted) from the bone marrow tissue of adults, but scientists are now discovering additional types of adult stem cells within other tissues of adult humans. Similar to human embryonic stem cells, adult stem cells can — under certain conditions — differentiate and proliferate into cell types specific to many of the human body's 210 different types of tissue.

For example, during 1980, Steven Teitelbaum and colleagues injected such cells from a donor into a 3.5-month-old girl who had the disease known as **osteopetrosis**, which almost always kills its victims in the first year of their life. The injected adult stem cells differentiated and proliferated and the girl is alive today.

During 2004, Nagy Habib injected such cells from a patient who was suffering from cirrhosis of the liver into the patient's own hepatic artery in the liver. The adult stem cells repopulated the liver and improved its function (i.e., reversed at least some of the liver cirrhosis).

See also CELL, STEM CELLS, MULTIPOTENT ADULT STEM CELLS, STEM CELL GROWTH FACTOR (SCF), DIFFERENTIATION

Adventitious From the Latin *adventitious* = "not properly belonging to."

The term can be utilized to refer to the following:

- Plant shoots emanating from sites other than typical ones (e.g., from a plant's leaves).
- A small amount of transgenic grain accidentally mixed into other grain, etc.

See also TRANSGENIC

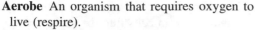

Aerobe An organism that requires oxygen to live (respire).

Aerobic Exposed to air or oxygen. An oxygenated environment.

Affinity Refers to the "attraction force" or "binding strength" between two entities (e.g., molecules).
See also AFFINITY CHROMATOGRAPHY, ANTIBODY AFFINITY CHROMATOGRAPHY, AFFINITY MATURATION

Affinity Chromatography A method of separating a mixture of proteins or nucleic acids (molecules) by specific interactions of those molecules with a component known as a **ligand**, which is immobilized on a support. If a solution of, say, a mixture of proteins is passed over (through) the column, **one** of the proteins binds to the ligand on the basis of specificity and high affinity (they fit together like a lock and key). If there is no naturally occurring "lock" on the desired protein molecule (to go with the ligand's "key"), then the scientist can add an **affinity tag** during the synthesis of the protein (e.g., in a cell-free gene expression system) to act as that protein molecule's "key."

The other proteins in the solution wash through the column because they are not able to bind to the ligand. Once the column is devoid of the other proteins, an appropriate wash solution is passed through the column, which causes the protein–ligand complex to dissociate. The protein is subsequently collected in a highly purified form.
See also CHROMATOGRAPHY, PROTEIN, NUCLEIC ACIDS, ANTIBODY AFFINITY CHROMATOGRAPHY, LIGAND (IN CHROMATOGRAPHY), AFFINITY, AFFINITY TAG, CELL-FREE GENE EXPRESSION SYSTEM

Affinity Maturation See B LYMPHOCYTES, AFFINITY

Affinity Tag Refers to a particular sequence (of amino acids) added to a given protein molecule (e.g., produced via recombinant methods, etc.). The **affinity tag** can later be utilized to make the recovery of *that protein* (out of a mixture of proteins) easier to accomplish (e.g., via chromatography or as part of the **tandem affinity purification tagging** process).

See also AFFINITY CHROMATOGRAPHY, AFFINITY, PROTEIN, AMINO ACID, SEQUENCE (OF A PROTEIN MOLECULE), LIGAND (IN CHROMATOGRAPHY), RIBOZYMES, TANDEM AFFINITY PURIFICATION TAGGING

AFGP Abbreviation for **antifreeze glycoprotein.**
See THERMAL HYSTERESIS PROTEINS

Aflatoxin The term that is used to refer to a group of related mycotoxins (i.e., metabolites produced by fungi that are toxic to animals and humans) produced by some strains of the fungi *Aspergillus flavus*, and *Aspergillus parasiticus* and, less often, by *Penicillium puberulum*. *Aspergillus flavus* and *Aspergillus parasiticus* are common fungi that typically live on decaying vegetation.

Corn earworm (*Helicoverpa zea*) and European corn borer (*Ostrinia nubilalis*) can be vectors (carriers) of *Aspergillus flavus*.

Aflatoxin B_1 is the most commonly occurring aflatoxin and is one of the most potent carcinogens known to man.

When dairy cattle eat aflatoxin-contaminated feed, their metabolism process converts the aflatoxin (e.g., aflatoxin B_1) into the mycotoxins known as aflatoxin M_1 and aflatoxin M_2, which soon appear in the cows' milk.

Consumption of aflatoxins by humans can also result in acute liver damage.
See also CARCINOGEN, TOXIN, FUNGUS, MYCOTOXINS, STRESS PROTEINS, P53 GENE, LIPOXYGENASE (LOX), PEROXIDASE, *HELICOVERPA ZEA (H. zea)*, BETA-CAROTENE, OH43, BRIGHT GREENISH-YELLOW FLUORESCENCE (BGYF), CORN, EUROPEAN CORN BORER (ECB)

A. flavus See *ASPERGILLUS FLAVUS*

AFLP Acronym for **amplified fragment length polymorphism**.
See AMPLIFIED FRAGMENT LENGTH POLYMORPHISM

AFM See ATOMIC FORCE MICROSCOPY

AFP Acronym for **antifreeze protein**.
See THERMAL HYSTERESIS PROTEINS

AG Abbreviation for the word **antigen**.
See ANTIGEN

Agar A complex mixture of polysaccharides obtained from marine red algae. It is also called agar-agar. Agar is used as an emulsion stabilizer in foods, as a sizing agent in fabrics, and as a solid substrate for the laboratory culture of microorganisms. Agar melts at 100°C (212°F) and when cooled below 44°C (123°F) forms a stiff and transparent gel. Microorganisms are seeded onto and grown (in the laboratory) on the surface of the gel.

See also POLYSACCHARIDES, CULTURE MEDIUM

Agarose A highly purified form of agar. Used as a stationary phase (substrate) in some chromatographic and electrophoretic methods.

See also CHROMATOGRAPHY, ELECTROPHORESIS, AGAR

Aging The process, affecting organisms and most cells, whereby each cell division (mitosis) brings that cell (or the organism composed of such cells) closer to its *final* cell division (i.e., death). Notable exceptions to this aging process include cancerous cells (e.g., in myelomas) and the single-celled organism; both of which are "immortal."

See also TELOMERES, MITOSIS, HYBRIDOMA, MYELOMA, CANCER

Aglycon A nonsugar component of a glycoside.

See also GLYCOSIDE

Aglycone The biologically active (molecular) form of molecules of isoflavones.

See also ISOFLAVONES, BIOLOGICAL ACTIVITY

Agonists Small protein or organic molecules that bind to certain cell proteins (i.e., receptors) at a site that is adjacent to the cell's "docking" site for protein hormones, neurotransmitters, etc. (i.e., receptor), to induce a conformational change in that cell's protein hormone or neurotransmitter, etc., receptor molecule, thereby enhancing its activity (i.e., effect on the cell).

See also RECEPTORS, ACTIVE SITE, CONFORMATION, CELL, HORMONE, ANTAGONISTS, NEUROTRANSMITTER, PPAR

Agraceutical See NUTRACEUTICALS, PHYTOCHEMICALS

Agriceuticals See NUTRACEUTICALS, PHYTOCHEMICALS

Agrobacterium tumefaciens A naturally occurring bacterium that is capable of inserting its DNA (genetic information) into plants,

resulting in a type of injury to the plant known as crown gall. In 1980, Marc van Montagu showed that *Agrobacterium tumefaciens* could alter the DNA of its host plants by inserting its own ("foreign") DNA into the genome of the host plants (thereby opening the way for scientists to insert virtually any foreign gene into plants via the use of *Agrobacterium tumefaciens*).

In 1983, Luis Herrera-Estrella created the first synthetic transgenic plant by inserting an antibiotic resistance gene into a tobacco plant.

During 2000, Weija Zhou and Richard Vierling proved that *Agrobacterium tumefaciens* is at least ten times more effective (i.e., at "infecting" plants by inserting DNA) **in space** (i.e., under conditions of weightlessness/microgravity) than it is on the surface of Earth. Among others, Monsanto Company has developed a way to stop *Agrobacterium tumefaciens* from causing crown gall while maintaining its ability to insert DNA into plant cells, and now uses *Agrobacterium tumefaciens* as a vehicle to insert desired genes into crop plants (e.g., insertion of the gene causing high production of CP4 EPSP synthase, thus conferring resistance to glyphosate-containing herbicide).

See also BACTERIA, DEOXYRIBONUCLEIC ACID (DNA), INFORMATIONAL MOLECULES, GENOME, TRANSGENIC (ORGANISM), PROTOPLAST, EPSP SYNTHASE, CP4 EPSPS, "SHOTGUN" METHOD, BIOLISTIC® GENE GUN, WHISKERS™, GENETIC ENGINEERING, GENE, BIOSEEDS, GLYPHOSATE, GLYPHOSATE-TRIMESIUM, GLYPHOSATE ISOPROPYLAMINE SALT, NOS TERMINATOR

AHG Antihemophilic globulin. Also known as factor VIII or antihemophilic factor VIII.

See also FACTOR VIII, GAMMA GLOBULIN

AI Acronym for **adequate intake**.

See also CHOLINE

AIDS See ACQUIRED IMMUNE DEFICIENCY SYNDROME (AIDS)

Alanine (Ala) A nonessential amino acid of the pyruvic acid family. In its dry, bulk form it appears as a white crystalline solid.

See also ESSENTIAL AMINO ACIDS

Albumin A protein that the liver synthesizes (i.e., "manufactures"). Most minerals and hormones utilized by the human body are first "attached" to a molecule of albumin before they are transported in the bloodstream to sites where they are needed in the body.

See also PROTEIN, HORMONE, SUPER-CRITICAL CARBON DIOXIDE

ALCAR Acronym for **Acetyl-L-carnitine.** See ACETYL CARNITINE

Aldose A simple sugar in which the carbonyl carbon atom is at one end of the carbon chain. A class of monosaccharide sugars; the molecule contains an aldehyde group.

See also MONOSACCHARIDES

Aleurone The layer ("skin") that covers the endosperm portion of a plant seed.

See also ENDOSPERM

AlfAFP Acronym for **alfalfa antifungal peptide.** See DEFENSINS

Algae A heterogeneous (i.e., widely varying) group of photosynthetic plants, ranging from microscopic single-cell forms to multicellular, very large forms such as seaweed. All of them contain chlorophyll and, hence, most are green, but some of them may be of different colors owing to the presence of other, overshadowing pigments.

Algorithm (in bioinformatics) Refers to a computational procedure that utilizes a combination of simple (e.g., mathematical) operations to process, analyze, and visualize (i.e., show pictorially) data about sequences (of DNA, RNA, proteins, etc.).

See also BIOINFORMATICS, SEQUENCE (OF A DNA MOLECULE), SEQUENCE (OF A PROTEIN MOLECULE), SEQUENCE MAP

Alicin A compound that is produced naturally by the garlic plant (*Allium sativum*) when the cells within garlic bulbs are broken open (e.g., during food preparation or consumption). Enzymes present within those garlic cells convert a precursor compound to alicin.

Research indicates that human consumption of alicin confers some specific health benefits (e.g., it is antithrombotic and reduces blood cholesterol levels, reduces or prevents coronary heart disease, enhances the immune system, etc.).

Alicin has also been shown to slow down the action of phase I detoxification enzymes (e.g.,

potentially reducing levels of some carcinogens within the human digestive system).

See also CELL, PHYTOCHEMICALS, ENZYME, INDUCIBLE ENZYMES, THROMBOSIS, CORONARY HEART DISEASE (CHD), CHOLESTEROL, CARCINOGEN, PHASE I DETOXIFICATION ENZYMES

Alkaline Hydrolysis A chemical method of liberating DNA from a DNA–RNA hybrid.

See also HYDROLYSIS, RIBONUCLEIC ACID (RNA), DNA–RNA HYBRID, DEOXYRIBONUCLEIC ACID (DNA)

Alkaloids A class of toxic compounds that are naturally produced by some organisms (e.g., certain ants, certain plants such as lupines and potatoes, and certain fungi such as ergot).

For example, the prickly yellow poppy (*Argemone mexicana*) naturally produces an alkaloid within the oil in its seeds.

Certain species of ants naturally produce alkaloids as a self-defense mechanism. Poison-dart frogs (*Dendrobates azureus*) and two species of New Guinea songbirds (*Pitohui dichrous* and *Ifrita kowaldi*) can tolerate these ant-produced alkaloids and they also acquire the self-defense toxin by eating those ants.

Another example is the moth *Utetheisa ornatrix*, whose larvae (caterpillars) feed on certain plants (*Crotalaria* spp.) that contain pyrrolizidine alkaloids. Because those alkaloids are extremely bitter tasting and toxic, spiders that normally prey on them refuse to eat these *Utetheisa ornatrix* even after they become adult moths. If those moths (which have consumed these pyrrolizidine alkaloids as larvae) get caught in the spider's web, the spider will cut it out of the web and release them.

Vinca alkaloids isolated from the specific plants that produce them have been utilized as cancer-treating (i.e., antitumor) drugs.

A chlorine-containing alkaloid named epibatine, isolated from the skin of the South American frog *Epipedobates tricolor*, has shown potential for use as a painkilling pharmaceutical that is 200 times more powerful than morphine.

See also TOXIN, FUNGUS, TREMORGENIC INDOLE ALKALOIDS, ERGOTAMINE, COLCHICINE

Allele From the Greek *allelon* = "mutually, each other."

The term refers to one of several alternate forms of a gene occupying a given locus on the chromosome, which controls expression (of the product) in different ways.

See also EXPRESS, GENE, CHROMOSOMES, LOCUS

Allelic Exclusion The expression in any particular manner of only one of the alleles (of the two inherited copies of each) in chromosomes owing to chromosomal inactivation. For example, only one allele of an **antibody gene** within a B lymphocyte (blast cell), coding for the expressed antibody (in response to antigenic stimulus), is involved in expression, because of chromosomal inactivation during blast transformation.

See also ALLELE, CODING SEQUENCE, GENE, CHROMOSOME, B LYMPHOCYTES, ANTIBODY, IMMUNOGLOBULIN, BLAST CELL, BLAST TRANSFORMATION

Allelopathy Refers to the secretion of certain chemicals (e.g., terpenoid compounds, etc.) by a plant in order to hinder the growth or reproduction of other plants growing near it. For example, the *Callistemon citrinus* bush secretes a chemical compound known as leptospermone, which falls from the bush and inhibits the growth of other plants near it.

In a similar manner, the fungus *Laccaria bicolor* secretes a chemical compound that paralyzes springtails (soil-dwelling insects) so that the fungus can engulf and digest them. The *Laccaria bicolor* fungus lives symbiotically among the roots of the eastern white pine tree, and this results in the **nitrogen within the springtails' bodies** (i.e., fertilizer) being delivered to the tree. In return, the tree roots supply the *Laccaria bicolor* fungus with certain carbohydrates that the fungus requires.

See also FUNGUS

Allergies (airborne) See MAST CELLS

Allergies (foodborne) The word was coined in 1906 by Clemens Freiherr von Piguet and refers to an IgE-mediated (aggressive) immune system response to antigens present on protein molecules in the particular food that a given person is allergic to. The antibodies (IgE) bind to these antigens and trigger a humoral immune response, which can cause vomiting, diarrhea, skin reactions (e.g., hives), blood pressure decline, wheezing, and respiratory distress. In severe cases, the immune response can cause death.

In some rare instances, the allergic reaction is mediated by sensitized T cells.

In some rare cases, the onset of a food allergy incident is induced by exercise (before or after eating a particular food).

The U.S. Food and Drug Administration (FDA) requires testing in advance to determine if a genetically engineered foodstuff has the potential to cause allergic reactions in humans before it (e.g., a modified crop plant) is approved by the FDA.

In general, the known food allergens (e.g., in peanuts, Brazil nuts, wheat, etc.) are protein molecules that are resistant to rapid digestion (e.g., because those protein molecules are too tightly "folded together" for digestive enzymes to access their chemical bonds and break them down). One potential way of genetically engineering allergenic crops (e.g., wheat) to make them less allergenic is to insert genes for extra production of thioredoxin.

Thioredoxin is a protein found in all living organisms that "targets" and breaks down the chemical bonds holding together a tightly-folded-together protein molecule (thereby making these protein molecules easier to digest). Future crops engineered to contain more thioredoxin than the traditional ones may be less allergenic.

See also PROTEIN, PROTEIN FOLDING, ANTIBODY, ANTIGEN, FOOD AND DRUG ADMINISTRATION (FDA), GENETIC ENGINEERING, IMMUNOGLOBULIN, HUMORAL IMMUNITY, MAST CELLS, LEUKOTRIENES, DIGESTION (WITHIN ORGANISMS), ORGANISM, REDUCED-ALLERGEN SOYBEANS

Allicin See ALICIN

Allogeneic Having a different set of genes (although belonging to the same species). For example, an organ transplant from one nonrelated human to another is allogeneic. An organ transplant from a baboon to a human would be xenogeneic.

See also GENE, SPECIES, XENOGENEIC ORGANS

Allosteric Enzymes Regulatory enzymes whose catalytic activity is modulated by the noncovalent binding of a specific metabolite (effector) at a site (regulatory site) **other** than the catalytic site (on the enzyme). Effector binding causes a three-dimensional conformation change in the enzyme and is the root of the modulation.

The term (allosteric) is used to differentiate this form of regulation from the type that may result from the competition between substrate and inhibitors at the catalytic site.

See also ENZYME, STERIC HINDRANCE, EFFECTOR, CONFORMATION, ACTIVE SITE

Allosteric Site The "site" on an (allosteric) enzyme molecule where, via noncovalent binding to the site, a given effector can increase or decrease that enzyme's catalytic activity. Such an effector is called an allosteric effector because it binds at a site on the enzyme molecule that is other ("allo") than the enzyme's catalytic site.

See also ALLOSTERIC ENZYMES, ACTIVATOR (of enzyme), CATALYTIC SITE, EFFECTOR, CONFORMATION, ENZYME, METABOLITE, CATALYST

Allosterism Refers to the deformation of a protein molecule's conformation (and, thus, its activity) that is caused when a ligand (e.g., effector) binds to that protein molecule (e.g., enzyme) at a spot (e.g., a "regulatory site" for the enzyme) other than the protein's **active site** (i.e., which is the "catalytic site" in an enzyme).

See also PROTEIN, CONFORMATION, LIGAND, EFFECTOR, ENZYME, ACTIVE SITE, CATALYTIC SITE, ALLOSTERIC SITE, ALLOSTERIC ENZYMES

Allotypic Monoclonal Antibodies Monoclonal antibodies that are isoantigenic.

See also MONOCLONAL ANTIBODIES (MAb), ANTIGEN

Allozyme See ALLOSTERIC ENZYMES

Aloe vera **L**. A "family" of short green plants (e.g., *Aloe barbadensis*) that grow in hot tropical climates, whose sap (juice) contains certain carbohydrates that naturally assist healing of human skin wounds. These carbohydrates "activate" macrophages, causing them to produce cytokines (that regulate the human immune system and the inflammatory responses that promote healing).

See also PHYTOCHEMICALS, CARBOHYDRATES (SACCHARIDES), MACROPHAGE, CYTOKINES

Alpha Amylase Inhibitor-1 A protein that is naturally produced in the seeds of the plant known as the common bean (*Phaseolus vulgaris*); it inhibits the amylase enzyme in the gut of the pest insect known as the pea weevil. Because the amylase enzyme is inhibited (i.e., prevented from helping digestion) by alpha amylase inhibitor-1, the seeds of the *Phaseolus vulgaris* plant are protected from depredation by the pea weevil.

See also AMYLASE INHIBITORS, PROTEIN, ENZYME, AMYLASE, WEEVILS

Alpha Galactosides The term refers to a "family" of polysaccharides (produced in plant seeds) composed (at the molecular level) of one sucrose unit linked by α 1,6 molecular bonds to several galactose units.

Alpha galactosides include raffinose, stachyose, and verbascose.

See also POLYSACCHARIDES, GALACTOSE (Gal), STACHYOSE

Alpha Helix (α-helix) A highly regular (i.e., repeating) structural feature that occurs in certain large molecules. First discovered in protein molecules by Linus Pauling in the late 1940s.

See also A-DNA, PROTEIN, PROTEIN FOLDING, PROTEIN STRUCTURE

α-Helix See ALPHA HELIX

Alpha Interferon Also written as α-interferon. One of the interferons, it has been shown to prolong life and reduce tumor size in patients suffering from Kaposi's sarcoma (a cancer that affects approximately 10% of people with acquired immune deficiency syndrome). It is also effective against hairy-cell leukemia and may work against other cancers. It has recently been approved by the U.S. FDA for use against certain types of sarcoma. Recent research indicates that injections of alpha interferon can limit the liver damage typically caused by hepatitis C, a viral disease.

See also INTERFERONS, CANCER, FOOD AND DRUG ADMINISTRATION (FDA)

Alpha Linolenic (α-Linolenic) Acid See LINOLENIC ACID

α-Linolenic Acid See LINOLENIC ACID

Alpha-Chaconine See CHACONINE

Alpha-Rumenic acid See CONJUGATED LINOLEIC ACID (CLA)

Alpha-Solanine See SOLANINE

Alpha-Synuclein A protein that is present in most cells of the brain.

Members of some families, who inherit a (mutated) gene (SNP) that codes for a (mutated) form of alpha-synuclein have a higher-than-average tendency to get Parkinson's disease.

See also PROTEIN, NEURON, CELL, PARKINSON'S DISEASE, GENE, MUTATION, SINGLE-NUCLEOTIDE POLYMORPHISMS (SNPs)

ALS A plant enzyme (also present in some microorganisms) known as **acetolactate synthase** or acetohydroxy acid synthase. ALS catalyzes (i.e., enables the occurrence of) one of the early chemical reaction steps in the synthesis ("manufacturing") of branched-chain amino acids (isoleucine, leucine, valine), which are required by plants to sustain life (i.e., to make needed proteins).

Herbicides that deactivate or destroy ALS are effective at killing plants (e.g., weeds).

See also ENZYME, GENE, ALS GENE, MICROORGANISMS, CATALYST, AMINO ACID, ISOLEUCINE (Ile), LEUCINE (Leu), VALINE (Val)

ALS Gene Gene that codes for (i.e., causes to be produced in microorganisms or in plants' chloroplasts) the critical-to-plants enzyme **acetolactate synthase (ALS)**. Also known as **acetohydroxy acid synthase**, ALS catalyzes (i.e., enables the occurrence of) one of the early chemical reaction steps in the synthesis ("manufacturing") of branched-chain amino acids (isoleucine, leucine, and valine) by plants. Because these branched-chain amino acids are required by plants to sustain life, herbicides that deactivate or destroy ALS are effective at killing plants (e.g., weeds).

See also GENE, HTC, MICROORGANISMS, CHLOROPLASTS, ENZYME, CATALYST, AMINO ACID, ISOLEUCINE (Ile), LEUCINE (Leu), VALINE (Val), STS SULFONYLUREA (HERBICIDE)-TOLERANT SOYBEANS

Alternative mRNA Splicing See ALTERNATIVE SPLICING

Alternative Splicing The process (during transcription) by which alternative exons (i.e., portion of gene that codes for a specific domain of a protein) within a given RNA molecule are combined (by RNA polymerase molecules known as snRNPs) to yield **different** mRNAs (messenger RNA molecules) from the same gene. Each such mRNA is known as a GENE TRANSCRIPT.

Other causes or sources of alternative splicing include:

- Varying translation start or stop site (on the mRNA during its translation), resulting in a given intron remaining in the mRNA transcript. For example, the COX-3 enzyme and the COX-1 enzyme are both produced from the COX-1 gene. The COX-3 enzyme results when **intron 1** is retained in the mRNA transcript.
- Frameshifting (i.e., a different set of triplet codons in the mRNA/transcript is translated by the ribosome).

Different body tissues and some diseases cause alternative splicing (i.e., resulting in **different** proteins being produced in *different* tissues or in *diseased* tissues) from a given gene.

See also TRANSCRIPTION, EXON, INTRON, DOMAIN (OF A PROTEIN), PROTEIN, GENE, ENZYME, RNA POLYMERASE, TRANSCRIPT, TRANSLATION, MESSENGER RNA (mRNA), CODING SEQUENCE, CODON, GENETIC CODE, FRAMESHIFT, RIBOSOMES, TRANSCRIPTOME, CENTRAL DOGMA (NEW), COX-1, COX-3, CYCLOOXYGENASE

Alu Family A set of dispersed and related genetic sequences, each about 300 base pairs (bp) long, in the human genome. At both ends of these 300 bp segments there is an A-G-C-T sequence. Alu1 is a restriction enzyme that recognizes this sequence and cleaves (cuts) it between the G (guanine) and the C (cytosine).

See also GENOME, RESTRICTION ENDONUCLEASES

Aluminum Resistance See CITRATE SYNTHASE (CSb) GENE, GENE, CITRIC ACID

A

Aluminum Tolerance See CITRATE SYN-THASE (CSb) GENE, GENE, CITRIC ACID

Aluminum Toxicity See CITRATE SYN-THASE (CSb) GENE, GENE, CITRIC ACID

Alzheimer's Disease Named after Alois Alzheimer who, in 1906, first described the amyloid β protein (AβP) plaques in the human brain that are caused by this disease. Alzheimer's disease causes certain proteins to misfold and aggregate in the brain, resulting in progressive memory loss and dementia in its victims as it kills the brain cells (neurons).

Some human haplotypes are more susceptible to Alzheimer's disease than others. Women tend to get Alzheimer's disease significantly more often than men of the same age. In North America, African-Americans tend to get Alzheimer's disease significantly more often than Caucasians.

Some drugs (e.g., tacrine, donepezil, etc.) appear to slow the progression of Alzheimer's disease (by increasing the availability of acetylcholine in the brain), but there is currently no way to stop the disease.

See also PROTEIN, PROTEIN FOLDING, AMYLOID PRECURSOR PROTEIN, AMYLOID β PROTEIN (AβP), AMYLOID β PROTEIN PRECURSOR (AβPP), NEURON, NEUROTRANSMITTER, ACETYLCHOLINE, OXIDATIVE STRESS, CURCURMIN, HAPLOTYPE, RAPID PROTEIN FOLDING ASSAY

AMD Acronym for **age-related macular degeneration.**

See LUTEIN, ANGIOGENESIS, LYCOPENE, BETA-CAROTENE, COMPLEMENT FACTOR H GENE

American Type Culture Collection (ATCC) An independent, nonprofit organization that was established in 1925 for the preservation and distribution of reference cultures.

See also CELL CULTURE, CULTURE, CULTURE MEDIUM, TYPE SPECIMEN, CONSULTATIVE GROUP ON INTERNATIONAL AGRICULTURAL RESEARCH (CGIAR)

Ames Test A simple bacterial-based test for carcinogens that was developed by Bruce Ames in 1961.

Although this test evaluates mutagenesis (i.e., causation of mutations) in the DNA of bacteria, its results have been utilized to approve, or not approve, certain compounds for consumption by humans.

See also BIOASSAY, BACTERIA, ASSAY, MUTUAL RECOGNITION AGREEMENTS (MRAs), GENOTOXIC CARCINOGENS, CARCINOGEN, PARP

Amino Acid There are 20 common natural amino acids and at least 2 uncommon natural amino acids, each specified by a different arrangement of 3 adjacent DNA nucleotides. These are the building blocks of proteins. Joined together in a strictly ordered chain, the sequence of amino acids determines the character of each protein (chain) molecule. The 20 common amino acids are: alanine, arginine, aspartic acid, glutamic acid, glutamine, glycine, histidine, isoleucine, leucine, phenylalanine, proline, serine, threonine, tryptophan, tyrosine, valine, cysteine, methionine, lysine, and asparagine. Note that virtually all of these amino acids (except glycine) possess an asymmetric carbon atom and thus are potentially chiral in nature.

One of the least common amino acids is selenocysteine, which is made by some *Archaea.*

See also PROTEIN, POLYPEPTIDE (PROTEIN), STEREOISOMERS, CHIRAL COMPOUND, MESSENGER RNA (mRNA), ESSENTIAL AMINO ACIDS, DEOXYRIBONUCLEIC ACID (DNA), ABSOLUTE CONFIGURATION, *ARCHAEA*

Amino Acid Profile Also known as "protein quality," this refers to a quantitative delineation of how much of each amino acid is contained in a given source of (livestock feed or food) protein. For example, of all protein meals, the amino acid profile of soybean meal is closest to the ideal profile of amino acids needed for human nutrition.

See also "IDEAL PROTEIN" CONCEPT, PROTEIN, AMINO ACID, SOYBEAN MEAL, LIPID RAFTS

Aminocyclopropane Carboxylic Acid Synthase/Deaminase See ACC SYNTHASE, ACC

AMP See ADENOSINE MONOPHOSPHATE (AMP)

Amphibolic Pathway A metabolic pathway used in both catabolism and anabolism.

See also ANABOLISM, CATABOLISM

Amphipathic Molecules Molecules bearing both polar and nonpolar domains (within the same molecule). Some examples of amphipathic molecules are wetting agents (SDS) and membrane lipids such as lecithin.
See also MICELLE, REVERSE MICELLE (RM), POLARITY (CHEMICAL)

Amphiphilic Molecules Also known collectively as amphiphiles. Molecules possessing distinct regions of hydrophobic ("water-hating") and hydrophilic ("water-loving") character within the same molecule. When dissolved in water above a certain concentration (known as the CMC), these molecules are capable of forming high-molecular-weight aggregates, or micelles.
See also CRITICAL MICELLE CONCENTRATION, HYDROPHOBIC, HYDROPHILIC, MICELLE, REVERSE MICELLE (RM)

Amphoteric Compound A compound capable of both donating and accepting protons and thus able to act chemically as either an acid or a base.

AMPK Acronym for **AMP-activated protein kinase**.
See AMP, PROTEIN KINASES

Amplicon A specific sequence of DNA that is produced by a DNA-amplification technology such as the polymerase chain reaction (PCR) technique.
See also DEOXYRIBONUCLEIC ACID (DNA), SEQUENCE (OF A DNA MOLECULE); POLYMERASE CHAIN REACTION (PCR) TECHNIQUE, NESTED PCR

Amplification The production of additional copies of a chromosomal sequence found as either intrachromosomal or extrachromosomal DNA.
See also *IN VITRO* SELECTION

Amplified Fragment Length Polymorphism Also known by its acronym **AFLP**, it is the "DNA marker" utilized in a **"genetic mapping"** technique that utilizes the specific sequence of bases (nucleotides) in a piece of DNA (from an organism). Because the specific sequence of bases in DNA molecules is different for **each** species, strain, variety, and individual (owing to DNA polymorphism), AFLP can be utilized to map these DNA molecules (e.g., to assist and speed up plant-breeding programs).

See also GENETIC MAP, SEQUENCE (OF A DNA MOLECULE), DEOXYRIBONUCLEIC ACID (DNA), GENOME, PHYSICAL MAP (OF GENOME), MARKER (DNA SEQUENCE), MARKER (GENETIC MARKER), POLYMORPHISM (CHEMICAL), NUCLEIC ACIDS, NUCLEOTIDE, GENETIC CODE, CAPILLARY ELECTROPHORESIS

Amplimer See AMPLICON

Amylase A term that is used to refer to a category of enzymes that catalyzes the chemical reaction in which amylose (starch) molecules are hydrolytically cleaved ("broken") into molecular pieces (e.g., the polysaccharides maltose, maltotriose, α-dextrin, etc.). For example:

- Amylases are produced within the digestive system of certain insects that feed upon starch-containing grains.
- α-Amylase is used to break up cornstarch molecules as the first step in the manufacture of fructose (sweetener for soft drinks).

Since 1857, amylase has been utilized to remove (amylose) starch from woven fabrics in the textile industry. Modern uses of some amylases include utilizing them to enable the substitution of barley grain for malt in the beer-brewing process.
See also ENZYME, STARCH, AMYLOSE, BARLEY, HYDROLYTIC CLEAVAGE, POLYSACCHARIDES, AMYLASE INHIBITORS, ALPHA AMYLASE INHIBITOR-1, DIGESTION (WITHIN ORGANISMS)

Amylase Inhibitors The term refers to compounds that chemically bind to an amylase (i.e., an enzyme that is produced within the digestive system of certain insects and other organisms), and thereby prevents the amylase from breaking down (i.e., digesting) any amylose (i.e., a carbohydrate present within many plants' seeds) consumed by these insects.
During 2004, South American researchers reported that coffee beans produced by plants (*Coffea arabica*) that had been genetically engineered to produce some amylase inhibitor in their beans were protected from depredation

by the pest insect known as the coffee berry borer (*Hypothenemus hampei*). That particular amylase inhibitor's gene had been isolated from the South American bean plant known as *Phaseolus coccineus*, in which it is naturally produced.

See also AMYLASE, ENZYME, PROTEIN, DIGESTION (WITHIN ORGANISMS), AMYLOSE, COFFEE BERRY BORER, GENE, GENETIC ENGINEERING, ALPHA AMYLASE INHIBITOR-1

Amyloid β Protein (AβP) Refers to the (short length) protein molecules that form into plaque within the brains and in brain blood vessels of victims of Alzheimer's disease.

See also PROTEIN, ALZHEIMER'S DISEASE, AMYLOID β PROTEIN PRECURSOR

Amyloid β Protein Precursor (AβPP) Refers to a collective set of protein molecules (e.g., prions) from which are derived/created Amyloid β Protein (AβP)

See also PROTEIN, PRION AMYLOID β PROTEIN (AβP)

Amyloid Plaques See ALZHEIMER'S DISEASE

Amyloid Precursor Protein A transmembrane (i.e., extends through cells' plasma membrane) protein (prion) within the brain cells of mammals. Under certain conditions, it can form the molecular derivative known as amyloid β-protein, a cause of Alzheimer's disease.

See also PROTEIN, CELL, PLASMA MEMBRANE, ALZHEIMER'S DISEASE

Amylopectin The form of starch (molecule) that consists of multibranched polymers, containing approximately 100,000 glucose units per molecule (polysaccharide).

See also STARCH, POLYMER, GLUCOSE (GLc), POLYSACCHARIDES, WAXY CORN

Amylose The form of starch that consists of unbranched polymers, containing approximately 4,000 glucose units per molecule (polysaccharide). It is present in potatoes at 23 to 29% content (the variation is thought to be caused by different growing conditions).

See also POLYMER, GLUCOSE (GLc), AMYLASE, POLYSACCHARIDES

Anabolism The phase of intermediary metabolism concerned with the energy-requiring biosynthesis of cell components from smaller precursor molecules.

See also CATABOLISM, ASSIMILATION, METABOLISM, CELL, PLASMA MEMBRANE

Anaerobe An organism that lives in the absence of oxygen and generally cannot grow in the presence of oxygen. The catabolic metabolism of anaerobic microorganisms reduces a variety of organic and inorganic compounds in order to survive (e.g., carbon dioxide, sulfate, nitrate, fumarate, iron, manganese); and anaerobes produce a large number of end products of metabolism (e.g., acetic acid, propionic acid, lactic acid, ethanol, methane, etc.).

See also CATABOLISM, METABOLISM, METABOLITE, REDUCTION (IN A CHEMICAL REACTION), ANAEROBIC

Anaerobic An environment without air or oxygen.

See also ANAEROBE

Analog Gene See ORTHOLOG

Analogue (Analog) A compound (or molecule) that is a (chemical) structural derivative of a "parent" compound. The word is also used to describe a molecule that may be structurally similar (but not identical) to another and that exhibits many or some of the same biological functions of the other.

For example, the large class of antibiotics known as the sulfa drugs are all analogs of the original synthetic chemical drug (known as Prontosil, a cure for streptococcal infections) discovered by the German biologist Gerhart Domagk. Domagk's (and others') discoveries made possible a program of further chemical syntheses based upon the original (sulfanilamide) molecular structure, which resulted in the large number of sulfonamide (also called "sulfa") drugs that are available today. All of the analogue (or analog) sulfa drugs, which were patterned after the original sulfanilamide molecular structure, may be called sulfanilamide analogues.

Today, analogues exist for various vitamins, amino acids, purines, sugars, growth factors, and many other chemical compounds. Research chemists produce analogues of various molecules in order to ascertain the biological role, or importance, of certain structures (within the molecule) in the molecule's function within a living organism.

See also BIOMIMETIC MATERIALS, RATIO-NAL DRUG DESIGN, HETEROLOGY, GIB-BERELLINS, QUANTITATIVE STRUC-TURE–ACTIVITY RELATIONSHIP (QSAR)

ANDA (to FDA) Acronym for **Abbreviated New Drug Application** (to the U.S. Food and Drug Administration).

See also NDA, "TREATMENT" IND REGU-LATIONS, FOOD AND DRUG ADMINIS-TRATION (FDA)

Angiogenesis Formation/development of new blood vessels in the body. Discovered, in the early 1980s, to be triggered and stimulated by angiogenic growth factors. For example, when heart arteries are clogged by arteriosclerosis, increased production of **granulocyte-mac-rophage colony-stimulating factor (GM-CSF)** can stimulate the development of new blood vessels (to sometimes restore blood flow).

Angiogenesis is required for malignant tumors to metastasize (spread throughout the body) because it provides the (newly created) blood supply that tumors require. For example, the gene that codes for the production of VEGF (vascular endothelial growth factor) is greatly upregulated by chemical signals that are pro-duced by hepatocarcinoma (HCC) tumors.

Angiogenesis is also crucial to the development of glaucoma and age-related macular degen-eration (AMD), a major cause of blindness in older people. In the case of AMD, the body's production of VEGF can cause creation and growth of blood vessels in front of the retina, which eventually leads to blindness. Recent research indicates that siRNA-based drugs might be able to prevent AMD via prevention of (over)production of VEGF by the body.

The drug thalidomide is also a potent inhibitor of angiogenesis, as are the proteins **angiosta-tin** and **endostatin**.

See also ANGIOGENIC GROWTH FAC-TORS, GRANULOCYTE-MACROPHAGE COLONY-STIMULATING FACTOR (GM-CSF), NITRIC OXIDE, ARTERIOSCLERO-SIS, TUMOR, CANCER, METASTASIS, GENE, UPREGULATION, VASCULAR ENDOTHELIAL GROWTH FACTOR (VEGF), SHORT INTERFERING RNA (siRNA), ANTIANGIOGENESIS, CHIRAL COMPOUND, ANGIOSTATIN, ENDOSTA-TIN

Angiogenesis Factors See ANGIOGENIC GROWTH FACTORS

Angiogenesis Inhibitors Refers to compounds (e.g., pharmaceuticals) that work to inhibit or stop angiogenesis (i.e., formation or develop-ment of new blood vessels). Because angiogen-esis is required for malignant tumors to grow or metastasize (spread), such compounds hold the potential to treat cancerous tumors.

For example, the biotechnology-derived angio-genesis inhibitor pharmaceutical known as Avastin® (bevacizumab) has been proven to be effective against metastatic colorectal cancer, some lung cancers, and some breast cancers. It acts by "starving" cancerous tumors of the blood supply (i.e., new blood vessels or feed-ers) that these tumors need to survive and grow.

See also ANGIOGENESIS, CANCER, TUMOR, METASTASIS, ANTIANGIO-GENESIS

Angiogenic Growth Factors Proteins that stimulate the formation of blood vessels (e.g., in tissue being formed by the body to repair wounds).

See also PROTEIN, VASCULAR ENDOTHE-LIAL GROWTH FACTOR (VEGF), FILLER EPITHELIAL CELLS, FIBROBLAST GROWTH FACTOR (FGF), MITOGEN, ANGIOGENIN, ENDOTHELIAL CELLS, TRANSFORMING GROWTH FACTOR-ALPHA (TGF-ALPHA), TRANSFORMING GROWTH FACTOR-BETA (TGF-BETA), PLATELET-DERIVED GROWTH FACTOR (PDGF), ANGIOGENESIS

Angiogenin One of the human angiogenic growth factors, it possesses potent angiogenic (formation of blood vessels) activity. In addi-tion to stimulating (normal) blood vessel for-mation, angiogenin levels are correlated with placenta formation and tumor growth (tumors require new blood vessels).

See also ANGIOGENIC GROWTH FAC-TORS, ANGIOGENESIS, TUMOR, GROWTH FACTOR

Angiostatin An antiangiogenesis (anti-blood-vessel-formation) human protein discovered by Judah Folkman. In combination with endostatin, it has been shown to cause certain cancer tumors in mice to shrink, via cutting off the creation of new blood vessels required to "feed" a growing tumor. Angiostatin acts

to halt the creation of new blood vessels by binding to ATP synthase (an enzyme needed to initiate new blood vessels).
See also PROTEIN, ANTIANGIOGENESIS, ENDOSTATIN, CANCER, ATP SYNTHASE, TUMOR

Angiotensin See ADIPOSE, INSULIN

Angstrom (Å) 10^{-8} cm (3.937×10^{-9} in.).

Anion See ION

Anneal The process by which the complementary base pairs in the strands of DNA combine.
See also BASE PAIR (bp), DEOXYRIBONUCLEIC ACID (DNA)

Annotation (in bioinformatics) Refers to the analysis and commentary that is appended to DNA sequences, protein sequences, etc., stored in databases. Such annotation can include:

- Known information about a given sequence's coding (or noncoding)
- Known information about the proteins coded for **by an analogous gene** that has already been sequenced and delineated in a **model organism's** DNA
- Known (or predicted) protein structure coded for by a gene
- Known (or predicted) domains of the protein
- Quaternary structure of the protein
- Known (or predicted) protein function (of the protein coded for by a gene)
- Common posttranslational modifications of the protein (e.g., addition of carbohydrate moieties, phosphorylation, acetylation, etc.)
- Known clinically observed effect on organism (of the protein coded for by a gene after **posttranslational modification of the protein**, etc.)

See also SEQUENCE (OF A DNA MOLECULE), SEQUENCE (OF A PROTEIN), BIOINFORMATICS, CODING SEQUENCE, PROTEIN, GENE, MODEL ORGANISM, HOMOLOGOUS (CHROMOSOMES OR GENES), FUNCTIONAL GENOMICS, DOMAIN (OF A PROTEIN), PHOSPHORYLATION, QUATERNARY STRUCTURE, POSTTRANSLATIONAL MODIFICATION OF PROTEIN

Anonymous DNA Marker Refers to a DNA marker with a clearly identifiable sequence variation (i.e., it is detectable by the specific variation in its DNA sequence whether or not it occurs in or near a coding sequence).
See also DEOXYRIBONUCLEIC ACID (DNA), SEQUENCE (OF A DNA MOLECULE), MARKER (DNA SEQUENCE), MICROSATELLITE DNA

Antagonists Molecules that bind to certain proteins (e.g., receptors, enzymes) at a specific (active) site on that protein. The binding suppresses or inhibits the activity (function) of that protein.
See also RECEPTORS, ACTIVE SITE, CONFORMATION, AGONISTS, ENZYME, ALLOSTERIC ENZYMES

Anterior Pituitary Gland See PITUITARY GLAND

Anthocyanidins Natural pigments (flavonoids) produced in blueberries (genus *Vaccinium*), blackberries (*Rubus fruticosus*), cranberries (*Vaccinium macrocarpon*), cherries (genus *Prunus*), black or purple carrots (*Daucus carota*), pomegranates (*Punica granatum* L), and some types of grapes.
Consumption of anthocyanidins by humans has been shown to be beneficial to eyesight, via promotion of the health of the retina. Within the human body, anthocyanidins act as antioxidants (i.e., "quenchers" of free radicals), so consumption of anthocyanidins apparently thereby reduces the risk of some cancers, coronary heart disease, eyesight loss, and cataracts.
See also PHYTOCHEMICALS, NUTRACEUTICALS, CAROTENOIDS, ANTIOXIDANTS, OXIDATIVE STRESS, CANCER, CORONARY HEART DISEASE (CHD), INSULIN, PROANTHOCYANIDINS, FOSHU

Anthocyanins See ANTHOCYANIDINS

Anthocyanosides Natural pigments (flavonoids) produced in bilberries (*Vaccinium myrtillus*) and certain other fruits. Consumption of anthocyanosides by humans has been shown to be beneficial to eyesight by aiding the health of retinal rhodopsin (a chemical within the retina). Within the human body, anthocyanosides act as antioxidants (i.e., "quenchers" of free radicals), so its consumption apparently reduces the risk of certain diseases (e.g., some cancers, eyesight loss, coronary heart disease, etc.).

See also PHYTOCHEMICALS, NUTRACEU-TICALS, FLAVONOIDS, ANTIOXIDANTS, OXIDATIVE STRESS, CANCER, CORO-NARY HEART DISEASE (CHD), FOSHU

Anti-idiotype Antibodies See ANTI-IDIO-TYPES

Anti-Idiotypes Antibodies to antibodies. In other words, if a human antibody is injected into rabbits, the rabbit's immune system will recognize the human antibody as foreign (regardless of the fact that they are antibodies) and produce antibodies against them. To the rabbit the foreign antibodies represent just another invader or nonself to be targeted and destroyed. Anti-idiotypes mimic antigens in that they are shaped to fit into the antibody's binding site (in lock-and-key fashion). As such, anti-idiotypes can be used to create vaccines that stimulate production of antibodies to the antigen (that the anti-idiotype mimics). This confers disease resistance (to the pathogen associated with that antigen) without the risk that a vaccine using attenuated pathogens entails (i.e., that the pathogen may "revive" and cause disease).

See also ANTIBODY, MONOCLONAL ANTI-BODIES (MAb), ANTIGEN, IDIOTYPE, PATHOGEN, ATTENUATED (PATHOGENS)

Anti-Interferon An antibody to interferon. Used for the purification of interferons.

See also ANTIBODY, INTERFERONS, AFFINITY CHROMATOGRAPHY

Anti-Oncogenes See ONCOGENES, ANTI-SENSE (DNA SEQUENCE)

Antiangiogenesis Refers to the impact of any compound that works to prevent angiogenesis (i.e., formation and development of new blood vessels). Because angiogenesis is required for malignant tumors to grow and metastasize (spread), antiangiogenesis was proposed as a means to combat cancer by Judah Folkman in 1970.

For example, the biotechnology-derived pharmaceutical known as Avastin® (bevacizumab) has been proved to be effective against metastatic colorectal cancer, some lung cancers, and some breast cancers. It acts by "starving" cancerous tumors of the blood supply (i.e.,

new blood vessels/feeders) that they need in order to survive and grow.

Because angiogenesis is required for embryonic development, antiangiogenic drugs inhibit proper development/growth of infants in the womb. Drugs that have been found to possess antiangiogenic properties include Avastin®, fumagillin, ovalicin, and thalidomide. The human proteins angiostatin and endostatin also have such properties.

See also ANGIOGENESIS, ANGIOGENIC GROWTH FACTORS, TUMOR, CANCER, METASTASIS, ANGIOSTATIN, ENDOSTA-TIN, GENISTEIN, RECEPTOR TYROSINE KINASE

Antibiosis Refers to the processes by which one organism produces a substance that is toxic or repellent to another organism (e.g., a parasite) that is attacking it. For example, certain varieties of corn or maize (*Zea mays L.*) naturally produce chemical substances in their roots that are toxic to the corn rootworm.

See also ANTIBIOTIC, *BACILLUS THURING-IENSIS (B.t.)*, CORN, CORN ROOTWORM

Antibiotic Coined by Selman Waksman during the 1940s, this term refers to organic compounds that are naturally formed and secreted by various species of microorganisms and plants. It has a defensive function and is often toxic to other species (e.g., penicillin, originally found to be produced by bread mold, is toxic to numerous human pathogens). Antibiotics generally act by inhibiting protein synthesis, DNA replication, synthesis of cell wall (cytoskeleton) constituents, inhibition of required cell (e.g., bacteria) metabolic processes, and nucleic acid (DNA and RNA) biosynthesis, hence, killing the (targeted bacteria) cells involved. Inorganic (e.g., certain metals) molecules may also have antibiotic properties.

See also PATHOGEN, MICROORGANISM, PROTEIN, NUCLEIC ACIDS, PENICILLIN G (BENZYLPENICILLIN), SYMBIOTIC, GRAM STAIN, GRAM NEGATIVE, ALLEL-OPATHY, BACTERIA, GRAM POSITIVE, CELL, ANTIBIOSIS, AUREOFACIN, *PHO-TORHABDUS LUMINESCENS*, BETA-LAC-TAM ANTIBIOTICS, METABOLISM, DEOXYRIBONUCLEIC ACID (DNA), CYTOSKELETON, PLASMA MEMBRANE, RIBONUCLEIC ACID (RNA), NISIN

A

A

Antibiotic Resistance A property of a cell (e.g., pathogenic bacteria) that enables it to avoid the effect of an antibiotic that had formerly killed or inhibited it. Ways in which this can occur include:

- By changing the structure of the cell wall (plasma membrane).
- By synthesis (manufacture) of enzymes to inactivate the antibiotic (e.g., penicillinases, which inactivate penicillin).
- By synthesis of enzymes to prevent the antibiotic from entering the cell.
- By active removal of the antibiotic from the cell. For example, the **membrane transporter protein** molecules known as **ABC transporters** are sometimes able to help pathogenic bacteria resist certain antibiotics by transporting out the antibiotic before it can kill the bacteria. The ABC transporter is a V-shaped molecule embedded in the (bacterial) cell's plasma membrane, with the "open end" of the "V" pointed toward the interior of the cell. When molecules of certain antibiotics (inside the cell) contact the ABC transporter molecule, the two "arms" of the ABC transporter **close around the antibiotic molecule, the ABC transporter flips over, and thereby sends the antibiotic molecule out through the exterior of the cell's plasma membrane**.
- By replacing some critical cell metabolic processes with new metabolic processes that bypass the antibiotic's (former) effect.

See also CELL, PATHOGEN, PATHOGENIC, BACTERIA, ANTIBIOTIC, PLASMA MEMBRANE, ENZYME, PENICILLINASES, METABOLISM, ABC TRANSPORTERS, *MYCOBACTERIUM TUBERCULOSIS*, GLYCOPROTEIN REMODELING

Antibody Also called immunoglobulin or Ig. A large defense protein that consists of two classes of polypeptide chains: light (L) chains and heavy (H) chains. A single antibody molecule consists of two identical copies of the L chain and two of the H chain. They are synthesized (i.e., made) by the immune system (B lymphocytes) of the organism. The antibody is composed of four proteins linked together to form a Y-shaped bundle of proteins (which looks somewhat like a slingshot, or like two hockey sticks taped together at the handles). The amino acid sequence that makes up the stem (H chains) of the Y (i.e., the handle of the taped-together hockey sticks) is similar for all antibodies. The stem is known as the Fc region of the antibody; it does not bind to antigen but has other regulatory functions.

The two arms of the Y are each made up of two side-by-side proteins called light chains and heavy chains (i.e., proteins are chains of amino acids), with identical antigen-binding (ab) sites on the tips of each arm. The antibody is thus bivalent in that it has two binding sites for antigen. Taken together, the two arms of the Y are known as the Fab portions of the antibody molecule. The Fab portions can be cleaved from the antibody molecule with papain (an enzyme that is also used as a meat tenderizer), or they can be produced via genetically engineered *Escherichia coli (E. coli)* bacteria.

When a foreign molecule (e.g., a bacterium, virus, etc.) enters the body, B lymphocytes are stimulated into becoming rapidly dividing blast cells, which mature into antibody-producing plasma cells. The plasma cells are triggered by the foreign molecule's epitopes (i.e., group or groups of specific atoms [also known as a hapten], that are recognized to be foreign by the body's immune system) into producing antibody molecules possessing antigen-binding (ab) sites (also called combining sites or determinants).

These fit into the foreign molecule's epitope. Thus, via the tips of its arms, the antibody molecule binds specifically to the foreign entity (antigen) that has entered the body. By this process it inactivates the foreign molecule or marks it for eventual destruction by other immune system cells.

System marking of the foreign molecule (e.g., pathogen or toxin) **for destruction** is accomplished by the fact that the stem of the Y (i.e., the Fc fragment) hangs free from the combined antibody–antigen clump, thereby providing a receptor for phagocytes, which roam throughout the body ingesting and subsequently destroying such "marked" foreign molecules. Research published during 2001 indicates that antibodies may also kill some pathogens themselves by catalyzing the formation of hydrogen peroxide from oxygen free radicals (singlet oxygen) and water. Hydrogen peroxide is highly reactive and could potentially kill pathogens when generated by an (attached) antibody. There are five classes of immunoglobulin: IgG, IgM, IgD, IgA, and IgE.

See also HUMORAL IMMUNITY, IMMUNO-GLOBULIN, PROTEIN, POLYPEPTIDE (PROTEIN), AMINO ACID, B LYMPHO-CYTES, BLAST CELL, ANTIGEN, HAPTEN, EPITOPE, COMBINING SITE, DOMAIN (OF A PROTEIN), SEQUENCE (OF A PROTEIN MOLECULE), *ESCHERICHIA COLIFORM (E. COLI)*, PATHOGEN, TOXIN, PHAGOCYTE, MACROPHAGE, MICRO-PHAGE, MONOCYTES, T CELLS, POLY-MORPHONUCLEAR LEUKOCYTES (PMN), CELLULAR IMMUNE RESPONSE, POLYMORPHONUCLEAR GRANULO-CYTES, GENETIC ENGINEERING, "MAGIC BULLET," ENGINEERED ANTI-BODIES, RECEPTORS, OXYGEN FREE RADICALS

Antibody Affinity Chromatography A type of chromatography in which antibodies are immobilized on the column material. The antibodies bind to their target molecules, whereas the other components in the solution are not retained. In this way, a separation (purification) is achieved.

See also ANTIBODY, CHROMATOGRAPHY, AFFINITY CHROMATOGRAPHY, AFFINITY

Antibody Arrays See PROTEIN MICROAR-RAYS

Antibody-Laced Nanotube Membrane See NANOTUBE

Antibody-Mediated Immune Response See HUMORAL IMMUNE RESPONSE

Anticoding Strand Refers to the single strand of DNA (double helix) that is transcribed. Sometimes called the **antisense strand** or the **template strand**.

See also DEOXYRIBONUCLEIC ACID (DNA), TRANSCRIPTION, ANTISENSE (DNA SEQUENCE)

Anticodon A specific sequence of three nucleotides in a transfer RNA (tRNA) that is complementary to a codon (also three nucleotides) for an amino acid in a messenger RNA.

See also CODON, TRANSFER RNA (tRNA), AMINO ACID, MESSENGER RNA (mRNA), NUCLEOTIDE

Antifreeze Proteins See THERMAL HYS-TERESIS PROTEINS

Antigen Also called an immunogen. Any large molecule or small organism whose entry into the body provokes synthesis of an antibody or immunoglobin (i.e., an immune system response).

See also HAPTEN, ANTIBODY, EPITOPE, CELLULAR IMMUNE RESPONSE, HUMORAL IMMUNITY

Antigenic Determinant See HAPTEN, EPI-TOPE, SUPERANTIGENS

Antihemophilic Factor VIII Also known as factor VIII or antihemophilic globulin (AHG).
See FACTOR VIII

Antihemophilic Globulin Also known as factor VIII or antihemophilic factor VIII.
See FACTOR VIII

Antioxidants Compounds (e.g., phytochemicals) that act to prevent lipids from oxidizing (e.g., to plaque) or breaking down (e.g., to carcinogenic compounds), or that act to capture and halt singlet oxygen (O) free radicals, which can damage DNA in cells (i.e., cause mutations). Because oxidation of lipids in the blood is the initial step in atherosclerosis, consumption of large amounts of certain antioxidants (e.g., flavonoids, melanoidins, etc.) may help prevent atherosclerosis.

Because oxidation reactions within the body often lead to formation of tissue-damaging free radicals (i.e., molecules containing an "extra" electron), consumption of antioxidants can help to prevent such tissue damage.

Evidence indicates that tissue damage due to free radicals may play a role in causing some forms of arthritis, coronary heart disease, diabetes, and cancers.

Synthetic analogues have also been manufactured (e.g., synthetic vitamins, etc.) that perform antioxidant functions similar to naturally occurring antioxidant phytochemicals.

See also OXIDATIVE STRESS, PHYTOCHEM-ICALS, LIPIDS, CARCINOGEN, CANCER,

A

ANALOGUES, OXIDATION, CORONARY HEART DISEASE, INSULIN, LYCOPENE, MUTAGEN, MUTATION, FLAVONOIDS, ISOFLAVONES, ATHEROSCLEROSIS, ASTAXANTHIN, HUMAN SUPEROXIDE DISMUTASE (hSOD), PEG-SOD (POLY-ETHYLENE GLYCOL SUPEROXIDE DIS-MUTASE), PLAQUE, PHYTATE, POLYPHE-NOLS, ELLAGIC ACID, BETA-CAROTENE, VITAMIN E, PROANTHOCYANIDINS, POLYUNSATURATED FATTY ACIDS (PUFA), CONJUGATED LINOLEIC ACID (CLA), CATECHINS, MELANOIDINS

Antiparallel Describes molecules that are parallel but point in opposite directions. The strands of the DNA double helix are antiparallel.

See also DOUBLE HELIX

Antiporter Refers to a membrane-transport system in which the transport of one substance in one direction (across a cell's membrane) is coupled to the transport of a second substance in the opposite direction. For example, the:

- *SOS1* gene in the *Arabidopsis thaliana* plant …
- *AtNHX1* gene in the *Arabidopsis thaliana* plant …

code for a plasma membrane antiporter (ion channel) that transports Na^+ (sodium) ions **out** (of plant's xylem tissue) while transporting H^+ ions **in**.

See also MEMBRANES (OF A CELL), CELL, MEMBRANE TRANSPORT, MEMBRANE TRANSPORTER PROTEIN, ION CHANNELS, GATED TRANSPORT, ABC TRANSPORTERS, *ARABIDOPSIS THALIANA*, VACUOLES, SALT TOLERANCE

Antisense (DNA sequence) A strand of DNA that produces a messenger RNA (mRNA) molecule which (when reversed end for end) has the same sequence as (i.e., is complementary to) the unwanted ("bad") mRNA. The sense (i.e., forward) and antisense (i.e., backward) mRNA strands hybridize (i.e., tightly bond to each other), which prevents the bonded pair from leaving the cell's nucleus, so that the bonded pair is rapidly degraded (destroyed) by nucleases within the cell nucleus.

In genetic targeting using antisense molecules (to block "bad" genes), these molecules are made to bind to a "bad" gene's (e.g., an oncogene) mRNA, thus canceling the (cancer-causing) message of the gene and preventing cells from following its (tumor growth) instructions. Another example would be the use of antisense DNA to block the gene that codes for production of polygalacturonase (an enzyme that causes ripe fruit to soften).

Physically, "antisense" is accomplished by removing a given gene from an organism's genome, reversing it (end for end), and reinserting it into the organism's genome.

See also DEOXYRIBONUCLEIC ACID (DNA), CODING SEQUENCE, GENE, GENOME, COMPLEMENTARY DNA (c-DNA), MESSENGER RNA (mRNA), GENETIC TARGETING, CANCER, POLYGALACTURONASE (PG), ONCO-GENES, SENSE, COSUPPRESSION, GENE SILENCING, HYBRIDIZATION (MOLECULAR GENETICS), NUCLEASE, ANTI-CODING STRAND

Antisense RNA See ANTISENSE (DNA SEQUENCE)

Antithrombogenous Polymers Synthetic polymers (i.e., plastics) that are used to make medical devices (e.g., catheters) that will be in contact with a patient's blood, and therefore must not initiate the coagulation process as synthetic polymers usually do. The natural anticoagulant heparin is incorporated into the polymer and is gradually released into the bloodstream by the polymer, thus preventing blood coagulation on the surface of the polymer.

See also POLYMER, THROMBOSIS

Antitoxin See POLYCLONAL ANTIBODIES, DIPHTHERIA ANTITOXIN

Antixenosis Refers to the effect of a chemical compound (e.g., produced within a plant) that causes relevant predators (e.g., plant-chewing insects) to prefer to attack **other** plants.

See also CORN EARWORM, CORN ROOTWORM, EUROPEAN CORN BORER (ECB)

AP Atrial peptide.

See ATRIAL PEPTIDES

APHIS Acronym for **Animal & Plant Health Inspection Service,** which is the agency of the U.S. Department of Agriculture that is responsible for regulating the field (outdoor)

testing of genetically engineered plants and certain microorganisms.

See COORDINATED FRAMEWORK FOR REGULATION OF BIOTECHNOLOGY, MICROORGANISM, GENETIC ENGINEERING

Aplastic Anemia An autoimmune disease of the bone marrow.

See also AUTOIMMUNE DISEASE

Apo A-1 Milano An apolipoprotein that was found to be naturally produced within the bodies of approximately 40 related people living in an Italian town near Milan. It prevented any buildup of plaque in their arteries.

When synthetic (i.e., made by scientists) *Apo A-1 Milano* was injected into the bloodstreams of people who were not related to that particular Italian family, it caused a **reduction** in the buildup of plaque in their arteries.

See also APOLIPOPROTEINS, PLAQUE

APO B-100 See LOW-DENSITY LIPOPROTEINS (LDLP), APOLIPOPROTEINS, VERY-LOW-DENSITY LIPOPROTEINS (VLDL)

APO-1/Fas See CD95 PROTEIN

Apoenzyme The protein portion of a holoenzyme. Many (but not all) enzymes are composed of functional "pieces." For example, a protein piece (chain) and another piece that is an organic or inorganic molecule. This other piece is known as a cofactor, and it may be removed from the enzyme under certain conditions. When this is done, the resulting inactive enzyme is known as an apoenzyme. The inactive apoenzyme becomes functionally active again if it is allowed to recombine with its cofactor.

See also COFACTOR, ENZYME, HOLOENZYME

Apolipoprotein B An apolipoprotein that is involved in human cholesterol metabolism.

See also CHOLESTEROL, LOW-DENSITY LIPOPROTEINS (LDLP), APOLIPOPROTEINS, VERY-LOW-DENSITY LIPOPROTEINS (VLDL)

Apolipoproteins The protein portion of lipoproteins (i.e., after the lipid portion is removed from those molecules).

See also LOW-DENSITY LIPOPROTEINS (LDLP), PROTEIN, LIPIDS, VERY-LOW-DENSITY LIPOPROTEINS (VLDL)

Apomixis A method of reproduction used by scientists to propagate (hybrid) plants without having to utilize sexual fertilization. By combining apomixis with tissue culture technology, Cai Detian, Ma Piugfu, and Yao Jialin were able to propagate rice varieties in 1994. In 1998, Dimitri Petrov, Phillip Sims, and Chester Deald were able to cause apomixis in corn (maize).

By "fixing" hybrid dominance, the need for (sexual) breeding is eliminated and the hybrid vigor is passed down via the seed from generation to generation.

See also ASEXUAL, GERM CELL, HYBRID VIGOR, TISSUE CULTURE, HYBRIDIZATION (PLANT GENETICS), CORN, F1 HYBRIDS

Apoptosis Also called "programmed cell death," it is a series of programmed steps that causes a cell to die via "self-digestion," without rupturing and releasing intracellular contents (e.g., nucleus, chromosomes, refractile bodies, etc.) into the local (i.e., surrounding tissue) environment. Manifestations of cell apoptosis include shrinkage of the cell's cytoplasm, chromatin condensation, and the presence of phosphatidyl serine on the exterior surface of the cell's plasma membrane.

If the normal cell apoptosis is prevented (e.g., by an enzyme that is present owing to disease) in the body, cells can grow uncontrollably (causing cancer). For example, people with chronic myelogenous leukemia (**CML**, also known as chronic myeloid leukemia) typically have 10–25 times as many white blood cells as normal.

See also CELL, CD95 PROTEIN, SIGNAL TRANSDUCTION, SIGNALING, REFRACTILE BODIES (RB), NUCLEUS, CHROMOSOMES, CHROMATIN, CYTOPLASM, *FUSARIUM*, GENE, p53 GENE, TUBULIN, CANCER, SELECTIVE APOPTOTIC ANTINEOPLASTIC DRUG (SAAND), REPLICON, HYPERSENSITIVE RESPONSE, SIGNAL TRANSDUCTION, SIGNAL TRANSDUCERS AND ACTIVATORS OF TRANSCRIPTION (STATS), MICRORNAs, GENE EXPRESSION CASCADE, ENZYME, WHITE BLOOD CELLS, PHILADELPHIA CHROMOSOME, GLEEVEC™, DNA FRAGMENTATION, RNase 1, GAMMA INTERFERON, CASPASES, POSTTRANSLATIONAL MODIFICATION

OF PROTEIN, MITOGEN-ACTIVATED PROTEIN KINASE CASCADE, PLASMA MEMBRANE, PHOSPHATIDYL SERINE

APP Acronym for **amyloid precursor protein.** See AMYLOID PRECURSOR PROTEIN

Approvable Letter (from the FDA) One of the final steps in the U.S. Food and Drug Administration's (FDA) review process for new pharmaceuticals. The letter precedes the final FDA clearance for marketing of the new compound.

See also FOOD AND DRUG ADMINISTRA-TION (FDA), IND, IND EXEMPTION

Aptamers Single-stranded RNA molecules that form extended three-dimensional structures which bind (i.e., "stick to") other specific molecules (e.g., proteins) and sometimes inactivate the molecules they bind to. The word aptamer is from the Latin *aptus* ("to fit").

During 2004, the U.S. Food and Drug Administration (FDA) approved for use as a pharmaceutical the aptamer Macugen™ (pegaptanib sodium), which is "pegylated" (i.e., joined with polyethylene glycol — PEG — to camouflage the aptamer molecule from the body's immune system so that it is not inactivated by the immune response before it can do its work). Macugen™ binds to vascular endothelial growth factor (VEGF) when injected into the eyeballs of people who are suffering from "wet" form of age-related macular degeneration (AMD). By doing so, Macugen™ prevents the VEGF from causing (more) growth of new blood vessels (i.e., in front of the retina), subsequent leakage of blood from which may cause further vision loss in AMD disease.

In 1992, Louis Bock and John Toole isolated aptamers that bind and inhibit the blood coagulation enzyme **thrombin**. Because thrombin is crucial to the formation of blood clots (coagulation), such aptamers may someday be useful for anticoagulant therapy (e.g., to prevent blood clots following surgery or heart attacks).

One current use of aptamers is as **capture agents** (i.e., ligands or other molecules that bind to proteins, which are attached to the microarray at specific/known locations).

See also ENZYME, OLIGONUCLEOTIDE, PROTEIN, INHIBITION, THROMBIN, THROMBUS, THROMBOSIS, VASCULAR ENDOTHELIAL GROWTH FACTOR (VEGF), PROTEIN MICROARRAYS, FOOD AND DRUG ADMINISTRATION (FDA), CAPTURE AGENT, IMMUNE RESPONSE

Aquaporins A class of plasma-membrane-spanning proteins that function as channels (for water movement into and out of cells) to allow cells to regulate cellular volume. Discovered by Peter C. Agre.

See also PLASMA MEMBRANE PROTEIN, CELL

Arabidopsis thaliana A small weed plant (*Cruciferae*) possessing 70,000 kilobase pairs in its genome, with very little repetitive DNA. This makes it an ideal model for studying plant genetics. At least two genetic maps have been created for *Arabidopsis thaliana* (one using yeast artificial chromosomes). Because of this, a large base of knowledge about it has been accumulated by the scientific community.

Arabidopsis thaliana was first genetically engineered in 1986. In 1994, researchers succeeded in transferring genes for polyhydroxylbutylate (PHB, a biodegradable plastic) production into *Arabidopsis thaliana*. Production of PHB requires the simultaneous expression of three genes (i.e., the PHB production process is "polygenic"), but researchers have only been able to insert a maximum of two genes; they have to insert two genes into one plant and the third gene into a second plant, and finally get the total of three genes in (offspring) plants via traditional breeding.

During 2001, Eduardo Blumwald and Hong-Xia Zhang inserted a salt-tolerance gene from *Arabidopsis thaliana* into a tomato (*Lycopersicon esculentum*) and thereby made the tomato plant resistant to salt in concentrations up to 200 m*M* (i.e., far higher than it could previously tolerate).

See also *BRASSICA*, GENE, EXPRESS, BASE PAIR (bp), KILOBASE PAIRS (Kbp), GENOME, GENETIC CODE, GENETIC MAP, GENETICS, TRAIT, POLYGENIC, DEOXYRIBONUCLEIC ACID (DNA), POLYHYDROXYLBUTYLATE (PHB), YEAST ARTIFICIAL CHROMOSOMES (YAC), MODEL ORGANISM, TOMATO, SALT TOLERANCE

Arachidonic Acid (AA) Also known as eicosatetraenoic acid. Arachidonic acid is one of the "omega-6" (n-6) highly unsaturated fatty acids (HUFA). It is synthesized (i.e., "manufactured") by the human body from linoleic acid (e.g., that obtained via consuming soybean oil). AA is present in human breast milk, and research indicates that it plays an important role in the brain and eye tissue development of infants. Arachidonic acid is a crucial precursor for prostaglandins and other eicosanoids. The COX-1 enzyme converts arachidonic acid to **constitutive prostaglandins,** and the COX-2 enzyme converts arachidonic acid to **inducible prostaglandins**.

See also CYCLOOXYGENASE, POLYUNSATURATED FATTY ACIDS (PUFA), N-6 FATTY ACIDS, FATTY ACIDS, UNSATURATED FATTY ACIDS, LINOLEIC ACID, SOYBEAN OIL, CONSTITUTIVE ENZYMES, INDUCIBLE ENZYMES, LEUKOTRIENES, ESSENTIAL FATTY ACIDS, EICOSANOIDS

Archaea Single-celled life forms that can live at extreme ocean depths (i.e., under high pressure) and in the absence of oxygen. *Archaea* were delineated and named by Carl Woese. Enzymes robust (i.e., sturdy) enough for industrial-process utilization have been isolated by scientists from some strains of *Archaea*.

Other *Archaea* strains are sometimes present in the rumen (i.e., "first stomach") of cattle and sheep. These *Archaea* produce methane gas by breaking down some of the feed consumed by the animals.

See also ENZYME, EXTREMOZYMES, CELL, ANAEROBE, ANAEROBIC, STRAIN

Arginine (Arg) An amino acid (commonly abbreviated as Arg). In dry, bulk form arginine is colorless, crystalline, and water soluble. It is an essential amino acid of the α-ketoglutaric acid family.

See also AMINO ACID, ESSENTIAL AMINO ACIDS, NITRIC OXIDE SYNTHASE

ARM Acronym for **antibiotic resistance marker**.

See MARKER (GENETIC MARKER)

ARMD Acronym for **age-related macular degeneration**.

See LUTEIN

ARMG Acronym for **antibiotic resistance marker gene**.

See also ANTIBIOTIC, ANTIBIOTIC RESISTANCE, GENE, MARKER (GENETIC MARKER), RECOMBINASE

Armyworm Caterpillars (pupae) of the lepidopteran insect *Pseudaletia unipuncta* species, most of which are harmful to crops (e.g., wheat, corn or maize, etc.) grown by humans.

Armyworms are susceptible to some of the "Cry" proteins (e.g., they are killed if they eat plants genetically engineered to contain Cry1A (b), Cry9C, or Cry1F proteins).

Armyworms are preyed upon by some species of ground beetles, sphecid wasps, toads, birds, etc.

See also PROTEIN, VOLICITIN, CRY PROTEINS, CRY1A (b) PROTEIN, CRY1F PROTEIN, CRY9C PROTEIN, CORN, WHEAT, FALL ARMYWORM

AroA Refers to the transgene (cassette) that was initially isolated and extracted from the genome of the *Agrobacterium* bacterial species (strain CP4) and inserted via genetic engineering techniques into a crop plant (e.g., soybean, *Glycine max* (L.)) in order to make it tolerant to glyphosate-based herbicides (and also sulfosate-based herbicides).

See also GENE, TRANSGENE, CASSETTE, GENOME, *AGROBACTERIUM TUMEFACIENS*, EPSP SYNTHASE, mEPSPS, CP4 EPSPS, SOYBEAN, HERBICIDE-TOLERANT CROP, GENETIC ENGINEERING, SOYBEAN PLANT, GLYPHOSATE, SULFOSATE

ARS See ARS ELEMENT

ARS Element A sequence of DNA that will support autonomous replication (sequence, ARS).

See also DEOXYRIBONUCLEIC ACID (DNA), SEQUENCE (OF A DNA MOLECULE)

Arteriosclerosis A group of diseases (including atherosclerosis) that is characterized by deposits of plaques on the inside of blood vessel walls (beginning in the late teenage years), a decrease in elasticity (i.e., "stretchiness"), and a thickening of the walls of the body's arteries.

See also ATHEROSCLEROSIS, CORONARY HEART DISEASE (CHD), PLAQUE, GRANULOCYTE-MACROPHAGE COLONY-STIMULATING FACTOR (GM-CSF),

C-REACTIVE PROTEIN (CRP), HOMOCYSTEINE

Arthritis See OSTEOARTHRITIS, RHEUMATOID ARTHRITIS, AUTOIMMUNE DISEASE

Ascites Liquid accumulation in the peritoneal cavity. Used as an input in one of the methods for producing monoclonal antibodies.

See also MONOCLONAL ANTIBODIES (MAb), PERITONEAL CAVITY/MEMBRANE, ANTIBODY

Ascorbic Acid A water-soluble vitamin and antioxidant.

See also VITAMIN, ANTIOXIDANTS

Asexual Denotes fertilization or reproduction by *in vitro* means (without sex).

See also *IN VITRO*, APOMIXIS, GERM CELL

Asian Corn Borer Also known by its Latin name *Ostrinia furnacalis*, it is an insect (originally from Asia) whose larvae (caterpillars) eat and bore into the corn or maize (*Zea mays* L.) plant. In doing so, they can act as vectors (i.e., carriers) of the fungi known as *Aspergillus flavus* (a source of aflatoxin), *Fusarium moniliforme* (a source of fumonisin), or *Aspergillus parasiticus* (a source of aflatoxin).

See also EUROPEAN CORN BORER (ECB), CORN, FUNGUS, AFLATOXIN, *FUSARIUM*, *FUSARIUM MONILIFORME*

Asparagine (Asp) An amino acid (commonly abbreviated as Asp). In dry, bulk form asparagine appears as a white, crystalline solid. It is found in high amounts in many plants.

See also AMINO ACID

Aspartic Acid A dicarboxylic amino acid found in plants and animals, especially in molasses from young sugarcane and sugar beets.

See also AMINO ACID

Aspergillus flavus See AFLATOXIN, PEROXIDASE, BETA-CAROTENE

Assay A test (specific technique) that measures a response to a test substance or the efficacy (effectiveness) of the test substance.

See also IMMUNOASSAY, BIOASSAY, LUMINESCENT ASSAY, MULTIPLEXED (ASSAY), MULTIPLEX ASSAY, HYBRIDIZATION SURFACES

Assimilation The formation of "self" cellular material from small molecules derived from food.

See also INSULIN-LIKE GROWTH FACTOR-1 (IGF-1), RIBOSOMES, MESSENGER RNA (mRNA)

Association Mapping See HAPLOTYPE, HAPLOTYPE MAP

Association of Biotechnology Companies (ABC) An American trade association of companies involved in biotechnology and services to biotechnology companies (e.g., accounting, law, etc.). Formed in 1984, the ABC tended to consist of the smaller firms involved in biotechnology (and service firms that worked for all biotechnology companies). In 1993, the ABC was merged with the Industrial Biotechnology Association (IBA) to form the Biotechnology Industry Organization (BIO).

See also INDUSTRIAL BIOTECHNOLOGY ASSOCIATION (IBA), BIOTECHNOLOGY INDUSTRY ORGANIZATION (BIO), BIOTECHNOLOGY

Astaxanthin A carotenoid pigment that is responsible for the characteristic pink coloring of salmon, trout, and shrimp, and the red color of lobsters. It is produced by the microorganisms in the natural diets of those aquatic animals.

Research has shown that astaxanthin (an antioxidant) helps to boost the immune systems of humans who consume it. In rodents, astaxanthin helps to reduce oral cancer, and it inhibits breast cancer in mice.

See also CAROTENOIDS, ANTIOXIDANTS, OXIDATIVE STRESS

AT-III A human blood factor that promotes clotting. A deficiency of AT-III can be inherited, result from certain surgical procedures, certain illnesses and, sometimes, from the use of certain oral contraceptives.

See also FACTOR VIII

ATCC See AMERICAN TYPE CULTURE COLLECTION (ATCC), TYPE SPECIMEN, ACCESSION (GERMPLASM)

Atherosclerosis One form of arteriosclerosis; it is characterized by deposition and buildup of fatty deposits (plaque) on the internal walls of the body's arteries, in addition to the decrease in elasticity of the arteries' walls that characterizes all forms of arteriosclerosis. When a piece of plaque breaks off a blood clot generally forms, and the clot often blocks blood flow through the artery, which causes a heart attack or stroke in the person.

See also ARTERIOSCLEROSIS, CORONARY HEART DISEASE (CHD), CHOLESTEROL, THROMBOSIS, THROMBUS, FLA-VONOIDS, OXIDATIVE STRESS, ANTI-OXIDANTS, PLAQUE

AtNHX1 Gene See ANTIPORTER, SALT TOLERANCE

Atomic Force Microscopy Refers to one type of scanning probe microscopy (SPM) that is particularly utilized for the study of biological systems. Developed in 1986, atomic force microscopy (AFM) can produce high-resolution three-dimensional images of a (biological) surface in aqueous environments without the need to stain the biological specimen.

In AFM, a very sharp probe (stylus) is carefully suspended in near proximity to the specimen surface via a high-precision device such as a cantilever, or a piezoelectric or magnetic/electrostatic process. When carefully moving the probe over the entire specimen surface, the force between the probe and the atoms of the specimen keeps the probe just above the specimen surface and thereby delineates the surface topography of the specimen at atomic-scale resolution. AFM can also be utilized for "dip-pen nanolithography."

See also DIP-PEN NANOLITHOGRAPY

Atomic Weight The total mass of an atom is equal to the sum of the isotope's number of protons and neutrons (in the atom's nucleus). The atomic weights of Earth's elements are based on the assignment of exactly 12.000 as the atomic weight of the carbon-12 isotope (variation of atom). The atomic (weight) theory was established as a framework in 1869 by Meyer and Mendeléev, but standard precise values were not adopted internationally until an "international commission on atomic weights" was formed in 1899 in response to an initiative by the German Chemical Society.

An element's atomic weight is the average of the atomic weights of all isotopes present on Earth, and so it does not come out to a whole number (with the exception of carbon) because of the existence of small amounts of isotopes that differ slightly with respect to the number of neutrons each contains.

See also MOLECULAR WEIGHT, ISOTOPE

ATP See ADENOSINE TRIPHOSPHATE (ATP)

ATP Synthase An enzyme complex that forms ATP from ADP and phosphate during oxidative phosphorylation in the inner mitochondrial membrane (in animals), in chloroplasts (in plants), and in cell membranes (in bacteria). This is an energy-producing reaction in that ATP is a high-energy compound used by cells to maintain their life.

ATP synthase is also present on the surface of endothelial cells (lining of blood vessels) where it helps to build new blood vessels (e.g., to replace tissue damaged by injury or disease). Under certain circumstances, it also creates new blood vessels that provide blood supply to tumors.

When separated from the cell's membrane, ATP synthase hydrolyzes (i.e., breaks down) ATP via a chemical process in which one subunit (designated γ) of ATP synthase rotates within the other (hollow) part of ATP synthase.

See also ENZYME, CHLOROPLASTS, ADE-NOSINE TRIPHOSPHATE (ATP), HYDROLYSIS, ADENOSINE DIPHOS-PHATE (ADP), MITOCHONDRIA, TUMOR, ENDOTHELIAL CELLS, ANGIOSTATIN

ATP Synthetase See ATP SYNTHASE

ATPase Adenosine triphosphatase, an enzyme that hydrolyzes (clips the bond between two phosphates) ATP to yield ADP, phosphate, and energy. The reaction is usually coupled to an energy-requiring process. ATP is hydrolyzed in the act of shivering, and the energy produced is converted into heat to increase body temperature. This type of heat production involves what is known as a futile cycle because the energy is converted to (and wasted as) heat rather than used in motion, etc.

See also ATP SYNTHASE, ENZYME, ADE-NOSINE TRIPHOSPHATE (ATP), ADE-NOSINE DIPHOSPHATE (ADP), FUTILE CYCLE, HYDROLYSIS, HYDROLYZE

Atrial Natriuretic Factor An atrial peptide hormone that may regulate blood pressure and electrolyte balance within the body. An example is a peptide hormone.

See also HORMONE, ATRIAL PEPTIDES, PEPTIDE

A

Atrial Peptides Endocrine components (proteins) that act to regulate blood pressure as well as water and electrolyte homeostasis within the body. Atrial peptides are made by the heart in response to elevated blood pressure levels; they stimulate the kidneys to excrete water and sodium into the urine, thus lowering blood pressure. They also slow the heart rate. An example is a peptide hormone.
See also ENDOCRINE HORMONES, HOMEOSTASIS, ELECTROLYTE

Attenuated (pathogens) Inactivated or rendered harmless (e.g., killed viruses used to make a vaccine). Some of the ways in which viruses and other pathogens may be attenuated are by heat, chemical, or radiation treatment.
See also PATHOGEN

Attenuation (of RNA) Premature termination of an elongating RNA chain.
See also RIBONUCLEIC ACID (RNA)

Aureofacin An antifungal antibiotic produced by a strain of *Streptomyces aureofaciens*. At least one company has incorporated the gene for this antibiotic (which acts against wheat take-all disease) into *Pseudomonas fluorescens*, which is then used to confer resistance to wheat take-all disease. This is done by allowing the bacteria to colonize the wheat's roots. In this way, the plant obtains the benefits of the antibiotic because the bacteria become a part of the plant.
See also *PSEUDOMONAS FLUORESCENS*, ENDOPHYTE, ANTIBIOTIC, *BACILLUS THURINGIENSIS (B.t.)*

Autogenous Control The action of a gene product (a molecule) that either inhibits (negative autogenous control) or activates (positive autogenous control) expression of the **gene that codes for it** (Greek *auto* = "self"). The presence of the product either causes or stops its own production.
See also GENE, EXPRESS

Autoimmune Disease A disease in which the body produces an immunogenic (i.e., immune system) response to some constituent of its own tissue. In other words, the immune system loses its ability to recognize some tissue or system within the body as "self" and targets and attacks it as if it were foreign. Autoimmune diseases can be classified into those in which predominantly one organ is affected (e.g., hemolytic anemia and chronic thyroiditis) and those in which the autoimmune disease process is diffused through many tissues (e.g., multiple sclerosis, systemic lupus erythematosus, and rheumatoid arthritis).

For example, multiple sclerosis is thought to be caused by T cells attacking acetylcholine receptors in the sheaths (myelin) that surround the nerve fibers of the brain and spinal cord. This eventually results in loss of coordination, weakness, and blurred vision. Arthritis is caused by immune system cells attacking joint tissues.

Certain bacterial infections (e.g., Lyme disease, salmonella, etc.) are followed by arthritis in approximately 10% of cases. The antigen (on the surface of these bacteria) that is targeted by the human immune system is similar (in its molecular shape) to a protein that is located on the surface of cells in human joint tissues.
See also THYMUS, SUPERANTIGENS, T CELLS, TUMOR NECROSIS FACTOR (TNF), MULTIPLE SCLEROSIS, MYO-ELECTRIC SIGNALS, ACETYLCHOLINE, LUPUS, INSULIN-DEPENDENT DIABETES MELLITIS (IDDM), DIABETES, ANTIGEN, BACTERIA, *SALMONELLA TYPHIMURIUM*, PROTEIN, CELL, RHEUMATOID ARTHRITIS, GLUTAMIC ACID DECARBOXYLASE (GAD)

Autologous Refers to two things that are derived from the same organism.
See also ORGANISM

Autonomous Replicating Segment See ARS ELEMENT

Autonomous Replicating Sequence See ARS ELEMENT

Autoradiography A technique to detect radioactively labeled molecules by creating an image on photographic film. The slab of gel or other material in which the molecules are held (suspended) is placed on top of a piece of photographic film. The two are then securely fastened together such that movement is eliminated and the film is exposed for a period of time. The exposed film is subsequently developed and the radioactive area is seen as a dark (black) area. Among other uses, autoradiography has been used to track the spread of (radioactively labeled) viruses in a living plant. After treatment (i.e., the radioactive labeling process), the whole plant (in a slab) is placed on top of a piece of photographic film. When the film is subsequently developed, the "picture" seen is of the plant, with darker areas indicating regions of greater virus concentration.

See also LABEL (RADIOACTIVE), VIRUS

Autosomes All chromosomes except the sex chromosomes. A diploid cell has two copies of each autosome.

See also CELL, CHROMOSOMES, DIPLOID

Autotroph An organism that can live on very simple carbon and nitrogen sources, such as carbon dioxide and ammonia.

See also HETEROTROPH

Auxotroph An auxotrophic mutant is a mutant defective in the synthesis of a given biomolecule. The biomolecule must be supplied to the organism if normal growth is to be achieved.

MUTATION, GENE, GENE DELIVERY (GENE THERAPY), ESSENTIAL FATTY ACIDS

Avidin A protein that is naturally present in egg white, oilseed protein (e.g., soybean meal), and grain (e.g., corn or maize). The protein is 70 kDa in mass (weight) and has a high affinity for biotin (i.e., it "sticks" tightly to the biotin molecule). Because grain-eating insects require biotin (a B-complex vitamin) to live, adding extra avidin to grain (e.g., via inserting a gene to cause overproduction of avidin in the grain kernels) may be a way to protect grain from insects (e.g., weevils in stored corn or maize).

See also PROTEIN, SOY PROTEIN, CORN, KILODALTON (kDa), BIOTIN, WEEVILS, VITAMIN, STREPTAVIDIN

Avidity (of an antibody) The "tightness of fit" between a given antibody's combining site and the antigenic determinant that it combines with. The firmness of the combination of antigen with antibody.

See also ANTIGENIC DETERMINANT, ANTIBODY, ANTIGEN, COMBINING SITE, POLYCLONAL RESPONSE, CATALYTIC ANTIBODY

Azadirachtin The pharmacophore (i.e., active ingredient) in secretions of the tropical neem tree, which confers resistance to insect depredations.

See also PHARMACOPHORE, NEEM TREE

Azurophil-Derived Bactericidal Factor (ADBF) Potent antimicrobial protein produced by neutrophils (a type of white blood cell).

See also LEUKOCYTES

B

B-DNA A helical form of DNA. B-DNA can be formed by adding water to (dehydrated) A-DNA. B-DNA is the form of DNA whose model was first constructed in 1953 by James Watson and Francis Crick. It is found in fibers of very high (92%) relative humidity and in solutions of low ionic strength. This corresponds to the form of DNA that is prevalent in the living cell.

Irradiation by gamma rays of B-DNA (in copper-containing solution) converts B-DNA to Z-DNA.

See also DEOXYRIBONUCLEIC ACID (DNA), A-DNA, ION, CELL, Z-DNA

B Cells B lymphocytes.

See LYMPHOCYTE, B LYMPHOCYTES, BLAST CELL

B Lymphocytes A class of white blood cells originating in the bone marrow and found in blood, spleen, and lymph nodes. They are the precursors of (blood) plasma cells (B cells) that secrete antibodies (IgG) directed against invading antigens (e.g., of pathogenic bacteria). By a complex "gene splicing" process, the B cells of the human body are able to produce more than one billion different IgG antibodies (i.e., able to bind onto and neutralize a billion different antigens). By a natural process known as affinity maturation, the immune system selects those B cells producing antibodies with greater affinity for the antigen of the invading pathogen to combat the invader.

Sometimes, B cells can go awry and contribute to causing the disease rheumatoid arthritis (e.g., by producing antibodies against the body's own tissue). The pharmaceutical Rituxan™ (rituximab) is a monoclonal antibody that can be utilized to inhibit the structural damage (to body joints) due to rheumatoid arthritis.

See also ANTIGEN, ANTIBODY, BLAST CELL, LYMPHOCYTE, PATHOGEN, BACTERIA, GENE SPLICING, IMMUNOGLOBULIN, ALLELIC EXCLUSION, RHEUMATOID ARTHRITIS, MONOCLONAL ANTIBODIES (MAb)

BAC Acronym for **bacterial artificial chromosomes**.

See BACTERIAL ARTIFICIAL CHROMOSOMES (BAC)

Bacillus licheniformis A (rod-shaped) bacterium that dwells in soil.

Various biotechnology companies have extracted a number of enzymes (e.g., amylases) from the wild-type *Bacillus licheniformis*, modified the relevant enzymes' genes via mutagenesis (to improve the activity or other properties of that enzyme), and today sell the improved enzymes produced via genetically engineered *Bacillus licheniformis*.

See also BACTERIA, ENZYME, AMYLASE, GENE, WILD TYPE, MUTATION BREEDING, GENETIC ENGINEERING

Bacillus subtilis (B. subtilis) A (rod-shaped) aerobic bacterium commonly used as a host in recombinant DNA experiments.

During the 1990s, research showed that corn (maize) plant tissues infected with the endophyte *Bacillus subtilis* were less likely to become infected with the fungus *Fusarium moniliforme*.

Other research has indicated the potential for prior infection of corn (maize) plant tissues to hinder any subsequent aflatoxin production in that plant by *Aspergillus flavus* fungus.

See also BACTERIA, HOST VECTOR (HV) SYSTEM, DEOXYRIBONUCLEIC ACID (DNA), CORN, ENDOPHYTE, FUNGUS, *FUSARIUM MONILIFORME*, AFLATOXIN

Bacillus thuringiensis (B.t.) Discovered by bacteriologist Ishiwata Shigetane on a diseased silkworm in 1901. Later discovered on a dead Mediterranean flour moth, and first named *Bacillus thuringiensis* by Ernst Berliner in 1915.

Today, *Bacillus thuringiensis* refers to a group of rod-shaped soil bacteria found all over the earth, which produce "Cry" proteins that are indigestible by — yet still "bind" to — specific insects' gut (i.e., stomach) lining (epithelium cell) receptors. Those Cry proteins are thereby toxic to certain classes of insects (corn borers, corn rootworms, mosquitoes, black flies, some types of beetles, etc.), but are harmless to all mammals. At least 20,000 strains of *Bacillus thuringiensis* are known.

Genes that code for the production of these Cry proteins that are toxic to insects have been inserted into vectors (i.e., viruses, other bacteria, and other microorganisms) by scientists since 1989 in order to confer insect resistance on certain agricultural plants (e.g., via expression of those *B.t.* proteins by one or more tissues of the transgenic plant). For example, the *B.t.* strain known as *B.t. kurstaki*, which is fatal when ingested by the European corn borer, was first (genetically) inserted into a corn plant (via vector) in 1991. *B.t. kurstaki* kills borers via perforation of that insect's gut by Cry (crystal-like) proteins that are coded for by the *B.t. kurstaki* gene. The vectors listed earlier in this paragraph are entities that can take up and carry the DNA into plants or other cells. Vectors are DNA-carrying vehicles.

See also ENDOPHYTE, CORN, GENE, *PSEUDOMONAS FLUORESCENS*, *AGRO-BACTERIUM TUMEFACIENS*, AUREOFA-CIN, EUROPEAN CORN BORER (ECB), COWPEA TRYPSIN INHIBITOR (CpTI), PROTEIN, "SHOTGUN" METHOD, COD-ING SEQUENCE, *FUSARIUM*, VECTOR, EXPRESS, GENETIC ENGINEERING, "EXPLOSION" METHOD, BIOLISTIC® GENE GUN, CRY PROTEINS, CRY1A (b) PROTEIN, CRY1A (c) ROTEIN, CRY9C PROTEIN, *B.t. KURSTAKI*, *B.t. TENEBRIO-NIS*, *B.t. ISRAELENSIS*, *B.t. TOLWORTHI*, ION CHANNELS

Bacillus Rod-shaped bacteria.
See also BACTERIA, *BACILLUS SUBTILIS (B. SUBTILIS)*, *BACILLUS THURINGIENSIS (B.t.)*, *BACILLUS LICHENIFORMIS*

Back Mutation Reverses the effect of a mutation that had inactivated a gene; thus, it restores the wild phenotype.
See also PHENOTYPE, MUTATION

Bacteria From the Greek *bakterion* = (stick), because the first bacteria viewed by humans (via crude microscopes) appeared to be stick shaped.

Any of a large group of microscopic organisms having round, rodlike, spiral, or filamentous unicellular or noncellular bodies that are often aggregated into colonies, enclosed by a cell wall or membrane (procaryotes), and lack fully differentiated nuclei. Bacteria may exist as free-living organisms in soil, water, and organic matter or as parasites in the live bodies of plants and animals.
See also BACTERIOLOGY

Bacterial Artificial Chromosomes (BAC)
Pieces of DNA (e.g., plant DNA) that have been cloned (made) inside living bacteria (e.g., by plant researchers who need to "manufacture" some pieces of plant DNA). They can be utilized as vectors (for genetic engineering) to carry (inserted) genes into certain organisms.
Some potential uses of BAC include:

- The manufacture of probes (i.e., sequences of DNA utilized to "find" complementary sequences within large pieces of DNA) via hybridization
- The manufacture of "DNA sequence markers" for use in marker-assisted selection (e.g., to guide choices made by commercial crop breeders, so that they can more quickly select plants bearing genes for a particular trait) to develop improved future crop varieties faster than was previously possible

See also BACTERIA, CLONE (A MOLECULE), SYNTHESIZING (OF DNA MOLECULES), CHROMOSOMES, YEAST ARTIFICIAL CHROMOSOMES (YAC), HUMAN ARTIFI-CIAL CHROMOSOMES (HAC), PROBE, MARKER-ASSISTED SELECTION, COM-PLEMENTARY DNA (c-DNA), HYBRIDIZA-TION (MOLECULAR GENETICS), DEOX-YRIBONUCLEIC ACID (DNA), SEQUENCE (OF A DNA MOLECULE), MARKER (DNA SEQUENCE), GENE, TRAIT, GENETIC ENGINEERING, VECTOR

Bacterial Expressed Sequence Tags These are ESTs (expressed sequence tags) that are based on sequenced or mapped bacterial genes instead of the genes of ("traditional" EST) *C.*

elegans nematode. They are utilized to "label" a given gene (i.e., in terms of that gene's function or protein).

See also EXPRESSED SEQUENCE TAGS (EST), BACTERIA, SEQUENCING (OF DNA MOLECULES), SEQUENCE (OF A DNA MOLECULE), MAPPING, *Caenorhabditis elegans (C. elegans)*

Bacterial Two-Hybrid System See TWO-HYBRID SYSTEMS

Bactericide See MICROBICIDE, BIOCIDE, ANTIBIOTIC

Bacteriocide See BACTERICIDE

Bacteriocins Proteins produced by many types of bacteria that are toxic (primarily) to other closely related strains of the particular bacteria that produce those proteins. Bacteriocins hold promise (e.g., after genetic engineering of the DNA responsible for their production) for possible future use as food preservatives (i.e., acting against bacterial species that cause food spoilage).

For example:

- The bacteriocin known as curvaticin 13, which is produced by *Lactobacillus curvatus* bacteria, inhibits the food-poisoning bacteria *Listeria monocytogenes*.
- The bacteriocin known as sakacin K, which is produced by *Lactobacillus sakei* bacteria, inhibits the food-poisoning bacteria *Listeria monocytogenes*.

However, the effectiveness of both curvaticin 13 and sakacin K is lessened by the presence of salt (e.g., in processed meat products), so salt resistance would be a desired property that may someday be engineered into those bacteriocins.

Nisin is also referred to as a bacteriocin, but it is active against many more species of bacteria than most of the bacteriocins.

See also PROTEIN, BACTERIA, BACTERIOLOGY, *BIFIDUS*, STRAIN, TOXIN, GENETIC ENGINEERING, DEOXYRIBONUCLEIC ACID (DNA), CODING SEQUENCE, COLICINS, LISTERIA MONOCYTOGENES, EXTREMOPHILIC BACTERIA, NISIN

Bacteriology The science and study of bacteria, a specialized branch of microbiology. Bacteria constitute a useful and essential group in the biological community. Although some bacteria prey on higher forms of life, relatively few are pathogens (disease-causing organisms). Life on Earth depends on the activity of bacteria to mineralize organic compounds and to capture the free nitrogen molecules in the air for use by plants. Also, bacteria are important industrially for the conversion of raw materials into products such as organic chemicals, antibiotics, cheeses, etc. Genetically engineered bacteria are starting to be used to produce high-value-added pharmaceuticals and specialty chemicals.

See also *ESCHERICHIA COLIFORM (E. COLI)*

Bacteriophage Discovered in 1917 by Felix d'Herelle, a bacteriophage (fr. bacteria eaters) is a virus that attaches to, injects its DNA into, and multiplies inside bacteria, which eventually causes bacteria to die. Often abbreviated as simply **phage**. Phage is also another name for virus.

As an example, bacteriophage lambda is commonly used as a vector in rDNA experiments in *Escherichia coli* and attaches to a specific receptor that, in the bacteria, also normally functions in sugar transport across the cell wall. Viruses come in many shapes and sizes.

See also *ESCHERICHIA COLIFORM (E. COLI)*, RECEPTORS, VIRUS, TRANSDUCTION (GENE), TRANSDUCTION (SIGNAL), TRANSFECTION, LAMBDA PHAGE, HOLINS

Bacterium See BACTERIA

Baculovirus A class of virus that infects lepidopteran insects (e.g., cotton bollworm or gypsy moth larva). Baculoviruses can be modified via genetic engineering to insert new genes into the larva, causing those larva to then produce proteins desired by humans (e.g., pharmaceuticals).

Baculoviruses are potentially very useful for pharmaceutical production because:

- The protein molecules produced are **glycosylated (i.e., have relevant oligosaccharides attached to them)**.
- Baculoviruses cannot infect vertebrate animals.

Thus, such pharmaceuticals are not even a theoretical pathogenic risk to humans.

See also VIRUS, GENETIC ENGINEERING, GENE, PROTEIN, GLYCOSYLATION, BACULOVIRUS EXPRESSION VECTORS (BEVs), PATHOGEN

Baculovirus Expression Vector (BEV) Refers to vectors (used by researchers to carry new genes into insect cells) in which the agent is a baculovirus (i.e., a virus that infects certain types of insect cells only). A genetically engineered BEV is commonly utilized to carry a new gene into the insect cells within a baculovirus expression vector system (BEVS) to induce cell culture production of a protein desired by humans.

A BEV could conceivably be used to make a genetically engineered insecticide that is specific to a targeted insect (i.e., it would not harm anything but that insect). For example, a BEV might be used to cause a cotton bollworm *adult* protein to be expressed when the bollworm is a *juvenile*, thus killing the bollworm before it has a chance to damage a cotton crop.

See also BACULOVIRUS, VIRUS, VECTOR, GENE, PROTEIN, CELL, GENETIC ENGINEERING, INSECT CELL CULTURE, BACULOVIRUS EXPRESSION VECTOR SYSTEM (BEVS)

Baculovirus Expression Vector System (BEVS) Refers to an insect cell culture system, invented in 1982 by Gale Smith and Max Summers, in which a genetically engineered baculovirus expression vector (BEV) is utilized to carry into the insect cells a gene that codes for a protein desired by humans.

See also INSECT CELL CULTURE, CELL, GENE, GENETIC ENGINEERING, CODING SEQUENCE

Bakanae See *FUSARIUM MONILIFORME*

BAR Gene A dominant gene from the *Streptomyces hygroscopicus* bacterium that codes for (i.e., causes production of) the enzyme **phosphinothricin acetyl transferase (PAT)**. When the BAR gene is inserted into a plant's genome (i.e., its DNA), it imparts resistance to glufosinate-ammonium-based herbicides.

Because the glufosinate-ammonium herbicides act via inhibition of glutamine synthetase (an enzyme that catalyzes the synthesis of glutamine), this inhibition (of enzyme) kills plants (e.g., weeds). That is because glutamine is crucial for plants to synthesize critically needed amino acids.

The BAR gene is often utilized by genetic engineers as a marker gene.

See also GENE, GENOME, GENETIC ENGINEERING, MARKER (GENETIC MARKER), DOMINANT ALLELE, ESSENTIAL AMINO ACIDS, HERBICIDE-TOLERANT CROP, GTS, SOYBEAN PLANT, CANOLA, CORN, GLUTAMINE, GLUTAMINE SYNTHETASE, PHOSPHINOTHRICIN, PHOSPHINOTHRICIN ACETYLTRANSFERASE (PAT), PAT GENE

Barley The domesticated plant *Hordeum vulgare*, whose grain is utilized by humans for various purposes:

- Feed barley varieties, utilized for feeding of livestock
- Malting barley varieties (containing beta-amylase in their seeds) were created via mutation breeding (i.e., bombardment of the seeds by ionizing radiation to cause random genetic mutations, followed by selection of the particular mutation in which maltose is produced by that barley plant in its seeds)

See also TRADITIONAL BREEDING METHODS, MUTATION, MUTATION BREEDING, AMYLASE

Barnase Abbreviation for *Bacillus amyloliquefaciens* **RNase**, it is an enzyme that catalyzes destruction of nucleic acids (which thus kills the cell that the barnase is in). When the gene that codes for barnase is inserted via genetic engineering into a given plant and activated only in that plant's pollen (i.e., the barnase is produced only in its pollen cells), that plant's male parts become sterile. For crop plants possessing both male and female parts (i.e., monoecious plants), such "male sterility" facilitates the development of hybrids, because self-pollination does not occur.

See also ENZYME, NUCLEIC ACIDS, CELL, GENE, GENETIC CODE, GENETIC ENGINEERING, GENETICS, HYBRIDIZATION

(PLANT GENETICS), F1 HYBRIDS, MONOECIOUS, RNase

Base (general) A substance with a pH in the range of 7 to 14 that will react with an acid to form a salt. Mild bases normally taste bitter and feel slippery.

See also ACID

Base (nucleotide) A segment of the DNA (and RNA) molecules, one of the four (repeating) chemical units that constitute DNA or RNA and that, according to their order and pairing (on the parallel strands of the DNA or RNA molecules), represent the different amino acids (i.e., within the protein molecule that each gene in the DNA codes for). The four bases that constitute DNA are adenine (A), cytosine (C), guanine (G), and thymine (T).

See also DEOXYRIBONUCLEIC ACID (DNA), RIBONUCLEIC ACID (RNA), POLYMER, CODING SEQUENCE, CONTROL SEQUENCES, EXPRESSION, AMINO ACID, PROTEIN, GENE, ADENINE, CYTOSINE, GUANINE, THYMINE, URACIL, BASE PAIR (bp)

Base Excision Sequence Scanning (BESS) A method that can be utilized to detect a "point mutation" in DNA (via rapid DNA sequence scanning).

See also BASE PAIR (bp), NUCLEOTIDE, DEOXYRIBONUCLEIC ACID (DNA), MUTATION, POINT MUTATION, EXCISION, SEQUENCING (OF DNA MOLECULES), SEQUENCE (OF A DNA MOLECULE)

Base Pair (bp) Two nucleotides that are in different nucleic acid chains and whose bases pair (interact) by hydrogen bonding. In DNA, the nucleotide bases are adenine (which pairs with thymine) and guanine (which pairs with cytosine).

See also DEOXYRIBONUCLEIC ACID (DNA), GENETIC CODE, INFORMATIONAL MOLECULES

Base Substitution Replacement of one base (within a DNA molecule) by another base.

See also BASE (NUCLEOTIDE), TRANSITION, TRANSVERSION

Basic Fibroblast Growth Factor (BFGF) See FIBROBLAST GROWTH FACTOR (FGF)

Basophilic Staining strongly with basic dye. For example, basophil leukocytes are polymorphonuclear leukocytes that stain strongly with (take up a lot of) basic dyes.

See also POLYMORPHONUCLEAR LEUKOCYTES (PMN)

Basophils Also called **basophilic leukocytes**. A type of white blood cell (leukocyte) produced by stem cells within the bone marrow that synthesizes and stores histamine and also contains heparin. When two IgE molecules of the same antibody "dock" at adjacent receptor sites on a basophil cell, the two IgE molecules capture an allergen between them. A chemical signal is sent to the basophil causing the basophil cell to release histamine, serotonin, bradykinin, and "slow-reacting-substance." Release of these chemicals into the body causes the blood vessels to become more permeable, which consequently causes the nose to run. These chemicals also cause smooth-muscle contraction, resulting in sneezing, coughing, wheezing, etc.

See also MAST CELLS, ANTIGEN, ANTIBODY, HISTAMINE, WHITE BLOOD CELLS, BASOPHILIC, LEUKOCYTES, POLYMORPHONUCLEAR LEUKOCYTES (PMN), STEM CELLS

BB T.I. See TRYPSIN INHIBITORS

BBB See BLOOD–BRAIN BARRIER (BBB)

BCA Acronym for **Bio–Bar Code Amplification**.

See BIO–BAR CODES

Bce4 The name of a promoter (region of DNA) that controls or enhances an oilseed plant's genes that code for components (e.g., fatty acids, amino acids, etc.) of that plant's seeds. The Bce4 promoter causes such genes to be expressed during one of the earliest stages of canola plant seed production, for instance.

See also PROMOTER, DEOXYRIBONUCLEIC ACID (DNA), GENE, POLYGENIC, PLASTID, EXPRESS, CANOLA, SOYBEAN PLANT, TRANSCRIPTION

Bcr-Abl Gene The gene (SNP) that causes the blood cancer **chronic myelocytic leukemia (CML)** in humans who possess it.

See also GENE, SINGLE-NUCLEOTIDE POLYMORPHISMS (SNPs), CANCER, GLEEVEC™

bcr-abl Genetic Marker See GENETIC MARKER, FLUORESCENCE *IN SITU* HYBRIDIZATION (FISH)

BESS Method See BASE EXCISION SEQUENCE SCANNING (BESS)

BESS T-Scan Method See BASE EXCISION SEQUENCE SCANNING (BESS)

Best Linear Unbiased Prediction (BLUP) A statistical (data) technique that is utilized by livestock breeders to determine the breeding (genetic trait) value of animals in a breeding program.

See also GENETICS, TRAIT, PHENOTYPE, GENOTYPE, EXPECTED PROGENY DIFFERENCES (EPD)

Beta-Carotene A phytochemical (vitamin precursor) that is naturally produced in carrots, other orange vegetables, apricots, cantaloupe, kiwi, papaya, and in the endosperm portion of the corn (maize) kernel. If the corn kernel seed coat is torn (e.g., via insect chewing), the beta-carotene inhibits growth of *Aspergillus flavus* fungi in the endosperm region of the kernel.

In 1970, an orange (-fruited) cauliflower was discovered growing in Bradford Marsh in Canada. It was the result of a natural mutation that caused beta-carotene to be produced in that cauliflower plant, at a level that was approximately 100 times higher than normal for cauliflower. Beta-carotene has been found to aid eyesight and to strengthen the immune system in people who consume it, and may help prevent lung cancer and heart disease.

Because beta-carotene is processed into vitamin A by the human body, consumption of this phytochemical can help prevent human diseases (e.g., in developing countries where vitamin A is scarce) that result from deficiency of vitamin A, e.g.:

- Coronary heart disease
- Certain cancers (e.g., cancer of prostrate, lungs, etc.)
- Childhood blindness
- Age-related macular degeneration, a leading cause of blindness in older people
- Various childhood diseases that often result in death, because of a weakened immune system

See also VITAMIN, GOLDEN RICE, AFLATOXIN, FUNGUS, OH43, PHYTOCHEMICALS, NUTRACEUTICALS, CAROTENOIDS, CANCER, CORONARY HEART DISEASE (CHD), ANTIOXIDANTS, AMD, DESATURASE

Beta-Conglycinin Abbreviated β-conglycinin. One of the (structural) categories of proteins that is produced in seeds of legumes. For example, it constitutes approximately 5% of soybeans. In general, β-conglycinin contains one quarter to one third as much cysteine (Cys) and methionine (Met) per unit of protein as does glycinin.

β-conglycinin has greater emulsifying capacity (in water) and emulsion stability than glycinin, so its presence can assist the manufacture of better protein-based (emulsion) drinks.

See also PROTEIN, CYSTEINE (Cys), METHIONINE (Met), GLYCININ, EMULSION

β-Conglycinin See BETA-CONGLYCININ

Beta-D-Glucuronidase See GUS GENE

Beta-Glucan See WATER-SOLUBLE FIBER

Beta-Glucuronidase See BETA-D-GLUCOURONIDASE

Beta-Lactam Antibiotics A category of antibiotics (e.g., penicillin G, ampicillin, etc.) that kill targeted bacteria by altering their essential cellular function of enzymatic controls that keep cell wall (peptido–glycan) synthesis (i.e., creation or repair) in balance with cell wall degradation, thereby causing cell wall breakdown and death of those bacteria (pathogens).

See also ANTIBIOTIC, PENICILLIN G, BACTERIA, CELL, ENZYME, PATHOGEN, bla GENE

Beta-Oxidation See CARNITINE

Beta-Secretase An enzyme that (in the human brain) is linked to presence of Alzheimer's disease.

See also ENZYME, ALZHEIMER'S DISEASE, AMYLOID β, PROTEIN PRECURSOR (AβPP)

Beta Cells Insulin-producing cells in the pancreas. If these cells are destroyed, childhood (also known as early-onset or type I) diabetes results.

See also ISLETS OF LANGERHANS, INSULIN, TYPE I DIABETES

Beta Conformation An extended, zigzag arrangement of a polypeptide (molecule) chain.

See also POLYPEPTIDE (PROTEIN)

Beta Interferon One of the interferons, it is a protein that was approved by the U.S. Food and Drug Administration (FDA) in 1993 for use in treating multiple sclerosis (MS).
See also INTERFERONS, FOOD AND DRUG ADMINISTRATION (FDA), PROTEIN

Beta Sitostanol See SITOSTANOL

β Sitostanol See BETA SITOSTANOL (β sitostanol)

Beta Sitosterol See SITOSTEROL

BEVS See BACULOVIRUS, BACULOVIRUS EXPRESSION VECTOR (BEV), BACULOVIRUS EXPRESSION VECTOR SYSTEM (BEVS)

BFGF Basic fibroblast growth factor.
See FIBROBLAST GROWTH FACTOR (FGF)

BGYF See BRIGHT GREENISH-YELLOW FLUORESCENCE (BGYF)

Bifidobacteria See *BIFIDUS*

Bifidus A family of bacterial species that live within the digestive systems of certain animals (e.g., humans, swine, etc.). Examples include *Bifidobacterium bifidum*, *Bifidobacterium longum*, *Bifidobacterium infantis*, *Bifidobactrium adolescentis*, and *Bifidobacterium acidophilus*. In general, bifidus bacteria help to promote good health of the host animals by several means:

- They produce organic acids (e.g., propionic, acetic, lactic), which make the host animal's digestive system more acidic. Because most pathogens (i.e., disease-causing microorganisms) grow zest at a neutral pH (i.e., neither acidic nor base/caustic), the growth rates of pathogens are thereby inhibited.
- They crowd out enteric pathogens, because bifidus bacteria grow fast in the acidic environment created by those organic acids.
- Some of the organic acids (e.g., propionic) produced by bifidus bacteria are able to pass through the outer cell membrane of pathogenic bacteria and fungi. Once inside those pathogens' cells, these acids dissociate and acidify the cell interior (which disrupts protein synthesis, growth, and replication of that pathogen).
- They produce bacteriocins, which are proteins that suppress growth of the pathogenic bacteria.
- They produce certain short-chain fatty acids, which are absorbed by the host animal (e.g., in the colon) and thereby result in a reduction of triglyceride (fat) levels in the host animal's bloodstream. This (triglyceride reduction) lowers the risk of coronary heart disease and thrombosis.

See also BACTERIA, SPECIES, ACID, BASE (GENERAL), PATHOGEN, CELL, PLASMA MEMBRANE, MICROORGANISM, FUNGUS, PROTEIN, RIBOSOMES, GROWTH (MICROBIAL), FRUCTOSE OLIGOSACCHARIDES, FATTY ACID, TRIGLYCERIDES, CORONARY HEART DISEASE (CHD), THROMBOSIS, PREBIOTICS, BACTERIOCINS, INULIN, TRANSGALACTOOLIGOSACCHARIDES

Bile A liquid (mixture) made by the liver to help digest fats (in the intestine) and facilitate intestinal absorption of certain fat-soluble vitamins and minerals. Bile consists primarily of water, cholesterol, lipids (fat), "natural detergents" (i.e., salts of bile acids such as cholic acid, chenodeoxycholic acid, etc.) that help break up fat globules in the intestines, and bilirubin.
See also BILE ACIDS, BILIRUBIN, FATS, DIGESTION (WITHIN ORGANISMS), FARNESOID X RECEPTOR (FXR), ENTEROCYTES

Bile Acids A family of acids (chenodeoxycholic acid, cholic acid, etc.) that are derived by the human liver from dietary cholesterol (i.e., from foods), and excreted into the bile by the liver. They help to emulsify (food-source) fats in the small intestine, as part of the crucial first step in the digestion of fats.
See also CHOLESTEROL, DIGESTION (WITHIN ORGANISMS), LECITHIN, FATS, LIPIDS, FARNESOID X RECEPTOR (FXR), ENTEROCYTES

Bilirubin A component (pigment) of red blood cells (i.e., erythrocytes) that is recovered (from old red blood cells) and recycled into making bile (a liquid that aids the digestive process) by the liver.

See also ERYTHROCYTES, BILE, DIGESTION (WITHIN ORGANISMS), ENDOTHELIUM

BIO See BIOTECHNOLOGY INDUSTRY ORGANIZATION (BIO)

Bioassay Determination of the relative strength or bioactivity of a substance (e.g., a drug). A biological system (such as living cells, organs, tissues, or whole animals) is exposed to the substance in question and the effect on the living test system is measured.

See also BIOLOGICAL ACTIVITY, ASSAY, BIOCHIP, MULTIPLEX ASSAY

Bio–Bar Codes Refers to oligonucleotides (DNA segments) located on the surface of:

- Nanoparticle probes — These are gold particles of 30-nm size to which have been attached one *antibody specific to a target protein molecule*, as well as thousands of (hybridized) single strands of a **specific DNA sequence**. Because each antibody binds to only one protein, these specific DNA sequences thereby serve as a *bar-code-like label specific to that protein*. During 2003, Chad Mirkin, Jwa-Min Nam, and C. Shad Thaxton created such "bar-coded" nanoparticle probes whose attached antibody was specific to the protein known as prostate-specific antigen (PSA). When utilized in conjunction with magnetic particles whose antibodies are also themselves specific to the same protein (i.e., PSA), these nanoparticle probes *jointly attach to that protein molecule along with the magnetic particles*. A magnetic field was utilized to remove the magnetic particle/nanoparticle probe agglomeration (from the solution mixture); then a dehybridization solution was used to remove the specific-to-PSA-molecule DNA segments for subsequent identification (e.g., via DNA microarray). Because the identification segments (of DNA) are thousands of times more numerous than

the analyte (i.e., protein molecules), Mirkin, Nam, and Thaxton named this process **bio-bar-code amplification**.

This nanoparticle probe or magnetic particle system can be utilized to simultaneously detect and identify **numerous different proteins** within a given sample, or **numerous different DNA segments** within a given sample.

- **"Phage-displayed Library" Peptides** — See the entry within this glossary for PHAGE DISPLAY.

See also OLIGONUCLEOTIDES, NANOMETERS (nm), NANOTECHNOLOGY, DEOXYRIBONUCLEIC ACID (DNA), ANTIBODY, PROTEIN, SEQUENCE (OF A DNA MOLECULE), PEPTIDE, PROSTATE-SPECIFIC ANTIGEN (PSA), PHAGE DISPLAY, MAGNETIC PARTICLES, HYBRIDIZATION (MOLECULAR GENETICS), DNA MICROARRAY, TARGET (OF A THERAPEUTIC AGENT)

Biochemistry The study of chemical processes in living things (systems). The chemistry of life and living matter. Despite the dramatic differences in the appearances of living things, the basic chemistry of all organisms is strikingly similar. Even tiny one-celled creatures carry out essentially the same chemical reactions that each cell of a complex organism (such as humans) carries out.

See also MOLECULAR BIOLOGY, MOLECULAR DIVERSITY

Biochips A term first used with regard to an electronic device that utilizes biological molecules as the "framework" for other molecules that act as semiconductors, and functions as an integrated circuit.

1. During the 1990s, this term also became commonly used to refer to various **"laboratories on a chip"**; e.g., to analyze very small samples of DNA, to assess the impact of pharmaceuticals — or pharmaceutical drug candidate molecules — on specific cells (i.e., attached to the biochip's surface) or on specific cellular

B

receptors (ligand–receptor response of cell), to size and sort DNA fragments (genes) via the (proportional) fluorescence of dyes intercalated in the DNA molecules, to detect presence of specific DNA fragment (gene) via hybridization to a probe (that was fabricated onto the chip), to size and sort protein molecules, (via various cells fabricated onto the chip), to assess pharmaceuticals via adhesion molecules attached to the chip, to detect specific pathogens or cancerous cells in a blood sample (e.g., by applying controlled electrical fields to cause those cells to collect at electrodes on the chip), to screen for compounds that act against a disease (e.g., by applying antibodies linked to fluorescent molecules, then measuring electronically the fluorescence that is triggered by antibody binding), to conduct gene expression analysis by measuring fluorescence of messenger RNA (specific to which particular gene is "turned on") when that mRNA hybridizes with DNA (from genome) on hybridization surface on chip, etc.

2. Shortly after the 1990s, several companies began to manufacture biochips capable of sequencing (i.e., determining the sequence of) DNA samples. Such biochips have all possible "DNA probes" (i.e., short sequences of DNA) attached to their surfaces. The sample (i.e., the unknown DNA molecule) is passed over the probe-covered surface of the biochip, where each relevant segment (within the large unknown DNA molecule) hybridizes with (i.e., "pairs" with) the short DNA probe attached to a known location on the surface of the biochip. Because the sequence of each DNA probe at each specified location on the biochip is known, that information (i.e., the probes' sequences that the unknown DNA molecule hybridized to) is then utilized to "assemble the complete sequence" of the unknown DNA molecule.

3. Sometimes it refers to an electronic device that uses biological molecules as the framework for other molecules that act as semiconductors, and functions as an integrated circuit. The future working parts of the science of bioelectronics, biochips may consist of two- or three-dimensional arrays of organic molecules used as switching or memory elements. One application will be to shrink currently existing biosensors in size. This would enable the biosensors to be implanted in the body or in organs and tissues for the sake of monitoring and controlling certain bodily functions. A future possibility is to try to provide sight for the blind using light-sensitive (e.g., protein-covered electrode) biochips implanted in the eyes to replace a damaged retina. For example, during 2001, Alan Chow implanted such biochips into several men whose retinas had been damaged by the disease **retinitis pigmentosa**.

See also BIOELECTRONICS, BIONICS, BIOSENSORS (ELECTRONIC), DEOXYRIBONUCLEIC ACID (DNA), RIBONUCLEIC ACID (RNA), GENE, RECEPTORS, HIGH-THROUGHPUT SCREENING (HTS), BIOINORGANIC, TARGET–LIGAND INTERACTION SCREENING, ANTIBODY, CHARACTERIZATION ASSAY, BIOASSAY, ASSAY, LUMINESCENT ASSAY, PROTEIN, LIGAND (IN BIOCHEMISTRY), MICROFLUIDICS, PROBE, PROTEOMICS, PROTEOME CHIP, BIORECEPTORS, HYBRIDIZATION (MOLECULAR BIOLOGY), FLUORESCENCE, ADHESION MOLECULE, GENE EXPRESSION ANALYSIS, PATHOGEN, BIOINFORMATICS, MICROARRAY (TESTING), HYBRIDIZATION SURFACES, MESSENGER RNA (mRNA), GENOMICS, QUANTUM DOT, QUANTUM WIRE, NANOCOMPOSITES, SEQUENCING (OF DNA MOLECULES)

Biocide Any chemical or chemical compound that is toxic to living things (systems). Literally

B

"biokiller" or killer of biological systems, it includes insecticides, bactericides, fungicides, etc. Most bactericides accomplish their task (i.e., killing bacteria) via massive lysis (disintegration) of bacterial cell walls (membranes). However, one (i.e., triclosan) kills bacteria by inhibiting enoyl-acyl protein reductase, a crucial enzyme utilized by bacteria in their synthesis of fatty acids.

See also BACTERICIDE, MICROBICIDE, LYSIS, BACTERIA, CELL, FATTY ACID, ENZYME, PROTEIN, ESSENTIAL FATTY ACIDS, ESSENTIAL NUTRIENTS

Biodegradable Describes any material that can be broken down by biological action (e.g., dissimilation, digestion, denitrification, etc.). The breakdown of material (e.g., animal carcasses, dead plants, even synthetic chemicals, etc.) is caused by microorganisms (bacteria, fungus, etc.).

The biodegradation process is often assisted (i.e., first step) by the actions of animals and insects (e.g., feeding on dead carcasses, which breaks down those carcasses for microorganisms). For example, the vulture and the yellow swallowtail butterfly often are the first to feed on the carcasses of dead alligators in the U.S. state of Florida, which helps to make the alligator's material (body tissue) more readily available to microorganisms (e.g., in the dung excreted by those first-step carcass feeders).

See also DIGESTION (WITHIN ORGANISMS), MICROORGANISMS, BACTERIA, FUNGUS, GLYCOLYSIS, METABOLISM, NITRIFICATION

Biodesulfurization The removal of organic and inorganic sulfur (a pollution source) from coal by bacterial and soil microorganisms.

See also BIOLEACHING, BIORECOVERY, BIOSORBENTS

Biodiversity Defined to be "the variability among living organisms from all sources, including terrestrial, marine/aquatic and the complexes of which they are a part" by the Convention on Biological Diversity.

See also CONVENTION ON BIOLOGICAL DIVERSITY

Bioelectronics Also called biomolecular electronics, it is the field in which biotechnology is crossed with electronics. The branch of biotechnology that deals with the electroactive properties of biological materials, systems, and processes together with their exploitation in electronic devices. For example, during 2003, Susan L. Lindquist utilized yeast prions (which self-assemble into fibers that are 60 to 300 nm long) to create **nanowires** by subsequently coating those fibers with gold or silver.

Bioelectronics will attempt to replace traditional semiconductor materials (e.g., silicon or gallium arsenide) with organic materials such as proteins (e.g., in biochips), or "hybrid" materials such as nanowires, or both.

See also BIONICS, QUANTUM WIRE, SELF-ASSEMBLY (OF A LARGE MOLECULAR STRUCTURE), NANOWIRE, PRION

Biofilm Refers to an integral layer of living microorganisms (e.g., on the surface of a vessel, on the surface of teeth, on the surface of an artificial joint or implant, etc.). Those microorganisms often differentiate in order that some of them perform different tasks necessary for the survival of the overall biofilm. For example, the microorganisms within the "bottom" layer might specifically differentiate or change in a manner that enables them to better adhere the entire biofilm onto the underlying substrate.

For example, the bacteria *Streptococcus mutans* can form a biofilm on the surface of teeth. Sometimes, the microorganisms that constitute a biofilm will act **collectively** to do something (e.g., "turning on" one or more pathways for production of specific chemical products from certain substrates). When enough of that species of microorganism are present, as determined via quorum sensing, those microorganisms collectively turn on a pathway for production of the product.

See also MICROORGANISM, BACTERIA, SUBSTRATE (STRUCTURAL), *STREPTOCOCCUS MUTANS*, QUORUM SENSING, PATHWAY, SUBSTRATE (CHEMICAL)

Biogenesis The theory that living organisms are produced only by other living organisms; that is, the theory of generation from preexisting life. It is the opposite of abiogenesis or spontaneous generation.

Biogeochemistry A branch of geochemistry that is concerned with biological materials and their relation to Earth's chemicals in an area.

Bioinformatics This term refers to the generation or creation, collection, storage (in databases), and efficient utilization of data or information from genomics (functional genomics, structural genomics, etc.), combinatorial chemistry, high-throughput screening, proteomics, and DNA sequencing research efforts in order to accomplish a (research) objective (e.g., to discover a new pharmaceutical or a new herbicide, etc.).

Examples of the data or information that is manipulated and stored include gene sequences, biological activity or function, pharmacological activity, biological structure, molecular structure, protein–protein interactions, and gene expression products, amounts, or timing.

See also GENOMICS, FUNCTIONAL GENOMICS, PHARMACOGENOMICS, STRUCTURAL GENOMICS, COMBINATORIAL CHEMISTRY, HIGH-THROUGHPUT SCREENING, PROTEOMICS, BIOCHIP, GENE, GENETIC MAP, GENETIC CODE, SEQUENCING (OF DNA MOLECULES), *IN SILICO* BIOLOGY, *IN SILICO* SCREENING, GENE EXPRESSION ANALYSIS, METAMODEL METHODS (OF BIOINFORMATICS)

Bioinorganic This term refers to the combination of "organic" materials (life) with inorganic materials to create useful materials. For example, Abalone shellfish make their shells via a combination of protein and calcium carbonate. Researchers are working on making semiconductor devices (chips) containing peptides, etc., attached to silicon or gallium arsenide.

See also PROTEIN, BIOCHIP, PEPTIDE, BIOSENSORS (ELECTRONIC), NANOCOMPOSITES

Bioleaching The biomediated recovery of precious metals from their ores. In the recovery of gold, for example, the microorganism *T. ferroxidans* may be used to cause the gold to leach out of the ore so that it may then be concentrated and smelted. Aluminum may be similarly bioleached from clay ores, using heterotropic bacteria and fungi.

See also BIORECOVERY, BIOGEOCHEMISTRY, BACTERIA, BIOSORBENTS

Biolistic® Gene Gun The word "biolistic" was coined from the words "biologic" and "ballistic" (pertaining to a projectile fired from a gun). Used to shoot pellets that are coated with genes (e.g., for desired traits) into plant seeds or plant tissues in order to get those plants to then express the new genes. The gun uses an actual explosive (.22-caliber blank) to propel the material. Compressed air or steam may also be used as the propellant. The Biolistic Gene Gun was invented in 1983–1984 at Cornell University by John Sanford, Edward Wolf, and Nelson Allen. The gun and its registered trademark are now owned by E. I. du Pont de Nemours and Company.

See also WHISKERS™, "SHOTGUN" METHOD, GENETIC ENGINEERING, GENE, BIOSEEDS, MICROPARTICLES

Biologic Response Modifier Therapy Refers to patient treatments (e.g., certain pharmaceuticals) that impact biological responses within an organism. For example, Avastin (bevacizumab) is a monoclonal antibody used in the treatment of certain cancers, which acts by inhibiting angiogenesis (formation of blood vessels within the body that "feeds" a growing tumor in response to chemical signals sent out by that tumor).

See also ORGANISM, CANCER, ANGIOGENESIS, TUMOR, ANTIANGIOGENESIS, MONOCLONAL ANTIBODIES (MAb), SIGNALING

Biological Activity The effect (change in metabolic activity upon living cells) caused by specific compounds or agents. For example, the drug aspirin causes the blood to thin, that is, to clot less easily.

See also BIOASSAY, PHARMACOPHORE, RETINOIDS

Biological Oxygen Demand (BOD) The oxygen used in meeting the metabolic needs of aerobic organisms in water containing organic compounds. Numerically, it is expressed in terms of the oxygen consumed in water at a temperature of 68°F (20°C) during a 5-d period. The BOD is used as an indication of the degree of water pollution.

See also METABOLISM

Biological Vectors See VECTORS

Biology From the two Greek words *bios* (life) and *logos* (word), it is the field of science encompassing the study of life.

See also GENETICS, CLADISTICS, ORGANISM, SPECIES

B

Bioluminescence The enzyme-catalyzed production of light by living organisms, typically during mating or hunting. This word literally means "living light." Bioluminescence was first identified and analyzed in 1947 by William McElroy.

For example, bioluminescence results when the enzyme luciferase comes into contact with adenosine triphosphate (ATP) or luciferin inside the photophores (organs which emit light) of the organism. Such production of light by living organisms is exemplified by fireflies, South America's railroad worm, and by many deep-ocean marine organisms.

Bioluminescence has been utilized by humans as a genetic marker (e.g., to cause a genetically engineered plant to glow as evidence that a gene was successfully transferred into that plant).

Another use of bioluminescence by humans is for the rapid detection of food-borne pathogenic bacteria (e.g., in a food-processing factory). One rapid test for bacteria uses two chemical reagents that first break down bacterial cell membranes, and then cause the ATP from those broken cells to luminesce. Another rapid test uses electrophoresis to first separate the sequences of bacteria's DNA (following its extraction from cell and enzymatic fragmentation) and cause those separated sequences to luminesce; then a camera is used to record the sequence-pattern light emission and compare that pattern to patterns of pathogenic bacteria previously stored in a database.

See also ENZYME, MARKER (GENETIC MARKER), BACTERIA, TOXIN, PATHOGENIC, *ESCHERICHIA COLIFORM 0157:H7 (E. COLI 0157:H7)*, CELL, LUMINESCENT ASSAY, ADENOSINE TRIPHOSPHATE (ATP), GENETIC ENGINEERING, ELECTROPHORESIS, POLYACRYLAMIDE GEL ELECTROPHORESIS (PAGE), SEQUENCE (OF A DNA MOLECULE), *PHOTORHABDUS LUMINESCENS*, RESTRICTION ENDONUCLEASES, NITRIC OXIDE, LUX GENE, QUORUM SENSING

Biomarkers Refers to various **proteins, metabolites, other compounds, genes,** or **biological events** that are indicative of a relevant biological condition (e.g., disease, predisposition to a disease, disease progression, disease regression, inflammation, etc.). For example, the presence of a specific antigen (e.g., the prostate-specific antigen or PSA) in the bloodstream some time (e.g., several years in the case of PSA) prior to its specific disease (e.g., prostate cancer in the case of PSA) makes that antigen useful as a **biomarker for presence of that disease**. Similarly, certain molecules (e.g., **C-reactive protein [CRP]** or **epidermal growth factor [EGF] receptor**) can function as biomarkers in pharmacogenomics (i.e., indicating whether a given pharmaceutical will be efficaceous in a specific person's body) owing to that person's haplotype.

The molecule **thiopurine S-methyl transferase** can be utilized as a biomarker in toxicogenomics (e.g., indicating likelihood for one haplotype **of pediatric leukemia patients** to suffer severe/life-threatening reactions to certain leukemia treatment drugs).

See also GENE, PROTEIN, METABOLITE, PHARMACOGENOMICS, PHARMACOGENETICS, HAPLOTYPE, TOXICOGENOMICS, ADME TESTS, ADME/Tox, C-REACTIVE PROTEIN (CRP), PROSTATE-SPECIFIC ANTIGEN (PSA), CANCER, MAGNETIC PARTICLES

Biomass All organic matter grown by the photosynthetic conversion of solar energy (e.g., plants) and organic matter from animals.

See also PHOTOSYNTHESIS, LOW-TILLAGE CROP PRODUCTION, NO-TILLAGE CROP PRODUCTION

BioMEMS Refers to MEMS that are designed to work within biological systems or organisms. Examples include microfluidic cell sorters, or a "biochip" possessing diverging nanometer-scale etched channels and a fluorescence detector. Via an electrical field that would drive electrophoretic separation of DNA (fragments), samples of DNA could be separated, sorted, or identified via fluorescence.

See also MEMS (NANOTECHNOLOGY), ORGANISM, ELECTROPHORESIS, MICROFLUIDICS, CELL SORTING, NANOMETERS (nm), FLUORESCENCE, BIOCHIP, NANOTECHNOLOGY

Biomimetic Materials Synthetic molecules or systems that are analogues of natural (i.e., made by living organisms) materials. For instance, molecules have been synthesized by humans that act chemically like natural proteins but are not as easily degraded by the digestive system (as are those natural protein molecules). Other systems such as reverse micelles and/or liposomes exhibit certain properties that mimic certain aspects of living systems.

See also PROTEIN, DIGESTION (WITHIN ORGANISMS), REVERSE MICELLE (RM), LIPOSOMES, ANALOGUE, BIONICS, BIOPOLYMER

Biomolecular Electronics See BIOELECTRONICS

Biomotors Refers to biologically based technologies or techniques utilized to "power" nanometer-size "machines" (e.g., "nanobots") in one way or another. For example, during 2000 Bernard Yurke and colleagues created a molecular-machine "tweezers" (grasper) consisting of three separate strands of DNA (i.e., two of them were hybridized separately to small complementary sequences near the two ends of the first DNA strand). The tweezers can then be closed (and/or opened) by sequentially adding other DNA strands (to the three) that:

- Hybridize to small complementary sequences on the second and third strands
- Hybridize to the fourth strand, causing it to unhybridize from the second and third strands

See also NANOTECHNOLOGY, BIOLOGY, NANOMETERS (nm), MOLECULAR MACHINES, DEOXYRIBONUCLEIC ACID (DNA), HYBRIDIZATION (MOLECULAR GENETICS), SEQUENCE (OF A DNA MOLECULE), COMPLEMENTARY (MOLECULAR GENETICS), SELF-ASSEMBLY (OF A LARGE MOLECULAR STRUCTURE)

Bionanotechnology Refers to the application of biotechnology within the fields of nanotechnology. Examples are the following:

- Using genetic engineering to create a "molecular template" on which is subsequently formed a nanotechnology device (e.g., a **nanowire**)

- Using genetic engineering to create specific molecules, which will subsequently self-assemble into a nanotechnology tool or device (e.g., a **nanofiber**)
- Using genetic engineering to create **nanobodies**, which could be utilized to "coat" an acid-sensitive pharmaceutical molecule, to enable that pharmaceutical to be orally administered

See also NANOTECHNOLOGY, GENETIC ENGINEERING, BIOTECHNOLOGY, TEMPLATE, NANOWIRE, SELF-ASSEMBLY (OF A LARGE MOLECULAR STRUCTURE), NANOFIBERS, DIRECTED SELF-ASSEMBLY, NANOBODIES, NANOCAPSULES, ORALLY ADMINISTERED, NANOTUBE, NANOSCIENCE

Bionics An interscience discipline for constructing artificial systems that resemble or have the characteristics of living systems. Bionics can encompass (in whole, or in part) bioelectronics, biosensors, biomimetic materials, biophysics, biomotors, and self-assembly (of a large molecular structure).

See also BIOLOGY, BIOELECTRONICS, BIOMIMETIC MATERIALS, BIOSENSORS (ELECTRONIC), BIOPHYSICS, BIOMOTORS

Biophysics An area of scientific study in which physical principles, physical methods, and physical instrumentation are used to study living systems or systems related to life. It overlaps with biophysical chemistry, which is more specialized in scope because it is concerned with the physical study of chemically isolated substances found in living organisms.

Biopolymer A high-molecular-weight organic compound found in nature, whose structure can be represented by a repeated small unit (i.e., monomer [links]). Common biopolymers include cellulose (long-chain sugars found in most plants and the main constituent of dried woods, jute, flax, hemp, cotton, etc.) and proteins in general and, specifically, collagen and gelatin.

See also MOLECULAR WEIGHT, PROTEIN, POLYMER

Bioreceptors Refers to fragments of DNA, antibodies, protein molecules, and cellular

B

probes (e.g., adhesion molecule) when they are attached to a synthetic surface (e.g., biochip) for purposes of analyzing biological substances.

See also HYBRIDIZATION SURFACES, BIOCHIPS, ANTIBODY, DEOXYRIBONUCLEIC ACID (DNA), PROTEIN, ADHESION MOLECULE, ORPHAN RECEPTORS, MICROARRAY (TESTING)

Biorecovery The use of organisms (including bacteria, plants, fungi, and algae) in the recovery of (collecting of) various metals or organic compounds from ores or garbage (other matrices).

See also BIOLEACHING, CONSORTIA, BIOSORBENTS, PHYTOREMEDIATION, METABOLIC ENGINEERING, BACTERIA, FUNGUS

Bioremediation The use of organisms (e.g., plants, bacteria, fungi, etc.) to consume or otherwise help remove (e.g., biorecovery) materials (e.g., toxic chemical wastes, metals, etc.) from a contaminated site (e.g., remove toluene from the land and ponds on the site of an old refinery, etc.).

See also BIORECOVERY, PHYTOREMEDIATION, METABOLIC ENGINEERING, BIOLEACHING, BIODESULFURIZATION, ORGANISM, BACTERIA, FUNGUS, ENDOPHYTE

Biosafety See CONVENTION ON BIOLOGICAL DIVERSITY (CBD)

Biosafety Protocol See CONVENTION ON BIOLOGICAL DIVERSITY (CBD), INTERNATIONAL PLANT PROTECTION CONVENTION (IPPC)

Bioseeds Plant seeds produced via genetic engineering of existing plants.

See also GENETIC ENGINEERING, BIOLISTIC® GENE GUN, HERBICIDE-TOLERANT CROP, PAT GENE, EPSP SYNTHASE, ALS GENE, CP4 EPSPS, GLYPHOSATE OXIDASE, CHOLESTEROL OXIDASE, HIGH-LYSINE CORN, ACURON™ GENE, HIGH-METHIONINE CORN, HIGH-PHYTASE CORN AND SOYBEANS, HIGH-STEARATE SOYBEANS, LOW-STACHYOSE SOYBEANS, LOX NULL, PLANT'S NOVEL TRAIT (PNT), "SHOTGUN" METHOD (TO INTRODUCE FOREIGN [NEW] GENES INTO PLANT

CELLS), *BACILLUS THURINGIENSIS (B.t.)*, *B.t. KURSTAKI*, *B.t. TENEBRIONIS*, *B.t. ISRAELENSIS*, CRY PROTEINS, CRY1A (b) PROTEIN, CRY1A (c) PROTEIN, CRY9C PROTEIN

Biosensors (chemical) Chemically based devices that are able to detect and measure the presence of certain molecules (e.g., DNA, antigens, glucose, active ingredients of pesticides, etc.). These devices are currently created in the following forms:

- A two-part diagnostic test that can detect the presence of trace amounts of specific chemicals (e.g., pesticides). The (chemical) biosensor consists of an immobilized enzyme (to bind the trace chemical) combined with a color reagent (to indicate visually the presence of the trace chemical).

- Carbon nanotubes onto which have been deposited a layer of glucose oxidase, with a layer of potassium ferricyanide adsorbed onto the glucose oxidase. Such coated nanotubes are placed into a tiny (permeable to glucose) dialysis capillary tube whose ends are then sealed. When the tube is inserted beneath the skin of, for example, a person with diabetes and subsequently illuminated with near-infrared light (which can pass through human tissue), the nanotubes fluoresce in a specific manner that is directly dependent on the glucose concentration (telling the diabetic patient when to inject insulin, for instance). That is because the body's glucose enters the semipermeable capillary; the glucose oxidase (enzyme) acts on the glucose to produce hydrogen peroxide, which then complexes with the ferricyanide so as to change the fluorescence properties of the nanotubes in a manner that is directly dependent on the concentration of glucose.

- A one-part test that can detect specific DNA segments in complex ("dirty," multiple-component) samples. The

B

biosensor consists of 13-nm gold particles onto which are attached numerous nucleotide "molecular chains." Each nucleotide chain contains 28 nucleotides. The 13 nucleotides that are closest to each gold particle serve as a "spacer," and solutions containing such (spaced) randomly distributed gold particles appear red in color when illuminated by appropriate light.

The 15 nucleotides that are farthest from each gold particle are chosen to be complementary to, and thus bind to (complementary) nucleotide sequences in the target (e.g., DNA) molecule. In the presence of the specific target molecule, a closely linked network of gold particles and double-stranded nucleotide molecular chains form (overcoming the 13-nucleotide spacer that previously held apart the gold particles). When double-stranded chains form (i.e., the target molecule is present), the distance between gold particles becomes less than the size of those particles, which makes the solution containing (bound) particles appear blue in color when illuminated by appropriate light.

See also ENZYME, IMMUNOASSAY, NANOCRYSTAL MOLECULES, NANO-TECHNOLOGY, DEOXYRIBONUCLEIC ACID (DNA), NANOMETERS (nm), ANTIGEN, GLUCOSE (GLc), DIALYSIS, SEQUENCE (OF A DNA MOLECULE), NUCLEOTIDE, POLYMER, COMPLEMENTARY DNA (c-DNA), DOUBLE HELIX, DUPLEX, SELF-ASSEMBLY, CARBON NANOTUBES, GLUCOSE OXIDASE, FLUORESCENCE, BIOCHIPS

Biosensors (electronic) Electronic sensors that are able to detect and measure the presence of biomolecules such as sugars or DNA segments. Some of these devices are currently created by the following means:

- Fusing organic matter (e.g., enzymes, antibodies, receptors, or nucleic acids) to tiny electrodes, yielding devices that convert natural chemical reactions into electric current to measure blood levels of certain chemicals (e.g., glucose or insulin), control functions in an artificial organ, monitor some industrial processes, act as a robot's "nose," etc.

- Fusing organic matter (e.g., segment of DNA, antibody, enzyme, etc.) onto the surfaces of etched silicon wafers, yielding devices that convert supramolecular interactions (e.g., nucleotide hybridization, enzyme–substrate binding, lectin–carbohydrate [sugar] interactions, antibody–antigen binding, host–guest complexation, etc.) into electric current via a charge-coupled device (CCD) detector that measures the shift in interference pattern caused by the change in refractive index that results when the (sensed) molecule tightly binds to the fused (electronic) organic matter. For such an etched-silicon-wafer biosensor, the nucleotide hybridization (binding) enables the detection of femtomolar (10^{15} mol) concentrations of DNA. If the (sensed) DNA segment is not complementary to the fused DNA segment, there is no significant change in the interference pattern.

A major goal is to build future generations of biosensors directly into computer chips. (Researchers have discovered that proteins can replace certain metals in semiconductors.) This would enable low-cost mass production via processes similar to those now used for existing semiconductor chips, with circuits built right into the sensor to process data picked up by the biological matter on the chip.

See also BIOCHIPS, QUARTZ CRYSTAL MICROBALANCES, BIOELECTRONICS, ENZYME, GENOSENSORS, RECEPTORS, ANTIBODY, BIOINORGANIC, INSULIN, COMBINATORIAL CHEMISTRY, SUBSTRATE (CHEMICAL), LECTINS, SUGAR MOLECULES, CARBOHYDRATES (SACCHARIDES), GLUCOSE (GLc), DEOXYRIBONUCLEIC ACID (DNA), NUCLEOTIDE, HYBRIDIZATION (MOLECULAR GENETICS), HYBRIDIZATION SURFACES,

ANTIGEN, COMPLEMENTARY DNA (c-DNA), GENE, NANOTECHNOLOGY, TEMPLATE

Biosilk A biomimetic, synthetic fiber produced by the following means:

1. Sequencing the "dragline silk" protein that is produced by the orb-weaving spider (*Nephila clavipes*)
2. Synthesizing the gene to code for the "dragline silk" protein (components), which are mostly glycine and alanine
3. Expressing the gene in a suitable host organism (e.g., yeast, bacteria, and plants) to cause production of the protein
4. Dissolving the protein in a suitable solvent, and then "spinning" the protein into fiber form by passing the liquid (dissolved protein) through a small orifice, followed by drying to remove the solvent

This results in biosilk fibers that are extremely strong.

See also BIOMIMETIC MATERIALS, BIOPOLYMER, PROTEIN, SEQUENCING (OF PROTEIN MOLECULES), GENE, GENE MACHINE, SYNTHESIZING (OF DNA MOLECULES), DEOXYRIBONU-CLEIC ACID (DNA), EXPRESS, GLYCINE (Gly), ALANINE (Ala), SUPERCRITICAL CARBON DIOXIDE

Biosorbents Microorganisms that, either by themselves or in conjunction with a support or substrate system (e.g., inert granules), effect the extraction (e.g., from ore) or concentration of desired (precious) metals or organic compounds by means of selective retention of those entities. Retention of organic compounds (e.g., gasoline) may be for the purpose of cleaning polluted soil.

See also BIORECOVERY, BIOLEACHING, CONSORTIA

Biosphere All the living matter on or in the earth, the oceans and seas, and the atmosphere. The area of the planet in which life is found to occur.

Biosynthesis Production of a chemical compound or entity by a living organism.

Biotechnology The means or way of manipulating life forms (organisms) to provide desirable products for humans' use. For example, beekeeping and cattle breeding could be considered to be biotechnology-related endeavors. The word biotechnology was coined in 1919 by Karl Ereky to apply to the interaction of biology with human technology.

However, usage of the word biotechnology in the U.S. has come to mean all parts of an industry that knowingly create, develop, and market a variety of products through the willful manipulation, on a molecular level, of life forms or utilization of knowledge pertaining to living systems. A common misconception is that biotechnology refers only to recombinant DNA (rDNA) work. However, recombinant DNA is only one of the many techniques used to derive products from organisms, plants, and parts of both for the biotechnology industry. A list of areas covered by the term biotechnology would more properly include recombinant DNA, plant tissue culture, rDNA or gene splicing, enzyme systems, plant breeding, meristem culture, mammalian cell culture, immunology, molecular biology, fermentation, and others.

See also GENETIC ENGINEERING, BIORECOVERY, RECOMBINANT DNA (rDNA), RECOMBINATION, DEOXYRIBONUCLEIC ACID (DNA), BIOLEACHING, GENE SPLICING, MAMMALIAN CELL CULTURE, FERMENTATION

Biotechnology Industry Organization (BIO) A U.S. trade association composed of companies and individuals involved in biotechnology and in services to biotechnology companies (e.g., accounting, law, etc.). Formed in 1993, the BIO was created by the merger of its two predecessor trade associations: the Association of Biotechnology Companies (ABC) and the Industrial Biotechnology Association (IBA). The BIO works with the government and the public to promote safe and rational advancement of genetic engineering and biotechnology.

See also BIOTECHNOLOGY, ASSOCIATION OF BIOTECHNOLOGY COMPANIES (ABC), INDUSTRIAL BIOTECHNOLOGY ASSOCIATION (IBA), JAPAN BIOINDUSTRY ASSOCIATION, SENIOR ADVISORY GROUP ON BIOTECHNOLOGY (SAGB)

Biotic Stresses The stress (e.g., to crop plants) caused by insects, bacteria, viruses, fungi, nematodes, and other living things that attack plants.
See also NEMATODES, FUNGUS, VIRUS, BACTERIA

Biotin A B-complex vitamin, also known as **vitamin H**, that is essential (i.e., required) for the life of many grain-eating insects and is also essential for many of the metabolic pathways (i.e., series of chemical reactions) involved in milk production by cattle. All of the predominant cellulolytic bacteria (i.e., those that break down cellulose molecules) within the rumen (first stomach) of cattle require biotin for them to be able to grow. Biotin (within certain molecules) acts as a coenzyme in carboxylation reactions, thereby playing a critical role in gluconeogenesis, fatty acid synthesis ("manufacture"), and protein synthesis reactions occurring within all animals.

Biotin binds very tightly to streptavidin (avidin). This property is utilized by some scientists to attach various molecules such as antibodies (e.g., to quantum dots, probes, etc.), utilizing the biotin–streptavidin to make a **molecular bridge**. Biotin enzymes are inhibited (i.e., blocked) by the protein avidin. Because insects must have biotin to live, avidin might be a useful ingredient to add to grain in order to protect it during storage from insects such as weevils.
See also VITAMIN, METABOLISM, INTERMEDIARY METABOLISM, PATHWAY, BACTERIA, CELLULOSE, LYSIS, ENZYME, COENZYME, WEEVILS, GLUCONEOGENESIS, FATTY ACID, PROTEIN, STREPTAVIDIN, MOLECULAR BRIDGE, QUANTUM DOT, ANTIBODY, PROBE

Biotinylation See STREPTAVIDIN

Biotransformation (of a biosynthesized product) See POSTTRANSLATIONAL MODIFICATION OF PROTEIN

Biotransformation (of an introduced compound) See the *biological means* portion of definition of PERSISTENCE.

bla Gene A gene that confers resistance to -lactam (beta-lactam) antibiotics (e.g., ampicillin).
See also GENE, BETA-LACTAM ANTIBIOTICS, MARKER (GENETIC MARKER)

Black-Layered (corn) An indicator of a corn plant's maturity. It refers to a distinctive dark line that forms in each corn kernel at maturity.
See also CORN

Black-Lined (corn) See BLACK-LAYERED (CORN)

Blast Cell A large, rapidly dividing cell that develops from a B cell (B lymphocyte) in response to an antigenic stimulus. The blast cell then becomes an antibody-producing plasma cell.
See also ANTIGEN, ANTIBODY, B LYMPHOCYTES, LYMPHOCYTE

Blast Transformation The process by which a B cell (B lymphocyte) becomes a blast cell.
See also ANTIBODY, LYMPHOCYTE, BLAST CELL

Blood Clotting See FIBRIN

Blood Derivatives Manufacturing Association A trade organization of firms involved in producing pharmaceuticals from collected blood.
See also SERUM, BUFFY COAT (CELLS), SEROLOGY

Blood Plasma See PLASMA

Blood Platelets See PLATELETS

Blood Serum See SERUM

Blood–Brain Barrier (BBB) The specialized layer of endothelial cells that lines all blood vessels in the brain. The BBB prevents most organisms (e.g., bacteria) and toxins from entering the brain via the bloodstream. However, the BBB does allow oxygen and needed nutrients (e.g., iron, glucose, tryptophan, etc.) to enter the brain from the bloodstream. For example, receptors that line BBB cell surfaces (on the bloodstream side of the BBB) latch onto transferrin molecules (which contain iron molecules) that pass by in the bloodstream. These transferrin receptors first bind to the (passing) transferrin molecules, transport them through the BBB via a process called vaginosis, and then release them (in order to supply needed iron to the brain cells). Factors such as aging, trauma, stroke, multiple sclerosis, and some infections will cause an increase in the permeability of the BBB.
See also ENDOTHELIAL CELLS, TOXIN, TRANSFERRIN, TRANSFERRIN RECEPTOR, CHELATING AGENT, GLUCOSE,

B

RECEPTORS, VAGINOSIS, HEME, BACTERIA, TRYPTOPHAN (Trp), SEROTONIN

Blue Biotechnology Term utilized in some countries to refer to **environmental improvement** applications of genetic engineering. One example would be bioremediation.

See also GENETIC ENGINEERING, BIOREMEDIATION

Blunt-End DNA A segment of DNA that has both strands terminating at the same base pair location, that is, fully base-paired DNA; no sticky ends.

See also STICKY ENDS

Blunt-End Ligation A method of joining blunt-ended DNA fragments using the enzyme T4 ligase that can join fully base-paired, double-stranded DNA.

See also LIGASE, DEOXYRIBONUCLEIC ACID (DNA), BASE PAIR (bp), BLUNT-END DNA

BLUP See BEST LINEAR UNBIASED PREDICTION (BLUP)

BOD See BIOLOGICAL OXYGEN DEMAND (BOD)

Boletic Acid See FUMARIC ACID ($C_4H_4O_4$)

Bollworms See *HELIOTHIS VIRESCENS (H. VIRESCENS), HELICOVERPA ZEA (H. ZEA), PECTINOPHORA GOSSYPIELLA, B.t. KURSTAKI*

Bone Morphogenetic Proteins (BMP) A family of proteinaceous growth factors (nine identified as of 1994) for bone tissue formation (e.g., at the site where a bone has been broken). BMPs stimulate "recruitment" of bone-forming cells (e.g., to the site of bone injury), which first form cartilage; then, that cartilage is mineralized to form bone.

See also GROWTH FACTOR, PERIODONTIUM, PROTEIN

Bovine Somatotropin (BST) Also called bovine growth hormone. A protein hormone produced in a cow's pituitary gland that increases the efficiency of the cow in converting its feed into milk, increases milk production in cows, and promotes cell growth in healing tissues of all ages of cattle; promotes body growth of young cattle.

See also PROTEIN, GROWTH HORMONE (GH), HORMONE, SOMATOMEDINS, SPECIES SPECIFIC

Bowman–Birk Trypsin Inhibitor See TRYPSIN INHIBITORS

bp Common abbreviation for base pair.

See also BASE PAIR (bp)

Bradyrhizobium japonicum A nitrogen-fixing strain of bacteria that lives symbiotically among the roots of the soybean plant, providing almost all of the nitrogen needed by the soybean plant.

See also BACTERIA, SYMBIOTIC, NODULATION, NITROGEN FIXATION, SOYBEAN PLANT, ISOFLAVONES, *RHIZOBIUM* (BACTERIA)

Brassica A fast-growing category of the mustard plant family, which also produces sulfur-based gases (a natural defense against certain fungi, nematodes, and insect pests). For example, Australian CSIRO scientists discovered in 1994 that sulfur-based isothiocyanates emitted by *Brassica* actively combat wheat take-all disease (a fungal disease that attacks the roots of the wheat plant).

See also *ARABIDOPSIS THALIANA*, WHEAT, WHEAT TAKE-ALL DISEASE, CANOLA, ALLELOPATY, FUNGUS, NEMATODES

Brassica campestre See *BRASSICA*

Brassica campestris See CANOLA, *BRASSICA*

Brassica napus See CANOLA, *BRASSICA*

Brazzein A protein that imparts a sweet taste to foods that contain it.

See also PROTEIN

BRCA 1 Gene See BRCA GENES

BRCA 2 Gene See BRCA GENES

BRCA Genes Oncogenes that when mutated can cause development of breast cancer or ovarian cancer. All humans possess BRCA genes of one sort or another (the acronym BRCA stands for breast cancer). However, the two specific BRCA genes most likely to lead to breast cancer (i.e., **BRCA 1**, discovered by Mary-Claire King, and **BRCA 2**) are present in only 2% of women who are of northern European ancestry, most Caucasian women in the U.S., and Askenazi Jews whose ancestors are from Central and Eastern Europe.

Those women possessing the **BRCA 1** gene in their genome (DNA) have a 20 to 40% chance of developing ovarian cancer (and a 50 to 85% chance of developing breast cancer) in their lifetime. Those women possessing the **BRCA 2** gene in their genome (DNA) have a 15 to 20% chance of developing ovarian cancer (and a 55 to 85% chance of developing breast cancer) in their lifetime.

See also GENE, MUTATION, CANCER, ONCOGENES, HER-2 GENE

Breeder's Rights See PLANT BREEDER'S RIGHTS

Bright Greenish-Yellow Fluorescence (BGYF) An indication of the presence of fungus (e.g., in a sample of grain) when light of an appropriate wavelength is shined on the sample. For example, when the fungus *Aspergillus flavus* infects cottonseed during boll development on the cotton plant, the resultant seed (when harvested) shows BGYF on its lint and linters. The fungus gains entry into the bolls typically via holes made by the pink bollworm (*Pectinophora gossypiella*).

See also MYCOTOXINS, AFLATOXIN, FUNGUS, *PECTINOPHORA GOSSYPIELLA*, FLUORESCENCE

Broad Spectrum See GRAM STAIN

Bromoxynil An active ingredient in some herbicides, it kills certain types of plants (weeds).
See also NITRILASE

Broth A fluid culture medium (for growing microorganisms).
See also MEDIUM, CULTURE MEDIUM

Brown Stem Rot (BSR) A plant disease that can be caused by the soilborne fungus *Phialaphora gregata* in the soybean plant (*Glycine max (L.) Merrill*). Some soybean varieties are genetically resistant to BSR.
See also FUNGUS, SOYBEAN PLANT, GENOTYPE, GENE, PATHOGENIC

BSE Bovine spongiform encephalopathy. A neurodegenerative disease of cattle.
See also PRION

BSP Biosafety protocol.
See also CONVENTION ON BIOLOGICAL DIVERSITY (CBD)

BSR See BROWN STEM ROT (BSR)

BST See BOVINE SOMATOTROPIN (BST)

B.t See *BACILLUS THURINGIENSIS (B.t.)*

B.t. israelensis One of the approximately 30 subspecies groupings within the approximately 20,000 different strains of the soil bacteria known (collectively) as *Bacillus thuringiensis (B.t.)*.

When eaten (e.g., owing to presence on food), the protoxin proteins produced by *B.t. israelensis* are toxic to mosquitoes and black fly (diptera) larvae.

See also *BACILLUS THURINGIENSIS (B.t.)*, PROTOXIN, ION CHANNELS

B.t. Kumamotoensis One of the approximately 280 subspecies groupings within the approximately 50,000 different strains of the soil bacteria known (collectively) as *Bacillus thuringiensis (B.t.)*.

When eaten (e.g., owing to presence on/in their food plants), the protoxin proteins produced by *B.t. kumamotoensis* are toxic to larvae of the insect known as the corn rootworm (*Diabrotica virgifera virgifera*).

See also *BACILLUS THURINGIENSIS (B.t.)*, PROTOXIN, ION CHANNELS, CORN, CORN ROOTWORM, STRAIN, BACTERIA

B.t.k. See *B.t. KURSTAKI*

B.t. kurstaki One of the approximately 30 subspecies groupings within the approximately 20,000 different strains of the soil bacteria known (collectively) as *Bacillus thuringiensis (B.t.)*.

When eaten (e.g., as part of a genetically engineered plant), the protoxin proteins produced by *B.t. kurstaki* are toxic to certain caterpillars (lepidoptera larvae), such as the European corn borer (pyralis).

See also *BACILLUS THURINGIENSIS (B.t.)*, PROTOXIN, CRY1A (b) PROTEIN, ION CHANNELS, EUROPEAN CORN BORER (ECB)

BtR-4 Gene See TOXICOGENOMICS

B.t. tenebrionis One of the approximately 30 subspecies groupings within the approximately 20,000 different strains of the soil bacteria known (collectively) as *Bacillus thuringiensis (B.t.)*.

When eaten (e.g., as part of a genetically engineered plant), the protoxin proteins produced by *B.t. tenebrionis* are toxic to certain insects.

See also *BACILLUS THURINGIENSIS (B.t.)*, PROTOXIN, GENETIC ENGINEERING, ION CHANNELS

B.t. tolworthi One of the approximately 30 subspecies groupings within the approximately 20,000 different strains of the soil bacteria known (collectively) as *Bacillus thuringiensis (B.t.)*.

B

When eaten (e.g., as part of a genetically engineered crop plant), the protoxin proteins produced by *B.t. tolworthi* are toxic to certain caterpillars (lepidoptera larvae), such as the European Corn Borer (pyralis).

See also *BACILLUS THURINGIENSIS (B.t.)*, PROTOXIN, CRY9C PROTEIN, GENETIC ENGINEERING, ION CHANNELS

Buffy Coat (cells) The layer of white blood cells (leukocytes) that separates out when blood is subjected to centrifugation.

See also ULTRACENTRIFUGE, LEUKOCYTES, PLASMA, BLOOD DERIVATIVES MANUFACTURING ASSOCIATION

Bundesgesundheitsamt (BGA) German Federal Health Organization. The German government agency that must approve new pharmaceutical products for sale within Germany, it is the equivalent of the U.S. Food and Drug Administration (FDA).

See also FOOD AND DRUG ADMINISTRATION (FDA), KOSEISHO, COMMITTEE FOR PROPRIETARY MEDICINAL PRODUCTS (CPMP), COMMITTEE ON SAFETY IN MEDICINES, MEDICINES CONTROL AGENCY (MCA), EUROPEAN MEDICINES EVALUATION AGENCY (EMEA)

BXN Gene See NITRILASE

C

C-DNA Also known as copy DNA. A helical form of DNA. It occurs when DNA fibers are maintained in 66% relative humidity in the presence of lithium ions. It has fewer base pairs per turn than B-DNA.

See also B-DNA, DEOXYRIBONUCLEIC ACID (DNA), BASE PAIR (bp), COMPLEMENTARY DNA (cDNA)

C. elegans See *CAENORHABDITIS ELEGANS*

c-kit Genetic Marker See GENETIC MARKER, FLUORESCENCE *IN SITU* HYRIDIZATION (FISH)

C-Reactive Protein (CRP) Discovered in 1929 by Oswald Avery, CRP is a general inflammation "biomarker" (protein molecule) produced in humans in the liver in response to certain bacterial infections or certain physical trauma (that cause inflammation). Elevated blood levels of CRP are related to the degree of risk of arteriosclerosis, coronary heart disease (CHD), heart attack, and stroke. Typical healthy humans (e.g., those not suffering an infection) tend to have blood CRP levels of less than 3 mg/l. Blood levels of CRP increase 1000-fold or more when the individual becomes infected. Aspirin and statin-type pharmaceuticals (e.g., pravastatin, simvastatin, atorvastatin, etc.) help to lower inflammation and bloodstream CRP levels. Consumption of -linolenic acid causes a decline in bloodstream CRP levels. Blood levels of CRP also decline when (overweight) people lose weight. Blood levels of CRP are increased by:

- Aging
- Obesity
- Type II diabetes
- Smoking and excessive alcohol consumption

See also BIOMARKERS, PROTEIN, BACTERIA, ARTERIOSCLEROSIS, CORONARY HEART DISEASE (CHD), HUMORAL IMMUNE RESPONSE, INTERLEUKIN-6 (IL-6), TYPE II DIABETES, LINOLENIC ACID

C Terminus See CARBOXYL TERMINUS (OF A PROTEIN MOLECULE)

C Value The total amount of DNA in a haploid genome.

See also DEOXYRIBONUCLEIC ACID (DNA), HAPLOID, GENOME

Caco-2 A cell line (i.e., cells propagated over time in cell culture) of human colon cells that is utilized by research scientists. When caco-2 cells are grown on suitable surfaces (in cell culture vessel), they differentiate and assume properties akin to intestinal mucosa cells.

Such cultured caco-2 cells are used to assess **absorption** of pharmaceutical candidate (chemical) compounds (e.g., the likelihood and rate for a given candidate compound to be absorbed into the body through cell membranes from the gastrointestinal tract).

Enough is now known of caco-2's absorption of each major category/type of chemical for such absorption to often be predicted *in silico* (i.e., via computer modeling).

See also CELL, DIFFERENTIATION, ADME TESTS, ABSORPTION, PLASMA MEMBRANE, PHARMACOKINETICS, PHARMACOGENOMICS, CELL CULTURE, ADME, ADMET, *IN SILICO* SCREENING, STRUCTURE–ACTIVITY MODELS, ADME/Tox

Cadherins A class of (cell surface) adhesion molecules that causes cells (e.g., in the lining of the intestine known as the epithelium) to "stick together" to form a continuous lining; also, cadherins sometimes function as cellular adhesion receptors. For example, the (food poisoning) pathogenic bacteria *Listeria monocytogenes* is able to infect humans via its use of the E-cadherin receptor located on the surface of intestinal epithelium cells. The bacteria's "key" (a bacterial membrane surface protein known as internaulin) is "inserted" into the E-cadherin ("lock"), which opens up the otherwise closed-to-bacteria intestinal epithelium. The bacteria then leave the intestine and infect the human body tissues.

See also ADHESION MOLECULE, CELL, RECEPTORS, LISTERIA MONOCYTOGENES, EPITHELIUM

Caenorhabditis elegans (C. elegans) The name of a nematode (microscopic roundworm) that is commonly utilized by scientists in genetics experiments. Because of this, a large base of knowledge about *C. elegans* genetics has been accumulated by the world's scientific community. For example, of the nearly 300 "disease-causing genes" in the human genome, more than half of them have an analogous gene within the *C. elegans* genome. *C. elegans* was one of the first organisms whose entire genome was sequenced.

Thus, one of the methodologies utilized by researchers to rapidly screen large numbers of chemical compounds for their potential use as pharmaceuticals is to do the following:

- Expose large numbers of *C. elegans* to the various chemical compounds that the researcher wants to investigate for potential pharmaceutical activity.
- Pass those large numbers of previously exposed *C. elegans*, suspended in liquid such as water, through a small transparent chamber where a focused laser beam is shined upon the roundworm's side (for its full length, as the roundworm passes by).
- Utilize expression-of-fluorescent-protein, autofluorescence, lectin (in the fluid) binding detected via laser reflectance, antibody (in the fluid) binding detected via laser reflectance, etc., as the basis for individual *C. elegans* to be "sorted" via tiny jets of air that blow into a container those *C. elegans* that show visible signs of having been changed by the particular chemical compound they were exposed to.
- Evaluate in detail (e.g., via conventional gene expression analysis, etc.) the specific impact of that particular

chemical compound on those *C. elegans* that had indicated an apparent change, so were sorted into the "likely target" receptacle.

See also NEMATODES, GENETICS, GENE, GENOME, GENE EXPRESSION, GENE EXPRESSION MARKERS, EXPRESSED SEQUENCE TAGS (EST), SEQUENCING (OF DNA MOLECULES), HIGH-THROUGHPUT SCREENING (HTS), HIGH-THROUGHPUT IDENTIFICATION, GENE EXPRESSION ANALYSIS, TARGET-LIGAND INTERACTION SCREENING, TARGET (OF A THERAPEUTIC AGENT), FLUORESCENCE, LECTINS, MODEL ORGANISM

Caffeine A chemical ($C_8H_{10}N_4O_2$) that is naturally produced in some plants (e.g., coffee tree) to repel predatory insects. It also acts as a stimulant (when consumed by humans), so is classified as a "phytochemical." Caffeine was first isolated chemically and named in 1819 by Friedlieb Ferdinand Runge.

Research done by Seymour Diamond during 2000 showed that caffeine consumption causes interactions within the human body with the synthetic chemical painkiller known as Ibuprofen. Consuming both together was shown to be more effective and faster in relieving pain than was consuming Ibuprofen alone.

See also PHYTOCHEMICALS

Calcium Channel Blockers Refers to:

- Drugs (e.g., verapamil, amlodipine, diltiazem, nifedipine, etc.) that are used to slow down calcium movement through cell membranes. This leads to dilation of the blood vessels and reduces the heart's workload. Blood vessels need calcium to contract (causing flow constriction and, hence, an increase in blood pressure), so the drug-induced shortage of available calcium causes the body's blood vessels to remain dilated (which results in lower blood pressure).
- Drugs such as Prialt™/ziconotide (an *N-type calcium channel blocker*), or Neurotonin™ and Lyrica™

(GABAergic calcium channel blockers) that act as powerful painkillers by slowing down calcium movement through certain cell membranes.

See also CELL, ION CHANNELS, MEMBRANE TRANSPORT

Calcium Oxalate A crystalline salt that is normally deposited in the cells of some species of plants. The presence of such oxalate inhibits absorption of calcium (present in spinach) in humans eating spinach. In many animals, calcium oxalate is excreted in the urine, or retained in the animal's body in the form of urinary calculi.

See also ABSORPTION, OXALATE, CELL

Callipyge (Means "beautiful buttocks" in Greek.)

An inherited trait in livestock (e.g., sheep) that results in thicker, meatier hindquarters. First identified as a genetic trait in 1983, this desirable trait results in a higher meat yield per animal.

See also TRAIT, GENOTYPE, PHENOTYPE, WILD TYPE

Callus An undifferentiated cluster of plant cells that is a first step in regeneration of plants from tissue culture.

See also SOMACLONAL VARIATION

Calorie The amount of heat (energy) required to raise the temperature of 1 g of water from 14.5°C (58°F) to 15.5°C (60°F) at a constant pressure of 1 atm. This unit measure of energy (i.e., 1 cal) is also frequently utilized to express the amount of energy contained within certain foods or animal feeds.

See also CARBOHYDRATES (SACCHARIDES), FATS, TME (N)

Calpain-10 A gene that increases the likelihood for development of diabetes in humans whose DNA carries that gene (i.e., approximately 80% of humans carry that gene).

See also DIABETES, INSULIN, INSULIN-DEPENDENT DIABETES MELLITIS (IDDM), GENE, DEOXYRIBONUCLEIC ACID (DNA)

Campesterol A phytosterol that is produced within the seeds of the soybean plant (*Glycine max (L.)*), among others. Evidence shows that human consumption of campesterol helps to reduce total serum (blood) cholesterol and low-density lipoproteins (LDLP) levels, and thereby lowers the risk of coronary heart disease (CHD). Evidence indicates that certain phytosterols (including campesterol) interfere with absorption of cholesterol by the intestines, and decrease the body's recovery and reuse of cholesterol-containing bile salts, which causes more (net) cholesterol to be excreted from the body.

See also PHYTOSTEROLS, PHYTOCHEMICALS, STEROLS, SOYBEAN PLANT, CHOLESTEROL, STIGMASTEROL, BETA-SITOSTEROL (B-SITOSTEROL), CORONARY HEART DISEASE (CHD)

Campestrol See CAMPESTEROL

Campsterol See CAMPESTEROL

Camptothecins See RUBITECAN

CaMV See CAULIFLOWER MOSAIC VIRUS 35S PROMOTER (CaMV 35S)

CaMV 35S See CAULIFLOWER MOSAIC VIRUS 35S PROMOTER (CaMV 35S)

Canavanine An uncommon amino acid. It is used in biology as an arginine (another amino acid) analogue. It is a potent growth inhibitor of many organisms.

See also AMINO ACID, BIOMIMETIC MATERIALS

Cancer The name given to a group of diseases characterized by uncontrolled cellular growth (e.g., formation of tumor) without any differentiation of those cells (i.e., into specialized and different tissues). Causes include consumption of carcinogens (e.g., certain mycotoxins), mutagens (e.g., certain radiation), some viruses (e.g., approximately 99% of human cervical cancer is caused by human papillomavirus), etc.

See also CARCINOGEN, ONCOGENES, TUMOR SUPPRESSOR GENES, TUMOR, VIRUS, TELOMERES, RETINOIDS, MUTAGEN, CELL, TELOMERASE, NEOPLASTIC GROWTH, CHEMOTHERAPY, DIFFERENTIATION, ORAL CANCER, MYCOTOXINS, RNase 1 GENE

Cancer Epigenetics See EPIGENETIC

CANDA Computer-Assisted New Drug Application. An application to the U.S. Food and Drug Administration (FDA) seeking approval of a drug that has undergone Phase 2 and Phase 3 clinical trials. A CANDA is submitted in the form of computer-readable (e.g., clinical) data that provide the FDA with a sophisticated database which allows the FDA reviewers to evaluate (e.g., statistically) the data themselves, directly.

See also NDA (to FDA), NDA (to Koseisho), FOOD AND DRUG ADMINISTRATION (FDA), MAA MARKETING AUTHORIZATION APPLICATION (MAA), PHASE I CLINICAL TESTING

Canola Historically, this term has referred to *Brassica napus* or *Brassica campestris* strains of the rapeseed plant, which were developed by plant breeders after the 1960s. This was because oil produced from rapeseed grown prior to 1971 contained 30 to 60% erucic acid (high dietary levels of which were associated with cardiac lesions in experimental animals via toxicology testing).

By 1974, canola varieties producing oil containing less than 5% erucic acid constituted virtually all of that year's Canadian rapeseed crop, and Canadian breeders continued to develop new canola varieties with ever-lower erucic acid content.

In 1982, Canada filed with the U.S. Food and Drug Administration (FDA) to have low-erucic-acid rapeseed (LEAR) oil affirmed to be GRAS (Generally Recognized As Safe), which the FDA did. LEAR was one of the first foodstuffs to be determined to be "substantially equivalent" under the OECD-defined criteria for "substantial equivalence" because LEAR was shown (in OECD petition) to be very similar to, and composed of the same basic components as, traditional rapeseed oil (and other commonly consumed vegetable oils) except for a lower level of erucic acid (the component of concern, per the preceding text). In 2002, a *Brassica juncea* canola variety was introduced for the first time ever, in Canada.

See also STRAIN, FATS, LAURATE, FATTY ACID, OLEIC ACID, GRAS LIST, ORGANIZATION FOR ECONOMIC COOPERATION AND DEVELOPMENT (OECD), GLUCOSINOLATES, *BRASSICA*, HIGH-STEARATE CANOLA

CAP Catabolite gene-activator protein, also known as CRP, catabolite regulator protein (or cyclic AMP receptor protein). The protein mediates the action of cyclic AMP (cAMP) on transcription in that cAMP and CAP must first combine. The cAMP-CAP complex then binds to the promoter regions of *Escherichia coli* and stimulates transcription of its operon. Because a cell component increases rather than inhibits transcription, this type of regulation of gene expression is called positive transcriptional control.

See also *ESCHERICHIA COLIFORM (E. COLI)*, CATABOLITE REPRESSION, TRANSCRIPTION, OPERON, TRANSCRIPTION ACTIVATORS

Capillary Electrophoresis A research technology or methodology that is utilized to electrophoretically separate ions (e.g., DNA/RNA/nucleic acids, protein molecules, etc.). That separation occurs inside a tiny capillary tube when a powerful electrical field is applied across the (length of) capillary tube, because the ions (in solution inside capillary tube) move at different speeds throughout the tube depending on their charges and their molecular size or weight. Optical detection systems are typically utilized to determine each of the ions (each molecule) as they emerge from the capillary tube. Capillary electrophoresis is utilized to perform DNA sequencing, biowarfare (pathogen) detection, heterozygote detection, mutation analysis (e.g., in site-directed mutagenesis efforts), single-nucleotide polymorphism (SNP) analysis, gene expression analysis, amplified fragment length polymorphism (AFLP) analysis/"fingerprinting," quantitation of PCR (products), quantitation of RT-PCR (products), etc.

See also ELECTROPHORESIS, ION, PROTEIN, ISOELECTRIC FOCUSING (IEF), MOLECULAR WEIGHT, NUCLEIC ACIDS, DEOXYRIBONUCLEIC ACID (DNA), PROTEIN, RIBONUCLEIC ACID (RNA), SEQUENCE (OF A DNA MOLECULE), GENE, SEQUENCING (OF DNA MOLECULES), PATHOGEN, HETEROZYGOTE, MUTATION, SITE-DIRECTED MUTAGENESIS (SDM), SINGLE-NUCLEOTIDE POLYMORPHISMS (SNPs), AMPLIFIED FRAGMENT LENGTH POLYMORPHISM, GENE EXPRESSION ANALYSIS, PCR, RT-PCR, ISOTACHOPHORESIS

Capillary Isotachophoresis See ISOTACHO-PHORESIS

Capillary Isotechophoresis See ISOTACHO-PHORESIS

Capillary Zone Electrophoresis See CAPILLARY ELECTROPHORESIS

Capsid The external protein coat of a virus particle that surrounds the nucleic acid. The individual proteins that make up the capsid are called capsomers or protein subunits. It has been discovered that resistance to certain viral diseases may be imparted to some plants by inserting the gene for production of the capsid protein coat into the plants (thereby preventing the virus from uncoating, which it must first do in order to infect the plants).

See also TOBACCO MOSAIC VIRUS (TMV), VIRUS, PROTEIN

Capsule An envelope surrounding many types of microorganisms. The capsule is usually composed of polysaccharides, polypeptides, or polysaccharide–protein complexes. These materials are arranged in a compact manner around the cell surface. Capsules are not absolutely essential cellular components.

See also MICROORGANISM, POLYSACCHARIDES, POLYPEPTIDE (PROTEIN), PROTEIN, CELL, GRAM NEGATIVE (G−), MANNANOLIGOSACCHARIDES (MOS), GRAM POSITIVE (G+)

Capture Agent Also known as a **capture molecule**.

See CAPTURE MOLECULE

Capture Molecule Also known as a **capture agent**. Refers to molecules such as ligands, receptors, aptamers, DNA segments, enzymes, antigens, antibodies, etc., which bind to specific molecules sought by a scientist (e.g., within a sample being analyzed via microarray testing).

See also MICROARRAY (TESTING), PROTEIN MICROARRAYS, DEOXYRIBONUCLEIC ACID (DNA), HYBRIDIZATION (MOLECULAR GENETICS), DNA CHIP, BIOCHIP, MAGNETIC PARTICLES, LIGAND (IN BIOCHEMISTRY), RECEPTORS, APTAMERS, ENZYME, ANTIGEN, ANTIBODY

CARB See CENTER FOR ADVANCED RESEARCH IN BIOTECHNOLOGY (CARB)

Carbetimer An antineoplastic (i.e., anticancer) low-molecular-weight polymer that acts against several types of cancer tumors, perhaps via stimulation of the patient's immune system. It has minimal toxicity.

Carbohydrate Engineering The selective, deliberate alteration or creation of carbohydrates (and the oligosaccharide side chains of glycoprotein molecules) by humans.

See also GLUCONEOGENESIS, GLYCOBIOLOGY, GLYCOFORM, GLYCOLIPID, GLYCOLYSIS, GLYCOPROTEIN, GLYCOSIDASES, RESTRICTION ENDOGLYCOSIDASES, GLYCOSIDE, GLYCOSYLATION

Carbohydrate Microarray See MICROARRAY (TESTING)

Carbohydrates (Saccharides) A large class of carbon-hydrogen-oxygen compounds. Monosaccharides are called simple sugars, of which the most abundant is D-glucose. It is both the major fuel for most organisms and constitutes the basic building block of the most abundant polysaccharides, such as starch and cellulose.

Whereas starch is a fuel source, cellulose is the primary structural material of plants. Carbohydrates are produced by photosynthesis in plants. Most, but not all, carbohydrates are represented chemically by the formula $Cx(H_2O)n$, in which n is three or higher. On the basis of their chemical structures, carbohydrates are classified as polyhydroxy aldehydes, polyhydroxy ketones, and their derivatives.

See also GLUCOSE (GLc), GLYCOGEN, MONOSACCHARIDES, OLIGOSACCHARIDES, POLYSACCHARIDES, SIALIC ACID

Carbon Nanotubes Refers to any tiny tube composed of carbon whose diameter is measured in nanometers.

There are several potential applications for the utilization of carbon nanotubes (CNTs) within fields of biotechnology.

For example, during 2003, Bruce J. Hinds and coworkers were able to incorporate numerous CNTs into a polymer membrane (film) in a manner such that the CNTs served as "pores" through which molecules possessing 1 to 10 nm "diameters" could pass from one side of the membrane to the other.

Such **nanotube membranes** hold significant potential utility as **molecular sieves** (e.g., to screen certain biochemicals out of solution or mixture), as the contact surface for certain biosensors (e.g., allowing in only the molecules **sought to be sensed**), etc.

For example, during 2004, Hongjie Dai and Paul A. Wender utilized single-walled carbon nanotubes (SWNTs) to "ferry" specific proteins (e.g., streptavidin) across the plasma membrane of certain cells, where the protein was able to then act on the cell's interior. Dai and Wender showed that those specific proteins (bound to biotin-"coated" carbon nanotubes) entered the cells via endocytosis. Some carbon nanotubes can also act as an "antenna" to receive electromagnetic radiation possessing wavelengths of several hundred nanometers length (i.e., visible light). That visible light's energy is converted by the carbon nanotubes into either electricity or thermal energy (i.e., to drive a chemical reaction in adjacent substrate). Thus, these carbon nanotubes may be utilized in the future to construct light-sensing biosensors.

See also NANOSCIENCE, NANOMETERS (nm), NANOTECHNOLOGY, SELF-ASSEMBLY (OF A LARGE MOLECULAR STRUCTURE), SINGLE-STRANDED DNA, POLYMER, BIOSENSORS (CHEMICAL), BIOSENSORS (ELECTRONIC), PROTEIN, STREPTAVIDIN, CELL, PLASMA MEMBRANE, BIOTIN, ENDOCYTOSIS, SUBSTRATE (CHEMICAL), ACTIVATION ENERGY

Carboxyl Terminus (of a protein molecule) Refers to the carboxyl group (-COOH) that is attached to one end of some protein molecules or one end of some amino acid molecules.

See also PROTEIN, AMINO ACID

Carcinogen A cancer-causing agent.

See also MUTAGEN, PROTO-ONCOGENES, AFLATOXINS, ANTIOXIDANTS

Carnitine A "vitamin-like" nutrient that occurs naturally in the cells within animals and is needed for the body to convert fatty acids to energy (which can then be used by the body's cells). Carnitine is essential to facilitate the transport of acyl-CoA enzyme (attached to a fatty acid molecule) into the cell's mitochondria, where the beta-oxidation of fatty acids occurs (thereby providing energy to the cell).

Before fatty acids can enter the mitochondria, they must be "activated" by a chemical reaction (which occurs on the outer mitochondrial membrane), in which acyl-CoA is attached to the fatty acid molecule via a chemical reaction that is driven by adenosine triphosphate (ATP) and is catalyzed by acyl-CoA synthetase. Adenosine monophosphate (AMP) is a by-product of that chemical reaction.

See also FATTY ACIDS, METABOLISM, ACYL-CoA, ENZYME, ACETYL CARNITINE, ACETYLCARNITINE TRANSFERASE, MITOCHONDRIA, PLASMA MEMBRANE, ACTIVATION ENERGY, ADENOSINE TRIPHOSPHATE (ATP), SYNTHASE, ADENOSINE MONOPHOSPHATE (AMP)

Carotenoids A general term for a group of plant-produced and microorganism-produced pigments ranging in color from yellow to red and brown that act as protective antioxidants in photosynthetic plants and in animals that consume carotenoids.

Approximately 600 carotenoids have been discovered and studied. The carotenes and the xanthophylls, orange to yellow in color, are the most common. Carotenoids are responsible for the coloration of certain plants (e.g., the carrot) and of some animals (e.g., the lobster). The carotenoid pigments are transferred to animals as an element in their foods. Carotenoids are composed of isoprene units (usually eight), which may be modified by the addition of other chemical groups on the molecule. The carotenes are of importance to higher animals because they are utilized in the formation of vitamin A.

Carotenoids act as antioxidants ("quenchers" of free radicals), so consumption of carotenoids apparently reduces the risk of some cancers, coronary heart disease, eyesight loss, and cataracts.

See also VITAMIN, BETA-CAROTENE, CANCER, CORONARY HEART DISEASE (CHD), ASTAXANTHIN, LYCOPENE, ANTIOXIDANTS, FREE RADICAL, OXIDATIVE STRESS, INSULIN, LUTEIN,

ZEAXANTHIN, GOLDEN RICE, PHOTO-SYNTHESIS, MICROORGANISM

Cartilage-Inducing Factors A and B Compounds produced by the body that also have immunosuppressive activity.

See also IMMUNOSUPPRESSIVE

Cascade A sequential series of events (e.g., gene expressions, chemical reactions, immune responses, etc.) that are initiated (i.e., "set off") by a specific first event (e.g., a signaling molecule "docking" at a receptor molecule, an antibody–antigen complex forming in the body, thrombin cleaving fibrinogen, etc.).

See also SIGNALING MOLECULE, SIGNAL TRANSDUCTION, RECEPTORS, PROTEIN SIGNALING, SYSTEMIC ACQUIRED RESISTANCE (SAR), HARPIN, COMPLEMENT (COMPONENT OF IMMUNE SYSTEM), COMPLEMENT CASCADE, THROMBIN, FIBRIN, GENE EXPRESSION CASCADE, R GENES, TRANSACTIVATING PROTEIN, VIRAL TRANSACTIVATING PROTEIN, KINASES, MITOGEN-ACTIVATED PROTEIN KINASE CASCADE

Caspases Refers to a "family" of cysteine proteases, which are coded for by certain genes (e.g., the **ced-3** gene) during cell apoptosis. As a result of apoptosis causing synthesis of several caspases, the (dying) cells cleave/destroy a variety of cellular proteins (i.e., the cell undergoes "self-digestion").

See also ENZYME, PROTEASE, CELL, GENE, APOPTOSIS, PROTEIN, PARP

Cassette A "package" of genetic material (containing more than one gene) that is inserted into the genome of a cell via gene splicing techniques. May include promoters, leader sequence, termination codon, etc.

See also GENE SPLICING, LEADER SEQUENCE, PROMOTER, GENETIC CODE, TERMINATION CODON (SEQUENCE), GENETIC ENGINEERING, TRANSGENE, GENOME

Catabolism Energy-yielding pathway. The phase of metabolism involved in the energy-yielding breakdown of nutrient (food) molecules.

See also DISSIMILATION, METABOLISM, PATHWAY, STEROLS

Catabolite Activator Protein See CAP

Catabolite Repression Common in bacteria. The decreased expression of catabolic enzymes as brought about by a catabolite such as glucose. For example, glucose is the preferred fuel source for certain bacteria and when present in the culture medium, it represses the formation of enzymes that are required for the utilization of other fuel sugars, such as β-galactosidase. Because glucose or other catabolites (other molecules derived from glucose) cause the repression, it is known as catabolite repression.

See also CAP, OPERON, GLUCOSE (GLc), ADENOSINE MONOPHOSPHATE (AMP), PATHWAY FEEDBACK MECHANISMS

Catalase An enzyme that catalyzes the very rapid decomposition of hydrogen peroxide to water and oxygen. Catalase is in the group of enzymes known as metalloenzymes because it requires the presence of a metal in order to be catalytically active. The metal (known as a cofactor) is, in the case of catalase, iron. Found in both plants and animals.

See also HYDROLYSIS, HUMAN SUPEROXIDE DISMUTASE (hSOD), PEG-SOD (POLYETHYLENE GLYCOL SUPEROXIDE DISMUTASE)

Catalysis Coined by Jons J. Berzelius in 1838, this term refers to the act of increasing the rate of a given chemical reaction via use of a catalyst. Almost all chemical reactions in biological systems (e.g., within an organism) are catalyzed by molecules known as enzymes. Enzymes typically increase the rate of a given biological or chemical reaction by at least a millionfold.

See also CATALYST, CATALYTIC SITE, ENZYME, METALLOENZYME

Catalyst From the Greek word "katalyein," which meant "to dissolve."

Any substance (entity), either of protein or of nonproteinaceous nature, that increases the rate of a chemical reaction without being consumed itself in the reaction. In the biosciences, the term "enzyme" is used for a proteinaceous catalyst. Enzymes catalyze biological reactions.

See also ENZYME, CATALYTIC SITE, ACTIVE SITE, CATALYTIC ANTIBODY, SEMISYNTHETIC CATALYTIC ANTIBODY, METALLOENZYME

C

Catalytic Antibody Discovered by Richard A. Lerner and Peter G. Shultz during the 1980s, these are antibodies produced by an organism's body in order to help catalyze certain chemical reactions (e.g., needed for certain body functions). Scientists have subsequently been able to cause organisms to produce an antibody in response to a carefully selected antigen (e.g., target molecule in bloodstream, or molecule involved in chemical reaction of interest) that itself catalyzes the "splitting" of a molecule in the bloodstream (e.g., heroin into two harmless small molecules) or mimics:

- Restriction endonucleases that cleave (cut) proteins or DNA molecules precisely at specific locations on those molecules
- Restriction endoglycosidases that are capable of cleaving oligosaccharides or polysaccharide molecules precisely at specific locations on those molecules
- Transition-state chemical complex in the chemical reaction that is to be catalyzed — resultant antibody acts both as an antibody (to the selected transition-state-complex antigen) and as a catalyst (for the chemical reaction possessing that selected-transition-state chemical complex)

This catalyst (enzyme) thus possesses the remarkable specificity of an antibody (i.e., specific only to the desired transition-state reactant), which holds the potential to yield chemical reaction products of greater purity than those achieved via current (less specific) catalysts.

Because the immune system will (in theory) produce an antibody to virtually every molecule of sufficient size to be detected by the immune system (i.e., 6 to 34 Å), it should be possible to raise catalytic antibodies for a large number of industrial chemical reactions that are currently catalyzed via conventional (less specific) catalysts. Commercial quantities of such antibodies would be produced via monoclonal antibody techniques (e.g., in bioreactors or fermentation vats).

See also OLIGOSACCHARIDES, CATALYST, ANTIBODY, ORGANISM, RESTRICTION ENDONUCLEASES, RESTRICTION ENDOGLYCOSIDASES, CELL, MONOCLONAL ANTIBODIES (MAb), ANTIGEN, TRANSITION STATE, PROTEIN, ACTIVATION ENERGY, SEMISYNTHETIC CATALYTIC ANTIBODY, ANGSTROM (Å), ABZYMES

Catalytic Domain See DOMAIN (OF A PROTEIN)

Catalytic RNA Discovered by Thomas R. Cech and Sidney Altman in 1983, this refers to an RNA (ribonucleic acid) molecule that acts to cleave ("cut") any other RNA.

See also RIBOZYMES, RIBONUCLEIC ACID (RNA)

Catalytic Site The site (geometric area) on an enzyme molecule (or other catalyst) that is actually involved in the catalytic process. The catalytic site usually consists of a small portion of the total area of the enzyme.

See also CATALYST, ENZYME, ACTIVE SITE, CATALYTIC ANTIBODY

Catechins Refers to a "family" of polyphenol chemical compounds (phytochemicals) that are naturally produced in most teas, red wines, apples, grapes, chocolate, etc. When consumed by humans, catechins have been shown to have beneficial antioxidant, anti-inflammatory, and antithrombotic effects.

See also POLYPHENOLS, PHYTOCHEMICALS, ANTIOXIDANTS, THROMBOSIS

Catecholamines Hormones (such as adrenalin) that are amino derivatives of a base structure known as catechol. Catecholamines are released into the bloodstream by exercise and act as natural tranquilizers.

See also ENDORPHINS, HORMONE

Cation See ION, CHELATION, CHELATING AGENT

Cauliflower Mosaic Virus 35S Promoter (CaMV 35S) A promoter (sequence of DNA) that is often utilized in genetic engineering to control expression of a (inserted) gene; i.e., synthesis of desired protein in a plant.

See also VIRUS, PROMOTER, DEOXYRIBONUCLEIC ACID (DNA), GENE, GENETIC ENGINEERING, PROTEIN

Caveolae Discovered during the 1950s by Eichi Yamada and George Palade. Named by Yamada, who thought they looked like small caves (**Latin caveola = "small caves"**).

See PLASMA MEMBRANE

CBA Acronym for **cell-based assay**.
See CELL-BASED ASSAYS

CBD See CONVENTION ON BIOLOGICAL DIVERSITY (CBD)

CBF1 A transcription factor (i.e., special protein) that is synthesized (i.e., manufactured) within certain plants (e.g., *Arabidopsis thaliana*, etc.) when that plant is exposed to cold temperatures. CBF1 then interacts with certain portions of the plant's DNA (i.e., regulatory sequences) to thus "switch on" the process of cold hardening (via proteins coded for by that plant's genes).
See also TRANSCRIPTION FACTORS, PROTEIN, SYNTHESIZING (OF PROTEINS), *ARABIDOPSIS THALIANA*, GENETIC CODE, CODING SEQUENCE, REGULATORY SEQUENCE, DEOXYRIBONUCLEIC ACID (DNA), COLD HARDENING

CCC DNA A covalently linked circular DNA molecule, such as a plasmid.
See also DEOXYRIBONUCLEIC ACID (DNA), PLASMID

CD4 EPSP Synthase See EPSP SYNTHASE, CP4 EPSPS

CD4 EPSPS See EPSP SYNTHASE, CP4 EPSPS

CD4 Protein An adhesion molecule (protein) embedded in the outer wall (envelope) of human immune system and brain cells, which functions as the receptor (door to entry into the cell) for the HIV (AIDS) virus. The gp120 envelope glycoprotein of the HIV (i.e., AIDS virus) directly interacts with the CD4 protein on the surface of helper T cells to enable the virus to invade the helper T cells.
See also T CELL RECEPTORS, ADHESION MOLECULE, GP120 PROTEIN, SOLUBLE CD4

CD4-PE40 A pharmaceutical discovered in 1988 by Ira Pastan and Bernard Moss that has shown potential to combat acquired immune deficiency syndrome (AIDS). CD4-PE40 is a conjugated protein (fusion protein) consisting of a CD4 protein (molecule) attached to pseudomonas exotoxin (a substance produced by pseudomonas bacteria that is toxic to certain living cells). The gp120 glycoprotein on the surface of the HIV (i.e., AIDS) virus attaches preferentially to the CD4 portion of this immunoconjugate, and the virus is inactivated by the pseudomonas exotoxin portion of this immunoconjugate.
See also PROTEIN, CD4 PROTEIN, FUSION PROTEIN, GP120 PROTEIN, SOLUBLE CD4, IMMUNOTOXIN, CONJUGATED PROTEIN, ACQUIRED IMMUNE DEFICIENCY SYNDROME (AIDS), HUMAN IMMUNODEFICIENCY VIRUS TYPE 1 (HIV-1), HUMAN IMMUNODEFICIENCY VIRUS TYPE 2 (HIV-2), RICIN, ABRIN

CD44 Protein One of the adhesion molecules (embedded in the surface of the linings of blood vessels) that assists the neutrophils on their journey from the bloodstream through the walls of blood vessels (e.g., to combat pathogens into adjacent tissues). Tumor cells also exploit CD44 molecules in order to metastasize (spread throughout the body's tissue from a single beginning tumor) via a similar (tumor cell) through blood vessel wall adhesion molecule mechanism.
See also ADHESION MOLECULE, CD4 PROTEIN, PROTEIN, NEUTROPHILS, PATHOGEN, TUMOR, CANCER, SOLUBLE CD4

CD95 Protein Also called APO-1/Fas, it is a transmembrane protein (embedded within the surface membrane of the cell) that transmits apoptosis ("programmed" cell death) "signal" into cells. Transduction of that apoptosis signal occurs when certain ligands or antigens (i.e., the APO-1/Fas antigen) bind to the extracellular (i.e., portion outside of cell membrane) part (i.e., receptor) of the CD95 protein.
See also APOPTOSIS, PROTEIN, CELL, SIGNAL TRANSDUCTION, SIGNALING, NUCLEAR RECEPTORS, ANTIGEN, RECEPTORS, *FUSARIUM*

cDNA See COMPLEMENTARY DNA (cDNA)

cDNA Array See MICROARRAY (TESTING)

cDNA Clone A DNA molecule synthesized ("made") from an mRNA sequence via sequential use of reverse transcriptase (acting on mRNA) and DNA polymerase. A collection of such cloned molecules, which represents all the genetic information expressed by a given cell or by a given tissue type, is referred to as a **cDNA library**.

See also DEOXYRIBONUCLEIC ACID (DNA), MESSENGER RNA (mRNA), COMPLEMENTARY DNA (cDNA), SEQUENCE (OF A DNA MOLECULE), REVERSE TRANSCRIPTASE, DNA POLYMERASE, CLONE (A MOLECULE), CELL, GENETIC CODE

cDNA Library See cDNA CLONE

cDNA Microarray See MICROARRAY (TESTING), COMPLEMENTARY DNA (cDNA)

CE Acronym for capillary electrophoresis. See CAPILLARY ELECTROPHORESIS

Cecrophins (Lytic Proteins) Proteins produced by certain white blood cells (called cytotoxic T lymphocytes [CTL] or killer T cells). The proteins allow lysis (i.e., bursting) of infected cells. Cecrophins are amphopathic (i.e., contain both a hydrophobic region and a hydrophilic region) and work by "worming" the hydrophobic portion into the cell membrane (so the hydrophobic portion of the cecrophin molecule is out of the water). This creates a transmembrane pore (i.e., a hole in the membrane) that is lined with the cecrophin's hydrophilic portion. Membranes function simply to separate various components. This separation is required for life to exist. When holes are introduced into cell membranes, water rushes into the targeted cell due to differences in osmotic pressure and the cell ruptures (explodes). T cecrophins are only able to lyse (i.e., burst) infected cells because only "sick" cells have a weakened cytoskeleton (located just inside the cell membrane), which cannot prevent the contents of the cell from spilling out through the pores (created by cecrophins).

See also HELPER T CELLS (T4 CELLS), PATHOGEN, COMPLEMENT, HYDROPHOBIC, HYDROPHILIC, COMPLEMENT CASCADE, LYSE, LYSIS

Cecropin A See CECROPIN A PEPTIDE

Cecropin A Peptide See CECROPHINS, PEPTIDE

Cell From the Latin word *cella*, which means "small room."

The fundamental self-containing unit of life. The living tissue of every multicelled organism is composed of these fundamental living units. Certain organisms may consist of only one cell, such as yeast or protein bacteria, protozoa, some algae, and gametes (the reproductive stages) of higher organisms. Larger organisms are subdivided into organs that are relatively autonomous but cooperate in the functioning of that plant or animal. Unicellular (i.e., single-cell) organisms perform all life functions within the single cell. In a higher organism (i.e., a multicellular organism), entire populations of cells (i.e., an organ) may be designated a particular specialized task (e.g., the heart to facilitate circulation). The cells of muscle tissue are specialized for movement and those of bone and connective tissue, for structural support.

Most cells are too small to be seen with the unaided eye. The egg yolk of birds is a single cell, so the egg yolk of an ostrich is the world's largest cell.

See also PLASMA MEMBRANE, GAMETE, GERM CELL, MICROBIOLOGY, OOCYTES

Cell Culture The *in vitro* (i.e., outside of body, in a test tube or vat) propagation of cells isolated from living organisms.

See also MAMMALIAN CELL CULTURE, INSECT CELL CULTURE, DISSOCIATING ENZYMES, HARVESTING ENZYMES

Cell Cytometry See CELL, CELL SORTING, FLUORESCENCE-ACTIVATED CELL SORTER (FACs), MAGNETIC PARTICLES

Cell Differentiation The process whereby descendants of a common parental cell achieve and maintain specialization of structure and function. In humans, for instance, all the different types of cells (e.g., muscle cells, bone cells, etc.) differentiate from the zygote (itself formed by union of the simple sperm and egg). In humans, the various blood cell types (e.g., red blood cells, white blood cells, etc.) differentiate from stem cells in the bone marrow. Cell differentiation is caused/triggered/assisted by micro-RNAs, colony-stimulating factors (CSFs), growth factors (GFs), and certain other proteins (e.g., hedgehog proteins).

See also STEM CELLS, STEM CELL ONE, DIFFERENTIATION, PROTEIN, HEDGEHOG SIGNALING PATHWAY, HEDGEHOG

PROTEINS, ERYTHROCYTES, LEUKO-
CYTES, COLONY-STIMULATING FAC-
TORS, GROWTH FACTORS, MITOGEN-
ACTIVATED PROTEIN KINASE CASCADE,
MICRORNAs

Cell Differentiation Proteins The various
growth factors and other proteins that
cause/assist in cell differentiation.

See also CELL DIFFERENTIATION,
HEDGEHOG PROTEINS

Cell Fusion The combining of cell contents of
two or more cells to become a single cell.
Fertilization is such a process (fusing of
gametes' cells).

See also GAMETE

Cell Motility Refers to **cell movement** (e.g.,
during an organism's early development,
repair of some tissues, cancer metastasis, etc.).

During some stages of a human baby's development in the womb, entire "sheets" of cells
will suddenly move significant distances to a
new location on the baby's body.

Also, when blood vessels get injured, the
injured cells release a signal. That signal
causes some of the endothelial smooth muscle
cells to "transform" from **contractile** phenotype (i.e., normal state, in which they help to
control blood pressure) to **synthetic** phenotype (i.e., which can move). The cells in synthetic state move to the site of the injury,
where they repair it by growing/dividing, and
then they return to the contractile state.

During metastasis, transforming growth factor-
beta (TGF-beta) exuded by a cancerous tumor
causes epithelial cells to "transform" to mesenchymal phenotype (thereby enabling subsequent cell motility).

The molecule **n-cofilin** plays a critical role in
the body's regulation of cell motility (e.g.,
helps to break down actin fibers, resulting in
cells moving during development, etc.).

See also CELL, PATHWAY, SIGNALING,
HEDGEHOG SIGNALING PATHWAY,
EMBRYOLOGY, ENDOTHELIUM, CAN-
CER, METASTASIS, TRANSFORMING
GROWTH FACTOR-BETA (TGF-BETA),
PHENOTYPE, CHOLESTEROL, ACTIN

Cell Recognition See ADHESION MOLE-
CULE, SIGNAL TRANSDUCTION,
RECEPTORS

Cell Signaling See SIGNALING

Cell Sorting A process utilized (e.g., by
researchers) to sort/separate different cells
(e.g., pathogens, cancerous vs. normal cells,
sperm that bear chromosomes for male vs.
female, etc.).

Some automated means of cell sorting include
"biochips" (utilizing controlled electrical
fields to collect specific cell types onto electrodes in the biochip), fluorescence-activated cell sorter (FACs) machines, magnetic
particles (e.g., attached to antibodies), etc.

See also CELL, PATHOGEN, CANCER,
CHROMOSOME, BIOCHIP, BIOMEMS,
FLUORESCENCE-ACTIVATED CELL
SORTER (FACs), MAGNETIC PARTICLES

Cell-Based Assays Refers to assays in which
whole cells (generally living) are probed.

See also ASSAY, BIOASSAY CELL, MULTI-
PLEXED (ASSAY), HIGH-CONTENT
SCREENING, FLOW CYTOMETRY,
WHOLE- ELL PATCH-CLAMP RECORDING

Cell-Free Gene Expression System Refers
to a (science researcher's) system of carefully
prepared compounds/vessels for the **expression of a given gene** without the use of any
cells. For example, a given gene can be transcribed in a research vessel (test tube) by addition of the proper RNA polymerase. The
resultant RNA is then translated via the proper
lysate (e.g., extracted from reticulocytes or
from wheat germ).

See also CELL, GENE, EXPRESS, TRAN-
SCRIPTION, TRANSLATION

Cell-Mediated Immunity See CELLULAR
IMMUNE RESPONSE

Cellular Adhesion Molecule See ADHE-
SION MOLECULE

Cellular Adhesion Receptors See ADHE-
SION MOLECULE, RECEPTORS, INTE-
GRINS, SELECTINS, CADHERINS

Cellular Affinity Tendency of cells to adhere
specifically to cells of the same type. This
property is lost in some cancer cells.

See also CELL, ADHESION MOLECULE,
CELL DIFFERENTIATION

Cellular Immune Response Also called cell-
mediated immunity. The immune response
of specialized cells, in contrast to the
response of soluble antibodies. The specialized cells that make up this group include
cytotoxic T lymphocytes (CTL), helper T

lymphocytes, macrophages, and monocytes. This system works in concert with the humoral immune response.

See also HUMORAL IMMUNITY, T CELLS, T CELL RECEPTORS, PHAGOCYTE, HELPER T CELLS (T4 CELLS), CYTO-KINES, MACROPHAGE

Cellular Oncogenes See PROTO-ONCO-GENES

Cellular Pathway Mapping Refers to the process of determining each of the pathways and pathway feedback mechanisms within a given cell's vital processes.

Cellular pathway mapping can be utilized to identify targets of therapeutic agents, identify cross-talk between some of the cell's pathways, and to identify "branched" pathways that, when perturbed by a potential therapeutical agent (e.g., pharmaceutical), could result in toxic side effects.

See also PATHWAY, CELL, PATHWAY FEED-BACK MECHANISM, TARGET (OF A THERAPEUTIC AGENT), VALIDATION (OF TARGET), TOXICOGENOMICS, METABOLITE PROFILING, HIGH-CON-TENT SCREENING, RNA INTERFER-ENCE (RNAi), METABONOMICS

Cellulase An enzyme that digests cellulose to simple sugars such as glucose.

See also ENZYME, DIGESTION (WITHIN CHEMICAL PRODUCTION PLANTS)

Cellulose A polymer of glucose units found in all plant matter; it comprises 40 to 55% of the cell wall in plant cells. Because of its presence in all plant cells, cellulose is the most abundant biological compound on Earth.

See also CARBOHYDRATES, GLUCOSE (GLC), CELL, VAN DER WAALS FORCES

Center for Advanced Research in Biotechnology (CARB) A protein engineering research consortium that was established in Rockville (MD) during 1989 by the U.S. Government, the University of Maryland, and local government.

See also PROTEIN ENGINEERING

Central Dogma (new) Coined by Shankar Subramaniam during 1999, it is a restatement of the (old) former "Central Dogma" that includes the fact that an organism's environment/activity also impact **when** and **how** and **how much** some of its genes are expressed

(e.g., to cause certain proteins to be "manufactured"). Environmental factors impacting gene expression include temperature, sunlight, humidity, consumption of some vitamins, presence of certain bacteria, presence of signal transducers and activators of transcription (STATs), etc. For example, the eggs of the saltwater crocodile (*Crocodylus porosus*) yield a larger fraction of male offspring when those eggs are incubated in the nest (made of rotting vegetation) at temperatures above 90°F (32°C) than when those eggs are incubated at temperatures below 90°F (32°C).

Recent research indicates that **physical exercise** changes the expression levels of some genes (within human skeletal muscles) involved in the body's metabolism of carbohydrates.

That (Central Dogma) restatement also expressly includes the fact that **more than one protein** can result from each gene in an organism's genome (e.g., owing to interactions **between** genes, interactions between genes and their protein products [e.g., STATs], interactions between genes and histones, and interactions between genes and some environmental factors). Mechanistically, this results in (different) proteins via:

- Alternative splicing of the mRNA transcript. For example, the COX-3 enzyme is produced in the human body when **intron 1** is retained in the mRNA transcript during transcription of the COX-1 gene. For example, a single intronic base substitution that is present within the IKAP gene (the allele responsible for the human disease known as *Familial Dysautonomia*) affects the splicing of the IKAP transcript (i.e., the mRNA segment that determines which protein is subsequently "manufactured" by relevant cells).
- Varying translation start or stop site (on the gene).
- Frameshifting (i.e., different set of triplet codons in the mRNA is translated).

- Contiguous genes.
- Recombination of some gene segments.

See also CENTRAL DOGMA (OLD), ORGANISM, MOLECULAR GENETICS, COMPLEMENTARY DNA (c-DNA), GENE, ALLELE, PROTEIN, ENZYME, REPLICATION (OF VIRUS), TRANSCRIPTION, TRANSLATION, DEOXYRIBONUCLEIC ACID (DNA), GENOME, RIBONUCLEIC ACID (RNA), MESSENGER RNA (mRNA), TRANSCRIPTION FACTORS, RIBOSOMES, SIGNAL TRANSDUCTION, SIGNAL TRANSDUCERS AND ACTIVATORS OF TRANSCRIPTION (STATs), PHOTOPERIOD, GENE EXPRESSION, ALTERNATIVE SPLICING, GENE SPLICING, SPLICING, SPLICE VARIANTS, FRAMESHIFT, CODON, INTRON, PHARMACOENVIROGENETICS, CYCLOOXYGENASE, METABOLISM, CARBOHYDRATES, TRANSCRIPTOME, ACTIVATOR (OF GENE), CONTIGUOUS GENES, EPIGENETIC, VITAMIN, HISTONES

Central Dogma (old) The historical organizing principle of molecular genetics; it states that genetic information flows from DNA to RNA to protein or, stated in another way: DNA makes RNA which makes protein. This principle was first stated by Watson and Crick. It is, however, not rigorously accurate as illustrated by the facts that:

- DNA (i.e., genes) "information flow" is influenced (e.g., timing, amounts, etc.) by some environmental factors (e.g., temperature, humidity, etc.).
- The enzyme reverse transcriptase produces ("makes") DNA using an RNA template.
- Prions do not contain any DNA.

See also MOLECULAR GENETICS, COMPLEMENTARY DNA (c-DNA), PROTEIN, ENZYME, REPLICATION (OF VIRUS), TRANSCRIPTION, TRANSLATION, DEOXYRIBONUCLEIC ACID (DNA), RIBONUCLEIC ACID (RNA), MESSENGER RNA (mRNA), PRION, TEMPLATE, CENTRAL

DOGMA (NEW), REVERSE TRANSCRIPTASES, RT-PCR, ACTIVATOR (OF GENE)

Centrifuge A machine that is used to separate heavier from lighter molecules and cellular components and structures.
See also ULTRACENTRIFUGE

Centromere A constricted region of a chromosome that includes the site of attachment to the mitotic or meiotic spindle.
See also CHROMOSOMES, MEIOSIS, CHROMATIN, MITOSIS, KARYOTYPE, KARYOTYPER

Cerebrose See GALACTOSE (Gal)

Cessation Cassette A three-gene cassette (genetic sequence construct) that, **when inserted into a plant** and when activated via tetracycline antibiotic, prevents the seeds produced by that plant from germinating. This is because the "cessation cassette" stops those resultant seeds from synthesizing a specific protein needed for seed germination.
See also CASSETTE, GENE, GENETIC ENGINEERING, PROTEIN, SYNTHESIZING (OF PROTEINS), SEQUENCE (OF A DNA MOLECULE), ANTIBIOTIC

CFH Protein Abbreviation for **complement factor H protein**.
See COMPLEMENT FACTOR H GENE

CFP Acronym for **cyan fluorescent protein**.
See VISIBLE FLUORESCENT PROTEINS

CFTR See CYSTIC FIBROSIS TRANSMEMBRANE REGULATOR PROTEIN (CFTR)

CGE Acronym for **control** of **gene expression**.
See GENETIC USE RESTRICTION TECHNOLOGIES

CGIAR See CONSULTATIVE GROUP ON INTERNATIONAL AGRICULTURAL RESEARCH (CGIAR)

cGMP Current Good Manufacturing Practices. The set of current, up-to-date methodologies, practices, and procedures mandated by the Food and Drug Administration (FDA), which are to be followed in the testing and manufacture of pharmaceuticals. The set of rules and regulations promulgated and enforced by the FDA to ensure the manufacture of safe clinical supplies. The cGMP guidelines are more fine-tuned and up-to-date (technologically speaking) than the more general GMP.

See also PHASE I CLINICAL TESTING, IND, GOOD MANUFACTURING PRACTICES (GMP)

Chaconine A neurotoxin that is naturally present at low levels within potatoes. As a result, chaconine is present at detectable levels in the bloodstream of humans who consume potatoes. When consumed by humans, chaconine acts as a plasma cholinesterase inhibitor.

See also TOXIN, SOLANINE, PLASMA, CHOLINESTERASE, INHIBITION

Chakrabarty Decision *Diamond vs. Chakrabarty*, U.S. Department of Commerce, 1980; a landmark case in which the U.S. Supreme Court held that the inventor of a "new" microorganism (*Burkholderia cepaci* bacteria) whose invention otherwise met the legal requirements for obtaining a patent, could not be denied a patent solely because the invention was alive. It essentially allowed the patenting of life forms.

Ananda Chakrabarty, a scientist, had modified the genes of *Burkholderia cepaci*, making it better able to break down petroleum and digest it.

See also U.S. PATENT AND TRADEMARK OFFICE (USPTO), MICROORGANISM, BACTERIA

Chalcone Isomerase An enzyme present within some plants (e.g., tomato) that can catalyze or increase production of certain flavonols (e.g., naringenin chalcone, quercitin glycosides, etc.), which act as antioxidants in the human body when they are consumed by humans. Because oxidation of certain lipids (e.g., low-density lipoproteins) in the bloodstream is the initial step in atherosclerosis disease, consumption of large amounts of such flavonols may help to prevent atherosclerosis (and some other diseases caused by oxidative stress).

See also FLAVONOLS, OXIDATION, LIPIDS, OXIDATIVE STRESS, ANTIOXIDANTS, ATHEROSCLEROSIS, QUERCITIN

Channel Blockers See CALCIUM CHANNEL BLOCKERS

Chaotropic Agent A substance that yields ions that can dissolve biological membranes/proteins and/or denature nucleic acids.

One example of a chaotropic agent is guanidium isothiocyanate.

See also ION, PLASMA MEMBRANE, DENATURATION, DENATURED DNA, NUCLEIC ACIDS

Chaperone Molecules See CHAPERONES

Chaperone Proteins See CHAPERONES

Chaperones Protein molecules inside living cells that assist with correct protein folding as the protein molecule emerges from the cell's ribosomes. Also, they help to convey those proteins to their ultimate destinations in the organism.

Later, when cellular protein molecules begin to "unfold" owing to age, heat, viruses, or exposure to certain chemicals or ultraviolet light, chaperones often cause those unfolded protein molecules to return to their correct (initial) conformation. Examples of such chaperone molecules include heat-shock protein 70, heat-shock protein 40, GroEL, and GroES.

See also LEADER SEQUENCE (PROTEIN MOLECULE), PROTEIN FOLDING, HEAT-SHOCK PROTEINS, PROTEIN, RIBOSOMES, CELL, CONFORMATION, VIRUS, CONGO RED

Chaperonins Protein molecules inside living cells that facilitate proper folding of the (new) protein molecules that are synthesized (i.e., "manufactured") in the cell's ribosomes.

See also PROTEIN, CO-CHAPERONIN, CHAPERONES, MOLECULAR CHAPERONES, PROTEIN FOLDING, RIBOSOMES, CELL, CONFORMATION

Characterization Assay See ASSAY, HIGH-THROUGHPUT SCREENING (HTS), BIO-ASSAY, BIOCHIPS

CHD Acronym for **coronary heart disease.**

See CORONARY HEART DISEASE (CHD), ATHEROSCLEROSIS, LOW-DENSITY LIPOPROTEINS (LDLP), CAROTENOIDS

Chelating Agent A molecule capable of "binding" metal atoms. The chelating agent or metal complex is held together by coordination bonds that have a strong polar character. One example of a common chelating agent is ethylenediamine tetraacetate (EDTA), which tightly and reversibly binds Mg^{2+} and other divalent cations (positively charged ions). If a chelate is allowed to bind to metal ions required for enzyme activity, the enzyme will be inactivated (inhibited). Cobalamin (vitamin B_{12}), EDTA, and the iron–porphyrin complex of heme (which provides the red color of blood) are other examples of chelates. See also EDTA, PHYTATE, LOW-PHYTATE SOYBEANS, LOW-PHYTYATE CORN, CHELATION, HEME, TRANSFERRIN

Chelation The binding of metal cations (metal atoms or molecules possessing a positive electrical charge) by atoms possessing unshared electrons (thus, the electrons can be "donated" to a bond with a cation). The binding of the metal (cation) to the (electron-excess) chelator atom (ligand) results in formation of a chelator/metal cation complex. The intra-atom bonds thus formed are given the name of coordination bonds. The properties of the chelator/metal cation complex frequently differ markedly from the "parent" cation. Both carboxylate and amino (molecular) groups readily bind metal cations. One of the most widely used chelators is EDTA (ethylenediamine tetraacetate). It has a strong affinity for metal cations possessing two (bi) or more positive (electrical) charges. Each EDTA molecule binds one metal cation. The EDTA molecule can be visualized as a "hand" (having only four fingers) that grasps the metal cation. Some enzymes (that require metal cations for their activity) are inactivated by EDTA (and other chelators) in that the chelators preferentially remove the metal from the enzyme.

See also ION, EDTA, LIGAND (IN BIOCHEMISTRY), CARBOHYDRATES, ENZYME, HEME, CHELATING AGENT, TRANSFERRIN, PHYTATE, LOW-PHYTATE CORN, LOW-PHYTATE SOYBEANS

Chemical Genetics Coined by Rebecca Ward and Tim Mitchison, this term refers to the creation and use of synthetic chemicals that act to either change the sequence (of amino acids in), change the conformation, block, or enhance the activity of a protein (or gene that codes for protein). This enables scientists to then determine the specific functions of specific protein molecules.

For example, during 2002, Henning D. Mootz and Tom W. Muir devised a methodology to use a dimerizer ligand to initiate protein splicing. When carefully devised, e.g., the dimerizer ligands are each bound to one half of an **intein**, which are themselves bound to **exteins**, the intein is thereby "popped out" of the center (of the protein molecule), and the two exteins (i.e., the two "end sequences" of the protein molecule after the intein is removed) are spliced together in a manner that is controlled (to yield the desired **new net protein** molecule).

See also GENOMICS, FUNCTIONAL GENOMICS, PROTEIN, GENE, GENETIC CODE, ZINC FINGER PROTEINS, COMBINATORIAL CHEMISTRY, CONFORMATION, GENOMIC SCIENCES, GENE FUNCTION ANALYSIS, SEQUENCE (OF A PROTEIN MOLECULE), LIGAND (IN BIOCHEMISTRY), INTEIN, EXTEIN

Chemiluminescence See LUMINESCENT ASSAYS, CHEMILUMINESCENT IMMUNOASSAY (CLIA)

Chemiluminescent Immunoassay (CLIA) An immunoassay (i.e., an antibody-based bioassay) that utilizes a signal that is generated by light-releasing chemical reactions (e.g., triggered by the binding of antibody to analyte).

See also IMMUNOASSAY, ANTIBODY, LUMINESCENT ASSAYS

Chemoautotroph A microorganism that obtains its energy from reactions between itself and inorganic (chemical) compounds. For example, certain *Archaea* microorganisms derive energy from chemicals present on the ocean floor where they live (e.g., in/near volcanoes, lava vents, etc.).

See also AUTOTROPH, *ARCHAEA*

Chemometrics An empirical methodology utilized to (inexpensively) infer a chemical quantity/value from (indirect) measurements of other physical/chemical values (which can be obtained inexpensively). The term chemometrics was coined in 1975 by Bruce Kowalski. One example of the use of chemometrics is to infer the TME (N) or "true metabolizable energy" of high-oil corn from its protein and oil (fat) content.

See also HIGH-OIL CORN, TME (N), PROTEIN, FATS

Chemopharmacology Therapy (to cure disease) by chemically synthesized drugs.

See also PHARMACOLOGY, CISPLATIN

C

Chemotaxis Sensing of, and movement toward or away from a specific chemical agent by living, freely moving cells (e.g., bacteria, macrophages, neutrophils, etc.).

For example, the bacteria *Clostridium botulinum* can sense and move away from nitric oxide (which can kill them).

See also CELL, BACTERIA, MACROPHAGE, NEUTROPHILS, ACTIN, NODULATION, NITRIC OXIDE

Chemotherapy When this term was first coined by Paul Ehrlich in 1905, it was defined as any therapy (to cure diseases) via chemically synthesized drugs.

Over time, the term has increasingly been utilized to refer to only application of such therapy to treat cancers.

See also CHEMOPHARMACOLOGY, CANCER, CISPLATIN, TAXOL, PACLITAXEL, TOXICOGENOMICS

Chimera An organism consisting of tissues or parts of diverse genetic constitution. An example of a chimera would be a centaur: the half-man, half-horse figure of Greek mythology. The word "chimera" is from the mythological creature by that name, which possessed the head of a lion, the body of a goat, and the tail of a serpent. The word chimera is very general and may be applied to any number of entities. For example, chimeric antibodies may be produced by cell cultures in which the variable, antigen-binding regions are of murine (mouse) origin, whereas the rest of the molecule is of human origin. It is hoped that this combination will lead to an antibody that, when injected into patients, would not elicit "rejection" and not give rise to a lesser immune response by the host against diseases the antibody is "aimed" at.

See also DEOXYRIBONUCLEIC ACID (DNA), GENETIC ENGINEERING, CHIMERIC DNA, CHIMERIC PROTEINS, CHIMERIC ANTIBODY, CHIMERAPLASTY, ORGANISM, ANTIBODY, ENGINEERED ANTIBODIES

Chimeraplasty A method utilized by man to introduce a gene (from same or another species) into the DNA of a living organism or cell via the "gene repair" mechanism. Scientists add the desired DNA (gene) to a cell, along with RNA, in a paired group known as a chimeraplast. The chimeraplast attaches itself to the cell's DNA at the site of the specific gene (to be changed) and "repairs" it by utilizing its (new) chimeraplast-DNA as a "template."

See also GENE REPAIR (DONE BY HUMANS), GENE, SPECIES, DEOXYRIBONUCLEIC ACID (DNA), DNA REPAIR, ORGANISM, CELL, CHIMERA, TEMPLATE, RIBONUCLEIC ACID (RNA)

Chimeric Antibody A (genetically engineered) antibody that combines characteristics of antibodies from two different sources. For example, the complementarity-determining (i.e., antigen-binding) portion of an animal antibody (e.g., raised against a specific antigen) with human monoclonal antibody.

See also ANTIBODY, ANTIGEN, AVIDITY, MONOCLONAL ANTIBODIES (MAb), CHIMERA, CHIMERIC PROTEINS, GENETIC ENGINEERING, HUMANIZED ANTIBODY

Chimeric DNA (Recombinant) DNA containing spliced genes from two different species. Transcription/translation of chimeric DNA results in synthesis (by ribosome) of a **chimeric protein** (also known as a fusion protein).

See also DEOXYRIBONUCLEIC ACID (DNA), GENE, TRANSCRIPTION, TRANSLATION, RIBOSOME, PROTEIN, CHIMERIC PROTEINS, GENE SPLICING, SPECIES, RECOMBINANT DNA (rDNA), GENETIC ENGINEERING, GENE FUSION

Chimeric Proteins Fused proteins from different species, produced from the chimeric DNA template.

See also CHIMERA, CHIMERIC DNA, DEOXYRIBONUCLEIC ACID (DNA), ANTIBODY, ENGINEERED ANTIBODIES, CHIMERIC ANTIBODY, GENE FUSION

Chinese Hamster Ovary Cells See CHO CELLS

Chiral Compound A chemical compound that contains an asymmetrical center and is capable of occurring in two nonsuperimposable mirror images. This phenomenon was first described by Louis Pasteur. "Chiral" is a word that is derived from the Greek *cheir* (meaning "hand"). For example, human hands may be used to illustrate chirality in that when the left and right hands are held one on top of the other, one thumb sticks out on one side while the other thumb sticks out on the other side. The point is that the same number and type of fingers and thumbs exist in both hands, but their arrangement in space may be different. So it is with the arrangement of a given molecule's (e.g., a drug's) atoms in three-dimensional space.

Approximately 40% of drugs on the market today consist of chiral compounds. In many chiral drugs, only one type of the molecule is beneficially biologically active (i.e., acts beneficially to control disease, reduce pain, etc.), whereas the other type of the drug molecule is either inactive or else causes undesired impacts (called "side effects" of the drug mixture). For example, one enantiomer of the drug thalidomide is a potent angiogenesis inhibitor, but the other enantiomer causes birth defects in babies of pregnant women taking it.

See also STEREOISOMERS, ANGIOGENESIS, OPTICAL ACTIVITY, ENANTIOMERS, *cis/trans* ISOMERISM

Chitin A water-insoluble polysaccharide polymer composed of *N*-acetyl-D-glucosamine molecular units, which forms the exoskeletons of arthropods (insects) and crustacea. Shellac is produced from chitin.

See also POLYSACCHARIDES, POLYMER, CHITINASE

Chitinase An enzyme that degrades (breaks down) chitin. It is one of the pathogenesis-related proteins produced by certain plants as a disease-fighting response to the entry into the plant of pathogenic (i.e., disease-causing) fungi.

It (chitinase) is also sometimes produced by certain fungi and actinomycetes that destroy the eggs (i.e., chitin-containing shells) of harmful roundworms.

See also CHITIN, ENZYME, STRESS PROTEINS, PATHOGENESIS-RELATED PROTEINS, FUNGUS, AFLATOXIN

Chloroplast Transit Peptide (CTP) A transit peptide that when fused to a protein acts to transport the protein into chloroplasts in a plant. Once (both are) inside the chloroplast, the transit peptide is cleaved off the protein and that protein is then free to do the task it was designed for. For example, the CP4

EPSPS enzyme in genetically engineered glyphosate-resistant soybean (*Glycine max* (L) Merrill) plant is transported into the soybean plant's chloroplasts by the CTP known as "N-terminal petunia chloroplast transit peptide." After both reach the chloroplast, the CTP is cleaved and degraded, so the CP4 EPSPS is then free to do its task (i.e., confer resistance to glyphosate).

See also PEPTIDE, CHLOROPLASTS, GATED TRANSPORT, VESICULAR TRANSPORT, TRANSIT PEPTIDE, FUSION PROTEIN, PROTEIN, SOYBEAN PLANT, CP4 EPSPS, EPSP SYNTHASE, HERBICIDE-TOLERANT CROP

Chloroplasts Specialized chlorophyll-containing photosynthetic organelles (plastids) in eucaryotic cells (i.e., the sites in which photosynthesis takes place in plants). Because there are approximately 100 chloroplasts within each plant cell, and each chloroplast contains approximately 100 copies of the plant's DNA, it is theoretically possible to have 10,000 copies (e.g., of a gene inserted via genetic engineering) coding for a given protein.

See also EUCARYOTE, ORGANELLES, CELL, PHOTOSYNTHESIS, CHLOROPLAST TRANSIT PEPTIDE (CTP), TRANSIT PEPTIDE, DEOXYRIBONUCLEIC ACID (DNA), GENE, GENETIC ENGINEERING, CODING SEQUENCE, PROTEIN

CHO Cells Abbreviation for **Chinese hamster ovary cells**. This refers to cell lines propagated/grown in cell culture (e.g., in petri dishes) that were originally removed from a Chinese hamster. Such cell culturing of CHO cells has been done by scientists since the 1960s to study genetics, gene expression, nutrition, etc. Some pharmaceutical proteins (e.g., etanercept) and some enzymes (e.g., PARP) are produced by CHO cells via large-scale cell culture (e.g., fermentation vats, which have internal substrates for the CHO cells).

See also CELL, CELL CULTURE, MAMMALIAN CELL CULTURE, GENE, GENE EXPRESSION, FUSION PROTEIN, ETANERCEPT, SUBSTRATE (STRUCTURAL), PARP

Cholera Toxin The toxin that is produced by the *Vibrio cholerae* (Latin America) bacteria, a source of food- and waterborne gastrointestinal disease.

The cholera toxin has a strong affinity for certain receptors that are present on the surface of gastrointestinal cells.

See also TOXIN, ENTEROTOXIN, CONJUGATE, IMMUNOCONJUGATE, RECEPTORS, G-PROTEINS

Cholesterol From the Greek word *chole* (bile); it is a sterol (sterol-lipid) that is an essential material for the creation of cell membranes and a "building block" for certain hormones (progesterone, estrogens, etc.) and acids used by the body. For example, the bile acids are made in the liver from cholesterol.

Cholesterol is also vital for normal embryonic development (e.g., of humans in the uterus) because it includes a crucial portion of the "hedgehog proteins" that direct tissue differentiation (of the mammal embryo into various organs, limbs, etc.).

However, deposition of (excess) oxidized cholesterol on the interior walls of blood vessels (in the form of plaque) can result in atherosclerosis and coronary heart disease (CHD), two often-fatal diseases.

See also HIGH-DENSITY LIPOPROTEINS (HDLPS), LOW-DENSITY LIPOPROTEINS (LDLP), CELL, STEROLS, PHYTOSTEROLS, HORMONE, SITOSTANOL, FRUCTOSE OLIGOSACCHARIDES, CHOLESTEROL OXIDASE, CORONARY HEART DISEASE (CHD), HIGH-OLEIC OIL SOYBEANS, STEROID, LIPIDS, HEDGEHOG PROTEINS, CAMPESTEROL, STIGMASTEROL, SITOSTEROL, SITOSTANOL, RESVERATROL, BILE ACIDS, ATHEROSCLEROSIS, PLAQUE, CYP46, APOE4, ALZHEIMER'S DISEASE

Cholesterol Oxidase An enzyme that catalyzes the breakdown of cholesterol molecules (causing oxygen consumption in the breakdown process). Because cholesterol molecules are essential for creation and maintenance of cell membranes and some hormones, an excess of cholesterol oxidase can be harmful (e.g., to certain insects).

When the gene (that codes) for cholesterol oxidase is inserted into the genome of the corn (maize) plant, it can enable that plant to resist many of the worm pests (e.g., corn earworm, European corn borer, corn rootworm, black cutworm, armyworm) that attack corn (maize) in the field.

When the gene (that codes) for cholesterol oxidase is inserted into the cotton plant, it can enable the plant to resist weevils and other sucking insects that attack cotton plants in the field.

See also ENZYME, GENE, GENETIC ENGINEERING, GENOME, CORN, CHOLESTEROL, *HELICOVERPA ZEA (H. ZEA)*, CORN ROOTWORM

Choline Formerly known as vitamin B_4, choline is an essential nutrient that takes part in many of the metabolism processes in the human body. Naturally present in egg yolks, organ meats, dairy products, soybean lecithin, spinach, and nuts, choline

- Is a major component of cell membranes
- Is required by the body to make phospholipids
- Promotes fat metabolism in the liver
- Is used by the liver to make certain choline-based compounds (necessary for the transport of fat from the liver to the rest of the body) and to synthesize high-density lipoproteins (i.e., HDLP, also known as "good" cholesterol

It is also utilized by the body in order to synthesize (i.e., "manufacture") acetylcholine, which is an important neurotransmitter (substance that transmits nerve impulses).

Because significant choline deficiency can cause liver carcinogenesis, cirrhosis, coronary heart disease, hypertension, and can also impair cell signaling, the U.S. government has defined choline to be an essential nutrient, and has formally established an **adequate intake (AI)** level per day for choline (550 mg/d for men and 425 mg/d for women, per NAS — 1998). In 1998, the U.S. Food and Drug Administration (FDA) authorized a formal **"nutrient content" claim (on labels)** for food products and dietary supplements containing appropriate amounts of choline (e.g., those containing soybean lecithin).

One active metabolite of choline is platelet activating factor (PAF), which is involved in the body's hormonal and reproductive functions. Choline is so important in proper infant development/growth that it is included in manufactured infant formula at the rate of at least 7 mg per 100 kcal.

See also LECITHIN, METABOLISM, METABOLITE, HIGH-DENSITY LIPOPROTEINS (HDLPS), ESSENTIAL NUTRIENTS, CELL, PLASMA MEMBRANE, PHOSPHOLIPIDS, HORMONE, SOYBEAN OIL, VITAMIN, ACETYLCHOLINE, CHOLINESTERASE, NEUROTRANSMITTER, FATS, CANCER, CORONARY HEART DISEASE (CHD), SIGNALING, HOMOCYSTEINE

Cholinesterase An enzyme that catalyzes the chemical reaction in which the neurotransmitter (i.e., substance that transmits nerve impulses) molecule **acetylcholine** is synthesized (i.e., "manufactured") from Ac-CoA and choline.

See also ENZYME, NEUROTRANSMITTER, AC-CoA, CHOLINE, LECITHIN, ALZHEIMER'S DISEASE, SOLANINE, CHACONINE

Chromatids Copies of a chromosome produced by replication within a living eucaryotic cell during the prophase (i.e., the first stage of mitosis). They are compact cylinders consisting of DNA coiled around flexible rods of histone protein.

See also CHROMATIN, EUCARYOTE, MITOSIS, CHROMOSOMES, REPLICATION (OF VIRUS), HISTONES, PROTEIN

Chromatin From the Greek word *chroma* = color.

Named by Walter Flemming in 1879 owing to the fact that chromatin's bandlike structures stained darkly, chromatin is the complex of DNA and (histone) protein of which the chromosomes are composed. Consisting of fibrous swirls of unraveled DNA molecules in the nucleus of the interphase (i.e., the prolonged period of cell growth between cell division phases) eucaryote cell, chromatin DNA gradually coils itself around flexible rods of histone protein during the prophase (i.e., the first stage of mitosis), forming two parallel compact cylinders (called chromatids) connected by a knotlike structure (called a centromere) at the middle. In appearance they are similar to two rolls of carpeting standing side by side that are tied together with rope at the middle. These (recently replicated) cylinders (that are joined at the middle) are homologous chromosomes (i.e., the genes of the two chromosomes are linked in the same linear order within the DNA strands of both chromosomes). While they are still joined at the middle, these paired chromosomes appear x-shaped when photographed by a karyotyper to produce a karyotype.

Chromatin is usually not visible during the interphase of a cell, but can be made more visible during all phases by reaction with basic stains (dyes) specific for DNA.

Chromatin modification is a term that refers to any (epigenetic) change in a cell's chromatin that impacts how (or if) a given gene is expressed.

See also CELL, BASOPHILIC, DEOXYRIBONUCLEIC ACID (DNA), PROTEIN, HISTONES, CHROMATIDS, CHROMOSOMES, MITOSIS, REPLICATION (OF VIRUS), CENTROMERE, KARYOTYPE, EUCARYOTE, KARYOTYPER, EPIGENETIC, EXPRESS, CHROMATIN REMODELING, CHROMATIN REMODELING ELEMENTS, SHORT INTERFERING RNA (siRNA)

Chromatin Modification See CHROMATIN

Chromatin Remodeling Refers to a reshaping (at molecular scale) of chromatin (i.e., organism's complex of DNA and histone protein) that **alters which specific genes in that organism's DNA subsequently get expressed**. Can be caused by short interfering RNA (siRNA), certain transcription activators, acetylation of histone, methylation of histone, etc.

See also CHROMATIN, DEOXYRIBONUCLEIC ACID (DNA), GENE, GENE EXPRESSION, EPIGENETIC, GENE SPLICING, SHORT INTERFERING RNA (siRNA), TRANSCRIPTION ACTIVATORS, HISTONES, METHYLATED

Chromatin Remodeling Elements See CHROMATIN REMODELING, TRANSCRIPTION ACTIVATORS, SHORT INTERFERING RNA (siRNA)

Chromatography Coined by Mikhail S. Tswett in 1906, this word refers to a process by which complex mixtures of different molecules may be separated from each other. This is accomplished by subjecting the mixture to many repeated partitionings between a flowing phase and a stationary phase. Chromatography constitutes one of the most, if not *the* most, fundamental separation techniques used in the biochemistry/biotechnology arena to date.

See also POLYACRYLAMIDE GEL ELECTROPHORESIS (PAGE), SUBSTRATE (IN CHROMATOGRAPHY), AFFINITY CHROMATOGRAPHY, BIOTECHNOLOGY, AGAROSE, GEL FILTRATION

Chromosomal Packing Unit See NUCLEOSOME

Chromosomal Translocation See JUMPING GENES

Chromosome Map See LINKAGE MAP

Chromosome Painting See FLUORESCENCE *IN SITU* HYBRIDIZATION (FISH)

Chromosome Walking A methodology for determining the location of, and sequencing, **a given gene** (within an organism's DNA) by sequencing (specific DNA sequences that overlap and span collectively) that gene's location within the organism's DNA.

See also GENE, DEOXYRIBONUCLEIC ACID (DNA), SEQUENCE (OF A DNA MOLECULE), ORGANISM, CHROMOSOMES

Chromosomes Discrete units of the genome carrying many genes, consisting of (histone) proteins and a very long molecule of DNA. Found in the nucleus of every plant and animal cell.

See also GENOME, GENE, GENETIC CODE, CHROMATIN, CHROMATIDS, KARYOTYPE, KARYOTYPER, PHILADELPHIA CHROMOSOME

Chronic Heart Disease See CORONARY HEART DISEASE (CHD)

Chymosin Also known as rennin. It is an enzyme used to make cheeses (from milk). Chymosin occurs naturally in the stomachs of calves and is one of the oldest commercially used enzymes. Chymosin (rennin) is chemically similar to renin, an enzyme that plays an important role in regulating blood pressure in humans.

See also RENIN

Cilia Protein-based structures that occur in certain cells of both the plant and animal world. Cilia are very tiny hairlike structures and occur in large numbers on the outside of certain cells. In higher organisms such as humans, they usually function to move extracellular material along the cell surface. An example is the "sweeping-out-of-foreign matter" action of cilia in the bronchial tubes in which very small particles are moved into the throat to be expelled or swallowed. Lower organisms may use cilia for locomotion (swimming). Cilia are used in the swimming motion of bacteria toward sources of nutrients in a process called chemotaxis. Cilia are shorter and occur in larger numbers per cell than flagella. Singular: cilium.

See also CHEMOTAXIS, MICROTUBULES, FLAGELLA

Ciliary Neurotrophic Factor (CNTF) A human protein that has been shown to help the survival of those cells in the nervous system that act to convey sensation and control the function of muscles and organs. CNTF was approved by the U.S. FDA to treat amyotrophic lateral sclerosis (also known as Lou Gehrig's disease) in 1992. Amyotrophic lateral sclerosis causes a victim's muscles to degenerate severely, and it affects approximately 30,000 people per year in the U.S. CNTF *might* prove useful for treating Alzheimer's disease and other human neurological diseases.

See also PROTEIN, CELL, NERVE GROWTH FACTOR (NGF), FOOD AND DRUG ADMINISTRATION (FDA)

cis-**Acting Protein** A *cis*-acting protein has the exceptional property of acting only on the molecule of DNA from which it was expressed.

See also *trans*-ACTING PROTEIN, DEOXYRIBONUCLEIC ACID (DNA)

Cisplatin A drug that is used in chemotherapy regimens against certain types of cancer tumors. Cisplatin works against (tumor) cells by binding to the cell's DNA and generating intrastrand cross-links (between the two strands of the DNA molecule). These intrastrand cross-links prevent replication and cause cell death.

See also CHEMOPHARMACOLOGY, CHE-MOTHERAPY, CANCER, DEOXYRIBO-NUCLEIC ACID (DNA), REPLICATION FORK, REPLICATION (OF DNA)

cis/trans Isomerism A type of geometrical isomerism found in alkenic systems in which it is possible for each of the doubly bonded carbons in a molecule to carry two different atoms or groups. Two similar atoms or groups may be on the same side (i.e., *cis*) or on opposite sides (i.e., *trans*) of a plane bisecting the alkenic molecule's carbons and perpendicular to the plane of the alkenic systems.

See also ISOMER, CHIRAL COMPOUND, *TRANS* FATTY ACIDS

cis/trans Test Assays (determines) the effect of relative configuration on expression of two (gene) mutations. In a double heterozygote, two mutations in the same gene show mutant phenotype in *trans* configuration, wild (phenotype) in *cis* configuration. The phenotypic distinction is referred to as the position effect.

See also GENE, PHENOTYPE, *cis*-ACTING PROTEIN, POSITION EFFECT, HETEROZYGOTE, MUTATION

Cistron Synonymous with **gene**, it refers to a specific DNA sequence that codes for the synthesis (by ribosome) of a single protein (polypeptide molecular chain).

See also GENE, DEOXYRIBONUCLEIC ACID (DNA), PROTEIN, RIBOSOME

Citrate Synthase The enzyme that is utilized (e.g., by plants) to synthesize (i.e., create) citric acid.

See also ENZYME, CITRIC ACID

Citrate Synthase (CSb) Gene A bacterial gene that is utilized by certain bacteria (e.g., *Pseudomonas*) to code for (i.e., cause to be produced by the bacterium possessing that gene) the enzyme known as citrate synthase, which is utilized to synthesize (i.e., create) citric acid. In 1996, Luis Herrera-Estrella discovered that inserting the CSb gene from *Pseudomonas aeruginosa* into certain plants caused them to produce up to ten times more citrate in their roots, and to release up to four times more citric acid from those roots into the surrounding soil (thus decreasing aluminum toxicity via chemically "binding" aluminum ions that are present in some soils). Such soil aluminum, which slows plant growth and

decreases crop yields, is present to a certain degree in approximately one third of Earth's arable land (e.g., in Colombia, it affects 70% of the arable land).

See also GENE, ENZYME, EXPRESS, CITRATE SYNTHASE, ION, CITRIC ACID

Citric Acid A tricarboxylic acid occurring naturally in plants, especially citrus fruits. It is used as a flavoring agent, as an antioxidant in foods, as an animal feed ingredient, and as a sequestering agent. The commercially produced form of citric acid melts at 153°C (307°F). Citric acid is found in all cells, and its central role is in the metabolic process. Some plants naturally release citric acid from their roots into the surrounding soil, in order for that citric acid to chemically "bind" aluminum ions that are present in some soils. Such aluminum, which slows plant growth and decreases crop yields, is present to a certain degree (which causes at least some crop yield reduction) in approximately one third of the world's arable land. For example, 70% of the agricultural land in Colombia possesses harmful amounts and conditions of aluminum likely to damage crops. Corn (maize) yields are reduced up to 80% by such aluminum in soils. Soybeans, cotton, and field bean yields are also reduced.

See also METABOLISM, ACID, CELL, CITRATE SYNTHASE, CITRATE SYNTHASE GENE, CITRATE SYNTHASE (Csb) GENE, CITRIC ACID CYCLE, METABOLITE, CELL, ION, SOYBEAN PLANT, CORN, PROBIOTICS

Citric Acid Cycle Also known as the tricarboxylic acid cycle (TCA cycle, because the citric acid molecule contains three [tri] carboxyl [acid] groups). Also known as the Kreb's cycle after H. A. Krebs, who first postulated the existence of the cycle in 1937 under its original name of "citric acid cycle." A cyclic sequence of chemical reactions that occurs in almost all aerobic (air-requiring) organisms. A system of enzymatic reactions in which acetyl residues are oxidized to carbon dioxide and hydrogen atoms and in which formation of citrate is the first step.

See also CITRIC ACID, CITRATE SYNTHASE, CITRATE SYNTHASE GENE, CITRATE SYNTHASE (Csb) GENE, ACID,

C

AEROBIC, METABOLISM, ENZYME, OXIDATION

CKR-5 Proteins See HUMAN IMMUNO-DEFICIENCY VIRUS TYPE 1 (HIV-1), HUMAN IMMUNODEFICIENCY VIRUS TYPE 2 (HIV-2), RECEPTORS, PROTEIN

CLA Abbreviation for **conjugated linoleic acid.**

See CONJUGATED LINOLEIC ACID (CLA)

Clades The taxonomic subgroups within cladistics.

See also CLADISTICS

Cladistics Initially popularized by Willi Hennig's 1950 book entitled *Phylogenetic Systematics*, cladistics is a system of taxonomic classification of organisms (and/or their specimens) that is based on (determined by) similar lines of selected shared traits.

See also CLADES, TYPE SPECIMEN, GENETICS, BIOLOGY, SPECIES, SYSTEMATICS, AMERICAN TYPE CULTURE COLLECTION (ATCC), TRAIT

CLIA Acronym for **chemiluminescent immunoassay.**

See CHEMILUMINESCENT ASSAY (CLIA)

Clinical Trial One of the final stages in the collection of data (for drug approval prior to commercialization) in which the new drug is tested in human subjects. Used to collect data on effectiveness, safety, and required dosage.

See also PHASE I CLINICAL TESTING, FOOD AND DRUG ADMINISTRATION (FDA), KOSEISHO, BUNDESGESUND-HEITSAMT (BGA), COMMITTEE ON SAFETY IN MEDICINES, COMMITTEE FOR PROPRIETARY MEDICINAL PRODUCTS (CPMP)

Clone (a molecule) To create copies of a given molecule by various methods.

See also POLYMERASE CHAIN REACTION (PCR), MONOCLONAL ANTIBODIES (MAb), COCLONING, ANTIBODY, cDNA CLONE

Clone (an organism) A group of individual organisms (or cells) produced from one individual cell through asexual processes that do not involve the interchange or combination of genetic material. As a result, members of a clone have identical genetic compositions. For example, many plants reproduce asexually (i.e., without sex) via a process known as apomixis.

Protozoa, bacteria, and some animals (e.g., the anemone *Anthopleura elegantissima*) can reproduce asexually (i.e., without sex) by a process called binary fission. In binary fission, a single-celled organism undergoes cell division. The result is two cells with identical genetic composition. When these two identical cells undergo division, the result is four cells with identical genetic composition. These identical offspring are all members of a clone. The word "clone" may be used either as a noun or a verb. Scientists have cloned some adult mammals via nuclear transfer in which the nucleus of an oocyte is removed and replaced with a nucleus taken out of another conventional somatic (adult's body) cell. That oocyte can then grow up to become a clone of the (adult) animal.

See also ORGANISM, APOMIXIS, BACTERIA, CELL, OOCYTES, SOMATIC CELLS

Clostridium A genus of bacteria. Most are obligate anaerobes and form endospores.

See also ANAEROBE, ENDOSPORE

CML Abbreviation for **chronic myelogenous leukemia** (also known as **chronic myeloid leukemia** or **chronic myelocytic leukemia**).

See GLEEVEC™

CMV See CYTOMEGALOVIRUS

CNTF See CILIARY NEUROTROPHIC FACTOR (CNTF)

CNTs Acronym for **carbon nanotubes**.

See CARBON NANOTUBES

Co-Chaperonin A protein molecule inside living cells that "works together" with applicable chaperonins to help ensure proper folding of the (new) protein molecules that are synthesized ("manufactured") in the cell's ribosomes.

See also CHAPERONINS, PROTEIN, PROTEIN FOLDING, CELL, RIBOSOMES, CONFORMATION

Colinearity Refers to when the DNA segments common to two different organisms (e.g., rice and maize/corn) are present in the same linear order within their respective DNA molecules (i.e., when one overlooks other **inserted or deleted segments**. Sometimes called **indels**).

See also DEOXYRIBONUCLEIC ACID (DNA), SEQUENCE (OF A DNA MOLECULE), ORGANISM, CORN, GENE

CoA See COENZYME A

Coccus A spherical bacterium.

See also *BACILLUS*

Cocloning (of molecules) The additional (accidental) cloning (i.e., copying) of extra molecular fragments, other than the desired one, that sometimes occurs when a scientist is attempting to clone a molecule.

See also CLONE (A MOLECULE), POLYMERASE CHAIN REACTION (PCR), Q-BETA REPLICASE TECHNIQUE

Codex Alimentarius See CODEX ALIMENTARIUS COMMISSION

Codex Alimentarius Commission An international regulatory body that is part of the United Nations' Food and Agriculture Organization (FAO). It is one of the three international SPS (sanitary and phytosanitary) standard-setting organizations that is recognized by the World Trade Organization (WTO). It was created in 1962 by the UN's FAO and the World Health Organization (WHO) and has 165 member nations.

In Latin, *Codex Alimentarius* means "food law" or "food code." The Codex Alimentarius Commission is responsible for execution of the Joint FAO/WHO Food Standards Program. The Codex Alimentarius standards are a set of international food mandates that have been adopted by the Commission. The Commission is composed of delegates from member country governmental agencies. The Codex Secretariat is headquartered in Rome, Italy.

The Commission periodically determines and then publishes a list of food ingredients and maximum allowable levels that it deems safe for human consumption (known as the *Codex Alimentarius*).

See also MAXIMUM RESIDUE LEVEL (MRL), SPS, INTERNATIONAL PLANT PROTECTION CONVENTION (IPPC), INTERNATIONAL OFFICE OF EPIZOOTICS (OIE), WORLD TRADE ORGANIZATION (WTO)

Coding Region See CODING SEQUENCE

Coding Sequence The region within a DNA molecule (i.e., between the start and stop codons) that encodes the amino acid sequence of a protein.

See also GENETIC CODE, INFORMATIONAL MOLECULES, GENE, MESSENGER RNA (mRNA), BASE (NUCLEOTIDE), CONTROL SEQUENCES, CODON

Codon A triplet of nucleotides (three nucleic acid units [residues] in a row) within messenger RNA (mRNA) that code for an amino acid (triplet code) or a termination signal.

See also GENETIC CODE, TERMINATION CODON (SEQUENCE), AMINO ACID, NUCLEOTIDE, INFORMATIONAL MOLECULES, MESSENGER RNA (mRNA), LEADER SEQUENCE (mRNA)

Coenzyme A nonproteinaceous organic molecule required for the action of certain enzymes. The coenzyme contains as part of its structure one of the vitamins. This is why vitamins are so critically important to living organisms. Sometimes, the same coenzyme is required by different enzymes that are involved in the catalysis of different reactions. By analogy, a coenzyme is like a part of a car such as a tire that can be identified in and of itself and which can, furthermore, be removed from the car. The car (enzyme), however, must of necessity have the tire in order to carry out its prescribed function. Coenzymes have been classified into two large groups: fat soluble and water soluble. Examples of a few water-soluble vitamins are: thiamin, biotin, folic acid, vitamin C, and vitamin B_{12}. Examples of fat-soluble vitamins are: vitamins A, D, E, and K.

See also ENZYME, CATALYST, HOLOENZYME, VITAMIN, POLYPEPTIDE (PROTEIN), BIOTIN

Coenzyme A A water-soluble vitamin known as pantothenic acid. A coenzyme in all living cells. It is required by certain condensing enzymes and functions in acyl-group transfer and in fatty-acid metabolism. Abbreviated CoA.

See also ENZYME, FATS, FATTY ACID

Coenzyme Q10 A name sometimes utilized for ubiquinone as dietary ingredient.

See also UBIQUINONE

Cofactor A nonprotein component required by some enzymes for activity. The cofactor may be a metal ion or an organic molecule called a coenzyme. The term "cofactor" is a general term. Cofactors are generally heat stable.

See also COENZYME, HOLOENZYME, MOLECULAR WEIGHT

Cofactor Recycle The regeneration of spent cofactor by an auxiliary reaction such that it may be reused many times over by a cofactor-requiring enzyme during a reaction.

See also COFACTOR, HOLOENZYME, ENZYME

Coffee Berry Borer Refers to the pest insect *Hypothenemus hampei*, which attacks berries of the coffee tree (*Coffea arabica*).

See also AMYLASE INHIBITORS

Cohesive Ends See STICKY ENDS

Cohesive Termini See STICKY ENDS

Colchicine Discovered in 1937, it is a chemical (alkaloid) that can be extracted from certain members of the lily family of plants (e.g., *Colchicum autumnale*, autumn crocus, or meadow saffron). It has sometimes been used as an anti-inflammatory agent to treat gout in humans. Colchicine has also been used by some plant breeders to induce mutations in crop plants (e.g., by soaking seeds in it) in order to create crop plant varieties with new traits. This happens because colchicine prevents chromosomes from separating during the anaphase of mitosis, thereby causing the cell to become tetraploid (i.e., four copies of each chromosome).

See also ALKALOIDS, MUTATION BREEDING, TRADITIONAL BREEDING METHODS, TRAIT, CHROMOSOMES, MITOSIS, TETRAPLOID

Cold Acclimation See COLD HARDENING

Cold Acclimatization See COLD HARDENING

Cold Hardening A process of acclimatization in which certain organisms produce specific proteins that protect them from freezing to death during the winter. Among other organisms, the common housefly, the *Arabidopsis thaliana* plant, the fruit fly *Drosophila*, and "no-see-em's" (i.e., *Culicoides variipennis*) can produce these proteins (e.g., during the gradually decreasing temperatures of a typical autumn season in North America). The amount of such proteins produced within their bodies is proportional to the severity and duration of the cold experienced.

For example, prior to cold hardening, *Culicoides variipennis* insects usually die after exposure for 2 h to a temperature of 14°F (10°C). If those insects are first exposed for 1 h to a temperature of 41°F (5°C), approximately 98% of them can then survive exposure for 3 d to a temperature of 14°F (10°C).

In certain plants, such exposure to cold causes oxidative stress, which then can initiate the activation of the mitogen-activated protein kinase (MAPK) cascade, resulting in production of several **stress responsive proteins** (e.g., heat-shock proteins). These "stress proteins" help protect such plants from cold temperatures.

See also ACCLIMATIZATION, PROTEIN, LOW-TILLAGE CROP PRODUCTION, NO-TILLAGE CROP PRODUCTION, DROSOPHILA, *ARABIDOPSIS THALIANA*, CBF1, TRANSCRIPTION FACTORS, LINOLEIC ACID, MITOGEN-ACTIVATED PROTEIN KINASE CASCADE, OXIDATIVE STRESS, STRESS PROTEINS

Cold Tolerance See COLD HARDENING

Cold-Shock Protein Refers to particular protein molecules that are expressed by cells in an organism exposed to low environmental temperatures to protect living cells (from freeze damage). For example, at low temperatures, *Escherichia coli* bacteria sometimes express spA, a cold-shock protein that protects them from (some) freeze damage.

See also COLD HARDENING, PROTEIN, ORGANISM, BACTERIA

Colicins Proteins produced by *Escherichia coli* (*E. coli*), which are toxic (primarily) to other closely related strains of bacteria. The particular *E. coli* bacteria that produce a given colicin are generally unaffected by the colicin that they produce.

See also BACTERIOCINS, BACTERIOLOGY, STRAIN, BACTERIA, PROTEIN, TOXIN, *ESCHERICHIA COLIFORM (E. COLI)*

Collagen The major structural protein in connective tissue. It is instrumental in wound healing (stimulated by fibroblast growth factor [FGF], platelet-derived growth factor, and insulin-like growth factor-1).

See also PROTEIN, FIBROBLAST GROWTH FACTOR (FGF), PLATELET-DERIVED GROWTH FACTOR (PDGF), INSULIN-LIKE GROWTH FACTOR-1 (IGF-1)

Collagenase An enzyme that catalyzes the cleavage of collagen. One example of this is when bacteria in the mouth cause production of collagenase that then cleaves (i.e., breaks down) the collagen that holds teeth in place. Some cancers use collagenase to break down connective tissues in the body they inhabit, enabling the cancers to form the (new) blood vessels that nourish those cancers and help them spread through the body. Collagenase may also be responsible indirectly for certain autoimmune diseases such as arthritis by breaking down the protective proteoglycan coat that covers cartilage in the body.

See also STROMELYSIN (MMP-3), PROTEOLYTIC ENZYMES, ENZYME, COLLAGEN, CANCER, AUTOIMMUNE DISEASE

Colony A growth of a group of microorganisms derived from one original organism. After a sufficient growth period, the growth is visible to the eye without magnification.

Colony Hybridization A technique using *in situ* hybridization to identify bacterial colonies carrying inserted DNA that is homologous with some particular sequence (probe).

See also DNA PROBE, HOMOLOGY, *IN SITU*, REGULATORY SEQUENCE

Colony-Stimulating Factors (CSFs) Specific glycoprotein growth factors required for the proliferation and differentiation of hematopoietic progenitor cells. Different CSFs stimulate the growth of different cells.

See also MACROPHAGE COLONY-STIMULATING FACTOR (M-CSF), GRANULOCYTE COLONY-STIMULATING FACTOR (G-CSF), GRANULOCYTE-MACROPHAGE COLONY-STIMULATING FACTOR (GM-CSF), EPIDERMAL GROWTH FACTOR (EGF), FIBROBLAST GROWTH FACTOR (FGF), HEMATOLOGIC GROWTH FACTORS (HGF), INSULIN-LIKE GROWTH FACTOR-1 (IGF-1), MEGAKARYOCYTE-STIMULATING FACTOR (MSF), NERVE GROWTH FACTOR (NGF), PLATELET-DERIVED GROWTH FACTOR (PDGF), TRANSFORMING GROWTH FACTOR-ALPHA (TGF-ALPHA), TRANSFORMING GROWTH FACTOR-BETA (TGF-BETA)

Combinatorial Biology A term used to describe the set of DNA technologies that are utilized to generate a large number of samples of new chemicals (metabolites) via creation of nonnatural metabolic pathways. The collection of samples thus generated is called a "library," and the samples are then tested for potential use (e.g., for therapeutic effect in the case of a pharmaceutical). These technologies enable greater efficiency in a pharmaceutical researcher's screening process for drug discovery.

See also COMBINATORIAL CHEMISTRY, TARGET, MOLECULAR DIVERSITY, METABOLISM, INTERMEDIARY METABOLISM, METABOLITE, RECEPTORS

Combinatorial Chemistry A term used to describe the set of technologies that are utilized to generate a large number of samples of (new) chemicals, which are then tested (screened) for potential use (e.g., for therapeutic effect in the case of a pharmaceutical). These large numbers of chemical samples thus generated are called a "library" and are screened (e.g., for therapeutic effect) via a variety of laboratory, biosensor, computational, receptor, or animal tests.

Combinatorial chemistry was made feasible by the fact that, during the 1980s, H. Mario Geysen developed a methodology to synthesize arrays of peptides on pin-shaped solid supports. In addition, Richard A. Houghten developed a technique for creation of peptide libraries in small mesh "bags" by solid-phase parallel synthesis, thereby enabling automation of the process (in the early 1990s). For a library used for new-drug (candidate) screening, high diversity in molecular structure among the chemicals (in the library) is desired in order to increase the efficiency of the screening process. One method used to measure diversity of the molecular structure among samples in a library is called "molecular fingerprinting." If two samples are identical in molecular structure, the "fingerprint" coefficient is 1.0. If two samples are totally dissimilar in molecular structure, the coefficient is 0. The diversity of a library is measured by comparing each sample's molecular structure to that of all the others in the library.

See also COMBINATORIAL BIOLOGY, TARGET, MOLECULAR DIVERSITY, RECEPTORS, BIOSENSORS (ELECTRONIC), PEPTIDE, SYNTHESIZING (OF PROTEINS), BIOCHIPS, HIGH-THROUGHPUT SCREENING, TARGET–LIGAND INTERACTION SCREENING

Combinatorics See COMBINATORIAL CHEMISTRY

Combining Site The site on an antibody molecule that locks (binds) onto an epitope (hapten).

See also ANTIBODY, EPITOPE, ENGINEERED ANTIBODIES, NANOBODIES, HAPTEN, CATALYTIC ANTIBODY

Commensal A term that literally means "**eating at the same table.**" It is used to refer to organisms such as the house mouse (*Mus musculus*), etc., that tend to thrive alongside or among humans.

For example, the numerous strains of salmonella bacteria can live within the intestine of an adult cow without harming it, but would be pathogenic (i.e., disease-causing) in a human's intestine. Another example is that the *E. coli 0157:H7* strain of *Escherichia coliform* bacteria can live within the digestive system of an adult cow without harming it, but would be pathogenic (i.e., disease-causing) in a human's digestive system. However, hundreds of **other** strains of *Escherichia coliform* bacteria live within the digestive system of humans without causing harm.

See also ORGANISM, MICROORGANISM, BACTERIA, *SALMONELLA TYPHIMURIUM*, *SALMONELLA ENTERITIDIS*, PATHOGEN, PATHOGENIC, STRAIN, *ESCHERICHIA COLIFORM (E. COLI)*, *ESCHERICHIA COLIFORM 0157:H7*

Commission E Monographs Documents published by the government of Germany that detail the proven safety and efficacy of certain phytochemical-containing herbs (approved by the German government). For example, consumption of **St. John's Wort** (a plant native to Europe) is approved in Germany for treatment of depressive mood disorders, anxiety, and nervous unrest.

See also PHYTOCHEMICALS

Commission of Biomolecular Engineering An agency of the French government established to oversee and regulate all genetic engineering activities in the country of France.

See also GENETIC ENGINEERING, IOGTR, RECOMBINANT DNA ADVISORY COMMITTEE (RAC), ZKBS (CENTRAL COMMITTEE ON BIOLOGICAL SAFETY), INDIAN DEPARTMENT OF BIOTECHNOLOGY, GENE TECHNOLOGY REGULATOR (GTR), GENE TECHNOLOGY OFFICE

Committee for Proprietary Medicinal Products (CPMP) The European Union's (EU's) scientific advisory organization dealing with new human pharmaceuticals' approval. Its recommendations (e.g., to either approve or not approve a new product) are usually adopted by the European Medicines Evaluation Agency (EMEA), to which the CPMP reports.

Within 60 d of a CPMP "approval for recommendation" being adopted by the EMEA, each of the EU's member countries must advise the EMEA of its progress toward a regulatory decision on that pharmaceutical's submission for approvals.

See also FOOD AND DRUG ADMINISTRATION (FDA), KOSEISHO, EUROPEAN MEDICINES EVALUATION AGENCY (EMEA), COMMITTEE ON SAFETY IN MEDICINES, BUNDESGESUNDHEITSAMT (BGA)

Committee for Veterinary Medicinal Products (CVMP) The European Union's (EU's) scientific advisory organization dealing with approvals of new medicinal products' intended use in animals. Its recommendations (e.g., to either approve or not approve a new product) are usually adopted by the European Medicines Evaluation Agency (EMEA).

See also COMMITTEE FOR PROPRIETARY MEDICINAL PRODUCTS (CPMP), FOOD AND DRUG ADMINISTRATION (FDA), KOSEISHO, COMMITTEE ON SAFETY IN MEDICINES, MEDICINES CONTROL AGENCY (MCA), EMEA, BUNDESGESUNDHEITSAMT (BGA)

Committee on Safety in Medicines The British government agency that must approve new pharmaceutical products for sale within the U.K. In concert with the

Medicines Control Agency (MCA), it regulates all pharmaceutical products in the U.K. It is the equivalent of the U.S. Food and Drug Administration.

See also FOOD AND DRUG ADMINISTRATION (FDA), MEDICINES CONTROL AGENCY (MCA), COMMITTEE FOR PROPRIETARY MEDICINAL PRODUCTS (CPMP), KOSEISHO, NDA (TO KOSEISHO), IND, BUNDESGESUNDHEITSAMT (BGA), EMEA

Community Plant Variety Office An agency of the European Union that was established by Council Regulation 2100/94, located in Angers, France. It applies UPOV rules across all countries of the European Union when a plant breeder registers a new plant variety at the Community Plant Variety Office. Thus, it confers and protects PLANT BREEDER'S RIGHTS (PBR) across the entire European Union analogous to the way the European Patent Office (EPO) confers patent rights (for patented inventions) across the entire European Union.

See also UNION FOR PROTECTION OF NEW VARIETIES OF PLANTS (UPOV), PLANT BREEDER'S RIGHTS (PBR), EUROPEAN PATENT OFFICE (EPO), PLANT VARIETY PROTECTION ACT (PVP)

Comparative Analysis See HOMOLOGOUS (CHROMOSOMES OR GENES)

Competence Factor See PLATELET-DERIVED GROWTH FACTOR (PDGF)

Complement (Component of Immune System) A group of more than 15 soluble proteins found in blood serum that interacts in a sequential fashion, in which a precursor molecule is converted into an active enzyme. Each enzyme uses the following molecule in the system as a substrate and converts it into its active (enzyme) form. This cascade of events and reactions leads ultimately to the formation of an attack complex that forms a transmembrane channel in the cell membrane (e.g., of a pathogen). It is the presence of the channel that leads to lysis (rupturing) of the cell.

See also PLASMA MEMBRANE, CELL, PATHOGEN, CASCADE, COMPLEMENT CASCADE, COMPLEMENT FACTOR H GENE, CECROPHINS, HUMORAL IMMUNITY, LYSE, LYSIS

Complement Cascade The precisely regulated, sequential interaction of proteins (in the blood) that is triggered by a complex of antibody and antigen to cause lysis of infected cells. The triggering of lysis by multivalent antibody–antigen complexes is mediated by the classical pathway, beginning with the activation of C1, the first component (protein) of the pathway. This activation step, in which C1 undergoes conversion from a zymogen to an active protease, results in sequential cleavage of the C4, C2, C3, and C5 components (proteins). C5b, a fragment of C5, then joins C6, C7, and C8 to penetrate the (cell) membrane bearing the antigen. Finally, the binding of some 16 molecules of C9 to this "bridgehead" produces large pores in the (cell) membrane, which cause the lysis and destruction of the target cell.

See also ANTIBODY, ANTIGEN, LYSIS, CELL, PLASMA MEMBRANE, COMPLEMENT, COMPLEMENT FACTOR H GENE, ZYMOGENS, CECROPHINS, CASCADE, PATHWAY

Complement Factor H Gene A gene that codes for production of complement factor H, a protein also known as **CFH protein**, which helps regulate the complement cascade of the human immune system. For example, CFH protein can bind (inflammation-) initiation factors such as C-reactive protein and can inactivate certain components of the complement cascade. Certain variants (alleles) of this gene in humans increase the probability of that person developing age-related macular degeneration (AMD) disease.

See also GENE, PROTEIN, CODING SEQUENCE, ALLELE, COMPLEMENT, COMPLEMENT CASCADE, INITIATION FACTORS, C-REACTIVE PROTEIN (CRP)

Complementary (Molecular Genetics) Refers to strands of DNA that will hybridize ("bind") to each other owing to one-to-one matchup of each strand's sequence of nucleotides. Any sequence (within the two strands) that does **not** match up one-to-one will not hybridize to the respective sequence (in adjacent strand).

See also MOLECULAR GENETICS, HYBRIDIZATION (MOLECULAR GENETICS), DEOXYRIBONUCLEIC ACID (DNA), DOUBLE HELIX, NUCLEOTIDE, MICROARRAY (TESTING), BIOMOTORS, SOUTHERN BLOT ANALYSIS

Complementary DNA (cDNA) A single-stranded DNA that is complementary to a strand of mRNA. The DNA is synthesized *in vitro* by an enzyme known as reverse transcriptase. Then, a second DNA strand is synthesized via the enzyme known as **DNA polymerase**. Complementary DNA is often utilized in hybridization studies and in microarrays (e.g., to detect or identify genes) because cDNAs usually do not contain **regulatory sequences** of DNA as the cDNA was copied from mRNA. cDNA is a DNA copy of mRNA (messenger RNA) and this "rebukes" the (old) Central Dogma.

See also DEOXYRIBONUCLEIC ACID (DNA), MESSENGER RNA (mRNA), CENTRAL DOGMA (OLD), ENZYME, DNA POLYMERASE, HYBRIDIZATION (MOLECULAR GENETICS), MICROARRAY (TESTING), GENE EXPRESSION ANALYSIS, REGULATORY SEQUENCE

Compound Q See TRICHOSANTHIN

Computational Biology See BIOINFORMATICS, *IN SILICO* BIOLOGY, RATIONAL DRUG DESIGN, DOCKING (IN COMPUTATIONAL BIOLOGY)

Computer-Assisted New Drug Application (also called computer-assisted NDA) See CANDA

Computer-Assisted Drug Design (CADD) See RATIONAL DRUG DESIGN

Con-Till An abbreviation that refers to **conservation tillage** farming practices.

See also CONSERVATION TILLAGE, LOW-TILLAGE CROP PRODUCTION, NO-TILLAGE CROP PRODUCTION, GLOMALIN

Configuration The three-dimensional arrangement in space of substituent groups in stereoisomers.

Confocal Microscopy Invented by Marvin Minsky in 1957, this refers to use of a special microscope used to scan (e.g., in tissue) **a two-dimensional plane** at varying depths. Today, this is typically done using laser beams that rapidly raster scan the sample via galvomirrors.

The resultant images can then be put together via a process known as volume rendering in order to yield a three-dimensional overall image.

Today, using visible fluorescent proteins to "label" some protein molecules of interest, it is possible to watch the movement and interactions of labeled proteins inside living cells via confocal microscopy.

Some confocal microscopes utilize FRET (fluorescence resonance energy transfer) to achieve better resolution or four-dimensional images.

See also VOLUME RENDERING, MULTIPLEX ASSAY, FLUORESCENCE, PROTEIN, LABEL (FLUORESCENT), VISIBLE FLUORESCENT PROTEINS, GREEN FLUORESCENT PROTEIN, FLUORESCENCE RESONANCE ENERGY TRANSFER (FRET)

Conformation The three-dimensional arrangement of substituent groups in a protein or other molecular structure (e.g., aptamer) that is free to assume different positions. The geometric form or shape of a protein in three-dimensional space.

See also NATIVE CONFORMATION, TERTIARY STRUCTURE, APTAMERS, EFFECTOR, PROTEIN FOLDING, PROTEOMICS, TRANSCRIPTOME, DISULFIDE BOND, STRUCTURE–ACTIVITY MODELS, RAMAN OPTICAL ACTIVITY SPECTROSCOPY

Congo Red A chemical dye that adheres to β-amyloid protein (which can lead to Alzheimer's disease when clumped together inside neurons). At high concentrations, Congo red can inhibit such clumping. Research indicates that when molecules of Congo red are chemically linked to relevant ligands for FKBP (a large cellular chaperone protein), this linked-together chemical entity "recruits" an FKBP protein molecule to insert itself between β-amyloid proteins, which could prevent clumping.

See also ALZHEIMER'S DISEASE, PROTEIN, CELL, NEURON, LIGAND (IN BIOCHEMISTRY), CHAPERONES

Conjugate A molecule created by fusing together (e.g., via recombination or chemically) two unlike (different) molecules. The purpose of this is to create a molecule in which one of the original molecules has one function, for example, a toxic, cell-killing function, whereas the other original molecule has another function, such as targeting the toxin to a specific site in the body, which might be cancerous cells.

For example, molecules of interleukin-2 (IL-2) have been fused with molecules of diphtheria toxin to create a conjugate that does the following:

- It enters leukemia and lymphoma cells. Because these two types of cancer cells possess IL-2 receptors on their surfaces, the IL-2 (targeting function) binds to that receptor and is internalized by the cell.
- The diphtheria toxin (killing function) then shuts down protein synthesis within the cancer cells.
- It then kills the cancerous cells.

This type of approach is widespread, and there are many different types of this category of conjugate. Another type of conjugate consists of enzymes used in the treatment of certain molecular diseases attached covalently to polyethylene glycol (PEG). In this case, the PEG greatly diminishes both the immunogenicity (the tendency to induce the body's immune reaction) and the antigenicity (the ability to react with preformed antibodies).

Another type of conjugate consists of various molecules (e.g., fluorophores, toxins, etc.) or nanoparticles (e.g., quantum dots) attached to antibodies. Such conjugated antibodies may be utilized as vectors to carry either small molecules of destructive toxins or imaging proteins (e.g., green fluorescent protein) or imaging particles (e.g., quantum dots) to specific sites (cells) within the body. Antibodies may be coupled to enzymes, toxins, or ribosome-inhibiting proteins as well as to radioisotopes. These conjugates are known collectively as immunoconjugates.

See also IMMUNOCONJUGATE, CONJU-GATED PROTEIN, "MAGIC BULLET,"

FUSION PROTEIN, MOLECULAR BRIDGE, RECOMBINATION, TOXIN, INTERLEUKIN-2 (IL-2), RICIN, ABRIN, RECEPTORS, RIBOSOMES, MESSENGER RNA (mRNA), DIPHTHERIA TOXIN, ANTIBODY, FLUORPOHORE, GREEN FLUORESCENT PROTEIN, QUANTUM DOT, ENZYME, NANOPARTICLES

Conjugated Linoleic Acid (CLA) Also known as alpha-rumenic acid or 9-cis, 11-trans C 18:1, it is naturally occurring n-6 polyunsaturated fatty acid (PUFA) discovered in 1979 by Michael W. Pariza. CLA consumption by humans has been linked to:

- Reduction in risk for atherosclerosis
- Reduction in blood triglyceride levels
- Reduction in body fat (adipose tissue) in obese humans
- Increase in lean body mass
- Reduction in risk for breast cancer, skin cancer, and some other types of cancer

CLA inhibits angiogenesis (i.e., formation of new blood vessels such as the ones needed for tumors to be able to grow) and exhibits powerful antioxidant properties (i.e., it "quenches" free radicals). Chemically, CLA consists of two linoleic acid molecules linked together by a chemical bond, so it is a dimer. Foods that are naturally highest in CLA content include beef, lamb, full-fat milk, butter, cheese, some creams, and full-fat yogurt. However, the natural level (3 to 7 mg per g of fat) is too small to have much beneficial impact. Feeding of soybean oil (in feed rations) to livestock has been proved to increase CLA content in the resultant meat. In 1998, T.R. Dhiman showed that feeding of soybean-oil-containing (i.e., whole) soybeans to dairy cattle also did increase the content of CLA in their milk.

Research conducted during the 1990s indicated that consumption of CLA (e.g., by humans, swine, rats, etc.) causes the bodies of those animals to change the way they utilize and store energy. Thus, the body requires less food to perform at the same level. The body also

C

tends to produce less body fat (adipose tissue) and more lean protein (e.g., muscle) tissue.

See also POLYUNSATURATED FATTY ACIDS (PUFA), FATS, LINOLEIC ACID, ATHEROSCLEROSIS, OXIDATIVE STRESS, ANTIOXIDANTS, SOYBEAN OIL, ADIPOSE, CANCER, VOLICITIN, OLIGOMER, TUMOR, ANGIOGENESIS

Conjugated Protein A protein containing a metal or an organic prosthetic group (e.g., heme group, carbohydrate, lipid group) or both. For example, a glycoprotein is a conjugated protein bearing at least one oligosaccharide group.

See also PROSTHETIC GROUP, GLYCOPROTEIN, PROTEIN, OLIGOSACCHARIDES, CONJUGATE, CD4-PE40

Conjugation A process akin to sexual reproduction occurring in bacteria; mating in bacteria. A process that involves cell-to-cell contact and the one-way transfer of DNA from the donor to the recipient. In contrast to some other DNA-transfer processes of bacteria, conjugation may involve the transfer of large portions of the genome. The discovery caused considerable controversy at the time.

See also TRANSFORMATION, BACTERIA, TRANSDUCTION (GENE), TRANSDUCTION (SIGNAL), DEOXYRIBONUCLEIC ACID (DNA), GENOME, SEXUAL CONJUGATION

Consensus Sequence The nucleotide sequence (within a DNA molecule) that gives the *most common* nucleotide at each position (along that sequence of the DNA molecule) for those instances (in certain organisms) in which a (usually small) number of variations in nucleotide sequences can occur (e.g., for a given nucleotide sequence such as a promoter sequence).

See also NUCLEOTIDE, DEOXYRIBONUCLEIC ACID (DNA), SEQUENCE (OF A DNA MOLECULE), GENETIC CODE, GENE, PROMOTER, PHARMACOGENOMICS

Conservation Tillage Refers to crop production (farming) techniques or practices such as **low-tillage crop production**, **no-tillage crop production**, etc., that avoid or minimize the disturbance of topsoil.

See also LOW-TILLAGE CROP PRODUCTION, NO-TILLAGE CROP PRODUCTION, DROUGHT TOLERANCE, GLOMALIN

Conserved A term used to describe the following:

- The number of genes that are present within the DNA of more than one species. For example, approximately 25% of the genes found within the human genome (DNA) are also found within the DNA of plants.
- A particular domain (region) of a molecule on the surface of a rapidly mutating microorganism (e.g., the influenza virus, the AIDS virus) that remains the same in all, or most, variations of that microorganism. If that *conserved* region is suitable to act as an antigen (hapten, epitope), it may be possible to create a successful vaccine against that microorganism, which would otherwise be unsuccessful because the rapid mutation would cause it (e.g., the AIDS virus) to appear to be "different" from the one (antigen) the vaccine was designed against.

See also DOMAIN (OF A PROTEIN), GP120 PROTEIN, SUPERANTIGENS, MUTATION, ACQUIRED IMMUNE DEFICIENCY SYNDROME (AIDS), ANTIGEN, HAPTEN, EPITOPE, VIRUS, GENE, DEOXYRIBONUCLEIC ACID (DNA), HIV-1 and HIV-2

Consortia Microorganisms that interact with each other (or at least "coexist peacefully") when growing together. An example of such interaction or coexistence would be bioleaching.

See also BIOLEACHING, BIORECOVERY, BIODESULFURIZATION, BIOSORBENTS

Constitutive Enzymes Enzymes that are part of the basic, permanent enzymatic machinery of the cell. They are formed at a constant rate and in constant amounts regardless of the metabolic state of the organism. For example, enzymes that function in the production of cell-usable energy (such as ATP) might be good candidates. And this, in fact, is the case with the enzymes of the glycolytic sequence, which is the most ancient energy-yielding catabolic pathway.

See also ENZYME, METABOLISM, CELL, PATHWAY

Constitutive Genes Expressed as a function of the interaction of RNA polymerase with the promoter, without additional regulation. They are also called "household genes" in the context of describing functions expressed in all cells at a low level.

See also GENE, RNA POLYMERASE, PROMOTER

Constitutive Heterochromatin The inert state of permanently nonexpressed sequences, usually satellite DNA.

See also EXPRESS, CODING SEQUENCE, DEOXYRIBONUCLEIC ACID (DNA), CHROMATIN

Constitutive Mutations Mutations (changes in DNA) that cause genes which are nonconstitutive (have controlled protein expression) to become constitutive (in which state the protein is expressed all of the time).

See also CONSTITUTIVE GENES, MUTATION, REGULATORY SEQUENCE, PROTEIN

Constitutive Promoter Refers to a promoter that is (present or acts at) a high level in all cells of an organism.

See also PROMOTER, CELL, ORGANISM

Construct See CASSETTE, TRANSGENE

Consultative Group on International Agricultural Research (CGIAR) An organization that is cosponsored by the Rome-based United Nations Food and Agriculture Organization (FAO), the United Nations Development Programme (UNDP), and the World Bank. The CGIAR is an association of 58 public and private donors that jointly support 16 international agricultural research centers that are located primarily in developing countries. Twelve of the research centers have collectively assembled 500,000 different preserved samples (i.e., germplasm) of major food, forage, and forest plant species into a gene bank. This is the world's largest internationally held collection of genetic resources and was legally placed under the auspices of the FAO in 1994 in order "to hold the collection in trust for the international community." Since 1970, CGIAR's collection

has supported research efforts to develop better varieties of staple foods consumed primarily in developing countries of the world.

See also AMERICAN TYPE CULTURE COLLECTION (ATCC), TYPE SPECIMEN, GERMPLASM

Contaminant By definition, it is any unwanted or undesired organism, compound, or molecule present in a controlled environment. Unwanted presence of an entity in an otherwise clean or pure environment.

See also ORGANISM

Contiguous Genes A "group" of genes that are situated together on an organism's chromosome and which often function **together as a unit** to express a trait in that organism.

See also LINKAGE, ORGANISM, GENE, CHROMOSOME, TRAIT

Continuous Perfusion A type of cell culture in which the cells (either mammalian or otherwise) are immobilized in a part of the system, and nutrients and oxygen are allowed to flow through the stationary cells, thus effecting nutrient and waste exchange. Ideally, the system incorporates features that retard the activity of proteolytic enzymes and reduce the need for anti-infective agents (e.g., antibiotics) and fetal bovine serum, which are required by most other cell culture systems. Continuous perfusion is used because, among other things, it eliminates the need to separate the cells from the culture medium when fresh medium is exchanged for old.

See also MAMMALIAN CELL CULTURE, ENZYME, PROTEOLYTIC ENZYMES

Control Sequences Those sequences of DNA that are adjacent to a gene (in genome) and "turn on" and "turn off" that gene.

See also SEQUENCE (OF A DNA MOLECULE), GENE, GENOME, PROMOTER, TERMINATION CODON (TERMINATOR SEQUENCE), BASE (NUCLEOTIDE), CODING SEQUENCE

Convention on Biological Diversity (CBD) The international treaty governing the conservation and use of biological resources around the world, that was signed by more than 150 countries at the 1992 United Nations Conference on Environment and Development.

Article 19.4 of the CBD called for the establishment of a "protocol on biosafety" to govern the transnational-boundary movement of non-indigenous living organisms.

See also MEA, CONSULTATIVE GROUP ON INTERNATIONAL AGRICULTURAL RESEARCH (CGIAR), INTERNATIONAL PLANT PROTECTION CONVENTION (IPPC), BIODIVERSITY, INTRODUCTION

Convergent Improvement See TRANS-GRESSIVE SEGREGATION

Coordinated Framework for Regulation of Biotechnology The regulatory "framework" through which the U.S. evaluates and approves new products derived via biotechnology. The Coordinated Framework assigns specific regulatory tasks to each of the U.S. government's applicable agencies (see following text).

For example, the U.S. Environmental Protection Agency (EPA) is assigned to evaluate and regulate all genetically modified pest protected (GMPP) new plants in terms of their impact on pests. The U.S. Food and Drug Administration (FDA) is assigned to evaluate and regulate all new food crops derived via biotechnology in terms of their potential food safety impact (e.g., allergenicity, toxicity, etc.). The U.S. Department of Agriculture (USDA) is assigned to evaluate and regulate all new plants derived via biotechnology in terms of field (i.e., outdoor) testing and in terms of potential environmental impacts such as weediness.

See also BIOTECHNOLOGY, FOOD AND DRUG ADMINISTRATION (FDA), GENETICALLY MODIFIED PEST PROTECTED (GMPP) PLANTS, ALLERGIES (FOODBORNE), APHIS

Coordination Chemistry See CHELATION

Copy DNA (C-DNA) See C-DNA

Copy Number The number of molecules (copies) of an individual plasmid or plastid that is typically present in a single (e.g., bacterial for *plasmid*, plant for *plastid*) cell. Each plasmid has a characteristic copy number value ranging from 1 to 50 or more. Higher copy numbers result in a higher yield of the protein encoded for by the plasmid gene in each cell.

See also PLASMID, PLASTID, PROTEIN, GENE, EXTRANUCLEAR GENES,

GENETIC CODE, MULTICOPY PLAS-MIDS

Corepressor A small molecule that combines with the repressor to trigger repression (the shutting down) of transcription.

See also TRANSCRIPTION

Corn The domesticated plant *Zea mays L.* also known as maize. A green, leafy (grain) plant that is one of the world's largest providers of edible starch and fructose (sugar) for humans' use. This summer annual plant varies in height from 2 ft (0.5 m) to more than 20 ft (6 m) tall. The seeds (kernels) are borne in cobs, ranging in size from 2 ft long to smaller than a man's thumb.

Owing to genetic variation (i.e., of different hybrids or varieties), the fraction of kernel that consists of recoverable starch varies between 42 and 73% for different corn varieties.

Owing to genetic variation (i.e., of different hybrids or varieties), the fraction of kernel that consists of protein varies between 8 and 10%, but that protein content can be increased by 10% via insertion of the **glutamate hydrogenase (GDH) gene** into corn plant.

Owing to genetic variation (i.e., of different hybrids or varieties), the fraction of kernel that consists of oil varies between 3.5 and 8.5% for different corn varieties. Grown widely in the world's temperate zones, corn is grown as far north as latitude 58° in Canada and Russia and as far south as latitude 40° in the Southern Hemisphere.

During the 1980s, scientists were able to insert genes from *Bacillus thuringiensis (B.t.)* bacteria into the corn plant in order to make it resistant to certain insects. During the 1990s, scientists were able to insert genes into the corn plant in order to make it tolerant to certain herbicides and to cause the corn plant to produce monoclonal antibodies (MAb). Some of the major economic pests of corn include the European corn borer (*Ostrinia nubilalis*), corn earworm (*Helicoverpa zea*), corn rootworm (*Diabrotica virgifera virgifera*), and beet armyworm (*Pseudaletia unipuncta*).

See also HYBRIDIZATION (PLANT GENETICS), *BACILLUS THURINGIENSIS (B.t.)*, PROTEIN, STRESS PROTEINS, MAYSIN, CRY PROTEINS, CRY1A (b) PROTEIN, CRY1A (c) PROTEIN, CRY9C PROTEIN, GENE, "STACKED" GENES, OPAGUE-2,

HIGH- METHIONINE CORN, HIGH-LYSINE CORN, *B.t. KURSTAKI*, VALUE-ENHANCED GRAINS, *HELICOVERPA ZEA (H. ZEA)*, CHLOROPLAST TRANSIT PEPTIDE (CTP), HERBICIDE-TOLERANT CROP, HIGH-OIL CORN, EUROPEAN CORN BORER (ECB), AFLATOXIN, *FUSARIUM*, ORN ROOTWORM, VOLICITIN, GA21, TRANSPOSON, GLUTAMATE DEHYDROGENASE, BLACK-LAYERED (CORN), MONOCLONAL ANTIBODIES (MAb), *PHOTORHABDUS LUMINESCENS*, CHOLESTEROL OXIDASE

Corn Borer See EUROPEAN CORN BORER (ECB), ASIAN CORN BORER

Corn Earworm See *HELICOVERPA ZEA (H. ZEA)*, CORN

Corn Rootworm A complex of several strains of beetles, it refers to the larval stage of the corn rootworm beetle (*Diabrotica virgifera virgifera*), which historically has laid its eggs on corn or maize (*Zea mays L.*) plants. When they hatch, the larvae must feed on the roots of the corn or maize plant in order to live. Adult corn rootworm beetles also feed on the leaves and silks of corn or maize plants. Some strains of *Bacillus thuringiensis (B.t.)* have proved to be effective against the corn rootworm when sprayed onto them or genetically engineered into the corn or maize plant.

In 1992, a new genetic variant of corn rootworm known as the "western phenotype" or Western corn rootworm (*Diabrotica virgifera virgifera* LeConte) was discovered in the U.S. It prefers to lay its eggs on soybean plants instead of corn plants. Other genetic variants include the "northern phenotype" or Northern corn rootworm (*Diabrotica barberi*) and the Mexican corn rootworm (*Diabrotica virgifera zeae*).

See also CORN, PHENOTYPE, SOYBEAN PLANT, STRAIN, *BACILLUS THURINGIENSIS (B.t.)*, GENETIC ENGINEERING, CRY3B (b) PROTEIN, *B.t. KUMAMOTOENSIS*, ANTIBIOSIS

Coronary Heart Disease (CHD) A disease of the heart and arteries in which (among other effects) cholesterol is deposited on the interior walls (lumen endothelium), where it can sometimes later break off and cause death (e.g., via "heart attack").

Risk factors (i.e., increased risk) for CHD include high blood levels of triglycerides, high levels of apolipoprotein B, high levels of LDLPs/VLDLs (the two lipoproteins that are most likely to deposit cholesterol on artery walls), and low levels of HDLPs (the lipoproteins that help to clear away cholesterol deposits from artery walls).

A human diet containing a large amount of certain phytosterols (e.g., CAMPESTEROL, BETA-SITOSTEROL, and STIGMASTEROL) has been shown to lower total serum (blood) cholesterol and low-density lipoproteins (LDLP) levels by approximately 10% and thereby lower the risk of CHD. A human diet containing a large amount of oleic acid causes lower blood cholesterol levels and can thus lower risk of CHD and atherosclerosis.

See also CHOLESTEROL, LOW-DENSITY LIPOPROTEINS (LDLP), SITOSTEROL, VERY-LOW-DENSITY LIPOPROTEINS (VLDL), HIGH-OLEIC OIL SOYBEANS, PHYTOSTEROLS, STEROLS, CAMPESTEROL, HIGH-DENSITY LIPOPROTEINS (HDLP), BETA-SITOSTEROL (B-SITOSTEROL), STIGMASTEROL, SERUM LIFETIME, LYCOPENE, ATHEROSCLEROSIS, RESVERATROL, LUMEN, ENDOTHELIUM, TRIGLYCERIDES, ENDOTHELIN, ADIPOSE, HOMOCYSTEINE

Corticotropin See ACTH (ADRENOCORTICOTROPIC HORMONE [CORTICOTROPIN])

Cortisol A steroid hormone that is utilized by the human body to regulate blood pressure (e.g., via increased water retention, by decreasing the kidney's water excretion rate). A deficiency of cortisol causes **Addison's disease**.

See also TRANSCRIPTION ACTIVATORS, GLYCYRRHIZIC ACID, STEROID, HORMONE, HOMEOSTASIS

Cosuppression A significant decrease ("silencing") in the expression of a gene (within an organism's genome or DNA) that (often) results when man **inserts and causes to be expressed** a homologous gene.

For example, **high-oleic oil soybeans** result when the **GmFad2-1** gene (which codes for native Δ 12 desaturase enzyme) is inserted and expressed in traditional varieties of soybeans. That is because the inserted gene "silences" itself and the endogenous **GmFad2-1 gene** (i.e., the one naturally or originally present in the soybean plant), which thus prevents formation of the Δ 12 desaturase enzyme (that normally causes most oleic acid within soybeans to be converted into polyunsaturated linolenic acid or linoleic acid).

See also GENE SILENCING, OLEIC ACID, LINOLEIC ACID, LINOLENIC ACID, EXPRESS, GENE, POSTTRANSCRIPTIONAL GENE SILENCING (PTGS), KNOCKOUT, GENOME, HOMOLOGOUS (CHROMOSOMES OR GENES), SOYBEAN PLANT, HIGH-OLEIC OIL SOYBEANS, Δ 12 DESATURASE, ANTISENSE (DNA SEQUENCE), FAD3 GENE, RNA INTERFERENCE (RNAi)

Cowpea Mosaic Virus (CpMV) A virus that infects cowpea (*Vigna unguiculata*) plants (known as black-eyed peas in the U.S.) but does not infect animals. Researchers have discovered how to cause CpMV to express certain animal virus proteins (i.e., antigens) on its surface via genetic engineering. These virus antigens have the potential to replace the antigens currently used in vaccines, which are fraught with problems owing to their production in animal cells, bacterial cells, or yeast cells. In addition, CpMV acts as an intrinsic natural adjuvant to the (animal virus) antigens, because it provokes an immune response itself.

See also VIRUS, COWPEA TRYPSIN INHIBITOR (CpTI), EXPRESS, PROTEIN, ADJUVANT (TO A PHARMACEUTICAL), IMMUNE RESPONSE, ANTIGEN

Cowpea Trypsin Inhibitor (CpTI) A chemical that is naturally coded for by a certain cowpea (*Vigna unguiculata*) plant gene. It kills certain insect larvae by inhibiting digestion of ingested trypsin by the larvae, thereby starving them to death.

See also TRYPSIN, TRYPSIN INHIBITORS, GENE, CODING SEQUENCE

COX See CYCLOOXYGENASE

COX-1 See CYCLOOXYGENASE

COX-2 See CYCLOOXYGENASE

COX-3 See CYCLOOXYGENASE

CP4 EPSP Synthase See CP4 EPSPS

CP4 EPSPS The enzyme 5-enolpyruvyl-shikimate-3-phosphate synthase that is naturally produced by an *Agrobacterium* species (strain CP4) of soil bacteria. CP4 EPSPS is essential for the functioning of that bacterium's metabolism biochemical pathway. CP4 EPSPS happens to be unaffected by glyphosate-containing or sulfosate-containing herbicides, so introduction of the CP4 EPSPS gene into crop plants (e.g., soybeans) makes them essentially impervious to glyphosate-containing or sulfosate-containing herbicides.

See also ENZYME, METABOLISM, GENE, GENETIC ENGINEERING, EPSP SYNTHASE, GLYPHOSATE, SULFOSATE, SOYBEAN PLANT, GLYPHOSATE OXIDASE, BACTERIA, CHLOROPLAST TRANSIT PEPTIDE (CTP), HERBICIDE-TOLERANT CROP, PATHWAY

CPMP See COMMITTEE FOR PROPRIETARY MEDICINAL PRODUCTS (CPMP)

CpDNA See CYTOPLASMIC DNA

CpMV See COWPEA MOSAIC VIRUS (CPMV)

CpTI See COWPEA TRYPSIN INHIBITOR (CPTI)

Cre-Lox System Refers to the use of a particular phage to accomplish a site-specific (on organism's DNA) insertion or deletion of a specific DNA fragment. Certain "knockouts" in transgenic organisms can be created via the Cre-Lox System.

See also PHAGE, ORGANISM, DEOXYRIBONUCLEIC ACID (DNA), DELETIONS, KNOCKOUT

Critical Micelle Concentration Also known as the CMC of a surfactant. It is the lowest surfactant concentration at which micelles are formed. That is, the CMC represents that concentration of surfactant at which the individual surfactant molecules aggregate into distinct, high-molecular-weight spherical entities called micelles. Or from another viewpoint, it represents the concentration of a surfactant above which micelles or reverse micelles will spontaneously form through the process of self-aggregation (self-assembly). For example, liposomes in a water solution will self-assemble into micelles or vesicles if their concentration is greater than the liposome's CMC.

See also MICELLE, REVERSE MICELLE (RM), LIPOSOMES

Cross Reaction When an antibody molecule (against one antigen) can combine with (bind to) a different (second) antigen. This sometimes occurs because the second antigen's molecular structure (shape) is very similar to that of the first.

See also ANTIBODY, ANTIGEN

Cross Reactivity See CROSS REACTION

Crossing Over The reciprocal exchange of material between chromosomes that occurs during meiosis. This event is responsible for genetic recombination. The process involves the natural breaking of chromosomes, the exchange of chromosome pieces, and the reuniting of DNA molecules.

See also LINKAGE, DEOXYRIBONU-CLEIC ACID (DNA), CHROMOSOMES, RECOMBINATION

Crown Gall See *AGROBACTERIUM TUME-FACIENS*

CRP Acronym for **C-reactive protein**.

See C-REACTIVE PROTEIN (CRP)

CRP Acronym for **catabolite regulator protein**.

See CAP

CRTL Gene See GOLDEN RICE, GENE

Cruciferae A taxonomic group ("family") of plants that includes canola, mustard, oilseed rape, etc.

See also *BRASSICA*

Cry Proteins A class of proteins produced by *Bacillus thuringiensis (B.t.)* bacteria (or plants into which a *B.t.* gene has been inserted). Cry (i.e., "crystal-like") proteins are toxic to certain categories of insects such as corn borers (e.g., *Ostrinia nubilalis*), corn rootworms (*Diabrotica virgifera virgifera*), armyworms (e.g., *Spodoptera frugiperda*), black cutworms (*Agostis ipsilon*), velvetbean caterpillar (*Anticarsia gemmatalis*), mosquitoes, black flies, tobacco hornworm, some types of beetles, etc., but harmless to mammals and most beneficial insects.

See also *BACILLUS THURINGIENSIS (B.t.)*, PROTEIN, BACTERIA, GENE, PROTOXIN, CORN, EUROPEAN CORN BORER (ECB), CORN ROOTWORM, ARMYWORM, TOBACCO HORNWORM, CRY1A (b) PROTEIN, CRY1A (c) PROTEIN, CRY3B (b)

PROTEIN, CRY9C PROTEIN, ION CHANNELS, COTTON, TOXICOGENOMICS

Cry1A (b) Protein One of the "Cry" (i.e., "crystal-like") proteins, it is a protoxin that when eaten by certain insects (e.g., *Lepidoptera* larvae such as the armyworm or tobacco hornworm or European corn borer) is toxic to those crop pest insects. However, if eaten by a mammal, the Cry1A (b) protein is digested within 1 min, harmlessly.

See also CRY PROTEINS, PROTEIN, *B.T. KURSTAKI*, PROTOXIN, EUROPEAN CORN BORER (ECB), ARMYWORM, TOBACCO HORNWORM, ION CHANNELS

Cry1A (c) Protein One of the "Cry" (i.e., "crystal-like") proteins.

See also CRY PROTEINS, ION CHANNELS

Cry1F Protein One of the "Cry" (i.e., "crystal-like" proteins), it is a protoxin that when eaten by European corn borer (*Ostrinia nubilalis*), southwestern corn borer (*Diatraea grandiosella*), black cutworm (*Agostis ipsilon*), fall armyworm (*Spodoptera frugiperda*), and western bean cutworm is toxic to them.

See also CRY PROTEINS, *BACILLUS THURINGIENSIS (B.t.)*, PROTOXIN, PROTEIN, EUROPEAN CORN BORER (ECB), ARMYWORM, ION CHANNELS

Cry3B (b) Protein One of the "cry" (i.e., "crystal-like") proteins, it is a protoxin that when eaten by certain insects (e.g., larvae of corn rootworm *Diabrotica virgifera virgifera*) is toxic to them.

See also PROTEIN, CRY PROTEINS, PROTOXIN, CORN ROOTWORM, ION CHANNELS, *B.T. KUMAMOTOENSIS*

Cry9C Protein One of the "Cry" (i.e., "crystal-like") proteins, it is a protoxin that when eaten by European corn borer (*Ostrinia nubilalis*), southwestern cornborer (*Diatraea grandiosella*), black cutworm (*Agostis ipsilon*), and some species of armyworm (e.g., *Spodoptera frugiperda*) is toxic to them.

See also CRY PROTEINS, *BACILLUS THURINGIENSIS (B.t.)*, *B. T. TOLWORTHI*, PROTOXIN, PROTEIN, EUROPEAN CORN BORER (ECB), ARMYWORM, ION CHANNELS

CSF See COLONY-STIMULATING FACTORS (CSFs)

CT Refers to conservation tillage practices of crop production.

See also LOW-TILLAGE CROP PRODUC-TION, NO-TILLAGE CROP PRODUC-TION, GLOMALIN

CTAB See HEXADECYLTRIMETHYLAM-MONIUM BROMIDE (CTAB)

CTNBio Acronym for Brazil's National Technical Commission on Biosafety, which is the Brazilian government's regulatory body for granting formal approval to a new genetically engineered plant (e.g., a genetically engineered crop to be planted). CTNBio is analogous to Germany's ZKBS (Central Commission on Biological Safety), Australia's GMAC (Genetic Manipulation Advisory Committee), Kenya's Biosafety Council, and India's Department of Biotechnology.

See also GMAC, RECOMBINANT DNA ADVISORY COMMITTEE (RAC), ZKBS (CENTRAL COMMISSION ON BIOLOGI-CAL SAFETY), GENETIC ENGINEERING, KENYA BIOSAFETY COUNCIL, INDIAN DEPARTMENT OF BIOTECHNOLOGY

CTP See CHLOROPLAST TRANSIT PEP-TIDE (CTP)

Culture Any population of cells (e.g., bacteria, algae, protozoa, virus, yeasts, plant cells, mammalian cells, etc.) growing on, or in, a medium that supports their growth. Typically used to refer to a population of the cells of a single species or a single strain. A medium that contains only one specific organism (e.g., *E. coli* bacteria) is known as a pure culture. A culture may be preserved (i.e., stored alive) via freezing, drying (in which the cells go dormant), subculturing on an agar medium, or other preservation methods.

See also CULTURE MEDIUM, TYPE SPEC-IMEN, LYOPHILIZATION, AMERICAN TYPE CULTURE COLLECTION (ATCC), SPECIES, STRAIN, CELL CULTURE, MAMMALIAN CELL CULTURE

Culture Medium Any nutrient system for the artificial cultivation of bacteria or other cells. It usually consists of a complex mixture of organic and inorganic materials. For example, the classic culture (growth) medium used for bacteria consists of nutrients (required by that bacteria) and agar to solidify or semisolidify the nutrient-containing mass.

See also MEDIUM, AGAR, CELL CULTURE, MAMMALIAN CELL CULTURE

Curcumin A compound (naturally found in some plants) that acts as an antioxidant in the body's tissues when consumed by humans. For example, curcumin is naturally produced in turmeric (*Curcuma longa*). Research indicates that lifelong consumption of curcumin might help to prevent or delay symptoms of Alzheimer's disease.

See also OXIDATIVE STRESS, ANTIOXI-DANTS, ALZHEIMER'S DISEASE

Curing Agent A substance that increases the rate of loss of plasmids during bacterial growth.

See also GROWTH (MICROBIAL), PLAS-MID

Current Good Manufacturing Practices See cGMP

Cut An enzyme-induced, highly specific break in both strands of a DNA molecule (opposite one another). The enzymes involved are called restriction enzymes.

See also RESTRICTION ENDONU-CLEASES, ENZYME, DEOXYRIBONU-CLEIC ACID (DNA)

CVD Acronym for **cardiovascular disease.**

See ATHEROSCLEROSIS, ARTERIOSCLE-ROSIS

Cyclic AMP A molecule of AMP (adenosine monophosphate) in which the phosphate group is joined to both the 3 and the 5 positions of the ribose, forming a cyclic (ring) structure. When cAMP binds to CAP, the complex is a positive regulator of procaryotic transcription.

See also ADENOSINE MONOPHOSPHATE (AMP), CAP, PROCARYOTES, TRAN-SCRIPTION, ADENYLATE CYCLASE

Cyclic Phosphorylation Synthesis (i.e., "manufacturing") of adenosine triphosphate (chemical reaction) that occurs during photosynthesis in plants. Also called PHOTOSYN-THETIC PHOSPHORYLATION (photophos-phorylation).

See also ATP SYNTHASE, ADENOSINE TRIPHOSPHATE (ATP), PHOTOSYNTHE-SIS, PHOTOSYNTHETIC PHOSPHORY-LATION

Cyclodextrin A macrocyclic (doughnut-shaped) carbohydrate ring produced enzymatically from starch. The external surface is hydrophobic, whereas the interior is hydrophilic in nature. The hole of the doughnut is large enough to accommodate guest molecules. Uses include solubilization, separation, and stabilization of molecules in the interior cavity of, or in association with, the cyclodextrin molecules.

For example, during 2005, Timothy Triche utilized cyclodextrins to carry some short interfering RNA (siRNA) into mouse tumors (after he attached a molecular tag-specific-to-tumors to the exterior of those cyclodextrins). After entry into the tumors, the siRNA inhibited their growth.

See also CARBOHYDRATES, SHORT INTERFERING RNA (siRNA), TUMOR

Cycloheximide Also called actidione. A chemical that inhibits protein synthesis by the 80S eucaryotic ribosomes; it does not, however, inhibit the 70S ribosomes of procaryotes. The chemical blocks peptide bond formation by binding to the large ribosomal subunits.

See also PROTEIN, RIBOSOMES

Cyclooxygenase Abbreviated COX, it refers to a "family" of enzymes (isozymes) that convert arachidonic acid to prostaglandins in the human body. There are at least three forms of cyclooxygenase:

- COX-1 (also known as PGHS-1) and COX-3, which convert arachidonic acid to **constitutive** prostaglandins, which help to maintain the tissues of the stomach, kidneys, and intestines. COX-1 is present in nearly all tissues of the body.
- COX-2 (also known as PGHS-2), which converts arachidonic acid to **inducible** prostaglandins, which can cause pain and inflammation in the body's joints when they accumulate there. COX-2 is generally not present in body tissues until those tissues are "inflamed" by monocytes or mast cells or "injured" (via mechanical shear and abrasion of endothelial cells).
- COX-3, which results when **intron 1** is retained in the mRNA transcript during transcription of the COX-1 gene (i.e., alternative slicing).

Aspirin and some other pain-relieving drugs (e.g., ibuprofen, indomethacin, etc.) chemically block the preceding activity of COX-1 and COX-2. Nexrutine (an extract from the *Phellodendron amurense* tree) and certain pain-relieving drugs (celecoxib, rofecoxib, etc.) chemically block the preceding activity of COX-2, while **not** blocking the (beneficial) COX-1. The pain-relieving drug acetaminophen chemically blocks the activity of COX-3, without blocking COX-1 or COX-2.

See also ENZYME, ISOZYMES, ARACHIDONIC ACID, PLATELETS, INDUCIBLE ENZYMES, SELECTIVE APOPTOTIC ANTINEOPLASTIC DRUG (SAAND), EICOSANOIDS, MONOCYTES, MAST CELLS, PROSTAGLANDINS, ENDOTHELIAL CELLS, PGHS, INTRON, TRANSCRIPTION, MESSENGER RNA (mRNA), GENE, CYCLOOXYGENASE, ALTERNATIVE SPLICING

Cyclosporin An immune-system-suppressing drug that was isolated from a mold in the mid-1970s by the Swiss firm F. Hoffmann-LaRoche. The drug is used to prevent (organ recipient's) immune system from "rejecting" a transplanted organ and typically must be taken by the organ recipient for the duration of his or her lifetime. Cyclosporin's mechanism of action is to prevent the divalent calcium cation (Ca^{2+}) from entering T lymphocytes to activate certain genes within those lymphocytes (that trigger the "rejection" process).

In 1996, Thomas Eisner reported that the mold *Tolypocladium inflatum*, from which cyclosporin is harvested, prefers a natural (wild) substrate of a deceased dung beetle.

During 2000, it was discovered that cyclosporin inhibits growth of the parasitic microorganism *Toxoplasma gondii* (which can cause loss of sight and neurological disease in humans).

See also T LYMPHOCYTES, FUNGUS, XENOGENEIC ORGANS, CATION, GENE, GRAFT-VERSUS-HOST DISEASE (GVHD), HUMAN LEUKOCYTE ANTIGENS (HLA), MAJOR HISTOCOMPATIBILITY COMPLEX (MHC), MICROORGANISM, GROWTH (MICROBIAL)

Cyclosporine See CYCLOSPORIN

CYP46 Gene A human gene that codes for a protein (within the brain) that is involved in the brain's usage and processing of cholesterol.

People whose DNA has a mutated version of the CYP46 gene are at higher-than-risk average of getting Alzheimer's disease.

See also GENE, PROTEIN, GENETIC CODE, CHOLESTEROL, MUTATION, APOE4, DEOXYRIBONUCLEIC ACID (DNA), HAPLOTYPE, ALZHEIMER'S DISEASE

Cysteine (Cys) An amino acid of molecular weight (mol wt) 121 Da. It is incorporated in many proteins. It possesses a sulfhydryl group (SH) that makes cysteine a mild reducing agent.

Cysteine can cross-link with another cysteine located on the same or on a different polypeptide chain to form disulfide bridges. The "free" cysteine group is called a *thiol group*.

High levels of cysteine content in certain genetically engineered corn (maize) kernels have been shown to inhibit in-field production of mycotoxins in corn (e.g., by several species of fungi that can be carried into corn plants by insects).

See also AMINO ACID, CYSTINE, DISULFIDE BOND, HOMOCYSTEINE, POLYPEPTIDE (PROTEIN), PROTEIN, MYCOTOXINS

Cystic Fibrosis See CYSTIC FIBROSIS TRANSMEMBRANE REGULATOR PROTEIN (CFTR)

Cystic Fibrosis Transmembrane Regulator Protein (CFTR) A protein, also known as **CF transmembrane conductance regulator** that regulates proper chloride ion transport across the cell membranes of human lung airway epithelial cells.

When the gene that codes for CFTR protein is damaged or mutated, the (mutant) CFTR protein fails to function properly (i.e., conducts chloride ions at a much slower rate), which causes mucus (and bacteria) to accumulate in the lungs. This lung disease is known as cystic fibrosis.

The SNP for cystic fibrosis was identified in 1989.

See also PROTEIN, GENE, ION, ION CHANNELS, DEOXYRIBOCYCLEIC ACID (DNA), INFORMATIONAL MOLECULES, GENOME, GENETIC CODE, RIBOSOMES, TRANSCRIPTION, SINGLE-NUCLEOTIDE POLYMORPHISMS (SNPs)

Cystine Two cysteine amino acids that are covalently linked via a disulfide bond. These units are important in biochemistry in that the disulfide bridges represent one important way in which the conformation of a protein is maintained in the active form. Cystine bridges lock in place the structure of the proteins in which they occur by disallowing certain types of (molecule) chain movement. When the disulfide bond is with a "free" cysteine (i.e., one that is not a part of the same protein molecule's amino acid backbone), the free cysteine is known as a *thiol group*. Cystine can be metabolized from methionine by certain animals (e.g., swine), but not vice versa.

See also CYSTEINE (Cys), AMINO ACID, CONFORMATION, PROTEIN, METHIONINE (Met), METABOLISM, DISULFIDE BOND

CystX Refers to a naturally occurring group of genes present in the genome (DNA) in some varieties of soybean plant that confers on those varieties some resistance to the soybean cyst nematode. Discovered via marker-assisted breeding and developed during the 1990s by Jamal Faghihi, John Ferris, Virginia Ferris, and Rick Vierling.

See also SOYBEAN PLANT, SOYBEAN CYST NEMATODES (SCN), GENE, MARKER-ASSISTED BREEDING

Cytochrome Any of the complex protein respiratory pigments (enzymes) occurring within plant and animal cells. They usually occur in mitochondria and function as electron carriers in biological oxidation. Cytochromes are involved in the "handing off" of electrons to each other in a stepwise fashion. In the process of handing off, other events take place that result in the production of energy that the cell needs and is able to use.

See also PROTEIN, ENZYME, MITOCHONDRIA, CELL

Cytochrome P450 A "family" of enzymes within the liver that contain an iron-heme cofactor. They catalyze many different biological hydroxylation reactions (i.e., metabolism of certain compounds). Essentially, the enzyme renders fat-soluble (hydrophobic)

molecules water soluble or **more water soluble** (by introduction of the hydrophilic hydroxyl group) so that the molecules may be removed (washed) from the body via the kidneys. These enzymes are being investigated for their potential as catalysts in the hydroxylation of specific (valuable) industrial chemicals.

See also CYTOCHROME, ENZYME, COFACTOR, HEME, HYDROXYLATION REACTION, METABOLISM, CYTOCHROME P450 3A4, CYTOCHROME P450 (CYP)

Cytochrome P450 (CYP) Refers to a class of liver enzymes (approximately 4000 known so far) that are responsible for the metabolism (breakdown) of more than 50% of human pharmaceuticals when those pharmaceuticals enter the bloodstream. For example, **cytochrome P450 3A4** catalyzes the breakdown of some pharmaceutical sedatives, the antihistamine terfenadine, antihypertensives, and the immunosuppressant cyclosporin. **CYP2D6** catalyzes such rapid breakdown of the pain reliever codeine that patients within the haplotype whose liver contains large amounts of CYP2D6 derive virtually no benefit from taking the standard dose of codeine.

Another example is that consumption of the pharmaceuticals tolbutamide, warfarin, or phenytoin can be riskier for people who possess a mutation (i.e., an SNP that codes for less or no expression of **CYP2C9**) within their liver tissue. That is because the CYP2C9 enzyme causes rapid metabolism of tolbutamide, warfarin, phenytoin (and some other pharmaceuticals), so the "typical dose" could result in higher-than-expected bloodstream levels of those pharmaceuticals in people possessing that particular SNP.

See also CYTOCHROME P450, CYTOCHROME P450 3A4, CYTOCHROME, ENZYME, METABOLISM, HAPLOTYPE, MUTATION, SNP, CODING SEQUENCE, EXPRESS, EXPRESSIVITY, PHARMACOGENETICS

Cytochrome P450 3A4 An enzyme within the liver that, in humans, catalyzes reactions involved in the metabolism (breakdown) of certain pharmaceuticals. Those pharmaceuticals include some sedatives, antihypertensives, the antihistamine terfenadine, and the immunosuppressant cyclosporin.

See also ENZYME, CYTOCHROME P450, METABOLISM, HISTAMINE, CYCLOSPORIN, METABOLIC PATHWAY, CYTOCHROME

Cytokines A large class of glycoproteins similar to lymphokines but produced by nonlymphocytic cells such as normal macrophages, fibroblasts, keratinocytes and a variety of transformed cell lines. They participate in regulating immunological and inflammatory processes and can contribute to repair processes and to the regulation of normal cell growth and differentiation.

Although cytokines are not produced by glands, they are hormone-like in their intercellular regulatory functions. They are active at very low concentrations and, for the most part, appear to function nonspecifically. For example, the cytokines stimulate the endothelial cells to express (synthesize and present) P-selectins and E-selectins on the internal surfaces (of blood vessels). These selectins protrude into the bloodstream, which causes passing white blood cells (leukocytes) to adhere to them, after which they leave the bloodstream by "squeezing" between adjacent endothelial cells. Cytokines are exemplified by the interferons.

See also INTERLEUKIN-1 (IL-1), LYMPHOKINES, INTERFERONS, GLYCOPROTEIN, PROTEIN, T CELLS, INTERLEUKIN-6 (IL-6), MACROPHAGE, LECTINS, FIBROBLASTS, HORMONE, ENDOTHELIAL CELLS, ENDOTHELIUM, SELECTINS, P-SELECTIN, ELAM-1, LEUKOCYTES, ADHESION MOLECULE, ERYTHROPOIETIN (EPO)

Cytolysis The dissolution of cells, particularly by destruction of their surface membranes.

See also LYSIS, CECROPHINS, LYSOZYME, MAGAININS, COMPLEMENT, COMPLEMENT CASCADE

Cytomegalovirus (CMV) A virus that infects different groups of people in varying amounts, depending on their behavior. For example, 40 to 90% of American heterosexuals and about 95% of homosexuals are infected with CMV. CMV normally produces a latent (nonclinical, nonobvious) infection, but when AIDS or other events cause immune system suppression, CMV produces a febrile (fever-causing) illness that is usually mild in nature but can become retinitis (eye infection).

CMV can be treated (to halt life- and sight-threatening infection) in immunocompromised patients (i.e., transplant patients and AIDS victims) with Ganciclovir™, an antiviral compound developed by Syntex; or Foscarnet™, a compound developed by Astra Pharmaceuticals.

In 1996, Stephen E. Epstein found that latent CMV may cause changes in artery wall cells that aid clogging of arteries in adults (especially following balloon angioplasty).

See also VIRUS, ACQUIRED IMMUNE DEFICIENCY SYNDROME (AIDS)

Cytopathic Damaging to cells.

Cytoplasm From the Greek words *kytos* = a "vessel to hold liquid" and *plasma* = "form."

Cytoplasm refers to the protoplasmic contents of the cell (e.g., plastids, mitochondria, etc.) not including the nucleus.

See also CELL, NUCLEUS, PROTOPLASM, CYTOPLASMIC DNA, PLASMA MEMBRANE, PLASTID, MITOCHONDRIA, CHLOROPLASTS

Cytoplasmic DNA The DNA within an organism (e.g., plant) that is not inside the cell's nucleus. Cytoplasmic DNA (i.e., located in the cells' mitochondria and the chloroplasts) is not transferred from plant to plant via pollen, as **nuclear DNA** is.

See also DEOXYRIBONUCLEIC ACID (DNA), ORGANISM, CELL, CYTOPLASM, NUCLEUS, MITOCHONDRIA, MITOCHONDRIAL DNA, CHLOROPLASTS

Cytoplasmic Membrane See PLASMA MEMBRANE

Cytosine A pyrimidine occurring as a fundamental unit (one of the bases) of nucleic acids.

See also NUCLEIC ACIDS, BASE (NUCLEOTIDE)

Cytoskeleton This term refers to the "structural framework" of cell and cytoplasm.

Some antibiotics work (e.g., kill a bacterial cell) via inhibition of **cytoskeleton building or repair** by relevant bacterial cells. During the late 1970s, scientists utilized fluorescent-labeled monoclonal antibodies to "show" (visually, under microscope) the existence of the cytoskeleton within cells. Components of a cell's cytoskeleton include microtubules, actin, etc.

See also CYTOPLASM, CELL, PLASMA MEMBRANE, BACTERIA, ANTIBIOTIC, LABEL (FLUORESCENT), MONOCLONAL ANTIBODIES (MAb), LABEL (FLUORESCENT), MICROTUBULES, ACTIN

Cytotoxic Poisonous to cells.

Cytotoxic Killer Lymphocyte See CYTOTOXIC T CELLS

Cytotoxic T Cells Also called **killer T cells**. T cells that have been created by stimulated helper T cells. The T refers to cells of the cellular system rather than to cells of the humoral system (B cells).

Cytotoxic T cells detect and destroy infected body cells by use of a special type of protein. The protein attaches to the infected cell's membrane and forms holes in it. This allows the uncontrolled leakage of ions out of the cell and water into it, causing cell death. In general, the loss of the integrity of the cell membrane leads to death. The cytotoxic T cells also transmit a signal to the (leaking) infected cells that causes the cell to "chew up" its DNA. This includes its own DNA as well as that of the virus.

See also CECROPHINS, MAGAININS, INTERLEUKIN-4 (IL-4), HELPER T CELLS (T4 CELLS), VIRUS, T CELLS, SUPPRESSOR T CELLS, PROTEIN, INTERLEUKIN-2 (IL-2), DEOXYRIBONUCLEIC ACID (DNA), PLASMA MEMBRANE, INSULIN-DEPENDENT DIABETES MELLITIS

CZE Acronym for **capillary zone electrophoresis.** See CAPILLARY ZONE ELECTROPHORESIS

D

D Loop A region within mitochondrial DNA in which a short stretch of RNA is paired with one strand of DNA, displacing the original partner DNA strand in this region. The same term is used also to describe the displacement of a region of one strand of duplex DNA by a single-stranded invader in the reaction catalyzed by RecA protein.

See also DEOXYRIBONUCLEIC ACID (DNA), MITOCHONDRIA, RIBONUCLEIC ACID (RNA), DUPLEX, DISPLACEMENT LOOP

Daffodil Rice See GOLDEN RICE

Daffodils Refers to the approximately 80 species of flowering plants within the genus *Narcissus*. Native to southern Europe and northern Africa, they are the source of "golden rice" and the Alzheimer's disease treatment compound **galantamine hydrobromide**.

See also GOLDEN RICE, ALZHEIMER'S DISEASE

Daidzein See ISOFLAVONES

Daidzen See ISOFLAVONES

Daidzin The β-glycoside form (isomer in which glucose is attached to the molecule at the 7 position of the A ring) of the isoflavone known as daidzein (aglycone form).

See also ISOFLAVONES, ISOMER, DAIDZEIN

Dalton A unit of mass very nearly equal to that of a hydrogen atom (precisely equal to 1.0000 on the atomic mass scale). Named after John Dalton (1766–1844), who developed the atomic theory of matter. One Dalton is 1.660×10^{24} g.

See also KILODALTON (kDa)

Data Mining Refers to a computational methodology utilized to search for relationships between, and **overall patterns among**, the myriad data within a (bioinformatics) database. Some "data-mining" techniques include neural network analysis, genetic algorithms (which improve themselves over time), volume rendering, etc.

See also BIOINFORMATICS, *IN SILICO* BIOLOGY, *IN SILICO* SCREENING, VOLUME RENDERING

DBT An acronym that is used by some to designate the **Indian Department of Biotechnology**.

See also INDIAN DEPARTMENT OF BIOTECHNOLOGY

DC Acronym for **dendritic cells**.

See DENDRITIC CELLS

ddRNAi Acronym for **DNA-directed RNA Interference**.

See DNA-DIRECTED RNA INTERFERENCE

Deamidation See POSTTRANSLATIONAL MODIFICATION OF PROTEIN

Deamination The removal of amino groups from molecules (e.g., in an animal's food) via the energy-consuming metabolism of "excess" amino acids eaten by that animal. For example, when livestock are fed more lysine (amino acid) than their body needs in a given day (i.e., the animals' bodies can only utilize the essential amino acids in precise amounts or ratios of their daily diet), the excess lysine is metabolized to urea and then excreted in their urine.

See also METABOLISM, AMINO ACID, ESSENTIAL AMINO ACIDS, LYSINE, IDEAL PROTEIN, "IDEAL PROTEIN" CONCEPT, PDCAAS, ACC SYNTHASE

Defective Virus A virus that by itself is unable to reproduce when infecting its host (cell) but can grow in the presence of another virus. The other virus provides the necessary molecular machinery that the first virus lacks.

Defensins A class of proteins that inhibits certain fungal diseases. These defensin proteins are produced as a natural defense by some plants.

For example, the alfalfa plant produces a defensin known as **alfAFP** (alfalfa antifungal peptide).

In addition to protecting the alfalfa plant from certain diseases, the alfAFP also inhibits a

fungal disease known as **potato early dying complex** (also called verticillium wilt), which is caused by the fungus *Verticillium dahliae*.
See also PROTEIN, PEPTIDE, FUNGUS

Deficiency Refers to the insufficiency (or total absence) of relevant forms of nutrients, enzymes, or environmental inputs (e.g., temperature, etc.) required for physiological functions. Such a deficiency can prevent or hinder an organism's development, growth, metabolism, or other physiological functions.
See also ENZYME, METABOLISM, FLUX, DIGESTION (WITHIN ORGANISMS), ESSENTIAL NUTRIENTS, ESSENTIAL AMINO ACIDS, ESSENTIAL FATTY ACIDS, ISOZYMES, IRON DEFICIENCY ANEMIA (IDA), ERGOTAMINE, INSULIN

Degenerate Codons Two or more codons that code for the same amino acid. For example, isoleucine is specified by the A-U-U, A-U-C, and A-U-A triplets. Because, in this case, more than one triplet codes for isoleucine, the codons are called degenerate.
See also GENETIC CODE, CODON

Dehydrogenases Enzymes that catalyze the removal of pairs of hydrogen atoms from their substrates.
See also SUBSTRATE (CHEMICAL), GLUTAMATE DEHYDROGENASE, ENZYME, DEHYDROGENATION

Dehydrogenation The removal of hydrogen atoms from molecules. When those molecules are the components of vegetable oils or fats, this results in a lower content (percentage) of "saturated" fats.
See also FATS, MONOUNSATURATED FATS, SATURATED FATTY ACIDS (SAFA), FATTY ACID

Deinococcus radiodurans A species of bacteria that is capable of surviving 1.5 million rd of gamma radiation (i.e., 3000 times the lethal radiation dose for humans), surviving long periods of dehydration, and surviving high doses of ultraviolet radiation.
Deinococcus radiodurans was discovered in 1956 in some canned meat.
See also BACTERIA, EXTREMOPHILIC BACTERIA

Delaney Clause Formerly part of U.S. federal law (1959 Delaney amendment to Food, Drug, and Cosmetic Act), it was eliminated during 1996. The Delaney Clause had set a zero-risk tolerance level for carcinogenic pesticide residues in processed foods.
See also CARCINOGEN

Deletions Loss of a section of the genetic material from a chromosome. The size of a deleted material can vary from a single nucleotide to sections containing a number of genes.
See also GENE, CHROMOSOMES, NUCLEOTIDE, CRE-LOX SYSTEM, MUTATION BREEDING

Delta 12 Desaturase An enzyme that is present within the soybean plant and in other oilseed crops (e.g., sunflower, canola, and maize or corn.).
Delta 12 desaturase ($\Delta12$) is involved in the synthesis "pathway" utilized by oilseed crops to synthesize (i.e., "manufacture") polyunsaturated fatty acids (e.g., linoleic acid and linolenic acid) from monounsaturated fatty acids (e.g., oleic acid) in seeds (while those seeds are developing).
See also ENZYME, DESATURASE, FATTY ACID, UNSATURATED FATTY ACID, MONOUNSATURATED FATTY ACIDS (MUFA), POLYUNSATURATED FATTY ACIDS (PUFA), PATHWAY, OLEIC ACID, LINOLEIC ACID, LINOLENIC ACID, SOYBEAN PLANT, HIGH-OLEIC SUNFLOWERS, CORN, CANOLA, COSUPPRESSION

Δ 12 Desaturase One of the desaturases (enzymes).
See also DELTA 12 DESATURASE, COSUPPRESSION, ENZYME, DESATURASE

Δ 15 Desaturase One of the desaturases (enzymes).
See also ENZYME, DESATURASE, DELTA 12 DESATURASE

Delta Endotoxins See CRY PROTEINS, PROTEIN

δ Endotoxins See DELTA ENDOTOXINS

Demethylase See METHYLATED

Demethylation See METHYLATED

Denaturation The loss of the native conformation of a macromolecule resulting, for instance, from heat, extreme pH (i.e., by acidity or basicity) changes, and chemical treatment. It is accompanied by loss of biological activity.

See also CONFORMATION, CONFIGURATION, MACROMOLECULES, LASER INACTIVATION, BIOLOGICAL ACTIVITY

Denatured DNA DNA that has been converted from the double-stranded to single-stranded form by a denaturation process such as heating the DNA solution. In the case of heat denaturation, the solution becomes very gelatinous and viscous.

See also DENATURATION, DEOXYRIBONUCLEIC ACID (DNA), DUPLEX

Denaturing Gradient Gel Electrophoresis One particular method of gel electrophoresis, which can be utilized to separate different segments of double-stranded DNA or RNA from each other.

In denaturing gradient gel electrophoresis (DGGE), a steadily increasing level of a DENATURING AGENT such as urea, formamide, etc., is present in the "path" of the DNA or RNA molecules as they are moved under the influence of the applied electrical field within the gel matrix (e.g., polyacrylamide gel). The denaturing agents cause the double-stranded DNA or RNA molecules to denature (e.g., "unwind" into single strands), which changes those DNA or RNA molecules' individual rates of movement through the gel, thereby enhancing their separation and ease of identification via the gel electrophoresis process.

See also DEOXYRIBONUCLEIC ACID (DNA), DOUBLE HELIX, POLYACRYLAMIDE GEL ELECTROPHORESIS (PAGE), DENATURATION, DENATURED DNA, DENATURING POLYACRYLAMIDE GEL ELECTROPHORESIS, SHORT INTERFERING RNA (siRNA)

Denaturing Polyacrylamide Gel Electrophoresis The use of PAGE (polyacrylamide gel electrophoresis) in order to separate and analyze DNA fragments (sequences) after that DNA is first denatured. This methodology can be utilized to scan DNA in order to detect point mutations.

See also POLYACRYLAMIDE GEL ELECTROPHORESIS (PAGE), POINT MUTATION, DENATURING GRADIENT GEL ELECTROPHORESIS, DEOXYRIBONUCLEIC ACID (DNA), DENATURED DNA, BASE EXCISION SEQUENCE SCANNING (BESS)

Dendrimers Polymers (i.e., molecules composed of repeating atomic units within the molecule) that repeatedly branch (while "growing," owing to addition of more atoms in a repeating pattern) until that branching is stopped by the physical constraint of contacting itself (i.e., having formed a complete, hollow sphere).

Research indicates that some dendrimers can encapsulate certain pharmaceuticals and subsequently deliver the pharmaceuticals into a person's bloodstream when those drug-containing dendrimers are spread on the surface of the skin.

Discovered during the 1970s by Donald Tomalia, dendrimers possess sites on their exterior surface to which genetic material (e.g., genes or other portions of DNA) can be "attached."

Dendrimers bearing such genetic material have been shown to be able to successfully transfer that genetic material into more than 30 types of living animal cells.

See also POLYMER, DENDRITIC POLYMERS, NANOCAPSULES, GENE, GENETIC ENGINEERING, GENE DELIVERY, INFORMATIONAL MOLECULES, CODING SEQUENCE, TUMOR SUPPRESSOR GENES, DEOXYRIBONUCLEIC ACID (DNA), GENETIC TARGETING, GENETICS

Dendrites Highly branched structures that extend from the (nucleus of) neurons to (synapse junctions with) other neurons (e.g., in human brain tissue). The primary purpose of dendrites is to "process" signals that are generated or received at the synapses (e.g., from the dendrites of adjoining neurons).

Neuron ribosomes are located in the dendritic spines, the dendrite projections that form synapses (i.e., the junctions between dendrites where "signal transfer" between neurons takes place). Thus, those ribosomes make the proteins that are crucial to learning and memory (e.g., accomplished via growth or changes of dendrites).

Messenger RNAs are synthesized (i.e., "manufactured") in the nucleus of the neuron, then transported on microtubules (filaments within neuron cell) to the ribosomes in the dendrites, where they cause manufacture of proteins (e.g., enzymes) in response to synapse activity (i.e., signals).

D

See also NEURON, CELL, NEUROTRANS-
MITTER, RIBOSOMES, PROTEIN,
ENZYME, MESSENGER RNA (mRNA),
MICROTUBULES, SYNAPSE

Dendritic Cells These are rare white blood
cells, which stimulate the human immune system lymphocytes (i.e., "naive" T cells) to
become **effector T cells** and combat certain
pathogens by "presenting" the **antigens of
those pathogens** to those T cells.

Dendrite cells are present within the lymph system (and some nonlymphoid tissues), and
their action of "presenting" **antigens (of some
tumors)** can cause the immune system to halt
certain types of cancer.

See also CELL, WHITE BLOOD CELLS,
LYMPHOCYTE, T CELLS, PATHOGEN,
ANTIGEN, IMMUNE RESPONSE, CAN-
CER, LEUKOCYTES, MAJOR HISTO-
COMPATIBILITY ANTIGEN — CLASS II,
MAJOR HISTOCOMPATIBILTY COM-
PLEX (MHC)

Dendritic Langerhans Cells A type of cell,
located in the mucous membranes of the
mouth and genital areas, that permits the
human immunodeficiency virus (i.e., the virus
that causes AIDS) to enter and infect the body,
even when there are no cuts or abrasions in
them.

See also HUMAN IMMUNODEFICIENCY
VIRUS TYPE 1 (HIV-1), HUMAN IMMUN-
ODEFICIENCY VIRUS TYPE 2 (HIV-2),
ACQUIRED IMMUNE DEFICIENCY SYN-
DROME (AIDS), ADHESION MOLECULE,
DENDRITIC POLYMERS

Dendritic Polymers Polymers (i.e., molecules
composed of repeating atomic units within the
molecule) that repeatedly branch (while
"growing" due to the addition of more atoms
in a repeating pattern) until that branching is
stopped (e.g., by physical constraints for those
polymers within living tissues). In the absence
of physical constraints, dendritic polymers
can continue branching (and growing) until
they form a complete (hollow) sphere. Such
spheres are potentially useful for protecting
and "delivering" a fragile pharmaceutical
molecule to specific tissues within the body.

See also POLYMER, DENDRIMERS

Denitrification The process (i.e., internal respiration) by which denitrifying bacteria (e.g.,

in soil) convert nitrates to gaseous nitrogen or
nitrous oxide, which then enters the atmosphere.

Reduction of nitrate to nitrites or into gaseous
oxides of nitrogen or even into free nitrogen
by organisms.

See also NITRATES, BACTERIA, RESPIRA-
TION, REDUCTION (IN A CHEMICAL
REACTION)

Denitrifying Bacteria See DENITRIFICA-
TION

De Novo Sequencing The sequencing of protein or DNA molecules via techniques that do
not depend on having in your possession some
preexisting knowledge of what the sequence
of that particular molecule is.

See also SEQUENCING (OF PROTEIN MOL-
ECULES), SEQUENCING (OF DNA MOL-
ECULES), SEQUENCE (OF A PROTEIN
MOLECULE), SEQUENCE (OF A DNA
MOLECULE)

Deoxynivalenol A mycotoxin (i.e., toxin that
is naturally produced by a fungus under certain conditions), which, under specific temperature or moisture conditions, is sometimes
produced by certain *Fusarium* fungi (e.g.,
Fusarium graminearum) growing in some
grains (e.g., wheat *Triticum aestivum* or corn
or maize *Zea mays* L.).

Deoxynivalenol is also known as DON, as well
as "vomitoxin," because certain animals
(especially swine) will often vomit after they
have consumed grain that contains deoxynivalenol, owing to its toxicity.

See also TOXIN, DON, MYCOTOXINS, FUN-
GUS, *FUSARIUM*

Deoxyribonucleic Acid (DNA) Discovered
by Frederick Miescher in 1869, it is the chemical basis for genes. The chemical building
blocks (molecules) of which genes (i.e.,
paired nucleotide units that code for a protein
to be produced by a cell's machinery, such as
its ribosomes) are constructed. Every inherited characteristic has its origin somewhere in
the code of the organism's complement of
DNA. The code is made up of subunits called
nucleic acids. The sequence of the four
nucleic acids is interpreted by certain molecular systems in order to produce the proteins
required by an organism. The structure of the
DNA molecule was elucidated in 1953 by

D

James Watson, Francis Crick, and Maurice Wilkins. The DNA molecule is a linear polymer made up of deoxyribonucleotide repeating units (composed of the sugar 2-deoxyribose, phosphate, and a purine or pyrimidine base). The bases are linked by a phosphate group, joining the 3' position of one sugar to the 5' position of the next sugar. Most molecules are double-stranded and antiparallel, resulting in a right-handed helix structure that is held together by hydrogen bonds between a purine on one chain and pyrimidine on the other chain. DNA is the carrier of genetic information, which is encoded in the sequence of bases; it is present in chromosomes and chromosomal material of cell organelles such as mitochondria and chloroplasts, and also in some viruses.

See also A-DNA, B-DNA, cDNA, Z-DNA, TRANSCRIPTION, ANTIPARALLEL, DOUBLE HELIX, MESSENGER RNA (mRNA), NUCLEOTIDE, PROTEIN, RIBOSOMES, GENETIC CODE, GENE, CHROMOSOMES, CHROMATIDS, CHROMATIN, MITOCHONDRIAL DNA, CYTOPLASMIC DNA, NUCLEAR DNA

Deprotection (of a peptide). See HF CLEAVAGE

Derepression The opposite of **repression (of gene transcription or translation)**. It typically occurs via removal of the **repressor protein** from the applicable site on relevant DNA (or RNA) molecule.

See also REPRESSION (of gene transcription or translation), REPRESSOR (PROTEIN), GENE, TRANSCRIPTION, TRANSLATION, DEOXYRIBONUCLEIC ACID (DNA)

Desaturase An enzyme "family" (group) that is present within the soybean plant and other oilseed crops (e.g., sunflower, canola, and corn or maize). One or more desaturases are involved in the synthesis "pathway" by which oilseed crops produce unsaturated fatty acids (e.g., linoleic acid). A desaturase is also involved in production of beta-carotene (in some plants).

See also ENZYME, FATS, STEAROYL-ACP DESATURASE, DELTA 12 DESATURASE, SOYBEAN PLANT, HIGH-OLEIC SUNFLOWERS, PATHWAY, LINOLEIC ACID, FATTY ACID, UNSATURATED FATTY ACID, GOLDEN RICE, BETA-CAROTENE

Desert Hedgehog Protein (Dhh) See HEDGEHOG PROTEINS

Desferroxamine Manganese An iron-chelating agent. It chemically binds to iron atoms in the blood, thus trapping the iron atoms. The molecule also acts as an hSOD mimic by capturing harmful oxygen free radicals in the blood before they damage the walls of blood vessels. Recent research indicates that desferroxamine manganese may be useful in blocking the onset of cataract.

See also HUMAN SUPEROXIDE DISMUTASE (hSOD), XANTHINE OXIDASE, LAZAROIDS

Desulfovibrio A genus of bacteria that reduces sulfate to H_2S (hydrogen sulfide). Energy is obtained by the oxidation of H_2 or organic molecules. Not a strict autotroph because CO_2 cannot be used as a sole carbon source.

See also REDUCTION (IN A CHEMICAL REACTION), AUTOTROPH

Dextran A polysaccharide produced by yeasts and bacteria as an energy storage reservoir (analogous to fat in humans). Consists of glucose residues, joined almost exclusively by alpha-1,6 linkages. Occasional branches (in the molecule) are formed by alpha-1,2, alpha-1,3, or alpha-1,4 linkages. Which linkage is used depends on the species of yeast or bacteria producing the dextran.

See also POLYSACCHARIDES

Dextrorotary (D) Isomer A stereoisomer that rotates the plane of plane-polarized light to the right (dextro = "right").

See also STEREOISOMERS, LEVOROTARY (L) ISOMER, POLARIMETER

DGGE Acronym for **denaturing gradient gel electrophoresis**.

See DENATURING GRADIENT GEL ELECTROPHORESIS

DHA See DOCOSAHEXANOIC ACID (DHA)

dHPLC Acronym for **denaturing high-pressure liquid chromatography**.

See HPLC, DENATURATION

Diabetes A group of diseases in which the body either does not synthesize (i.e., "manufacture") insulin, or else its tissues are insensitive to the insulin that it does synthesize.

D

Approximately 5 to 10% of all people with diabetes are unable to synthesize insulin (e.g., because their insulin-making tissue was destroyed by autoimmune disease). Approximately 90 to 95% of all people with diabetes are insensitive to the insulin their body synthesizes. One of the many impacts of diabetes is an increase in the sorbitol content within cells, which causes swelling of certain cells because of osmotic pressure. When cells thus swell in the lens of the eye, it can lead to diabetic cataracts.

See also PANCREAS, INSULIN, INSULIN-DEPENDENT DIABETES MELLITUS (IDDM), FLUX, CELL, AUTOIMMUNE DISEASE, BETA CELLS, N-3 FATTY ACIDS, CALPAIN-10, TYPE I DIABETES, TYPE II DIABETES, HAPTOGLOBIN, OSMOTIC PRESSURE

Diacylglycerols Molecules that consist of two fatty acids attached to a glycerol "backbone." Research during the 1990s indicated that consumption of vegetable oils (e.g., used in frying foods) containing primarily diacylglycerols (vs. typical triacylglycerols) is less likely to result in its being deposited as body fat (adipose tissue).

See also FATTY ACID, SATURATED FATTY ACIDS (SAFA), UNSATURATED FATTY ACID, ADIPOSE, TRIACYLGLYCEROLS

Diadzein See DAIDZEIN, ISOFLAVONES

Dialysis The separation of low-molecular-weight compounds from high-molecular-weight components in a solution by diffusion through a semipermeable membrane, frequently utilized to remove salts; also used to remove biological effectors (such as nicotinamide adenine dinucleotides, nucleotide phosphates, etc.) from polymeric molecules such as protein, DNA, or RNA. Commonly used membranes have a molecular weight cutoff (threshold) of around 10,000 Da, but other membrane pore sizes are available.

See also HOLLOW FIBER SEPARATION, ACTIVE TRANSPORT

Diamond v. Chakrabarty See CHAKRABARTY DECISION

Diastereoisomers Four variations of a given molecule, consisting of a pair of stereoisomers about a second asymmetric carbon atom for each of the two isomers of the first asymmetric carbon atom.

See also STEREOISOMERS, CHIRAL COMPOUND

DICER See RNA INTERFERENCE (RNAi)

Dicer Enzymes A "family" of RNAse III dsRNA-specific nucleases (i.e., nucleic-acid-digesting enzymes).

See RNA INTERFERENCE (RNAi)

Differential Display A technique of **gene expression analysis** in which two different tissues (or *same* tissue under two different conditions) are compared in terms of proteins expressed.

See also GENE, GENE EXPRESSION, GENE EXPRESSION ANALYSIS, GENETIC CODE, EXPRESS, PROTEIN, GENE EXPRESSION PROFILING, MICROARRAY (TESTING)

Differential Splicing A cellular process in which numerous mRNA molecules can be created by the joining of different exons (i.e., RNA sequence fragments) within a single RNA molecule.

See also CELL, TRANSCRIPTION, MESSENGER RNA (mRNA), SPLICING, RIBONUCLEIC ACID (RNA), SPLICE VARIANTS, SPLICING JUNCTIONS

Differentiation Refers to processes by which cells of a single type (e.g., stem cells, embryonic stem cells, etc.) become multiple, different types of (specialized) cells.

See also CELL, CELL DIFFERENTIATION, EPIGENETIC, STEM CELLS, STEM CELL ONE, STEM CELL GROWTH FACTOR (SCF), TOTIPOTENT STEM CELLS, COLONY-STIMULATING FACTORS (CSFs), EMBRYONIC STEM CELLS, HUMAN EMBRYONIC STEM CELLS, HEDGEHOG SIGNALING PATHWAY, HEDGEHOG PROTEINS, GRANULOCYTE-MACROPHAGE COLONY-STIMULATING FACTOR (GM-CSF), MULTIPOTENT, ADULT STEM CELL, MULTIPOTENT ADULT STEM CELL, RETINOID X RECEPTOR (RXR), MICRORNAs

Digestion (within chemical production plants) Breakdown of feedstocks by various processes (chemical, mechanical, and biological) to yield their desired building-block components for inclusion as raw materials in subsequent chemical or biological processes.

Digestion (within organisms) The enzyme-enhanced hydrolysis (breakdown) of major nutrients (food) in the gastrointestinal system to yield their building-block components (to the organism), such as amino acids, fatty acids, or other essential nutrients.

See also HYDROLYSIS, FATS, PROTEIN, AMINO ACID, ESSENTIAL AMINO ACIDS, ESSENTIAL NUTRIENTS, FATTY ACID, ESSENTIAL FATTY ACIDS, LIPASE, IDEAL PROTEIN CONCEPT, ENZYME, PROTEASES, PROTEOLYTIC ENZYMES, ABSORPTION, TRYPSIN, LECITHIN, PROTEIN-DIGESTIBILITY-CORRECTED AMINO ACID SCORING (PDCAAS)

Diglycerides See TRIGLYCERIDES

Dimeric RNase III Ribonucleases Also sometimes known as dicer enzymes.

See RNA INTERFERENCE (RNAi)

Dip-Pen Lithography See DIP-PEN NANO-LITHOGRAPHY

Dip-Pen Nanolithography Refers to the use of atomic force microscopy (AFM) to apply very small amounts of specific molecules to very precise locations (e.g., probes on the surface of a **microarray**, or DNA or thiol molecules on the individual "pieces" of a **self-assembling molecular structure**).

See also ATOMIC FORCE MICROSCOPY, MICROARRAY (TESTING), SELF-ASSEMBLY (OF A LARGE MOLECULAR STRUCTURE), DIRECTED SELF-ASSEMBLY, PROBE, DEOXYRIBONUCLEIC ACID (DNA), THIOL GROUP

Diphtheria Antitoxin Discovered by Emil von Behring in 1900.

See ANTITOXIN, ENTEROTOXIN

Diploid The state of a cell in which each of the chromosomes, except for the sex chromosomes, is always represented twice (46 chromosomes in humans); in contrast to the haploid state, in which each chromosome is represented only once.

See also DIPLOPHASE, CHROMOSOMES, HOMOZYGOUS, TRIPLOID

Diplophase A phase in the life cycle of an organism in which the cells of the organism have two copies of each gene. When this state exists, the organism is said to be diploid.

See also DIPLOID, GENE, HOMOZYGOUS, CELL

Direct Transfer Refers to methods of inserting a gene directly into a cell's DNA without the use of a vector. One example of direct transfer is electroporation.

See also GENE, GENETIC ENGIEERING, VECTORS, CELL, DEOXYRIBONUCLEIC ACID (DNA), ELECTROPORATION

Directed Evolution See DNA SHUFFLING

Directed Self-Assembly Refers to use of:

1. Carefully preplanned synthetic molecular components that can be caused to self-assemble via affinity or hybridization to each other of DNA or thiol-molecular segments attached to the relevant synthetic molecular components.

2. An atomic force microscope stylus tip to apply specific molecular (e.g., thiol-, DNA, etc.) segments to surfaces such as metals, oxides, etc., in order for those preapplied DNA segments to thereby direct (via hybridization to each other) the assembly of nanometer-scale structures such as gene chips, catalysts, nanoscale circuits, etc.

See also DEOXYRIBONUCLEIC ACID (DNA), HYBRIDIZATION (MOLECULAR GENETICS), DIP-PEN NANOLITHOGRAPHY, SELF-ASSEMBLING MOLECULAR MACHINES, NANOMETER (nm), TEMPLATE, CATALYST, GENE CHIPS, SELF-ASSEMBLY (OF A LARGE MOLECULAR STRUCTURE), THIOL GROUP

Disaccharides Carbohydrates consisting of two covalently linked monosaccharide units, hence "di" for "two."

See also OLIGOSACCHARIDES, MONOSACCHARIDES, POLYSACCHARIDES

Displacement Loop The unique DNA molecular structure that is created when the (normally) double-stranded DNA molecule takes up or incorporates an inserted third strand of DNA or RNA.

See also DEOXYRIBONUCLEIC ACID (DNA), DUPLEX, D LOOP, RIBONUCLEIC ACID (RNA)

Dissimilation The breakdown of food material to yield energy and building blocks for cellular synthesis.

See also DIGESTION (WITHIN ORGAN-ISMS)

Dissociating Enzymes See HARVESTING ENZYMES

Distribution See ADME TESTS, PHARMA-COKINETICS

Disulfide Bond An important type of covalent bond formed between two sulfur atoms of different cysteines in a protein molecule (or one each in two different protein molecules). Disulfide bonds (linkages or bridges) contribute to holding proteins together and also help provide the internal structure (conformation) of the protein molecule.

See also PROTEIN, CYSTEINE, CYSTINE, CONFORMATION, TERTIARY STRUC-TURE

Disulphide Bond See DISULFIDE BOND

Diversity (within a species) Refers to the genetic variation that exists within a population (of organisms) in a species. For example, black cattle and white cattle, or both toxic and nontoxic strains or serotypes of *Escherichi coliform (E. coli)* bacteria. This diversity is due to one or more single-nucleotide polymorphisms (SNPs) in each individual's genome (DNA) within the population of organisms.

See also SPECIES, SINGLE-NUCLEOTIDE POLYMORPHISMS (SNPs), POLYMOR-PHISM (GENETIC), NUCLEOTIDE, ORGANISM, STRAIN, SEROTYPES, *ESCHERICHIA COLIFORM (E.COLI)*, *ESCHERICHIA COLIFORM 0157:H7 (E. COLI 0157:H7)*

Diversity Biotechnology Consortium A non-profit U.S. organization that was formed in August 1994 by a group of research institutions and companies. The Consortium's first president was Stuart A. Kauffman of the Santa Fe Institute. The Consortium's purpose is to further the use of molecular diversity as a tool in drug design and in the study of mutating viruses.

See also MOLECULAR DIVERSITY, RATIO-NAL DRUG DESIGN, DIVERSITY ESTI-MATION (OF MOLECULES), MOLECU-LAR BIOLOGY, VIRUS, MUTATION, MUTANT, SITE-DIRECTED MUTAGENE-SIS (SDM), COMBINATORIAL CHEMIS-TRY, COMBINATORIAL BIOLOGY

Diversity Estimation (of molecules) See COMBINATORIAL CHEMISTRY

DNA See DEOXYRIBONUCLEIC ACID (DNA)

DNA Analysis See DNA PROFILING

DNA Bridges Large segments of DNA whose sequence (i.e., composition) is known or mapped entirely. Those sequences are then utilized by scientists to piece together (i.e., in "bridging" the DNA segments) and assemble a (more) complete map (e.g., of an organism's chromosome or genome).

See also DEOXYRIBONUCLEIC ACID (DNA), GENETIC MAP, SEQUENCE (OF A DNA MOLECULE), CHROMOSOME, GENOME, SEQUENCE MAP, SHOTGUN SEQUENCING

DNA Chimera One DNA molecule composed of DNA from two different species.

See also CHIMERA

DNA Chip See BIOCHIPS, MULTIPLEXED ASSAY, GENE EXPRESSION ANALYSIS, PROTEOMICS, NANOPARTICLES

DNA Fingerprinting See DNA PROFILING

DNA Fragmentation The cleavage (i.e., "chewing up") of DNA (within a cell) at inter-nucleosomal sites on that DNA molecule.

DNA fragmentation during cellular apoptosis prevents the (aberrant) cell's DNA from causing any further problems in the organism's body.

See also DEOXYRIBONUCLEIC ACID (DNA), CELL, NUCLEOSOME, APOPTO-SIS

DNA Glycosylase Refers to a category of enzymes (within cells) that initiate repair of cell's (damaged) DNA under certain circumstances.

See also ENZYME, CELL, DEOXYRIBONU-CLEIC ACID (DNA)

DNA Gyrase An enzyme, also known as **helix unwinding protein,** that works to "relax" the tension within a supercoiled DNA molecule.

See also ENZYME, DEOXYRIBONUCLEIC ACID (DNA), HELIX, DOUBLE HELIX, SUPERCOILING, POSITIVE SUPERCOIL-ING, DNA TOPOISOMERASE, PROTEIN

DNA Helicase See HELICASE

DNA Ligase Discovered during the 1960s by Baldomero Olivera, it is an enzyme that creates a phosphodiester bond between the 3' end of one DNA segment and the 5' end of another while they are base-paired to a template strand. The enzyme seals (joins) the ends of single-stranded DNA in a duplex DNA chain. DNA ligase constitutes a part of the DNA repair mechanism available to the cell.

See also NICK, LIGASE, DEOXYRIBONU-CLEIC ACID (DNA), GENE REPAIR (NAT-URAL), DUPLEX

DNA Marker See MARKER (DNA MAR-KER)

DNA Melting Temperature See MELTING TEMPERATURE (OF DNA) (Tm)

DNA Methylase Refers to a category of enzymes (within a cell) that catalyze the addition of methyl groups (-CH3) to DNA molecules. The methyl groups (-CH3) thereby inactivate relevant genes in the cell's DNA.

See also ENZYME, CELL, CATALYST, GENE, DNA METHYLATION

DNA Methylation Refers to a process resulting in a DNA molecule that is saturated with methyl groups (i.e., methyl submolecule groups CH3 have attached themselves to the DNA molecule's "backbone" at all possible locations on that DNA molecule). DNA methylation is used by healthy cells for the following:

- "Turn off" certain genes when those particular genes are not needed (e.g., they turn off genes involved in juvenile development after the organism reaches adulthood).
- Prevent the spread or activation of potentially harmful nucleic acids (e.g., certain transposable elements) within the organism's genome.

DNA methylation (of cell genes that would normally prevent inappropriate cell division or proliferation) also occurs in some cancers.

See also DEOXYRIBONUCLEIC ACID (DNA), METHYLATED, CELL, GENE, IMPRINTING, CANCER, TRANSCRIP-TION, GENETIC CODE, MESSENGER RNA (mRNA), P53 GENE, TUMOR SUP-PRESSOR GENES, EPIGENETIC, SHORT INTERFERING RNA (siRNA)

DNA Microarray Initially developed by Patrick Brown during the 1980s, these microarrays enable analysis of the levels of expression of genes in an organism, or comparison of gene expression levels (e.g., between diseased and nondiseased tissues) via hybridization of messenger RNA (mRNA) to its counterpart DNA sequence when biological samples containing DNA (e.g., in liquid) are passed over the array surface.

To manufacture the DNA microarray, cellular mRNA is used to make segments of complementary DNA (cDNA) in lengths of approximately 500 to 5000 base pairs long, using the reverse transcriptase polymerase chain reaction (RT-PCR). These cDNA segments are then attached to a nylon or glass surface at **known** spots, so when hybridization of sample DNA occurs, the location of the spot tells what DNA was in the sample.

Another way to manufacture another type of DNA microarray is to similarly attach oligonucleotides or peptide nucleic acids of known sequence (composition) at known spots on the nylon or glass surface and pass the biological sample containing DNA (e.g., in liquid) over that surface to identify the DNA in the sample, by the spot it hybridizes to.

See also GENE, ORGANISM, BIOCHIPS, MICROFLUIDICS, DEOXYRIBONU-CLEIC ACID (DNA), MESSENGER RNA (mRNA), HYBRIDIZATION (MOLECU-LAR GENETICS), EXPRESS, GENE EXPRESSION ANALYSIS, PROTEOMICS, MICROARRAY (TESTING), MULTI-PLEXED ASSAY, OLIGONUCLEOTIDE, NUCLEIC ACIDS, SEQUENCE (OF A DNA MOLECULE), BIOINFORMATICS

DNA Polymerase Discovered in 1956 by Arthur Kornberg, it is an enzyme that catalyzes the synthesis of DNA. It does this by catalyzing the addition of deoxyribonucleotide residues to the free 3'-hydroxyl end of a DNA molecular chain, starting from a mixture of the appropriate triphosphorylated bases, which are dATP, dGTP, dCTP, and dTTP. This chemical reaction is reversible, and hence DNA polymerase also functions as an exonuclease.

See also ENZYME, EXONUCLEASE, TAQ DNA POLYMERASE, DEOXYRIBONU-CLEIC ACID (DNA), SYNTHESIZING (OF DNA MOLECULES)

DNA Probe Also called gene probe or genetic probe. Short, specific (complementary to desired gene) artificially produced segments of DNA used to combine with and detect the presence of specific genes (or shorter DNA segments) within a chromosome. If a DNA probe of known composition and length is mingled with pieces of DNA (genes), from a chromosome, the probe will cling to its exact counterpart in the "chromosomal DNA pieces" (genes), forming a stable double-stranded hybrid. The presence of this (now) "labeled" probe is detected visually or with the aid of another detection instrument. Because the composition of the DNA probes is known, scientists can riffle through a chromosome, spotting segments of DNA (i.e., genes) that seem to be linked to genetic diseases.

See also MUSCULAR DYSTROPHY (MD), PROBE, POLYMERASE CHAIN REACTION (PCR), GENE, POLYMERASE CHAIN REACTION (PCR) TECHNIQUE, CHROMOSOMES, DOUBLE HELIX, DUPLEX, HYBRIDIZATION (MOLECULAR GENETICS), HYBRIDIZATION SURFACES, DEOXYRIBONUCLEIC ACID (DNA), HOMEOBOX, RAPID MICROBIAL DETECTION (RMD), SOUTHERN BLOT ANALYSIS

DNA Profiling Invented in 1985 by Alec Jeffreys, it is a technique used by forensic (i.e., crime-solving) chemists to match biological evidence (e.g., a blood stain) from a crime scene to the person (e.g., the assailant) involved in that particular crime. DNA profiling involves the use of RFLP (restriction oligonucleotide/polymerase fragment length polymorphism) analysis or ASO/PCR (allele-specific chain reaction) analysis to analyze the specific sequence of bases (i.e., nucleotides) in a piece of DNA taken from the biological evidence. Because the specific sequence of bases in DNA molecules is different for each individual (owing to DNA polymorphism), a criminal's DNA can be matched to that of the evidence to prove guilt or innocence. Biological evidence may include among other things blood, hair, nail fragments, skin, and sperm.

See also DEOXYRIBONUCLEIC ACID (DNA), RESTRICTION FRAGMENT LENGTH POLYMORPHISM (RFLP) TECHNIQUE, POLYMORPHISM (CHEMICAL), POLYMERASE CHAIN REACTION (PCR) TECHNIQUE, ALLELE, NUCLEOTIDE, NUCLEIC ACIDS, OLIGOMER, GENETIC CODE, INFORMATIONAL MOLECULES, OLIGIONUCLEOTIDE, CODON, NANOPARTICLES

DNA Repair Refers to the several ways in which damaged DNA gets repaired within living cells. Some examples include:

- The mismatch-repair system
- The "SOS" repair system
- The CHK1 and CHK2 signaling pathways
- MAPKAP kinase-2 (sometimes called CHK3 signaling pathway)
- DNA photolyase enzymes, which harness light energy to repair DNA that has been damaged by ultraviolet light
- Editing

See also CELL, DEOXYRIBONUCLEIC ACID (DNA), DNA LIGASE, MISMATCH REPAIR, SOS REPAIR SYSTEM, SOS RESPONSE (IN *ESCHERICHIA COLI* BACTERIA), GENE REPAIR (NATURAL), UBIQUITIN, SIGNALING, PATHWAY, PHOTOLYASES, EDITING

DNA Shuffling Refers to a process in which humans break apart a DNA segment (e.g., a gene), shuffle the order of (i.e., change the order of) the relevant nucleotides within that sequence, and then recombine those nucleotides into an intact DNA segment. When repeated DNA shuffling is coupled to a gene expression and assessment or improvement process (e.g., each new "shuffled" DNA segment is expressed, and the resultant protein is evaluated against a desired goal) incorporating feedback to the DNA shuffling process, the process is sometimes called **directed evolution**.

For example, during 2003, Linda A. Castle and coworkers utilized this process to increase the activity of a GAT enzyme 10,000-fold.

See also DEOXYRIBONUCLEIC ACID (DNA), GENE, GENETIC CODE, NUCLEOTIDE, SEQUENCE (OF A DNA MOLECULE), EXPRESS, PROTEIN, GENE EXPRESSION ANALYSIS, ENZYME, ACTIVE SITE, TURNOVER NUMBER, GAT

DNA Synthesis See SYNTHESIZING (OF DNA MOLECULES)

DNA Typing See DNA PROFILING

DNA Vaccines Products in which "naked" genes (i.e., pieces of bare DNA) are used to stimulate an immune response (e.g., either a cellular immune response, humoral immune response, or otherwise raising antibodies against the pathogen from which the naked genes have arisen or have been derived).

See also DEOXYRIBONUCLEIC ACID (DNA), IMMUNE RESPONSE, CELLULAR IMMUNE RESPONSE, HUMORAL IMMUNITY, ANTIBODY, "NAKED" GENE, PATHOGEN, DNA VECTOR

DNA Vector A vehicle (such as a virus) for transferring genetic information (DNA) from one cell to another.

See also BACTERIOPHAGE, RETROVIRUSES, VECTOR

DNA-Dependent RNA Polymerase See RNA POLYMERASE

DNA-Directed RNA Interference Abbreviated **ddRNAi**, this refers to when a scientist makes RNA interference occur by causing cellular genes to code for production of the relevant **shRNA (i.e., short hairpin RNA**, a dsRNA that the cell's dicer enzymes turn into the siRNA strands that cause RNA interference).

See also RNA INTERFERENCE (RNAi), CELL, GENE, CODING SEQUENCE, RIBONUCLEIC ACID (RNA), SHORT INTERFERING RNA (siRNA), DICER ENZYMES, dsRNA, SHORT HAIRPIN RNA

DNA–RNA Hybrid A double helix that consists of one chain of DNA hydrogen-bonded to a chain of RNA by means of complementary base pairs.

See also HYBRIDIZATION (MOLECULAR GENETICS), HYBRIDIZATION (PLANT GENETICS), DOUBLE HELIX

DNase Deoxyribonuclease, an endonuclease enzyme "family" that degrades (cuts up) DNA molecules. DNase I is produced and secreted by the salivary glands, intestines, liver, and pancreas of animals. It has optimal activity (i.e., its greatest ability to cut up DNA molecules) at neutral pH (i.e., neither acidic nor basic). DNase II has optimal activity between pH 4.6 and 5.5 (i.e., in slightly acidic solutions).

See also ENZYME, DEOXYRIBONUCLEIC ACID (DNA), ENDONUCLEASES, PANCREAS, ACID, BASE (GENERAL)

Docking (in computational biology) Refers to utilization of specific (molecular visualization) software to "create" (*in silico*) and to **test via simulation a large number of the (theoretical) ways in which a given molecule (e.g., a new pharmaceutical candidate compound) could bind** (as ligand) to an enzyme molecule, receptor molecule, DNA molecule, etc.

See also RATIONAL DRUG DESIGN, COMPUTATIONAL BIOLOGY, *IN SILICO* SCREENING, *IN SILICO* BIOLOGY, ENZYME, RECEPTORS, DEOXYRIBONUCLEIC ACID (DNA)

Docosahexanoic Acid (DHA) One of the "omega-3" (n-3) highly unsaturated fatty acids (HUFA), DHA is important in the development of the human infant's brain, spinal cord, and retina tissues. DHA aids optimal brain and nervous system development in human infants and is required for optimal brain function throughout life. DHA comprises 40% of the polyunsaturated fatty acids in human brain tissue and 60% of all fatty acids in human eye tissue. DHA is naturally present in human breast milk and fish oil.

The human body converts linolenic acid (e.g., from consumption of soybean oil) to the two HUFA, **DHA** and **eicosapentanoic acid (EPA)**.

Research indicates that consumption of DHA also helps to reduce the risk of heart disease (by lowering blood pressure) and depression (via its effect in the brain).

See also POLYUNSATURATED FATTY ACIDS (PUFA), HIGHLY UNSATURATED FATTY ACIDS (HUFA), N-3 FATTY ACIDS, FATTY ACIDS, UNSATURATED FATTY ACIDS, ESSENTIAL FATTY ACIDS, LINOLENIC ACID, SOYBEAN OIL, EICOSANOIDS, EICOSAPENTANOIC ACID (EPA)

Domain (of a chromosome) May refer either to a discrete structural entity defined as a region within which supercoiling is independent of other domains or to an extensive region, including an expressed gene that has heightened sensitivity to degradation by the enzyme DNAse I.

D

See also GENE, EXPRESS, ENZYME, DNase

Domain (of a protein) A discrete continuous part of the amino acid sequence that can be equated with a particular function.

See also EXON, COMBINING SITE, EPITOPE, IDIOTYPE, PROTEIN, p53 PROTEIN, MINIMIZED PROTEINS

Dominant (gene) See DOMINANT ALLELE

Dominant Allele Discovered by Gregor Mendel in the 1860s, it is a gene that produces the same phenotype when it is heterozygous as it does when it is homozygous (i.e., a trait, or protein, is expressed even if only one copy of the gene is present in the genome).

See also GENETICS, RECESSIVE ALLELE, HETEROZYGOTE, HOMOZYGOUS, PHENOTYPE, GENOTYPE, GENOME

DON Abbreviation for the mycotoxin **deoxynivalenol**, which is produced by certain *Fusarium* fungi (e.g., *Fusarium graminearum*). DON is also known as "vomitoxin," because it can cause some animals to vomit if they consume it.

See also MYCOTOXINS, DEOXYNIVALENOL, FUSARIUM, FUNGUS, VOMITOXIN

Donor Junction The junction between the left 5' end of an exon and the right 3' end of an intron.

See also EXON, INTRON

Double Helix The natural coiled conformation of two complementary, antiparallel DNA chains. This structure was first put forward by Watson and Crick in 1953.

See also DEOXYRIBONUCLEIC ACID (DNA)

Down Promoter Mutations Those mutations that decrease the frequency of initiation of transcription. Down promoter mutations lead to the production of less mRNA than is the case in the nonmutated state.

See also mRNA, MUTATION, TRANSCRIPTION, DOWNREGULATING

Downregulating Phrase utilized to refer to regulatory sequences, chemical compounds (e.g., transcription factors), mutations (e.g., down promoter mutations), etc., that cause a given gene to express **less** of the protein that it normally codes for.

See also GENE, GENE EXPRESSION, REGULATORY SEQUENCE, TRANSCRIPTION FACTORS, DOWN PROMOTER MUTATIONS, PROTEIN, CODING SEQUENCE, TRANSCRIPTIONAL REPRESSOR, NEGATIVE CONTROL, RIBOSWITCHES, MICRORNAs, METHYLATED

DPN Acronym for **Dip-pen nanolithography**. See DIP-PEN NANOLITHOGRAPHY

DREs Acronym for **DNA regulatory elements**. See also DEOXYRIBONUCLEIC ACID (DNA), REGULATORY SEQUENCE, REGULATORY GENES, DOWNREGULATING

Drosophila The name of a type of fly (*Drosophila melanogaster*) that reproduces rapidly and is commonly utilized in genetics experiments; owing to its short life cycle (14 d) and simple genome (four chromosome pairs). Because of this, a large base of knowledge about *Drosophila* genetics has been accumulated by the world's scientific community. For example, of the nearly 300 "disease-causing" genes in the human genome, more than half of them have an analogous gene in the *Drosophila* genome. *Drosophila* was one of the first organisms to have its entire genome sequenced by man.

See also GENETICS, GENOME, GENETIC CODE, GENETIC MAP, CHROMOSOMES, COLD HARDENING, HOMEOBOX, SEQUENCING (OF DNA MOLECULES), GENE

Drought Tolerance Refers to a given crop's or plant's ability to survive a prolonged period of little or no rainfall. This may result from:

- The plant possessing a **drought tolerance trait** either inherently or because it was genetically engineered (e.g., insertion of genes to produce trehalose or to reduce level of vitamin C in stoma-containing leaf tissues).

- The crop possessing greater drought tolerance as a result of its being genetically engineered to possess a new trait allowing farmers to utilize husbandry practices that conserve topsoil moisture. For example, genetically engineered herbicide-tolerant soybeans enable U.S. farmers to utilize conservation tillage practices (e.g., no-tillage or low-tillage crop production) on most U.S. soybean hectares or acres, which results in the overall U.S. soybean crop's being more drought-tolerant than before.

See also DROUGHT TOLERANCE TRAIT, GENE, TRAIT, GENETIC ENGINEERING, TREHALOSE, HERBICIDE-TOLERANT CROP, SOYBEAN PLANT, CONSERVATION TILLAGE, NO-TILLAGE CROP PRODUCTION, LOW-TILLAGE CROP PRODUCTION

Drought Tolerance Trait Refers to the polygenic trait (resulting from multiple genes), whereby a given plant is able to survive a prolonged period of little or no rainfall.

For example, during the 1990s, Monty Jones crossed the Asian rice variety *Oryza sativa* with the African variety *Oryza glaberrima*. The result was NERICA ("new rice for Africa") variety, a drought-resistant rice.

In the future, it is hoped that genetic engineering can be utilized to transfer the **nine genes that confer drought resistance on the South African resurrection plant** (*Xerophyta viscosa*) into the corn or maize plant.

See also TRAIT, GENE, POLYGENIC, GENETIC ENGINEERING, CORN, TREHALOSE, DROUGHT TOLERANCE

dsDNA Acronym for the **double-stranded structure of DNA molecule**.

See also DEOXYRIBONUCLEIC ACID (DNA), DOUBLE HELIX

dsRNA Acronym for the **double-stranded structure of RNA molecule**. Among its other functions, dsRNA can induce degradation of its counterpart (i.e., "matching") mRNA, thereby causing RNA interference.

It has been shown that dsRNA can induce methylation of DNA in some species.

See also RIBONUCLEIC ACID (RNA), DOUBLE HELIX, RNA INTERFERENCE (RNAi), DNA METHYLATION

Duchenne Muscular Dystrophy (DMD) Gene See MUSCULAR DYSTROPHY (MD)

Duplex The double-helical structure of DNA (deoxyribonucleic acid).

See also DOUBLE HELIX, DEOXYRIBONUCLEIC ACID (DNA)

Dynamics Term used to refer to the study of changes in genetics (of a given population of organisms) over time.

See also GENETICS, ORGANISM

D

E

EAA See ESSENTIAL AMINO ACIDS

EAA See EXCITATORY AMINO ACIDS (EAAs)

Early Development This refers to the period of a phage infection before the start of DNA replication.

See also PHAGE, BACTERIOPHAGE, DEOXYRIBONUCLEIC ACID (DNA)

Early vs. Late Genes Those genes transcribed early in a bacteriophage-mediated infection process as compared to those genes transcribed sometime later. May require different "p factors" (sigma) for the recognition of promoters.

See also GENE, PROMOTER

Early vs. Late Proteins During viral infection, viral-specific proteins are synthesized at characteristic times after infection. They are called "early" and "late." Often under positive control of bacterial and viral sigma factors.

See also EARLY VS. LATE GENES, PROTEIN

Earthworms *Eisenia foetida* These worms live in the soil, and consume up to 10 t of organic matter (e.g., old crop plant stalks, husks, etc.) per acre (i.e., approx. 0.4 ha) per yr. In so doing, earthworms make the soil more fertile, because the process breaks down that organic matter into soil (i.e., when excreted by the earthworms). Earthworm tunnels also help aerate soil, which fosters healthy plant root systems.

See also LOW-TILLAGE CROP PRODUCTION, GLOMALIN, NO-TILLAGE CROP PRODUCTION

ECB See EUROPEAN CORN BORER (ECB)

E. coli See *ESCHERICHIA COLIFORM (E. COLI)*

E. coli 0157:H7 See *ESCHERICHIA COLIFORM 0157:H7 (E. COLI 0157:H7)*

Ecology The study of the interrelationships between organisms and their environment.

See also HABITAT

Ectodermal Adult Stem Cells Certain stem cells present within the bodies of adult organisms, which can be differentiated (via chemical signals) to give rise to cells of skin, hair, tooth enamel, mucous membranes, and some glandular tissues.

See also STEM CELLS, MULTIPOTENT ADULT STEM CELLS, CELL, ORGANISM, SIGNALING

Edible Vaccines Edible substances, bearing antigens, that cause activation of an animal's immune system via the animal's GALT (gut-associated lymphoid tissues). These "edible vaccines" are derived from transgenic plants (e.g., grains, tubers, fruits, etc.) or eggs (i.e., via the activation of the hen's immune system to cause the hen to secrete desired molecules into the eggs it lays).

See also GUT-ASSOCIATED LYMPHOID TISSUES (GALT), PEYER'S PATCHES, ANTIGEN, CELLULAR IMMUNE RESPONSE, MOLECULAR PHARMING,™ HUMORAL IMMUNITY, PLANTIGENS

Editing A term with several different meanings:

- In transcription — the process that removes the intron sequences during synthesis of mRNA from DNA and joins together the exon sequences.
- During DNA recombination — the process of ligating two segments of DNA together.
- During one type of gene therapy — the process of utilizing zinc finger proteins (coupled with relevant nucleases) to "correct" a "wrong" DNA sequence (e.g., a disease-causing SNP) within cells of a living organism.

See also DEOXYRIBONUCLEIC ACID (DNA), GENE, TRANSCRIPTION, MESSENGER RNA (mRNA), SEQUENCE (OF A DNA MOLECULE), INTRON, EXON, SPLICEOSOMES, GENETIC CODE, DNA

REPAIR, GENE REPAIR, RECOMBINA-
TION, RECOMBINANT DNA, LIGATION,
ZINC FINGER PROTEINS, GENE THER-
APY, SINGLE-NUCLEOTIDE POLYMOR-
PHISMS (SNPs)

EDTA Ethylenediamine tetraacetate. An
organic molecule that owing to the chemical
groups it contains and their juxtaposition
within that molecule, is able to chelate (bind)
certain other molecules such as divalent metal
cations. EDTA thus inhibits some enzymes
requiring such ions for activity.

See also CHELATION, COFACTOR,
CHELATING AGENT

EETI Acronym for **Ecballium elaterium
trypsin inhibitors**, a category of trypsin
inhibitors naturally present in some plants
(e.g., squash).

See also TRYPSIN INHIBITORS, KNOTTINS

EFA See ESSENTIAL FATTY ACIDS

Effector A class of (usually small) molecules
that regulates the activity of a specific protein
(e.g., enzyme) molecule by binding to a specific site on the protein. Control of (existing)
enzyme molecules may be achieved by combination of the effector with the enzyme. The
effector molecule may either physically block
the active site on the enzyme molecule or alter
its three-dimensional conformation. That conformation change results in a change in the
enzyme's catalytic activity.

Effector is a general term. Effector molecules
may be activators (cause an *increase* in the
enzyme's catalytic activity) or inhibitors (cause
a *decrease* in the enzyme's catalytic activity).

A special class of effector, known as an allosteric effector, binds to the enzyme molecule
at a site other than the enzyme's active site
(thereby activating or inhibiting).

See also PROTEIN, ENZYME, CONFORMA-
TION, ALLOSTERIC ENZYMES, ALLO-
STERIC SITE, ACTIVE SITE, FEEDBACK
INHIBITION, CATALYTIC SITE

Effector T Cells See DENDRITIC CELLS

EGF See EPIDERMAL GROWTH FACTOR
(EGF)

EGF Receptor A protein embedded in the
surface of the membranes of skin cells. The
receptor consists of: (1) an outside (of the cell
membrane) enzyme that recognizes epidermal growth factor (EGF) and binds to it and

(2) an enzyme on the inside of the cell membrane, which is of the tyrosine kinase class.
When free EGF comes in contact with an
EGF receptor, they bind (in a lock-and-key
fashion), and then enter the cell (through the
cell membrane) together (where EGF then
stimulates growth or division of cell via *ras*
protein and *ras* gene). The EGF receptor (and
receptors in general) is similar to a butler who
allows the EGF (a guest) to enter the cell
(home).

EGF receptor is also (over)expressed in the
plasma membranes of the cells of some tumors
in colorectal cancer, head and neck cancers,
lung cancer, pancreatic cancer, and some other
cancers.

See also ONCOGENES, PROTEIN, PLASMA
MEMBRANE, TRANSMEMBRANE PRO-
TEINS, *ras* GENE, *ras* PROTEIN, RECEP-
TORS, SIGNAL TRANSDUCTION, CAN-
CER

EGFR See EGF RECEPTOR

EHEC See ENTEROHEMORRHAGIC *E.
COLI*

EIA See ENZYME IMMUNOASSAY (EIA)

Eicosanoids A group of chemical compounds,
containing twenty carbon atoms in their
"molecular backbone," that the human body
synthesizes (i.e., "manufactures") from
arachidonic acid, docosahexanoic acid, or
other n-3 and n-6 fatty acid starting materials.
The term **eicosanoids** is from the Greek word
eicosa meaning "twenty."

One subgroup of eicosanoids is that of the prostaglandins (cyclic fatty acids that act as hormones in the body). For example, the COX-1
enzyme converts arachidonic acid to **constitutive prostaglandins**, and the COX-2
enzyme converts arachidonic acid to **inducible prostaglandins**.

Other subgroups of eicosanoids are that of the
leukotrienes (lipid mediator molecules involved
in the body's inflammation processes), the pros-
tacyclins, and the thromboxanes.

See also ARACHIDONIC ACID (AA),
DOCOSAHEXANOIC ACID (DHA),
CYCLOOXYGENASE, CONSTITUTIVE
ENZYMES, INDUCIBLE ENZYMES,
PROSTAGLANDINS, HORMONE, COX-1,
COX-2, LEUKOTRIENES, FATTY ACID,
n-3 FATTY ACIDS, n-6 FATTY ACIDS

Eicosapentaenoic Acid (EPA) See EICOSA-PENTANOIC ACID (EPA)

Eicosapentanoic Acid (EPA) One of the "omega-3" (n-3) polyunsaturated fatty acids (PUFA), EPA is important for the development of the human brain, retina tissue, and the prevention of high blood pressure, coronary heart disease (CHD), and some cancers.

The human body converts linolenic acid (e.g., from consumption of soybean oil) to the two highly unsaturated fatty acids (HUFA) — eicosapentanoic acid (EPA) and docosahexanoic acid (DHA).

See also N-3 FATTY ACIDS, POLYUNSATURATED FATTY ACIDS (PUFA), UNSATURATED FATTY ACIDS, ESSENTIAL FATTY ACIDS, CORONARY HEART DISEASE (CHD), CANCER, HIGHLY UNSATURATED FATTY ACIDS (HUFA), LINOLENIC ACID, SOYBEAN OIL, STEARIDONIC ACID

Eicosatetraenoic Acid See ARACHIDONIC ACID (AA)

ELAM-1 Also known as E-selectin, it is a selectin molecule that is synthesized by endothelial cells after (adjacent) tissue is infected. ELAM-1 molecules then help leukocytes to leave the bloodstream to fight the infection.

See also SELECTINS, LECTINS, ADHESION MOLECULES, LEUKOCYTES

Elastase An enzyme secreted by neutrophils (white blood cells that engulf pathogens) that catalyzes the cleavage (breakdown) of specific proteins that function to provide elasticity to certain tissues.

May be indirectly responsible for some autoimmune diseases, such as arthritis (which results from breakdown of cartilage tissue). Elastase may also be indirectly responsible for the emphysema (caused by loss of lung elasticity) that results from prolonged smoke inhalation.

When α-1 antitrypsin (anti-elastase) efficacy is reduced (via smoke), the now-unrestrained excess elastase destroys alveolar walls in the lungs by digesting elastic fibers and other connective tissue proteins.

See also LEUKOCYTES, NEUTROPHILS, PROTEOLYTIC ENZYMES

Electrolyte Any compound (e.g., salt, acid, base, etc.) that in aqueous solution dissociates into ions (charged atom-sized particles). Electrolytes may either be strong (completely or nearly completely dissociated) or weak (only partially dissociated).

See also ION

Electron Carrier A protein, such as a flavoprotein or cytochrome, that can gain and lose electrons reversibly and functions in the transfer of electrons from one carrier to another until the electron is taken up by a final molecule or atom such as oxygen.

See also PROTEIN, CYTOCHROME

Electron Microscopy (EM) A technique for greatly magnifying and visualizing very small entities such as viruses and even large molecules. The technique uses beams of electrons instead of light rays. Because of the physics involved, beams of electrons permit much greater magnification than is possible with a light microscope. Electron microscopes have been used to examine the structures of viruses, bacteria, pollen grains, molecules, etc.

See also VIRUS, BACTERIA, LABEL (RADIOACTIVE)

Electropermeabilization See ELECTROPORATION

Electrophoresis A technique for separating molecules based on the differential movement of charged particles through a matrix when subjected to an electric field. The term is usually applied to large ions of colloidal particles dispersed in water. The most important use of electrophoresis (currently) is in the analysis of proteins and then a technique known as gel electrophoresis is used.

Because the proportion of proteins varies widely in different diseases, electrophoresis can be used for diagnostic purposes.

Electrophoresis, through agarose or other gel matrices, is a common way to separate, identify, and purify plasmid DNA, DNA fragments resulting from digestion (of DNA) with restriction endonucleases, and RNA. Electrophoresis is also used to study bacteria and viruses, nucleic acids, and some types of molecules, including amino acids.

See also PROTEIN, AMINO ACID, BIOLUMINESCENCE, POLYACRYLAMIDE GEL ELECTROPHORESIS (PAGE), TWO-DIMENSIONAL (2-D) GEL ELECTROPHORESIS, CAPILLARY ELECTROPHORESIS, CHROMATOGRAPHY, GEL, AGAROSE, PLASMID, DEOXYRIBONU-

E

CLEIC ACID (DNA), RESTRICTION ENDONUCLEASES, RIBONUCLEIC ACID (RNA), BACTERIA, VIRUS, BIOMEMS

Electroporation A process that can be utilized to introduce a foreign gene into the genome of an organism. For example:

- In 1995, the U.S. company Dekalb Genetics Corp. received a patent for producing genetically engineered corn by introduction of a foreign gene into corn plant cells via electroporation.
- During 2005, Richard Heller and Adil Daud were able to deliver into human melanoma (skin cancer) tumor cells a gene that codes for production of interleukin-12 (IL-12) via electroporation. Because IL-12 helps stimulate the human immune system to try to combat melanoma, it is hoped that this will someday become a way to treat melanoma.

Electroporation, also called electroporesis, or electropermeabilization, uses a brief direct current electrical pulse to cause formation of "micropores" (tiny holes) in the surface of cells (or protoplasts, in the case of plants; e.g., suspended in a solution containing DNA sequences [genes]). After the genes enter the cell via the temporarily created micropores, the electrical pulse ceases, and the micropores close so that the genes cannot leave the cell. The cell then incorporates some of the new genetic material (genes) into its genetic complement (genome) and produces whatever product (i.e., a protein) the newly introduced gene codes for.

See also CODING SEQUENCE, GENETIC ENGINEERING, VECTOR, BIOLISTIC® GENE GUN, "EXPLOSION" METHOD, AGROBACTERIUM TUMEFACIENS, GENE, GENOME, CELL, CORN, PROTOPLAST, DEOXYRIBONUCLEIC ACID (DNA), PROTEIN, INTERLEUKIN-12 (IL-12), CANCER, TUMOR, MELANOMA, GENE DELIVERY

Electroporesis See ELECTROPORATION

ELISA (test for proteins) An enzyme-linked immunosorbent assay (hence the acronym) that can readily measure less than a nanogram (10^9 g) of a protein. This assay is more sensitive than simple immunoassay (tests) because one of the two antibodies used to bind and quantitate (measure) the protein's antigen, based on two concurrent epitopes within the protein, is attached to an enzyme. The enzyme can rapidly convert an added colorless substrate into a colored product or a nonfluorescent substrate into an intensely fluorescent product (thus enabling finer quantitation).

See also ABSORBANCE (A), IMMUNOASSAY, PROTEIN, ANTIGEN, ENZYME, NANOGRAM (ng), FLUORESCENCE

Elite Germplasm Refers to germplasm that is adapted (selectively bred) and optimized to new surroundings (i.e., environment). For example, corn or maize (*Zea mays* L.), which is native to the country of Mexico, has been adapted and optimized to grow in field conditions in many countries.

See also GERMPLASM, INTROGRESSION, MARKER-ASSISTED SELECTION, CORN

Ellagic Acid A naturally occurring plant phenol (phytochemical) that has been shown to possess general antioxidant properties and to help inhibit some cancers when consumed by humans.

Research also indicates that human consumption of ellagic acid inhibits growth of certain pathogenic bacteria such as *Salmonella*, *Campylobacter*, etc.

Ellagic acid is naturally present in red raspberries, strawberries, pomegranate (*Punica granatum* L.), etc.

See also PHYTOCHEMICALS, POLYPHENOLS, ANTIOXIDANTS, OXIDATIVE STRESS, CANCER, BACTERIA, PATHOGEN, SALMONELLA

Ellagic Tannin See ELLAGIC ACID

EM See ELECTRON MICROSCOPY (EM)

EMAS Acronym for **ecomanagement and audit scheme**.

Embryo Rescue Refers to the tissue culture techniques and technologies that are utilized to enable the fertilized embryo resulting from a "wide cross" (between two non-sexually-compatible plant species) to grow and mature into a seed-producing plant.

See also TRADITIONAL BREEDING METHODS, WIDE CROSS, TISSUE CULTURE

Embryology The study of the early stages in the development of an organism. In these stages, a single highly specialized cell, the egg, is transformed into a complex many-celled organism resembling its parents.

See also CELL, ORGANISM, ANTIANGIO-GENESIS, GAMETE, HEDGEHOG SIGNALING PATHWAY, IMPRINTING, MICRORNAs, INSULIN-LIKE GROWTH FACTOR-2 (IGF-2)

Embryonic Stem Cells See HUMAN EMBRYONIC STEM CELLS

EMEA See EUROPEAN MEDICINES EVALUATION AGENCY (EMEA)

Emulsion From the Latin *emulgere,* meaning to *"milk out."*

It is a stable dispersion of one liquid in a second, immiscible (i.e., nonmixable) liquid. For example, milk is an emulsion of oil (fat) in water and latex paint is an emulsion of paint resin in water.

Certain ingredients (e.g., β-conglycinin protein) help enable a greater content of the first liquid to be dispersed in the second liquid and make a given emulsion more stable (i.e., prevents the two liquids from separating over an extended period of time).

See also PROTEIN, BETA-CONGLYCININ

Enantiomers From the Greek word *enantios,* which means "opposite."

Enantiomers are a pair of nonidentical, mirror-image molecules. This means that both molecules are made up of the same atoms, that is, they have the same molecular formula, but the constituent groups that are attached to a carbon atom can be arranged in two different ways (forms) around the carbon atom. This gives rise to an asymmetric molecule that can exist in either of two mirror-image forms whose mirror images are not superimposable. A pair of these molecules is known as enantiomers. The four attached groups are all different from each other.

See also RACEMATE, OPTICAL ACTIVITY, CHIRAL COMPOUND, ENANTIOPURE

Enantiopure Refers to a compound (e.g., a pharmaceutical) that consists of only *one* of that compound's two possible enantiomers. Sometimes expressed in relative terms. For example, 98% enantiopure would refer to a compound that consists of 98% (of) desired enantiomer.

See also ENANTIOMERS, CHIRAL COMPOUND, RACEMATE, OPTICAL ACTIVITY

Endergonic Reaction A chemical reaction with a positive standard free-energy change (i.e., an "uphill" reaction). An (heat) energy-requiring reaction. A nonspontaneous reaction at ambient temperature.

See also EXERGONIC REACTION, FREE ENERGY

Endocrine Glands Glands that secrete their products (hormones) into the blood, which then carries them to their specific target organs. For example, adrenalin, produced in the adrenal glands, is carried to the heart (and other muscles) when needed during periods of stress. The endocrine glands are the pituitary, thyroids, adrenals, pancreas, ovaries (in females), and testes (in males). Endocrine glands are found in some invertebrates as well as in vertebrates.

See also HORMONE, ENDOCRINE HORMONES

Endocrine Hormones These are the products secreted by the endocrine glands. They help control long-term bodily processes, such as growth, lactation, sex cycles, and metabolic adjustment. The endocrine system and the nervous system are interdependent and often referred to collectively as the neuroendocrine system. For example, the juvenile hormone, found in insects and annelids, affects sexual maturation. There is currently great interest among scientists in the potential use of such hormones in the control of destructive insects.

See also ENDOCRINE GLANDS, HORMONE, PHEROMONES

Endocrinology The branch of science that studies the endocrine glands, hormones, and hormone-like substances.

See also ENDOCRINE GLANDS, HORMONE, ENDOCRINE HORMONES

Endocytosis Also called **receptor-mediated endocytosis**. The import of substances (e.g., hormones, viruses, and toxins) into a cell via specific receptor/ligand binding. The chemical entity under consideration binds to receptors located in the plasma (cell) membrane, which then invaginates (infolds), hence taking up the entity via "endosomes" (formed by pinching-off of infold to form a "bag") into vesicles located within the cell.

E

It is one route to deliver essential metabolites to cells (e.g., low-density lipoprotein), and it is a means to modulate the cell's responses to many protein hormones and growth factors (e.g., insulin, epidermal growth factor, and nerve growth factor). It is a route by which certain proteins targeted for destruction can be taken up and delivered to the cell's lysosomes. For example, phagocytic cells have receptors enabling them to take up **antigen–antibody complexes** for subsequent destruction by the phagocytic cell. This route is also a means exploited by certain viruses and toxins to gain entry into cells through the otherwise impervious cell membranes (e.g., used by the AIDS virus and the Semliki Forest virus). Disorders of endocytosis can lead to disease states (e.g., high cholesterol levels in the blood of people whose low-density lipoprotein receptors are impaired).

Drugs (e.g., certain painkillers) can be targeted to specific receptors via receptor mapping (RM) and receptor fitting (RF) for greater efficacy.

Certain drugs (e.g., streptavidin) can be delivered into the interior of specific cells via biotin-"coated" carbon nanotubes (to which the streptavidin binds until the cell is entered, whereupon it is released).

See also CELL, INVASIN, ADHESION MOLECULE, CD4 PROTEIN, EXOCYTOSIS, T CELL RECEPTORS, SIGNAL TRANSDUCTION, VAGINOSIS, RECEPTORS, RECEPTOR FITTING (RF), HIGH-DENSITY LIPOPROTEINS (HDLPS), LOW-DENSITY LIPOPROTEINS (LDLP), RECEPTOR MAPPING (RM), SIGNALING, NUCLEAR RECEPTORS, STREPTAVIDIN, CARBON NANOTUBES

Endodermal Adult Stem Cells Certain stem cells present within (adult) bodies of organisms that can be differentiated (via chemical signals) to give rise to cells of tongue, tonsils, the bladder/urethra, digestive tract, liver, pancreas, lung tissues, etc.

See also STEM CELLS, MULTIPOTENT ADULT STEM CELLS, CELL, ORGANISM, SIGNALING

Endoglycosidase An enzyme capable of hydrolyzing (i.e., breaking) interior bonds in the oligosaccharide molecular branches of a glycoprotein molecule. That is, the enzyme is capable of cutting a sugar-to-sugar bond anywhere within the sugar polymer molecule (depending, of course, on the specificity of the enzyme). This is in contrast to an exoglycosidase, which must cut away at the polymer from the outside, that is, from the free end, one unit (or section as the case may be) at a time.

See also EXOGLYCOSIDASE, GLYCOPROTEIN, ENZYME, OLIGOSACCHARIDES, RESTRICTION ENDOGLYCOSIDASES, HYDROXYLATION REACTION

Endometrium The lining of the uterus.

Endonucleases A class of enzymes capable of hydrolyzing (breaking) the interior phosphodiester bonds of DNA or RNA chains. As opposed to cleavage (by exonucleases) at the terminal bonds (ends) of a chain.

See also ENZYME, DNase 1, DNase 2, EXONUCLEASE, ENDOGLYCOSIDASE

Endophyte A microorganism (fungus or bacteria) that lives inside vascular tissues of plants (in spaces between plant cells). At least one company has incorporated the gene for a protein toxic to insects (taken from *Bacillus thuringiensis*) into an endophyte to confer insect resistance on a crop plant.

During 2002, Regina Redman and Russell Rodriguez discovered that certain fungi (that live inside a grass that grows in hot soils adjacent to magma-heated geysers) impart heat tolerance to the grass they live in. Redman, Rodriguez, and Joan Henson were later able to show that when these fungi were inserted into tomato and watermelon seedlings, those plants and roots were able to withstand far higher temperatures than before.

During 2004, Daniel van der Lelie and other researchers incorporated a gene enabling certain bacteria to break down (biodegrade) toluene into the endophytic bacteria that naturally colonize yellow lupine. Such colonized plants could be useful for bioremediation of toluene-polluted land sites.

When endophyte-infested fescue grass is fed to cattle, sheep, horses, or rabbits, it is generally toxic to those animals owing to mycotoxins or alkaloids produced by that endophyte.

See also MICROORGANISM, BACTERIA, *BACILLUS THURINGIENSIS (B.t.)*, FUNGUS,

PROTEIN, THERMODURIC, MYCOTOX-
INS, TREMORGENIC INDOLE ALKA-
LOIDS, BIOREMEDIATION

Endoplasmic Reticulum (ER) Discovered in
1963 by George Palade, the ER is a highly
specialized, complex network of branching,
intercommunicating tubules (surrounded by
membranes) found in the cytoplasm of most
animal and plant cells. The two types of ER
recognized are the rough ER and smooth ER.
ER that is covered with many ribosomes is
called rough, and the ER without or with fewer
ribosomes attached is called smooth. This
nomenclature is due to the appearance of the
ER under a high-magnification microscope.
The rough ER is very well developed to facilitate cells carrying on abundant protein synthesis, because proteins are synthesized (manufactured) in ribosomes.
See also CELL, CYTOPLASM, RIBOSOMES,
FATS, LIPIDS, PLASMA MEMBRANE,
PROTEIN, PHOSPHOLIPIDS, GERL

Endorphins Discovered during the 1970s by
U.S. and Scottish scientists, these are hormones produced in the brain that act as natural
painkillers. For example, runners and long-
distance walkers achieve something of a
"high" because of endorphins released by the
brain during long runs or walks.
See also ENKEPHALINS, CATECHOLA-
MINES, HORMONE

Endosome See ENDOCYTOSIS

Endosperm The interior portion of a plant
seed, beneath the outer hull (the portion that
people tend to eat, in food crops). In grains
(e.g., rice or corn or maize), the endosperm
consists primarily of starch (carbohydrate). In
legumes (e.g., beans), the endosperm contains
mainly protein, a small amount of carbohydrates and, sometimes, vegetable oil.
See also STARCH, CORN, SOYBEAN
PLANT, CARBOHYDRATES (SACCHA-
RIDES), SOYBEAN OIL, ALEURONE

Endospore A highly resistant, dormant inclusion body formed within certain bacteria. To
kill spores, temperatures above boiling are
usually needed. For this, pressure cookers and
autoclaves are required. Endospores have survival value because the spore can remain in a
nongrowing state for long periods of time and
then, under appropriate conditions, can be
induced to germinate and regenerate the original cell. Endospore formation may be viewed
as being akin to hibernation, that is, a kind of
"bacterial hibernation."
See also BACTERIA

Endostatin An **antiangiogenesis** human protein discovered by Judah Folkman. In concert
with angiostatin, it causes certain cancer
tumors to shrink.
See also PROTEIN, ANTIANGIOGENESIS,
ANGIOSTATIN, CANCER

Endothelial Cells These are the flat, roughly
plate-shaped cells that line the surface of all
blood vessels, the heart, and lymphatics within
the body. Endothelial cells possess transmembrane (i.e., through the cell membrane) molecules known as adhesion molecules, which
selectively allow the passage (from bloodstream
to tissues) of some molecules (e.g., leukocytes,
monocytes, hormones, etc.).
Endothelial cells are packed much tighter
together in the capillaries that provide blood
to the brain. This tighter packing limits the
size and kind of molecules that can pass into
the brain. This blood–brain barrier serves to
protect the sensitive brain tissue from pathogens or harmful molecules (e.g., toxins).
See also ENDOTHELIUM, VASCULAR
ENDOTHELIAL GROWTH FACTOR
(VEGF), ADHESION MOLECULES,
MONOCYTES, MITOGEN, SELECTINS,
BLOOD–BRAIN BARRIER (BBB), LEC-
TINS, ELAM-1, ATP SYNTHASE, OXIDA-
TIVE STRESS, CYCLOOXYGENASE

Endothelial Nitric Oxide Synthase (eNOS)
An enzyme within certain endothelial cells that
synthesizes ("manufactures") nitric oxide in
response to a number of different stimuli such as
certain hormones, certain neurotransmitters (e.g.,
bradykinin, acetylcholine, etc.), or the stress on
blood vessels due to high blood pressure.
See also NITRIC OXIDE SYNTHASE,
ENDOTHELIAL CELLS, ENZYME,
NITRIC OXIDE, ACETYLCHOLINE

Endothelin A "family" of peptides that cause
arteries to contract (which consequently
causes blood pressure to increase).
Research indicates that overproduction of
endothelin-1 can combine with plaque deposits (on interior walls of arteries) to clog those
arteries.

E

See also PEPTIDE, ATRIAL PEPTIDES, PLAQUE, CORONARY HEART DISEASE (CHD), POLYPHENOLS

Endothelium The layer of epithelial cells that line blood vessels throughout the body. The layer selectively allows the passage (from bloodstream to tissues) of nutrients, hormones, and other molecules that are essential for tissue growth and function. The endothelium is involved in the recovery and recycling of old red blood cells. It also produces:

- Nitric oxide, which causes neighboring smooth-muscle (blood vessel) cells to relax so that those (neighboring) blood vessels dilate, and the body's blood pressure is lowered
- Two compounds that prevent blood clotting: prostacyclin and Von Willebrand factor

See also ENDOTHELIAL CELLS, VASCULAR ENDOTHELIAL GROWTH FACTOR (VEGF), SELECTINS, LECTINS, ADHESION MOLECULES, NITRIC OXIDE, NITRIC OXIDE SYNTHASE, BILIRUBIN

Endotoxin A lipopolysaccharide (fat–sugar complex; poison, also known as LPS) that forms an integral part of the cell wall of Gramnegative bacteria. It is only released when the cell is ruptured. It can cause, among other things, septic shock and tissue damage. Pharmaceutical preparations are routinely tested for the presence of endotoxins. This is one reason why pharmaceuticals must be prepared in a sterile environment.

See also SEPSIS, BACTERIA, LIPIDS, POLYSACCHARIDES, TOXIN, CHOLERA TOXIN, GRAM NEGATIVE (G), GOOD MANUFACTURING PRACTICES (GMP)

Engineered Antibodies Chimeric monoclonal antibodies that are produced via genetic engineering of human antibody-producing cells (clones). For example, the genes coding for antilymphoma binding sites from a rat have been inserted into human antibody-producing cells to yield rat (antigen) binding sites mounted on human antibody "stems."

See also CHIMERIC PROTEINS, MONOCLONAL ANTIBODIES (MAb), ANTIBODY, GENETIC ENGINEERING, COMBINING SITE, LYMPHOCYTE, SEMISYNTHETIC CATALYTIC ANTIBODY

Enhanced Nutrition Crops See NUTRIENT ENHANCED™

Enhancer Refers to a specific sequence within the DNA of a eucaryotic organism that **enhances transcription** of (promoter of) a given gene. A given gene or promoter's enhancer may be located up to several thousand base pairs distant from that promoter.

See also DEOXYRIBONUCLEIC ACID (DNA), SEQUENCE (OF A DNA MOLECULE), GENE, PROMOTER, EUCARYOTE, ORGANISM, TRANSCRIPTION, EXPRESSIVITY, BASE PAIR (bp)

Enkephalins A class of hormones produced in the brain that act as natural painkillers. Discovered by John Hughes and Hans Kosterlitz in 1975, they are some of the endorphins.

See also ENDORPHINS

Enolpiruvil Shikimate See EPSP SYNTHASE

Enolpyruvil Shikimate See EPSP SYNTHASE

Enoyl-acyl Protein Reductase An enzyme that is utilized by bacteria in their synthesis ("manufacture") of fatty acids.

See also ENZYME, PROTEIN, BACTERIA, FATTY ACID, ESSENTIAL FATTY ACIDS

Ensiling The fermentation of (usually chopped-up) agricultural vegetation in order to preserve it. It is carried out for 1 to 2 weeks using either indigenous microorganisms (e.g., *Lactobacillus* spp.) or introduced microorganisms (to speed up the process, to yield product containing more nutrients for livestock, etc.) in the absence of oxygen (to prevent the growth of aerobic mold fungi).

When indigenous microorganisms are used, *Lactobacillus* spp. become the dominant microorganisms present, and heat is generated by the microorganisms within the vegetative mass (optimum temperature is 25 to 30°C, which is 77 to 86°F). Lactic acid is produced by the microorganisms, which inhibits the growth of bacteria that would normally putrefy the vegetation.

See also FERMENTATION, MICROORGANISM, AEROBIC, FUNGUS, OPTIMUM TEMPERATURE

Enterocytes Specialized cells within the ileum (lining the intestines) that recover and reclaim bile acids from the intestinal (food) mass. The process is as follows:

- Bile acids trigger the expression within enterocytes of IBABP (ileal bile-acid-binding protein), a cytosolic-binding protein.
- IBABP causes translocation or transport of the bile acid molecules into the portal circulation (carried to the liver).
- When these bile acids reach the liver, they activate FXR (farnesoid X receptors), which represses transcription of the genes involved in bile acid creation. This prevents overproduction of bile acids in the body.

See also CELL, DIGESTION (WITHIN ORGANISMS), BILE, BILE ACIDS, RECEPTORS, FARNESOID X RECEPTOR (FXR), GENE, TRANSCRIPTION, REPRESSION (OF GENE TRANSCRIPTION/TRANSLATION)

Enterohemorrhagic *E. coli* The several dozen (approximately 60 known) serotypes (strains) of *E. coli* bacteria that cause internal hemorrhaging in humans who ingest them. The toxin produced by these bacteria attacks the human kidney, which often leads to kidney failure or death.

See also *ESCHERICHIA COLI 0157:H7 (E. COLI 0157:H7)*, TOXIN, SEROTYPES, ENTEROTOXIN

Enterotoxin The category (i.e., intestinally active) of toxins, produced by certain bacterial strains or serotypes, which attack the body's internal organs. For example, the serotype of *Escherichia coliform* bacteria known as *E. coli 0157:H7* attacks the kidneys and other internal organs of humans, also causing internal bleeding and sometimes death.

See also TOXIN, BACTERIA, *ESCHERICHIA COLIFORM 0157:H7*, ENTERPHEMORRHAGIC *E. COLI*, SEROTYPES, CHOLERA TOXIN

Enzyme An organic, protein-based catalyst that is not itself used up in the reaction. It is naturally produced by living cells to catalyze biochemical reactions. Each enzyme is highly specific with regard to the type of chemical reaction that it catalyzes and to the substances (called substrates) on which it acts. This specific catalytic activity and its control by other biochemical constituents are of primary importance in the physiological functions of all organisms. Although all enzymes are proteins, they may, and usually do, contain additional nonprotein components called coenzymes that are essential for catalytic activity.

See also APOENZYME, CATALYST, COENZYME, HOLOENZYME, SUBSTRATE (CHEMICAL), PROTEIN, HORMONE, EXTREMOZYMES, TURNOVER NUMBER

Enzyme Denaturation The loss of enzyme (catalytic) activity because of loss of the correct functional structure of the protein. Denaturation may be caused by factors such as exposure to heat and organic solvents and degradation of the enzyme molecule by proteases, oxygen, and acid or alkaline pH.

See also ENZYME, CONFORMATION, DENATURATION, EXTREMOZYMES

Enzyme Derepression Commonly known as induction (of an enzyme). Initially, a repressor protein is bound to a specific region of DNA. This binding inhibits transcription to mRNA, thus blocking the synthesis of the protein (enzyme) specified by the mRNA. When present, the inducer molecule binds to the repressor protein and inactivates it. Thus, the inhibition caused by the repressor protein is overcome and mRNA can be synthesized, which consequently leads to synthesis of the mRNA-specified protein (enzyme). The word "derepression" is sometimes used because the repressor protein is, by itself, active in repressing protein (enzyme) synthesis. Its repressive action is mitigated (derepressed) by the inducer molecule. Hence, derepression (or unrepression) of repression equals induction.

See also CONTINUOUS PERFUSION, ENZYME REPRESSION, ENZYME, REPRESSION (OF AN ENZYME)

Enzyme Immunoassay (EIA) See ELISA

Enzyme Repression Inhibition of enzyme synthesis caused by the availability of the product of that enzyme. On a molecular level, a repressor molecule (which could be, for example, the amino acid arginine) combines with a specific repressor protein that is present in the cell. This repressor molecule–repressor protein complex is then able to bind to a specific region of DNA at the initial end of the gene, which is called the operator region. It is in this region that the synthesis of mRNA is initiated. The repressor "roadblock" thus stops the synthesis of mRNA and, therefore, the synthesis of the protein is also blocked.

See also ENZYME, REPRESSION (OF AN ENZYME), ENZYME DEPRESSION

Enzyme-Linked Immunosorbent Assay See ELISA

Eosinophils Polymorphonuclear leukocytes made in the bone marrow. They circulate in the blood for a number of hours (three to eight) and then migrate into the tissue where they reside. They kill parasites too large to be phagocytized, by secreting substances that kill the parasites (hookworms, trichinosis, etc.). They also inhibit histamine release from mast cells and secrete chemicals that neutralize histamine. Allergy causes an increase in eosinophils. GM-CSF stimulates eosinophil production.

See also POLYMORPHONUCLEAR LEUKOCYTES (PMN), BASOPHILS, ANTIGEN, CELLULAR IMMUNE RESPONSE

EPD See EXPECTED PROGENY DIFFERENCES

Epidermal Growth Factor (EGF) A protein of 53 amino acids that greatly increases growth and reproduction of epidermal (skin) cells.

This protein also increases:

- Growth of wool in sheep
- Growth in more than 50% of human tumors

High concentrations of epidermal growth factor are found in human tears. EGF was discovered by Stanley Cohen.

See also PROTEIN, EGF RECEPTOR, GROWTH FACTOR, NERVE GROWTH FACTOR (NGF), AMINO ACID, FILLER EPITHELIAL CELLS, TUMOR

Epidermal Growth Factor Receptor See EGF RECEPTOR, HER-2 RECEPTOR, HER-2 GENE

Epigenetic Refers to mechanisms "in control" of (changing) gene expression (and interaction) primarily during development (e.g., of embryonic organism), which **do not require changes in actual gene or DNA sequences to occur**. From the Greek *epi* meaning "upon," this term more broadly refers to all the **nonclassical genetic/heredity** sources of a given organism's phenotype. For example:

- As a plant embryo develops into a seedling (juvenile in the case of an animal), different genes are expressed (or silenced) in that organism. For example, during 2002, researchers discovered that feeding certain compounds to pregnant inbred (yellow-colored) laboratory mice will cause their offspring to have **brown**-colored fur. When it results from consumption of certain foods or compounds, it is referred to as **nutritional epigenetics**.

- As a result of certain diseases afflicting the organism, different genes within the organism's DNA are silenced (or expressed). For example, hypoxia (e.g., occurring during tuberculosis or certain cancers) has been shown to result in epigenetic events within the bodies of relevant patients. When it results from cancer, it is referred to as **cancer epigenetics**.

- As an organism (especially during its embryo stage) interacts with its environment, some of those environmental impacts (e.g., temperature) cause certain genes to be expressed (or silenced). For example, the eggs of the saltwater crocodile (*Crocodylus porosus*) yield a larger fraction of male offspring when they are incubated (in the nest) at temperatures above 90°F (32°C) than when incubated at temperatures below 90°F (32°C).

- As an organism passes from the juvenile stage to later life stages. For example, the female honeybee (*Apis mellifera*) "switches on/off" approximately 40%

of her total genes as she matures from being a "nurse bee" (taking care of pupae while she is a juvenile) to being a "forager bee." During times in which the honeybee colony is in need of more forager bees (i.e., adults), the juveniles **mature faster** (to forager bees) than during normal times.

Epigenetic events include gene silencing, DNA methylation, chromatin remodeling, chromatin modification, histone modification, and gene imprinting.

At least one type of epigenetic regulation is caused by changes in the (molecular-scale) shape of an organism's chromatin. Such "chromatin remodeling" can be caused by introduction (into cell) of certain short interfering RNA (siRNA), certain transcription activators, etc.

See also GENE, EXPRESSION, PHENOTYPE, DEOXYRIBONUCLEIC ACID (DNA), HEREDITY, GENE SILENCING, DIFFERENTIATION, DNA METHYLATION, CHROMATIN, CHROMATIN REMODELING, HISTONES, SHORT INTERFERING RNA (siRNA), GENE IMPRINTING, IMPRINTING, ORGANISM, CENTRAL DOGMA (NEW), CANCER, CELL, HEDGEHOG SIGNALING PATHWAY

Epimerase An enzyme capable of the reversible interconversion of two epimers.

See also ENZYME, EPIMERS

Epimers Two stereoisomers differing in configuration.

See also CONFIGURATION, STEREOISOMERS

Episome (of a bacterium) An independent genetic element (DNA) that occurs inside a bacterium in addition to the normal bacterial cell genome. The episome can replicate either as an autonomous unit or as one integrated into the host genome. The F (fertility) factor is an episome.

See also GENOME, PLASMID, BACTERIA, DEOXYRIBONUCLEIC ACID (DNA)

Epistasis Interaction between nonallelic genes in which the presence of a certain allele at one locus prevents expression of an allele at a different locus.

See also ALLELE, GENE, EXPRESS, LOCUS

Epithelial Projections Projections that anchor the epidermis (surface skin) to the dermis (subsurface tissue). Growth of these projections is increased by epidermal growth factor during the wound-healing process.

See also EPIDERMAL GROWTH FACTOR (EGF)

Epithelium The prefix "epi" means on, above, or upon. The term refers to the membranous cellular tissue that covers a free surface or lines a tube or cavity of an animal body. It serves to enclose and protect the other tissues, produces secretions and excretions, and functions in assimilation.

See also ASSIMILATION, CADHERINS, ION CHANNELS

Epitope Also called antigenic determinant. The specific group of atoms (on an antigen molecule) that is recognized by (that antigen's) antibodies (thereby causing an immune response).

See also ANTIBODY, ANTIGEN, IDIOTYPE, HUMORAL IMMUNE RESPONSE

EPO See ERYTHROPOIETIN, EUROPEAN PATENT OFFICE

EPPO See EUROPEAN PLANT PROTECTION ORGANIZATION

EPSP Synthase Enolpyruvyl-shikimate phosphate synthase. An enzyme produced by virtually all plants and internally transported into their cells' chloroplasts; it is essential in a plant's metabolism biochemical pathway and for the biosynthesis (i.e., creation) of the aromatic (ring-shaped molecule) amino acids tyrosine, phenylalanine, and tryptophan, which are needed for plants to live.

Some (glyphosate-containing and sulfosate-containing) herbicides kill unwanted plants (e.g., weeds) by inhibiting EPSP synthase. By incorporating a gene that causes (over) production of CP4 EPSP synthase into several crops (e.g., soybeans, cotton, etc.), scientists have been able to help those crops to survive postemergence applications of glyphosate-containing herbicide. Additional resistance to glyphosate-containing and sulfosate-containing herbicides can be conferred on plants via incorporation into plants of a gene (GO) that causes those plants to produce glyphosate oxidase.

E

See also ENZYME, METABOLISM, GENE, PAT GENE, BAR GENE, GENETIC ENGINEERING, SOYBEAN PLANT, CORN, GLYPHOSATE, GLYPHOSATE OXIDASE, CP4 EPSPS, HERBICIDE-TOLERANT CROP, SULFOSATE, mEPSPS, CHLOROPLASTS, CHLOROPLAST TRANSIT PEPTIDE (CTP), TARGET (OF A HERBICIDE OR INSECTICIDE)

EPSPS See EPSP SYNTHASE, CP4 EPSPS, mEPSPS

ER See ENDOPLASMIC RETICULUM

erb B-2 Gene A designation that is sometimes utilized for the **Her-2/neu** gene.
See HER-2 GENE

ERBB2 Gene A designation that is sometimes utilized for the **Her-2/neu** gene.
See HER-2 GENE

Ergotamine A mycotoxin (i.e., metabolite produced by a fungus, which is toxic to animals and humans) produced by the fungus (*Claviceps spp.*) known as ergot. Ergotamine is an alkaloid vasoconstrictor, so its consumption can lead to severe constriction of blood vessels in the brain and extremities, causing hallucinations and dry gangrene. Humans whose bodies are deficient in vitamin A are especially vulnerable to ergotism ("ergot poisoning").
See also MYCOTOXINS, TOXIN, FUNGUS, VITAMIN

Erwinia caratovora A species of bacteria that can cause significant postharvest losses to potato farmers when it infects potatoes and causes "soft rot" (spoilage).
See also BACTERIA, SPECIES

Erwinia uredovora See GOLDEN RICE

Erythrocytes (Red Blood Cells) Hemoglobin-containing cells (manufactured in the bone marrow) that transport the oxygen from the lungs to the body tissues where it is needed.

Erythropoiesis The formation of red blood cells (erythrocytes) from pluripotent stem cells. Stimulated by the protein erythropoietin that is secreted by the kidneys.
People with damaged kidneys or with myeloma typically do not produce enough erythropoietin, so they often become anemic.
See also STEM CELLS, ERYTHROPOIETIN (EPO), PLURIPOTENT STEM CELLS

Erythropoietin (EPO) A glycoprotein cytokine produced in the kidneys that stimulates pluripotent stem cells in the bone marrow to differentiate, then increase the number of red blood cells. Erythropoietin can be used to help correct a variety of anemias.
See also GLYCOPROTEIN, CYTOKINES, ERYTHROCYTES, STEM CELLS, DIFFERENTIATION, PLURIPOTENT STEM CELLS

Escherichia coli See *ESCHERICHIA COLIFORM (E. COLI)*

Escherichia coli 0157:H7 (E. coli 0157:H7) See *ESCHERICHIA COLIFORM 0157:H7*

Escherichia coliform (E. coli) Named after Theodor Escherich, who isolated it in 1885, it is a bacterium that commonly inhabits the human intestine as well as the intestine of other vertebrates (i.e., animals possessing a skeleton). The most thoroughly studied of all bacteria, *Escherichia coli* is used in many microbiological experiments. It has historically been considered the workhorse of genetic engineering research, and genetically engineered versions have been used to produce human proteins (e.g., insulin).
One of the more exotic uses of genetically engineered *Escherichia coli* was to make indigo dye (originally discovered in 1983, using indole or tryptophan as starting materials). In 1993, Burt D. Ensley and coworkers at Amgen discovered a way to genetically engineer *Escherichia coli* to produce indigo from glucose starting material. *Escherichia coli* has 4288 genes.
See also BACTERIA, GENETIC ENGINEERING, GENE, RECOMBINANT DNA (rDNA), *ESCHERICHIA COLIFORM 0157:H7*, TRYPTOPHAN

Escherichia coliform 0157:H7 The particular strain (serotype) of *Escherichia coliform (E. coli)* bacteria that causes often-fatal diarrhea, internal bleeding, and kidney damage in humans. Children are more susceptible to *E. coli 0157:H7* than adults, because children possess more of the receptors (on cells inside the digestive tract) that are utilized by *E. coli 0157:H7* to enter the body from the digestive tract.
Although cattle were susceptible to *E. coli 0157:H7*'s toxins prior to the 1980s, they

eventually developed resistance. So the cattle could carry these bacteria without getting sick and transmit *E. coli 0157:H7* to humans whenever conditions allowed (e.g., when *E. coli 0157:H7*–infected cattle are slaughtered and people consume the meat without first heating it to a high enough temperature to kill the *E. coli 0157:H7*). Some varieties of *E. coli 0157:H7* are resistant to the antibiotics tetracycline and streptomycin.

In 1996, researchers at Cornell University, NY, discovered that nonambulatory cows (that could not walk) were approximately four times as likely as other cows to test positive for *E. coli 0157:H7*. Other research in Canada indicates that fasting of cattle (common occurrence for nonambulatory cows) tends to alter the pH inside the cow's rumen (stomach) in a way that encourages the proliferation of *E. coli 0157:H7* instead of the bacteria that normally populate the rumen.

See also *ESCHERICHIA COLIFORM (E. COLI)*, BACTERIA, SEROTYPES, TOXIN, RECEPTORS, BIOLUMINESCENCE, STRAIN, ENTEROTOXIN, COMMENSAL

E-Selectin See ELAM-1

Essential Amino Acids Those amino acids that cannot be synthesized by humans and most other vertebrates and therefore must be obtained from the diet. They are phenylalanine, valine, threonine, tryptophan, isoleucine, methionine, histidine, arginine, leucine, and lysine (glycine and proline for poultry).

See also AMINO ACID, LYSINE (Lys), METHIONINE (Met), SOY PROTEIN, OPAGUE-2, PROTEIN-DIGESTIBILITY-CORRECTED AMINO ACID SCORING (PDCAAS)

Essential Fatty Acids The group of polyunsaturated fatty acids of plants that are required in the human diet, because the human body cannot synthesize (i.e., "manufacture") them, yet must have them for proper functioning (e.g., of the body's metabolism, immune system function, etc.). These include linoleic acid, linolenic acid, arachidonic acid, docosahexanoic acid, etc.

If humans and other higher animals do not consume enough essential fatty acids per day, they suffer decreased growth rates, increased susceptibility to infection, impaired reproduction, kidney damage, and other adverse physiological effects.

See also FATTY ACID, SOYBEAN OIL, LECITHIN, FATS, ESSENTIAL NUTRIENTS, POLYUNSATURATED FATTY ACIDS (PUFA), LINOLEIC ACID, LINOLENIC ACID, DOCOSAHEXANOIC ACID (DHA), ARACHIDONIC ACID (AA)

Essential Nutrients Chemical compounds in foods that are required for (the consuming organism's) life, growth, or tissue repair and cannot be synthesized by that organism.

See also ESSENTIAL AMINO ACIDS, ESSENTIAL FATTY ACIDS, ESSENTIAL POLYUNSATURATED FATTY ACIDS, VITAMIN

Essential Polyunsaturated Fatty Acids See ESSENTIAL FATTY ACIDS

EST See EXPRESSED SEQUENCE TAGS (EST)

Establishment Potential Refers to a formal estimate of the likelihood for a given pest (e.g., weed, insect, disease, etc.) to successfully establish a permanent (reproducing) population within a specific **"pest-free area"** (e.g., country or region where **that pest** has not previously been established).

Determination of **establishment potential** requires reliable biological information (e.g., life cycle, host range if any, climate tolerance, epidemiology, etc.). For example, a pest that requires tropical temperatures or humidity to reproduce is not likely to have a significant **establishment potential** in a cold and dry country.

See also INTERNATIONAL PLANT PROTECTION CONVENTION (IPPC), PEST RISK ANALYSIS (PRA), QUARANTINE PEST, INTRODUCTION

Estrogen A female sex hormone, secreted by the ovaries, that promotes estrus and helps to regulate the pituitary gland's production of luteinizing hormone (LH) and follicle-stimulating hormone (FSH).

Estrogen causes proliferation of breast tissue (cells) and is also responsible for the development of female secondary sex characteristics (e.g., smaller body size, lack of facial hair, higher pitch voice in humans).

Research indicates that lack of estrogen (e.g., in postmenopausal women) makes humans more

E

prone to colon cancer and heart disease, but less prone to the "hormone-dependent" cancers (e.g., ovarian cancer, uterine cancer, etc.).

See also HORMONE, PITUITARY GLAND, FOLLICLE-STIMULATING HORMONE (FSH), SELECTIVE ESTROGEN EFFECT, TESTOSTERONE, LUTEINIZING HORMONE (LH), HYPOTHALAMUS, CANCER, CELL

Etanercept See FUSION PROTEIN, CHO CELLS

Ethylene A plant hormone that is synthesized ("manufactured") by some plants to induce ripening (of their fruit and seeds).

See also PLANT HORMONE, ACC SYNTHASE, ACC, SAM-K GENE

Etiological Agent (of a disease) The microorganism (or other agent) that causes the disease.

See also PATHOGEN, ETIOLOGY

Etiology The science (study) of the cause (source) of a disease.

See also PATHOGEN, ETIOLOGICAL AGENT

Eucaryote Also spelled eukaryote.

A cell characterized by compartmentalization (by membranes) of its extensive internal structures, or an organism made up of such cells. For example, eucaryotes possess a distinct membrane-surrounded nucleus containing the DNA. Eucaryotic cells (e.g., human cells) are much larger and more complex than procaryotic cells (e.g., bacteria). The cells of all higher organisms, both plant and animal, are eucaryotic, so those higher (complex) organisms are often referred to as eucaryotes.

Most eucaryotic organisms cannot survive temperatures greater than 131°F (55°C). However, one called the Pompeii worm (*Alvinella pompejana*) can withstand long-term exposure in water up to a temperature of 176°F (80°C).

See also PROCARYOTES, CELL, THERMOPHILE, DEOXYRIBONUCLEIC ACID (DNA), PLASMA, MEMBRANE, MICROTUBULES

Eugenics First formulated by Francis Galton, who was a cousin of Charles Darwin; eugenics is the concept that a species can be "improved" by encouraging reproduction of only those organisms in that species that possess "desired" traits.

This belief became popular in a number of countries during the early 20th century. Margaret Sanger, founder of America's Planned Parenthood organization, referred to African-Americans as "human weeds" and called for "more children from the fit, less from the unfit." Based on Charles Darwin's written assertion that "the civilized races of man will almost certainly exterminate and replace the savage races," a number of large genocides were committed by some national governments.

See also GENETICS, GENE, TRAIT, GENOTYPE, HEREDITY, HERITABILITY, GENOME

Eukaryote See EUCARYOTE

Euploid A cell carrying an exact multiple of the haploid chromosome number. For example, a diploid possesses twice the haploid number of chromosomes.

See also HAPLOID, DIPLOID, CHROMOSOMES

European Corn Borer (ECB) Also known as pyralis (*Pyralidae*), Latin (Linnaean) name *Ostrinia nubilalis*; it is an insect whose larvae (caterpillars) eat and bore into the corn or maize plant (*Zea mays* L.). In doing so, they can act as vectors (i.e., carriers) of the fungi known as *Aspergillus flavus* (a source of aflatoxin) or *Fusarium moniliforme* (a source of fumonisin) or *Aspergillus parasiticus* (a source of aflatoxin).

Full-grown ECB larvae overwinter by sheltering inside a variety of vegetative materials (e.g., plant stalks lying on top of soil in some fields).

ECB control can be effected by some of the following methods:

- Spraying of conventional synthetic chemical pesticides
- Spraying of pesticides produced via promulgation of *Bacillus thuringiensis (B.t.)* bacteria
- Incorporating a (protoxin) gene from *Bacillus thuringiensis (B.t.)* into the DNA of the corn plant so that the plant itself produces B.t. protoxin

As part of integrated pest management (IPM), farmers can utilize:

- Corn possessing *Bacillus thuringiensis (B.t.)* genes to control populations of ECB without applying insecticides

- The parasitic *Euplectrus comstockki* wasp to help control the ECB. When that wasp's venom is injected into ECB larva, it stops the larva from molting (and thus maturing)
- Other additional methods, alone or in conjunction with the preceding methods

See also CORN, FUNGUS, AFLATOXIN, INTEGRATED PEST MANAGEMENT (IPM), *BACILLUS THURINGIENSIS (B.t.), B.t. KURSTAKI, FUSARIUM, FUSARIUM MONILIFORME*, ASIAN CORN BORER, PROTOXIN, VOLICITIN

European Medicines Evaluation Agency (EMEA) A London-based agency of the European Union (EU) that began operation in 1995. It coordinates drug licensing and safety matters throughout the nations of the EU. Its licensing and approval process is compulsory throughout the EU.

See also COMMITTEE FOR PROPRIETARY MEDICINAL PRODUCTS (CPMP), MEDICINES CONTROL AGENCY (MCA), FOOD AND DRUG ADMINISTRATION (FDA), KOSEISHO, BUNDESGESUND-HEITSAMT (BGA), COMMITTEE ON SAFETY IN MEDICINES, COMMITTEE FOR VETERINARY MEDICINAL PRODUCTS (CVMP)

European Patent Convention An international patent treaty signed in 1973 by which the countries of Europe agreed to recognize and honor the patents granted by each country, and also those patents granted by the European Patent Office (EPO). Plant varieties or animal breeds were initially excluded from patentability by the European Patent Convention. In 1998, the European Parliament removed that exclusion.

See also EUROPEAN PATENT OFFICE (EPO), U.S. PATENT AND TRADEMARK OFFICE (USPTO), PLANT'S NOVEL TRAIT (PNT), PLANT BREEDER'S RIGHTS (PPR), UNION FOR PROTECTION OF NEW VARIETIES OF PLANTS (UPOV)

European Patent Office (EPO) The Munich (Germany)-based agency of the European Union (EU) — established in 1977 — that is responsible for common patent protection matters for all of the (EU) member countries, plus the non-EU countries of Switzerland and Liechtenstein. The EPO originally did not allow a "plant or animal breed" to be patented, whereas its U.S. counterpart — the U.S. Patent and Trademark Office (USPTO) — does allow patenting of microbes, plants, and animals (e.g., those which have been genetically engineered by man). In 1998, the European Parliament removed that exclusion, and in 1999 the European Patent Court issued a ruling that caused the European Patent Convention to allow patents on novel plants, thus making the two patent systems compatible.

See also EUROPEAN PATENT CONVENTION, MICROBE, GENETIC ENGINEERING, BIOTECHNOLOGY, AMERICAN TYPE CULTURE COLLECTION (ATCC), U.S. PATENT AND TRADEMARK OFFICE (USPTO), PLANT'S NOVEL TRAIT (PNT), PLANT BREEDER'S RIGHTS (PBR), UNION FOR PROTECTION OF NEW VARIETIES OF PLANTS (UPOV), COMMUNITY PLANT VARIETY OFFICE

European Plant Protection Organization (EPPO) One of the international SPS standard-setting organizations that develops plant health standards, guidelines, and recommendations (e.g., to prevent transfer of a plant disease or plant pest from one country to another). Its secretariat is in Paris (France).

EPPO is one of the organizations within the International Plant Protection Convention (IPPC), and it covers the countries of Europe.

See also INTERNATIONAL PLANT PROTECTION CONVENTION (IPPC), NORTH AMERICAN PLANT PROTECTION ORGANIZATION (NAPPO), SPS, PLANT'S NOVEL TRAIT (PNT), PLANT BREEDER'S RIGHTS (PBR)

Event Refers to each instance of a genetically engineered organism. For example, the same gene inserted by man into a given plant genome at two different locations (i.e., loci) along that plant's DNA would be considered two different "events." Alternatively, two different genes inserted into the same locus of two same-species plants would also be considered two different "events."

Generally speaking, the world's regulatory agencies confer new biotech-derived product approvals in terms of events.

See also GENETIC ENGINEERING, GENETICALLY ENGINEERED ORGANISM (GEO), GENE, DEOXYRIBONUCLEIC ACID (DNA), LOCUS, LOCI, GENOME, MUTUAL RECOGNITION AGREEMENTS (MRAs)

Excision The cutting out of a piece of damaged or defective DNA by enzymes. DNA damage might be constituted by the presence of a thymine dimer, which inactivates that part of the DNA. The region of the dimer is cut out and it is then repaired.

See also RECOMBINATION, GENOME, INFORMATIONAL MOLECULES

Excitatory Amino Acids (EAAs) Amino acids present in the brain (when released by certain immune system cells), which can kill brain cells when in excess (can result from strokes, which cause the release of too many EAAs in the brain). Another source of harmful EAAs (e.g., glutamate) is the disease known as multiple sclerosis.

Some spiders paralyze their prey with venom that contains a substance that blocks the action of EAAs. (Thus, pharmaceuticals based on an active ingredient in that venom may someday be used to prevent brain damage in stroke and in multiple sclerosis victims.)

See also AMINO ACID, MULTIPLE SCLEROSIS, CELL, IMMUNE RESPONSE

Exclusion Chromatography See GEL FILTRATION

Exergonic Reaction A chemical reaction with a negative standard free-energy change (i.e., a "downhill" reaction). A reaction that releases energy (exothermic, i.e., in the form of heat).

See also ENDERGONIC REACTION, FREE ENERGY

Exobiology Extraterrestrial biology.

Exocytosis The releasing of an entity that was bound inside an "endosome" (e.g., inside a cell).

See also ENDOCYTOSIS

Exoglycosidase An enzyme that hydrolyzes (cuts) only a terminal (i.e., end) bond in the oligosaccharide (molecular) branches of a glycoprotein.

See also ENDOGLYCOSIDASE, GLYCOPROTEIN, RESTRICTION ENDOGLYCOSIDASES

Exon The segment of a eucaryotic gene that is transcribed into an mRNA (messenger RNA) molecule; it codes for a specific domain of a protein.

See also DEOXYRIBONUCLEIC ACID (DNA), PROTEIN, EUCARYOTE, MESSENGER RNA (mRNA), GENE, HOMEOBOX, TRANSCRIPTION, EDITING

Exonuclease An enzyme that hydrolyzes (cuts) only a terminal phosphodiester bond of a nucleic acid.

See also HYDROLYZE

Exotic Germplasm Germplasm that has not been adapted (selectively bred) to the environment intended (for its offspring via selective breeding by man).

See also GERMPLASM, INTROGRESSION, HYBRIDIZATION (PLANT GENETICS)

Exotoxin Proteins (toxins) produced by certain bacteria that are released by the bacteria into their surroundings (growth medium). Produced by primarily Gram-positive bacteria. The diphtheria toxin was the first one discovered. Other exotoxins cause botulism, tetanus, gas gangrene, and scarlet fever. Exotoxins are generally more potent and specific in their actions than endotoxins.

See also ENDOTOXIN, TOXIN, GRAM POSITIVE (G+)

Expected Progeny Difference (EPD) Numerical rankings of (livestock) parental genetics in terms of an animal's genetic impact on progeny's four following commercial traits:

- Number of progeny born alive
- Weight of progeny at weaning age
- Number of days required to reach slaughter weight when fed adequately
- Carcass lean meat vs. fat percentages

EPDs allow a farmer to estimate differences in performance of future offspring (of a given parent) vs. offspring produced by parents of average genetic value. For example, a boar (male pig) possessing an EPD of 4 for "number of days required to reach slaughter weight" produces offspring that reach slaughter weight in four fewer days (of feeding time) than offspring that are sired by a boar possessing an EPD of 0.

See also GENETICS, TRAIT, PHENOTYPE, GENOTYPE, BEST LINEAR UNBIASED PREDICTION (BLUP)

"Explosion" Method (to introduce foreign [new] genes into plant cells) A technique for gene-into-cell introduction in which the gene (genetic material) is driven into plant cells by the force of an explosion (vaporization) of a drop of water (to which the gene and gold particles have been added). The explosion is caused by application of high-voltage electricity to the drop of gene-laden water; the water then vaporized explosively, driving the "shot" (gold particles) and genetic material through the cell membrane. The plant cell then heals itself (reseals the hole through which the gene entered), incorporates the new gene into its genetic complement, and produces whatever product (e.g., a protein) the newly introduced gene codes for.

See also AGROBACTERIUM TUMEFACIENS, CODING SEQUENCE, GENETIC ENGINEERING, VECTOR, "SHOTGUN" METHOD, GENE, GENOME, RIBOSOMES

Express To translate the cell's genetic information stored in the DNA (géne) into a specific protein (synthesized by the cell's ribosome system).

Certain proteins (i.e., when present in relevant cells) regulate the expression (e.g., increase/decrease/timing) of some genes.

See also GENE EXPRESSION CASCADE, RIBOSOMES, GENE, DEOXYRIBONUCLEIC ACID (DNA), CELL, TRANSCRIPTION, TRANSLATION, MESSENGER RNA (mRNA), TRANSCRIPTION UNIT, PROTEIN, COSUPPRESSION, GENE EXPRESSION ANALYSIS, FUNCTIONAL GENOMICS, SPLICE VARIANTS

Expressed Sequence Tags (EST) Molecular tags consisting of a DNA sequence approximately 200 base pairs long that are utilized to "label" a given gene (i.e., in terms of that gene's function/protein). Physically, the EST was historically composed of cRNA (i.e., the gene's "message" after the "junk DNA"

[introns] have been **edited out**), produced by the analogous gene in (simple) **model organisms** such as (traditionally) *Caenorhabditis elegans* nematode, which has been sequenced and mapped.

Functions of the "labeled" genes were (at least initially) inferred from (known function) *C. elegans* genes.

See also GENE, INTRON, PROTEIN, COMPLEMENTARY DNA (cDNA), DEOXYRIBONUCLEIC ACID (DNA), JUNK DNA, BEST, CAENORHABDITIS ELEGANS (*C. ELEGANS*), SEQUENCING (OF DNA MOLECULES), SEQUENCE (OF A DNA MOLECULE), MAPPING, MODEL ORGANISM, EXPRESS, BACTERIAL EXPRESSED SEQUENCE TAGS (BEST), GENE EXPRESSION ANALYSIS, SERIAL ANALYSIS OF GENE EXPRESSION (SAGE)

Expression Analysis See GENE EXPRESSION ANALYSIS, MICROARRAY (TESTING)

Expression Array See MICROARRAY (TESTING)

Expression Profiling See GENE EXPRESSION ANALYSIS

Expressivity The intensity with which the effect of a gene is realized in the phenotype. The degree to which a particular effect is expressed by individuals.

See also PHENOTYPE, EXPRESS, RIBOSOMES

Extension (in nucleic acids) The nucleic acid strand elongation (lengthening) that occurs in a polymerization reaction.

See also NUCLEIC ACIDS, POLYMER

Extranuclear Genes Genes that reside within the cell but *outside* the nucleus. Generally, extranuclear genes reside in the organelles such as mitochondria and chloroplasts.

See also GENE, CELL, NUCLEUS, COPY NUMBER, ORGANELLES, CHLOROPLASTS, MITOCHONDRIA

Extremophilic Bacteria Bacteria that live and reproduce outside (either colder or hotter) the typical temperature range of 40°F (4°C) to 140°F (60°C) that bacteria tend to be found in. Other extremes are high pressure (e.g., at the ocean bottom), salt saturation, (e.g., the Dead Sea), pH lower than 2 (e.g., coal deposits), pH higher than 11 (e.g., sewage sludge), high levels of radiation, etc.

E

See also BACTERIA, THERMOPHILIC BAC-
TERIA, THERMOPHILE, THERMODU-
RIC, *DEINOCOCCUS RADIODURANS*

Extremozymes Enzymes within the microorganisms (e.g., extremophilic bacteria) that populate extreme environments. Because extremozymes can catalyze reactions under high
pressure, high temperatures, etc., they are
increasingly being used as catalysts for industrial
processes.

See also EXTREMOPHILIC BACTERIA,
ENZYME, ARCHAEA, PHYTOMANU-
FACTURING

Ex Vivo **(testing)** The testing of a substance by
exposing it to (excised) living cells (but not
to the whole, multicelled organism) in order
to ascertain the effect of the substance (e.g.,
pharmaceutical) on the biochemistry of the
cell.

See also *IN VITRO, IN VIVO*

Ex Vivo **(therapy)** Removal of cells (e.g., certain blood cells) from a patient's body and
alteration of those cells in one or more therapeutic ways, followed by reinsertion of the
altered cells into the patient's body.

See also *IN VITRO, IN VIVO*

E

F

F1 Hybrids The first-generation offspring of crossbreeding; also known as first filial hybrids. They tend to be more healthy, productive, and uniform than their parents.
See also GENETICS, HYBRIDIZATION (PLANT GENETICS)

F-Box Proteins Proteins produced ("manufactured") within some eucaryotic cells that play an essential role in the degradation (i.e., breakdown) of cellular regulatory proteins after they have "completed their job" in the cell.
See also PROTEIN, CELL, EUCARYOTE

FABP Acronym for **fatty acid binding protein**.
See FATTY ACID BINDING PROTEIN

Facilitated Folding Refers to the improvement in protein molecular folding (e.g., into its native conformation, etc.) of certain protein molecules, when those molecules:

- Fuse with other relevant partner "folding facilitator" molecules such as SUMO (small ubiquitin-related modifier), etc.
- Partner with chaperone molecules, chaperonins, etc., as the newly formed protein molecules emerge from ribosomes within the cell.
- Partner with certain heat-shock proteins (e.g., HSP 90, HSP 70, etc.) — also called stress proteins — after stresses such as heat, age, exposure to ultraviolet light, certain viruses, or exposure to certain chemicals cause some protein molecules in cells to begin to "unfold."

See also CELL, PROTEIN, FUSION PROTEIN, PROTEIN FOLDING, CONFORMATION, NATIVE CONFORMATION, SMALL UBIQUITIN-RELATED MODIFIER, CHAPERONES, CHAPERONINS, RIBOSOMES, HEAT-SHOCK PROTEINS, STRESS PROTEINS

FACS See FLUORESCENCE-ACTIVATED CELL SORTER (FACS)

Factor IX A protein factor in the blood serum that is instrumental in the **cascade** of chemical reactions (involving 17 blood components) that leads to clot formation following a cut or other wound to body tissue.
A deficiency of factor IX is the cause of the disease known as **hemophilia B** (approximately 15% of all hemophilia patients).
See also FIBRIN, FIBRONECTIN, PROTEIN, CASCADE, FACTOR VIII

Factor VIII Also known as antihemophilic globulin (AHG) or antihemophilic factor VIII. A protein factor in the blood serum that is instrumental in the "cascade" of chemical reactions (involving 17 blood components in the **intrinsic pathway**) that leads to clot formation following a cut or other wound to body tissue. Also, a deficiency of AHG is the cause of the classical type of hemophilia sometimes known as **hemophilia AM** (approximately 85% of all hemophilia patients).
See also FIBRIN, PROTEIN, FIBRONECTIN, CASCADE, PATHWAY, FACTOR IX

Facultative Anaerobe An organism that will grow under either aerobic or anaerobic conditions.
See also AEROBE, ANAEROBE, ORGANISM

Facultative Cells Cells that can live either in the presence or absence of oxygen.
See also AEROBE, ANAEROBE

FAD See FLAVIN ADENINE DINUCLEOTIDE (FAD)

Fad Genes Refers to genes that code for the synthesis ("manufacturing") in plants of a specific **fatty acid desaturase** enzyme.
See also GENE, Fad3 GENE, ENZYME, FATTY ACID, DESATURASE, Δ 12 DESATURASE, DELTA 12 DESATURASE

Fad3 Gene A gene naturally found with the soybean plant (*Glycine max* (L.)) DNA, which codes for (i.e., causes production of) the ω-desaturase, an enzyme within the pathway in which the soybean plant synthesizes ("manufactures") oleic acid within the vegetable oil produced in the soybean.

Specifically, the ω-desaturase enzyme converts linoleic acid to linolenic acid in that pathway, so by increasing expression of the *Fad 3* gene in a (genetically engineered) soybean plant, a scientist could cause that soybean plant to produce soybean oil comprised of as much as 50% linolenic acid.

See also GENE, EXPRESS, Fad GENES, SOYBEAN PLANT, DEOXYRIBONUCLEIC ACID (DNA), ENZYME, PATHWAY, SOYBEAN OIL, FATTY ACID, OLEATE, OLEIC ACID, HIGH-OLEIC-OIL SOYBEANS, COSUPPRESSION, DESATURASE, Δ 12 DESATURASE, DELTA 12 DESATURASE, LINOLENIC ACID, LINOLEIC ACID, GENETIC ENGINEERING, HIGH-LINOLENIC-OIL SOYBEANS

Fall Armyworm Caterpillars (pupae) of the Lepidopteran insect *Spodoptera frugiperda*, which are harmful to certain crops grown by humans.

Fall armyworms are susceptible to **some** of the "Cry" proteins.

See also PROTEIN, CRY PROTEINS, ARMYWORM, INSECT CELL CULTURE

FAME Acronym for **fatty acid methyl esters**, i.e., the compounds that result when fatty acid molecules are reacted with compounds containing methyl submolecule groups (CH_3).

This acronym also refers to a method of identifying species of microorganisms (e.g., during the investigation of a disease outbreak) based on the fatty acid composition of the microorganism's cell wall (membrane). Such cell walls can contain up to 115 different fatty acids in varying amounts or ratios.

The cell wall of the microorganism of interest is broken down, and its fatty acids are converted to FAMEs as detailed in the preceding text. Then, the FAMEs are analyzed using a gas chromatograph to yield a "fingerprint" unique to each species or strain of microorganism.

See also FATTY ACID, MICROORGANISM, SPECIES, STRAIN

FAO Food and Agriculture Organization of the United Nations.

See also CONSULTATIVE GROUP ON INTERNATIONAL AGRICULTURAL RESEARCH (CGIAR), CODEX ALIMENTARIUS COMMISSION

Farnesoid X Receptor (FXR) Refers to nuclear receptors, primarily in enterohepatic system (e.g., cells within liver) for bile acids. When certain bile acids (e.g., chenodeoxycholic acid, cholic acid, etc.) "dock" at the FXR, they "turn on" the BSEP (bile salt efflux pump), a bile acid transporter that increases the flow of the bile acids into the body's bile (where they are utilized in the digestive system to help render fats and fat-soluble vitamins easily absorbable).

See also BILE ACIDS, NUCLEAR RECEPTORS, VITAMIN

Farnesyl Transferase An enzyme utilized by the *ras* gene (to help "signal" certain cells to divide or grow).

See also *ras* GENE, GENE, ENZYME, CELL, SIGNALING MOLECULE

Fats Energy storage substances produced by animals and some plants (e.g., soybeans), which consist of a combination of fatty acids and glycerol that form predominantly triglyceride molecules (although some diglyceride molecules are often present in fats). The structure of triglyceride molecules consists of three fatty acids attached to a glycerol **molecular backbone**, so "triglyceride" molecules are more accurately called TRIACYLGLYCERIDES, but **triglyceride** is the term most often used. Two separate components of plant cells are involved in the synthesis (i.e., "manufacturing") of plant fats (lipids), the **plastid** and the **endoplasmic reticulum**. Synthesis of fatty acids begins in the plastid, where AcCoA is first carboxylated (thereby becoming malonyl-CoA) via the enzyme **acetyl-CoA carboxylase**. Next, a group of seven related enzymes (known as FATTY ACID SYNTHETASES) catalyzes synthesis of palmityl-CoA (which is a long molecule possessing 18 carbon atoms in its "molecular backbone"), although shorter-length molecules result when a specific **ACP (acyl carrier protein)** thioesterase enzyme is present in plastid (e.g., $C_{16:0}$ACP), which results in fatty acids of various **"carbon chain" length**. After the palmityl-CoA is elongated (i.e., made a longer molecule via addition of carbons to its **molecular backbone**) to become the (stearate-like) molecule OLEOYL-ACP in a chemical reaction catalyzed by a **palmioyl elongase enzyme**, the oleoyl-ACP is transported to the plant's endoplasmic reticulum. In the endoplasmic reticulum, the oleoyl-ACP is either further elongated (via the addition of more carbon atoms to the fatty acid's **molecular carbon chain "backbone"**) or it is further desaturated (i.e., via desaturase-catalyzed removal of hydrogen atoms from that fatty acid molecule). Stearic acid (also known as stearate) is desaturated to become oleic acid, which can be desaturated to become linoleic acid, which can be desaturated to become linolenic acid.

Three of the resultant fatty acid molecules are then chemically attached to a **glycerol-3-phosphate** molecule (with the cleaved-off phosphate atom "recycled" in the endoplasmic reticulum for further utilization in the energy cycle of the cell).

The content levels of individual fatty acids in animal fat vary somewhat with the diet of the animal, and vary somewhat in plant fat (also known as vegetable oil) with the plant's growing conditions. No natural fat is either totally saturated or unsaturated.

When eaten, fats are generally not absorbed directly through the intestinal wall.

They are first emulsified, then hydrolyzed by the lipase enzyme. The components (i.e., fatty acids, cholesterol, monoacylglycerol, phospholipids, etc.) form micelles that pass through the intestinal wall and are absorbed by the body. Such emulsification and micelle formation is aided by the nutrient lecithin (a component in soybeans).

When fats are oxidized in cells, they provide energy for the body. Some of the energy is released as heat and some is stored in the form of adenosine triphosphate (ATP), which "fuels" metabolic processes.

See also FATTY ACID, HYDROLYSIS, HYDROLYTIC CLEAVAGE, HYDROLYZE, LIPASE, MONOUNSATURATED FATS, SATURATED FATTY ACIDS, TRIGLYCERIDES, TRIACYLGLYCEROLS, DIACYLGLYCEROLS, MICELLE, CELL, METABOLISM, DIGESTION (WITHIN ORGANISMS), CHOLESTEROL, LIPIDS, LECITHIN, SOYBEAN OIL, FREE FATTY ACIDS, OXIDATIVE STRESS, PLASTID, ACP, OXIDATION (OF FATS, OILS, OR LIPIDS), PLASMA MEMBRANE, ENZYME, AcCoA, ENDOPLASMIC RETICULUM, FATTY ACID SYNTHETASE, THIOESTERASE, DESATURASE, MITOCHONDRIA, LAUROYL-ACP THIOESTERASE, STEAROYL-ACP DESATURASE, ADIPOCYTES, ADENOSINE TRIPHOSPHATE (ATP), BILE ACIDS, PHOSPHATE TRANSPORTER GENES, PHOTOSYNTHESIS, OLEOSOMES, STEARATE (STEARIC ACID), OLEIC ACID, LINOLEIC ACID, LINOLENIC ACID (α-LINOLENIC ACID), CONJUGATED LINOLEIC ACID (CLA)

Fatty Acid A long-chain aliphatic acid found in natural fats and oils. Fatty acids are abundant in cell membranes and (after extraction and purification) are widely used as industrial emulsifiers, for example, phosphatidylcholine (lecithin). In general, fats possessing the highest levels of saturated fatty acids tend to be solid at room temperature, and those fats possessing the highest levels of unsaturated fatty acids tend to be liquid at room temperature. That rule of thumb was the original "dividing line" between compounds called *fats* and *oils*, respectively. In general, saturated fatty acids tend to be more stable (resistant to oxidation and thermal breakdown) than unsaturated fatty acids.

Fatty acids in biological systems (e.g., produced by plants in oilseeds, etc.) tend to contain an even number, typically between 14 and 24, of carbon atoms in their molecular "backbone." The molecular backbone (alkyl chain) may be saturated (no double bonds) or it may contain one or more double bonds. The configuration of the double bonds in most unsaturated fatty acids is *CIS*.

See also ESSENTIAL FATTY ACIDS, LAURATE, PHYTOCHEMICALS, SATURATED FATTY ACIDS, LECITHIN, SOYBEAN OIL, UNSATURATED FATTY ACID, MONOUNSATURATED FATS, POLYUNSATURATED FATTY ACIDS (PUFA), LPAAT PROTEIN, STEAROYL-ACP DESATURASE, SOYBEAN OIL, CANOLA, FATS, OLEIC ACID, *trans* FATTY ACIDS, ENOYL-ACYL PROTEIN REDUCTASE, OXIDATION (OF FATS,

F

OILS, OR LIPIDS), LIPIDS, MITOCHON-
DRIA, ADIPOCYTES, OLEOSOMES,
DELTA 12 DESATURASE, LINOLEIC
ACID, LINOLENIC ACID, FATTY ACID
SYNTHETASE, CARNITINE, BIOTIN

Fatty Acid Binding Protein Refers to certain protein molecules present within animal cells, which bind to specific fatty acids
(after they come through the cell's plasma
membrane) and help transport those fatty
acids to their needed destinations within the
cell.

For example, oleic acid molecules are transported to the nucleus of some cells (e.g., in
human breast tissue), where the oleic acid
molecules bind to the cell's DNA in a manner that reduces overexpression of the Her-
2/neu gene (in those women whose breast
cells overexpress Her-2/neu gene) and
thereby confer some protection against
breast cancer.

See also PROTEIN, TRANSPORT PROTEINS,
FATTY ACID, CELL, NUCLEUS, DEOX-
YRIBONUCLEIC ACID (DNA), PLASMA
MEMBRANE, INTRACELLULAR TRANS-
PORT, MEMBRANE TRANSPORT, TRAN-
SCRIPTION FACTORS, EXPRESS,
EXPRESSIVITY, CANCER, HER-2/NEU
GENE, DOWNREGULATING

Fatty Acid Methyl Esters Abbreviated **FAME**.
See FAME

Fatty Acid Synthetase A group of seven
related enzymes that catalyze synthesis (i.e.,
"manufacturing") of fatty acids within the
soybean plant (*Glycine max* (L.) Merrill).

See also ENZYME, CATALYZE, FATTY
ACID, SOYBEAN PLANT, DESATURASE,
FATS, OLEOSOMES, PATHWAY, DELTA 12
DESATURASE

FC Acronym for **flow cytometry**.
See FLOW CYTOMETRY

**Federal Coordinated Framework for Regu-
lation of Biotechnology** The legal framework created by the U.S. government in
1986, which divided regulation of biotechnology among the U.S. Department of Agriculture, the U.S. Environmental Protection
Agency, and the U.S. Food and Drug
Administration.

See also FOOD AND DRUG ADMINISTRA-
TION

**Federal Insecticide Fungicide and Rodenti-
cide Act (FIFRA)** A law enacted by the U.S.
Congress in 1972. During 1994, the U.S.
Environmental Protection Agency (EPA) proposed that the substances produced by plants
(e.g., genetically engineered crops) for their
defense against pests and diseases would be
regulated by EPA under FIFRA.

See also TOXIC SUBSTANCES CONTROL
ACT (TSCA), GENETICALLY ENGI-
NEERED MICROBIAL PESTICIDES
(GEMP), WHEAT TAKE-ALL DISEASE,
BACILLUS THURINGIENSIS (B.t.)

Feedback Inhibition Inhibition of the first
enzyme in a metabolic pathway by the end
product of that pathway. This is a method of
shutting down a metabolic pathway producing
a product that is no longer needed.

See also METABOLISM, ENZYME, EFFEC-
TOR

Feedstock Raw materials used for the production of chemicals or growth substrates of
microbes (e.g., yeasts or bacteria that require
a solid phase to which to attach themselves).

Fermentation A term first used with regard to
the foaming that occurs during the manufacture of wine and beer. The process dates back
to at least 6000 B.C., when the Egyptians
made wine and beer by fermentation. From
the Latin word *fermentare,* meaning "to cause
to rise." The term "fermentation" is now used
to refer to so many different processes that
fermentation is no longer accepted for use in
most scientific publications. Three typical definitions are as follows:

1. A process in which chemical
changes are brought about in an
organic substrate through the actions
of enzymes elaborated (produced) by
microorganisms.

2. The enzyme-catalyzed, energy-
yielding pathway in cells by which
"fuel" molecules such as glucose
are broken down anaerobically (in
the absence of oxygen). One product of the pathway is always the
energy-rich compound adenosine
triphosphate (ATP). The other products are of many types: alcohol,
glycerol, and carbon dioxide from

yeast fermentation of various sugars; butyl alcohol, acetone, lactic acid, and acetic acid from various bacteria; and citric acid, gluconic acid, antibiotics, and vitamin B_{12} and B_2 from mold fermentation. The Japanese utilize a bacterial fermentation process to make the amino acid, L-glutamic acid, a derivative of which is widely used as a flavoring agent.

3. An enzymatic transformation of organic substrates (feedstocks), especially carbohydrates, generally accompanied by the evolution of gas. A physiological counterpart of oxidation, permitting certain organisms to live and grow in the absence of air, used in various industrial processes for the manufacture of products such as alcohols, acids, and cheese by the action of yeasts, molds, and bacteria. Alcoholic fermentation is the best known example. Also known as zymosis. The leavening of bread depends on the alcoholic fermentation of sugars. The dough rises because of the production of carbon dioxide gas that remains trapped within the viscous dough.

See also ZYMOGENS, SUBSTRATE (CHEMICAL), ADENOSINE TRIPHOSPHATE (ATP), MICROORGANISM, ENZYME, FEEDSTOCK, CARBOHYDRATES (SACCHARIDES)

Ferritin An iron–protein complex (a metalloprotein) that occurs in living tissues. Functions in iron storage in the spleen. Dietary sources include the soybean plant.
See also HEMOGLOBIN, METALLOPROTEIN, SOY PROTEIN

Ferrobacteria Also called iron bacteria, it is a group of bacteria that oxidize iron as a source of energy. The oxidized iron in the form $Fe(OH)_3$ is then deposited in the environment by secretion from the bacterium. The energy obtained from these reactions is used to carry on processes in which the basic substances needed by the bacterium are manufactured. These bacteria are commonly found in seepage waters of coal- and iron-mining areas, where iron compounds abound.

Ferrobacteria are not disease producers (i.e., pathogenic), but they are important as scavengers. Sometimes, they create a nuisance by multiplying so profusely in iron water pipes that they stop the flow of water. Ferrobacteria have been active over long periods of geologic time. For example, the great Mesabi iron (ore) seam of Lake Superior region is thought to be a product of ferrobacterial activity.
See also PATHOGEN

Ferrochelatase A mitochondrial enzyme that catalyzes the incorporation of iron into the protoporphyria molecule.
See also MITOCHONDRIA, ENZYME, CATALYST, PORPHYRINS

Ferrodoxin An iron- and sulfur-containing protein important in the electron-transfer processes of photosynthesis in plants. It also plays a role in the metabolism of some bacteria and was first found in an anaerobic bacterium.
See also PHOTOSYNTHESIS, METABOLISM

Fertility Factor (F) A type of transmissible (i.e., can enter other cells) plasmid that is often found in *Escherichia coli (E. coli)*.
See also PLASMID, VECTOR, *ESCHERICHIA COLIFORM (E. COLI)*

Fertilization The union of the (haploid) male and (haploid) female germ cells (sex cells or gametes) to produce a diploid zygote. Fertilization marks the start of the development of a new individual (organism), the beginning of cell differentiation.
See also GERM CELL

FFA Acronym for **free fatty acids**.
See FREE FATTY ACIDS

FGF See FIBROBLAST GROWTH FACTOR (FGF)

FGMP See FOOD GOOD MANUFACTURING PRACTICE (FGMP)

FHB Acronym for **fusarium head blight**.
See *FUSARIUM*

FIA Refers to immunodiagnostic tests that are based on fluorescence tracers (labels).
See also IMMUNOASSAY, FLUORESCENCE, RADIOIMMUNOASSAY

Fibrin The ordered fibrous array of fibrin monomers, called a fibrin–platelet clot (blood clot), which spontaneously assembles from fibrin monomers (formed by the thrombin-catalyzed conversion of fibrinogen into fibrin).

F

Fibrinogen itself is the product of a controlled series of zymogen activation steps (enzymatic cascade) triggered initially by substances that are released from body tissues as a consequence of trauma (harm) to them.

See also FIBRONECTIN, ZYMOGENS, CASCADE, LIPOPROTEIN-ASSOCIATED COAGULATION (CLOT) INHIBITOR (LACI)

Fibrinogen See FIBRIN, LIPOPROTEIN-ASSOCIATED COAGULATION (CLOT) INHIBITOR (LACI)

Fibrinolytic Agents Bloodborne compounds that activate fibrin in order to dissolve blood clots.

See also TISSUE PLASMINOGEN ACTIVATOR (tPA), THROMBOLYTIC AGENTS, FIBRIN

Fibroblast Growth Factor (FGF) First described in the mid-1970s by Dr. Gospodarowicz and fellow researchers at the University of California, San Francisco. It is a protein that stimulates the formation and development of blood vessels and fibroblasts (precursors to collagen, the connective tissue "glue" that holds cells together). FGF also is mitogenic (causes cells to divide and multiply) for both fibroblasts and endothelial cells and attracts these two cell types (i.e., is chemotactic). Dr. Gospodarowicz named the FGF originally derived from bovine (cow) brain tissue to be acidic FGF and that from bovine pituitary tissue to be basic FGF. This was due to their identical *biological* activity but differing isoelectric points (i.e., the former being acidic and the latter being basic). Basic FGF is, however, ten times more "potent" than acidic FGF in most bioassays.

See also ANGIOGENIC GROWTH FACTORS, PROTEIN, FIBROBLASTS, PITUITARY GLAND, COLLAGEN, MITOGEN, ENDOTHELIAL CELLS, CHEMOTAXIS, BIOLOGICAL ACTIVITY, BIOASSAY, ACID, BASE (GENERAL)

Fibroblasts Cells that are precursors to the connective tissue cells found in the skin. They make structural proteins such as collagen, which gives skin its strength. Because fibroblasts do not express antigens on their cell surfaces (free standing, separated), fibroblasts possess potential for use in making artificial

organs (e.g., artificial pancreas for diabetics), because the recipient immune system cannot recognize the fibroblast cells as foreign.

See also CELLULAR IMMUNE RESPONSE, HUMORAL IMMUNITY, GRAFT-VERSUS-HOST DISEASE (GVHD), XENOGENEIC ORGANS, CELL, MULTIPOTENT, FIBROBLAST GROWTH FACTOR (FGF), COLLAGEN

Fibronectin An adhesive glycoprotein that forms a link between the epithelial cells and the connective tissue matrix (essential for blood clotting). Research has indicated that fibronectin may solve the problem of getting new cells to stick to existing tissue once a growth factor has caused them to grow (e.g., when a growth factor is administered after a serious wound to a tissue).

See also FIBRIN, GLYCOPROTEIN, GROWTH FACTOR, ORGANOGENESIS

Field Inversion Gel Electrophoresis (FIGE) A chromatographic procedure for the separation of a mixture of molecules by means of a two-dimensional electrical field applied across a gel matrix containing those molecules. For example, FIGE is commonly used to separate mixtures of large DNA molecules by their size and (electrical) charge. FIGE can be used to separate (resolve) DNA molecules up to 2000 Kbp in length.

See also TWO-DIMENSIONAL (2-D) GEL ELECTROPHORESIS, CHROMATOGRAPHY, ELECTROPHORESIS, KILOBASE PAIRS (Kbp), POLYACRYLAMIDE GEL ELECTROPHORESIS (PAGE), DEOXYRIBONUCLEIC ACID (DNA)

FIFRA See FEDERAL INSECTICIDE FUNGICIDE AND RODENTICIDE ACT (FIFRA)

Filler Epithelial Cells Skin cells that initially form under a scab in the wound-healing process in response to stimulation by epidermal growth factor (EGF).

See also EPIDERMAL GROWTH FACTOR (EGF)

Filopodia See MOTOR PROTEINS, ACTIN

Finger Proteins See ZINC FINGER PROTEINS

Fingerprinting See PEPTIDE MAPPING ("FINGERPRINTING"), COMBINATORIAL CHEMISTRY

FIONA Acronym for **fluorescence imaging with 1-nm accuracy**.
See FLUORESCENCE, FLUORESCENCE MAPPING, MULTIPLEXED ASSAY, NANOMETERS (nm)

Firefly Luciferase–Luciferin System See FLUORESCENCE, LUCIFERASE, LUCIFERIN

First Filial Hybrids See F1 HYBRIDS

FISH Acronym for **fluorescence *in situ* hybridization**.
See also FLUORESCENCE *IN SITU* HYBRIDIZATION (FISH), *IN SITU*

Flagella A protein-based, flexible, whiplike organ of locomotion found on some microorganisms with which they are able to swim. Flagella are usually very long and there are usually only one or two per cell. The tails of sperm cells are examples of flagella. Flagella are used in the swimming motion of bacteria toward sources of nutrients in a process called chemotaxis. The singular is flagellum.
See also MICROTUBULES, CILIA, CHEMOTAXIS, BACTERIA, PROTEIN

Flanking Sequence A segment of DNA molecule that either precedes or follows the region of interest on the molecule.
See also DEOXYRIBONUCLEIC ACID (DNA)

Flavin Also known as lyochrome. One of a group of pale yellow, greenly fluorescing biological pigments widely distributed in small quantities in plant and animal tissues. Flavins are synthesized only by bacteria, yeast, and green plants; for this reason, animals are dependent on plant sources for riboflavin (vitamin B_2), the most prevalent member of the group.

Flavin Adenine Dinucleotide (FAD) The coenzyme of some adenine dinucleotide (AD) oxidation–reduction enzymes; it contains riboflavin.
See also FLAVIN, ENZYME, COENZYME, OXIDATION–REDUCTION REACTION

Flavin Mononucleotide (FMN) Riboflavin phosphate, a coenzyme of certain oxidoreduction enzymes.
See also COENZYME

Flavin Nucleotides Nucelotide coenzymes (FMN and FAD) containing riboflavin.
See also FLAVIN MONONUCLEOTIDE (FMN), FLAVIN ADENINE DINUCLEOTIDE (FAD)

Flavin-Linked Dehydrogenases Dehydrogenases are enzymes (involved in removing hydrogen atoms from their substrate) that require one of the riboflavin coenzymes, FMN or FAD, in order to function.
See also DEHYDROGENASES, FLAVIN MONONUCLEOTIDE (FMN), FLAVIN ADENINE DINUCLEOTIDE (FAD), SUBSTRATE (CHEMICAL)

Flavinoids See FLAVONOIDS

Flavonoids A category of phytochemicals that are typically beneficial to the health (e.g., lower blood cholesterol levels) of humans who consume them. Hundreds of flavonoids are naturally produced by plants that are common human foods. For example, the three isoflavones (genistein, daidzein, and glycitein) produced in seeds of the soybean plant (*Glycine max* (L.) Merrill) are flavonoids, and they confer several health benefits on humans who consume them.

Coffee, tea, and chocolate products contain a number of antioxidant flavonoids (i.e., polyphenols). Because oxidation of lipids (e.g., low-density lipoproteins) in the bloodstream is the initial step in atherosclerosis disease, consumption of large amounts of coffee may help to prevent atherosclerosis. Research conducted by Joe Vinson in 1999 indicated that high coffee consumption by humans reduced oxidation of lipids in the bloodstream by 30%.

Cranberries (*Vaccinium macrocarpon*) contain a number of antioxidant flavonoids, and research indicates that consumption of large amounts on a regular basis may inhibit development of breast cancer. Blueberries (*Vaccinium ashei, Vaccinium corymbosum*, etc.) contain a number of flavonoids, and research indicates that consumption of large amounts on a regular basis helps to prevent urinary tract infections, strengthen eyesight, improve memory, inhibit certain cancers, and inhibit some physical aspects of the aging process.

Other subcategories of flavonoids are flavones, flavonols, flavanols, aurones, chalcones, etc.
See also PHYTOCHEMICALS, ISOFLAVONES, SOYBEAN PLANT, QUERCETIN, ATHEROSCLEROSIS, OXIDATION, ANTIOXIDANTS, OXIDATIVE STRESS, CANCER, LIPIDS, ANTHOCYANIDINS,

F

PROANTHOCYANIDINS, FLAVONOLS, POLYPHENOLS, CHOLESTEROL

Flavonols A group of phytochemicals consisting of a subcategory of the **flavonoid "family"** of phytochemicals. Flavonols are typically beneficial to the health of humans who consume them and are typically found in citrus fruits such as grapefruit, oranges, etc. However, at least two flavonols (quercitin glycoside and naringenin chalcone) are found in tomato peels.

See also PHYTOCHEMICALS, FLAVONOIDS, CHALCONE ISOMERASE

Flavoprotein An enzyme containing a flavin nucleotide as a prosthetic group.

See also PROSTHETIC GROUP

Flesh-Eating Infection A colloquialism for **necrotizing fasciitis**.

See also *STREPTOCOCCUS*

FLK-2 Receptors See TOTIPOTENT STEM CELLS

Flora The microorganisms found in a given situation, e.g., reservoir flora (the microorganisms present in a given municipal water reservoir) or intestinal flora (the microorganisms found in the intestines).

Floury-2 A gene in corn or maize (*Zea mays* L.) that (when present in the DNA of a given plant) causes the plant to produce seed that contains higher-than-traditional levels of the amino acids methionine and tryptophan.

See also GENE, CORN, METHIONINE (Met), HIGH-METHIONINE CORN, ESSENTIAL AMINO ACIDS, VALUE-ENHANCED GRAINS, DEOXYRIBONUCLEIC ACID (DNA)

Flow Cytometry See CELL SORTING, FLUORESCENCE-ACTIVATED CELL SORTER (FACS), MAGNETIC PARTICLES

Fluorescence The reaction in which certain molecules (known as fluorophores) upon absorption of a specific amount of light of specific wavelength emit (reradiate) light energy possessing a longer wavelength than the original light absorbed. All cells will naturally fluoresce, at least a bit.

Human colon cancer cells and precursor cells fluoresce much more (and emit much more red light when they fluoresce) than noncancerous cells, which may lead to a new and better means of early detection.

See also FLUOROPHORE, CELL, FLUORESCENCE MAPPING, CANCER, FIA, BRIGHT GREENISH-YELLOW FLUORESCENCE (BGYF), IMMUNOSENSOR, BIOCHIP, NEAR-INFRARED SPECTROSCOPY (NIR)

Fluorescence-Activated Cell Sorter (FACS) A machine or MEMS/lab-on-a-chip that is used to sort specific cells from a mixed group of cells (e.g., to remove only the cells of one type of tissue, or cells into which a new gene has been inserted via genetic engineering techniques, etc.).

Fluorescence *In Situ* Hybridization (FISH) A method for detecting the presence of particular genes (e.g., in a biological sample), which utilizes a number of fluorescein-"tagged" DNA probes. When those DNA probes hybridize to each of their respective particular genes (i.e., that they were selected to be complementary to), each DNA probe's "tag" fluoresces at a different wavelength (different "color"), thereby indicating positively the presence in the sample of that particular gene.

During August 2002, the U.S. Food and Drug Administration (FDA) approved use of **information from a FISH test** (for detection of the overexpression of HER-2 gene in women) to guide the administration of the humanized monoclonal antibody (trastuzumab), which the FDA had approved for use in conjunction with chemotherapy, etc., against metastatic breast cancers. The FISH test (an application of pharmacogenomics) helps to detect the approximately 35% of patients for whom trastuzumab will be effective.

Another use of such **genetic markers** is for the selection of the human haplotypes (patient groups) utilized in Phase I or Phase II clinical tests of new pharmaceutical candidate compounds. For example, the pharmaceutical known as Gleevec™ showed near 100% efficacy in clinical trials for:

- **Chronic myelogenous leukemia** disease when all patients in the patient group consisted of the haplotype possessing the genetic marker (gene) known as **bcr-abl**
- **Gastrointestinal stromal tumors (GIST)** when all patients in the

patient group consisted of the haplo-type possessing the genetic marker (gene) known as **c-kit**

See also GENE, GENETIC MARKER, HAP-LOTYPE, FLUORESCENCE, PROBE, DNA PROBE, COMPLEMENTARY (MOLECULAR GENETICS), HYBRID-IZATION (MOLECULAR GENETICS), HER-2 GENE, HER-2 RECEPTOR, CAN-CER, PHARMACOGENOMICS, PHAR-MACOGENETICS, MONOCLONAL ANTIBODIES (MAb), METASTASIS, LABEL (FLUORESCENT), FOOD AND DRUG ADMINISTRATION (FDA), TRAS-TUZUMAB, HUMANIZED ANTIBODY, PHASE I CLINICAL TESTING, PHASE II CLINICAL TESTS, GLEEVEC™

The desired cells are first labeled with a specific fluorescent dye or a gene for a fluorophore (e.g., green fluorescent protein) is inserted, and then the cells are passed through a flow chamber that is illuminated by a laser beam, which causes the labeled cells to fluoresce (i.e., glow). The molecules of the fluorescent dye, which "stick" to only one type of cell in the mixture, contain chromophores that can be elevated to an excited, unstable state by irradiation with specific wavelengths of light. The chromophores remain in the excited state for a maximum of 10^{-9} sec before releasing their energy by emitting light and returning to their unexcited "ground" state. This fluores-cence ("glow") is a measurable property, and the FACS machine utilizes it to separate the desired cells from the rest of the mixture.

See also BASOPHILIC, GENE, GENETIC ENGINEERING, CELL, FLUORESCENCE, FLUOROPHORE, CELL SORTING, LABEL (FLUORESCENT), GREEN FLUORES-CENT PROTEIN, LAB-ON-A-CHIP, MEMS (NANOTECHNOLOGY)

Fluorescence Mapping Refers to use of a spe-cial microscope or light of selected wavelength (i.e., to induce fluorescence of "targets") in order to scan (e.g., in tissue) **two-dimensional planes** at varying depths to thoroughly **"map" in three dimensions** all of the molecules of interest that fluoresce (e.g., when a pharma-ceutical compound binds to each "target" mol-ecule, such as a cell receptor).

See also FLUORESCENCE, MULTIPLEXED ASSAY, CONFOCAL MICROSCOPY, CELL, RECEPTORS, FIONA

Fluorescence Multiplexing See FLUORES-CENCE MAPPING, MULTIPLEXED ASSAY

Fluorescence Polarization (FP) A technol-ogy that can be utilized to detect the presence or the behavior of single molecules — or a single molecular species — within:

- Living cells (without killing the cell).
- Biological fluids (without disrupting or destroying other compounds in those biological fluids). For example, FP immunoassays have been exten-sively utilized since 1980 to measure the concentration of drugs in biolog-ical samples being evaluated in clin-ical laboratories.

In FP, plane-polarized light of **specific (to rel-evant molecule) wavelength** is utilized to cause that specific molecule to fluoresce. If the molecule remains stationary, the (fluoresc-ing) molecule emits light in the **same** plane as the original light.

See also CELL, IMMUNOASSAY, GENE EXPRESSION PROFILING, HIGH-THROUGHPUT SCREENING (HTS), SIN-GLE-NUCLEOTIDE POLYMORPHISMS (SNPs)

Fluorescence Resonance Energy Transfer (FRET) Refers to (fluorescence-induced) resonance that occurs when two different molecular (fluorescent) labels are in very close proximity to each other. That resonance causes (the two in combination) to emit a third color (wavelength), but the two revert (to orig-inal two colors) when some events, such as the following, move the two labels apart:

- A ligand "docking" at a cell's recep-tor (e.g., resulting in signal transduc-tion that releases from the receptor a labeled-chemical-signal molecule within the cell)
- A change in ion concentration (e.g., thereby causing two fluorophore-labeled molecules to move apart)

FRET can be utilized as a microscopy tool by scientists to obtain quantitative information

F

about the binding or other molecular interactions between enzymes, other proteins, lipids, DNA, and RNA. Via fluorescent labeling (e.g., with green fluorescent protein), FRET microscopy has been used to trace the movement of protein molecules inside living cells and to delineate the functioning and organization within cells.

See also FLUORESCENCE, FLUOROPHORE, LABEL (FLUORESCENT), GREEN FLUO-RESCENT PROTEIN, LIGAND (IN BIO-CHEMISTRY), CELL, RECEPTORS, SIGNAL TRANSDUCTION, ION, ENZYME, PRO-TEIN, LIPIDS, DEOXYRIBONUCLEIC ACID (DNA), RIBONUCLEIC ACID (RNA)

Fluorescent Real-Time PCR See REAL-TIME PCR (TESTING)

Fluorogenic Probe See MOLECULAR BEA-CON

Fluorophore Refers to any substance that is fluorescent.

See also FLUORESCENCE

Flux Refers to the specific biochemical reactions or cascades (and amounts or rate of metabolite production) in a given metabolic pathway.

For example, the human disease diabetes results in elevated levels of glucose in the bloodstream. Such elevated glucose levels cause the body's metabolism to begin increasing the flux through the **polyol pathway** (of metabolism). In nondiseased individuals, the polyol pathway is used very little, if at all. However, this massive increase in flux in the polyol pathway results in accumulation of the **reduced form** of the cofactor NADH (nicotinamide adenine dinucleotide, reduced) and thereby an increase in the ratio of NADH to NAD (its oxidized form). That higher ratio of NADH/NAD adversely impacts many of the biochemical pathways that NADH has a critical role in. Some pathogens (e.g., bacteria) are able to resist certain antibiotics via a change in their flux.

Metabolic flux analysis refers to the research methodology utilized to comprehensively evaluate an organism's metabolic biochemical pathways and their responses to environmental and genetic inputs.

See also METABOLISM, METABOLIC PATH-WAY, FLUX, METABOLITE, METABOLIC ENGINEERING, CASCADE, FEEDBACK INHIBITION, COFACTOR, DEFICIENCY, OXIDATION (CHEMICAL REACTION), REDUCTION (IN A CHEMICAL REAC-TION), OXIDATION–REDUCTION REAC-TION, GLUCOSE (GLc), ANTIBIOTIC RESISTANCE

Follicle-Stimulating Hormone (FSH) A protein hormone used in conventional medical therapy in an attempt to increase production of sperm in men (inside the follicles of the testes).

See also THYROID-STIMULATING HOR-MONE (TSH), GRAVE'S DISEASE, PRO-TEIN, HORMONE, PITUITARY GLAND

Food and Drug Administration (FDA) The federal agency charged with approving all pharmaceutical and food ingredient products sold within the U.S.

In 1992, prior to approval of any of the biotechnology-derived food crop plants, the FDA decided that food crops produced via "biotechnological (i.e., recombinant) technologies" must meet the same rigorous safety standards as those created via "traditional breeding methods" — both categories of which are regulated by the FDA.

Historically, new food crops created via "traditional breeding technologies" (e.g., crossing with wild type in order to confer disease resistance, increased yield, etc., on the resultant domesticated plant varieties or strains) have sometimes contained unexpectedly high levels of known (and naturally occurring) toxins (e.g., solanine, a naturally occurring toxin in potatoes and some other plants, and psoralene, a naturally occurring toxin in celery; etc.).

See also KOSEISHO, COMMITTEE FOR PROPRIETARY MEDICINAL PRODUCTS (CPMP), COMMITTEE FOR VETERINARY MEDICINAL PRODUCTS (CVMP), COM-MITTEE ON SAFETY IN MEDICINES, WILD TYPE, STRAIN, "TREATMENT" IND REGULATIONS, KEFAUVER RULE, IND, IND EXEMPTION, RECOMBINANT DNA (rDNA), PHASE I CLINICAL TEST-ING, EUROPEAN MEDICINES EVALUA-TION AGENCY (EMEA), MEDICINES CONTROL AGENCY (MCA), BUNDESGE-SUNDHEITSAMT (BGA), TRADITIONAL BREEDING METHODS, SOLANINE, PSO-RALENE

Food Good Manufacturing Practice (FGMP) The Food and Drug Administration's (FDA's) approval mechanism for a process to manufacture a given food or food additive. It is implemented instead of specific regulations (such as those used to dictate processes, such as beef packing, in simple food manufacture) owing to the newness of the technology and may later be superseded (because of further advances in the technology).

See also FOOD AND DRUG ADMINISTRATION (FDA)

Footprinting A technique used by researchers to determine precisely *where* (on DNA molecule) certain DNA-binding proteins make specific contact with that DNA molecule. For example, certain types of drugs act by binding tightly to certain DNA molecules in specific locations (e.g., in order to halt cancerous growth of cells, etc.).

See also DEOXYRIBONUCLEIC ACID (DNA), PROTEIN, GENOTOXIC

For Treatment IND See "TREATMENT" IND REGULATIONS

Formaldehyde Dehydrogenase An enzyme that catalyzes the oxidation of formaldehyde to formic acid (formate at intracellular pH). It requires NAD (i.e., nicotinamide adenine dinucleotide) as an electron acceptor. It is important in the metabolism of methanol.

See also METABOLISM, ENZYME, NAD (NADH, NADP, NADPH), CATALYST

Forward Mutation A mutation from the wild (natural) type to the mutant (type).

See also MUTATION, WILD TYPE

FOS See FRUCTOSE OLIGOSACCHARIDES

FOSHU A Japanese government designation meaning "Foods of Specified Health Use." Introduced in the early 1980s, these are foods or food ingredients that meet the following specific criteria:

- Must improve human nutrition and health.
- A benefit to human health and nutrition must be proven for that food or ingredient.
- An appropriate daily dose (i.e., amount to be consumed) must be confirmed by doctors or dietitians.

- The food or ingredient must guarantee balanced nourishment.
- The active component (e.g., phytochemical) must be scientifically confirmed regarding (1) its quantitative and qualitative definition and (2) its chemical and physical features.
- The active component must not lower nutritional value (e.g., of the food it is added to).
- The food or ingredient must be consumed in a normal fashion (i.e., eaten or drank, not as pill or powder form).
- The active component must be of natural origin.

Some of the foods or ingredients designated "FOSHU" are those containing polyphenols, anthocyanins, and diacylglycerols.

See also NUTRACEUTICALS, PHYTOCHEMICALS, MANNANOLIGOSACCHARIDES, FRUCTOSE OLIGOSACCHARIDES, ANTHOCYANINS, POLYPHENOLS, DIACYLGLYCEROLS

Foundation on Economic Trends A small organization that lobbies against agricultural biotechnology.

See also BIOTECHNOLOGY

FP Acronym for **fluorescence polarization**.

See FLUORESCENCE POLARIZATION (FP)

Frameshift A shift (displacement) of the reading frame in a DNA or RNA molecule.

Frameshifts generally result from the addition or deletion of one or more nucleotides to or from the DNA or RNA molecule.

See also READING FRAME, CODON, GENETIC CODE, MUTATION, DEOXYRIBONUCLEIC ACID (DNA), NUCLEOTIDE, RIBONUCLEIC ACID (RNA), CENTRAL DOGMA (NEW)

Free Energy The component of the total energy of a system that can do work at a constant temperature and pressure. Also known as Gibbs' free energy.

Free energy is a key variable calculated and monitored for different (proposed) drug molecules or drug–target interactions during **rational drug design** activities (e.g., molecular modeling).

See also RATIONAL DRUG DESIGN, TARGET (OF A THERAPEUTIC AGENT), ACTIVATION ENERGY

Free Fatty Acids (F.F.A.) Individual fatty acid molecules within a vegetable oil, which exist in an **uncombined-with-glycerine** molecular state. The presence of F.F.A. can be caused by naturally occurring noncombination (e.g., in some varieties of oilseeds), sprouting of the oilseeds prior to processing into vegetable oil, or breakdown of the fat (oil) during processing or usage.

See also FATS, FATTY ACID, SATURATED FATTY ACIDS, UNSATURATED FATTY ACID

Free Radical Sometimes called **reactive oxygen species**, **singlet oxygen**, or **oxygen free radical**.

Term utilized to refer to an oxygen (atom) bearing an "extra" electron. Because of this, it possesses a large amount of energy, and in a biological system (i.e., inside the body of an organism), it can damage body tissues when it "discharges" that energy.

For example, during 2001, researchers showed that an excess of free radicals within tissues of diabetic organisms is a major factor in the development of the vascular and nerve damage typically found in late stage diabetes.

See also OXIDATIVE STRESS, ANTIOXIDANTS, HUMAN SUPEROXIDE DISMUTASE (hSOD), CAROTENOIDS, CONJUGATED LINOLEIC ACID (CLA), DIABETES, INSULIN, HAPTOGLOBIN, NEUTROPHILS

FRET Acronym for **fluorescence resonance energy transfer**.

See FLUORESCENCE RESONANCE ENERGY TRANSFER (FRET)

Fructan A general term utilized to refer to any carbohydrate in which **fructosyl–fructose (molecule)** linkages constitute the majority of the molecule's glycosidic bonds (i.e., between atoms in the molecule).

See also CARBOHYDRATES (SACCHARIDES), OLIGOSACCHARIDES, FRUCTOSE OLIGOSACCHARIDES, GLYCOSIDE

Fructooligosaccharides See FRUCTOSE OLIGOSACCHARIDES

Fructose Oligosaccharides A "family" of oligosaccharides, some of which help to foster the growth of bifidobacteria in the lower colon of monogastric animals (e.g., humans, swine, etc.). These bifidobacteria generate certain short-chain fatty acids, which are absorbed by the colon and result in a reduction of triglyceride (fat) and cholesterol levels in the bloodstream, thereby lowering risk of coronary heart disease and thrombosis. Research indicates that they also promote absorption of calcium from foods (in the large intestine). Fructose oligosaccharides are classified as a "water-soluble fiber" (e.g., by the European Union's government food regulatory agencies), because humans cannot digest them.

See also BIFIDOBACTERIA, *BIFIDUS*, INULIN, FOSHU, OLIGOSACCHARIDES, NUTRACEUTICALS, CHOLESTEROL, HIGH-DENSITY LIPOPROTEINS (HDLPs), LOW-DENSITY LIPOPROTEINS (LDLPs), BACTERIA, FATTY ACID, PREBIOTICS, MANNANOLIGOSACCHARIDES (MOS), CORONARY HEART DISEASE (CHD), TRIGLYCERIDES, THROMBOSIS

Fumarase (Fum) An enzyme that catalyzes the hydration (addition of hydrogen atoms) of fumaric acid to maleic acid, as well as the reverse dehydration reaction (removal of hydrogen atoms).

See also ENZYME, CATALYST

Fumaric Acid ($C_4H_4O_4$) A dicarboxylic organic acid produced commercially by chemical synthesis and fermentation, it is the *trans* isomer of maleic acid and a colorless crystal with a melting point of 87°C (191°F). It is used to make resins, paints, varnishes, and inks, in food, as a mordant (dye fixer or stabilizer), and as a chemical intermediate. Also known as boletic acid.

See also ACID, ISOMER, BOLETIC ACID

Fumonisins A "family" of mycotoxins that are primarily produced by the fungi *Fusarium moniliforme, Fusarium verticillioides,* and *Fusarium proliferatum* (e.g., in insect-damaged corn or maize and wheat).

Consumption of fumonisins by horses and swine can be fatal and consumption by other animals (including humans) can result in tumors (e.g., cancer of the esophagus in humans).

See also MYCOTOXINS, FUNGUS, *FUSARIUM*, *FUSARIUM MONILIFORME*, EUROPEAN CORN BORER (ECB), CANCER, P53 GENE

Functional Foods Refers to foods that provide health benefits beyond basic nutrition.

See also NUTRACEUTICALS, PHYTOCHEMICALS, FOSHU

Functional Genomics Study of, or discovery of, what traits or functions (generally via proteins expressed) are conferred on an organism by given (gene) sequences. The timing and location of the expression of those genes is also impacted sometimes by external and environmental factors such as temperature, sunlight, humidity, the presence of signal transducers and activators of transcription (STATs), etc. Also impacting the functions or traits are interactions among genes, signaling cascades, and response–reaction mechanisms within the body of that organism.

Typically, functional genomic study follows after discovery of gene sequences found via structural genomics study.

Some methods utilized to determine which traits or functions result from which genes are the following:

- Site-directed mutagenesis (SDM), to compare two same-species organisms possessing two different genes at the same site on the genome
- Antisense DNA sequence, to compare two same-species organisms (one of which has gene at same site "turned off" via antisense DNA)
- Reporter gene, to compare two same-species organisms (with two different genes at same site on genome) via a "reporter" gene adjacent to gene or site, to detect presence of desired trait or function
- Chemical genetics, to compare two same-species organisms (one of which has gene at same site on DNA molecule at least partially inactivated by a specific chemical)
- "Silencing" or "knocking out" a particular gene via other methods than antisense or chemical genetics, to compare

See also GENOMICS, TRAIT, GENE, GENOTYPE, PHENOTYPE, POLYGENIC, EXPRESS, STRUCTURAL GENE, STRUCTURAL GENOMICS, DEOXYRIBONUCLEIC ACID (DNA), SEQUENCE (OF A DNA MOLECULE), PLEIOTROPIC, GENETIC CODE, EXPRESSED SEQUENCE TAGS, INFORMATIONAL MOLECULES, POINT MUTATION, SITE-DIRECTED MUTAGENESIS (SDM), ANTISENSE (DNA SEQUENCE), REPORTER GENE, METHYLATION, ZINC FINGER PROTEINS, DNA METHYLATION, POSITIONAL CLONING, CHEMICAL GENETICS, GENE SILENCING, *DROSOPHILA, CAENORHABDITIS ELEGANS*, CENTRAL DOGMA (NEW), TRANSCRIPTION FACTORS, SIGNAL TRANSDUCERS AND ACTIVATORS OF TRANSCRIPTION (STATs), GENE EXPRESSION ANALYSIS, GENE FUNCTION ANALYSIS, PATHWAY, PATHWAY FEEDBACK MECHANISMS, CASCADE

Functional Group A molecule, or portion of a molecule, that will react with other molecules. For example, "hedgehog proteins" must first add a cholesterol molecule (to themselves) before they can carry out their task of directing or controlling tissue differentiation development (into various organs, limbs, etc.) during mammal embryo.

An "acetyl (functional) group" must be added to a choline molecule in order for the body to have the critical neurotransmitter acetylcholine.

See also PROTEIN, PEPTIDE, HEDGEHOG PROTEINS, CHOLESTEROL, ACETYL CHOLINE, NEUROTRANSMITTER, SIGNAL TRANSDUCTION

Functional Protein Microarrays Refers to the category of protein microarrays in which the **capture agents** are themselves protein molecules so that such microarrays can evaluate the following:

- Protein–protein interactions
- Protein–ligand interactions
- How some protein molecules modify other proteins (e.g., how tyrosine kinases will phosphorylate some proteins)

See also PROTEIN MICROARRAYS, PROTEIN, CAPTURE AGENT, PROTEIN INTERACTION ANALYSIS, PROTEIN–PROTEIN

F

INTERACTIONS, TARGET–LIGAND INTERACTION SCREENING, PROTEIN TYROSINE KINASES, PHOSPHORYLATION

Fungicide Any chemical compound that is toxic to fungi.

See also BIOCIDE, FUNGUS

Fungus (plural: fungi) Any of a major group of saprophytic and parasitic plants that lack chlorophyll and flowers, including molds, toadstools, rusts, mildews, smuts, ergot, mushrooms *Aqaricus bisporus*, and yeasts.

Under certain conditions (e.g., temperature, humidity, etc.), some fungi can produce mycotoxins via their metabolism.

See also RUSTS, *APERGILLUS FLAVUS*, MYCOTOXINS, *FUSARIUM*, *FUSARIUM GRAMINEARUM*, AFLATOXIN, FUMONISINS, VOMITOXIN, DON, ERGOTAMINE, METABOLISM, RICE BLAST

Furanocoumarins See PSORALENE

Furanose A sugar molecule containing the five-membered furan ring.

See also SUGAR MOLECULES

Furocoumarins A term that is sometimes utilized to refer to furanocoumarins.

See FURANOCOUMARINS

Fusaric Acids See *FUSARIUM MONILIFORME*

Fusarium A genus of fungus that infests certain grains (e.g., wheat *Triticum aestivum*, corn or maize *Zea mays L.*, etc.) during growing seasons in which climate (e.g., high humidity, cool weather) and other conditions combine to enable rapid growth and proliferation of the fungus.

In wheat, the (*Fusarium graminearum,* head blight) fungus infestation, also known as "scab," causes the wheat plant to weaken and to produce empty seed heads, which reduces yield.

In corn (maize), the (*Fusarium graminearum*) fungus infestation, also known as *Gibberella zeae* or "Gibberella ear rot," ruins grain kernels, which reduces yields.

As a by-product of their metabolism, some of the *Fusarium* types (species) produce deoxynivalenol (also known as DON or "vomitoxin" — produced by *Fusarium graminearum*), zearalenone, and fumonisins (a group of very potent mycotoxins that are produced by *Fusarium moniliforme* and *Fusarium proliferatum* and *Fusarium verticillioides* fungi). Fumonisin B_1 is the most prevalent *Fusarium*-produced mycotoxin in corn (maize). Its presence can cause livestock to refuse to eat infested feed, decrease reproductive efficiency in swine, and even kill horses (via equine leukoencephalomalacia).

When consumed by humans, fumonisin B_1 induces cell death via apoptosis, and the tissues that are adjacent to killed cells respond with cell replication or proliferation to replace the lost cells.

Fumonisin B_1 inhibits the enzyme ceramide synthetase (that is crucial to the biosynthetic pathway for the creation of sphingolipids in cells), resulting in accumulation of sphinganine in cells and decreases ceramides and complex sphingolipids. These internal changes signal the cells, especially liver and kidney cells, to die via apoptosis ("programmed cell death").

Maximum fumonisin content allowed in flour (for U.S. bread) is one part per million. Maximum fumonisin content allowed in U.S. malting barley (*Hordeum vulgare*) is zero.

In 1997, Iowa State University research showed that *B.t.* corn varieties (that express the *B.t.* protoxin in the corn ears) have significantly less ear mold caused by *Fusarium* fungi. That is because the European corn borer (ECB) is a vector (carrier) of *Fusarium*.

See also FUNGUS, MYCOTOXINS, TOXIN, METABOLISM, FUMONISINS, ZEARALENONE, APOPTOSIS, ENZYME INHIBITION, LIPIDS, VOMITOXIN, DON, DEOXYNIVALENOL, *BACILLUS THURINGIENSIS (B.t.)*, EUROPEAN CORN BORER (ECB), CD95 PROTEIN, SOYBEAN CYST NEMATODES (SCN), *FUSARIUM MONILIFORME*, *FUSARIUM GRAMINEARUM*

Fusarium graminearum A fungus, also sometimes known as *Gibberella zeae*, that can infect wheat (*Triticum aestivum*) or corn/maize (*Zea mays L.*) under certain growing season conditions.

In wheat, this fungus infestation, also known as "scab," causes the wheat plant to weaken and to produce empty seed heads, which reduces yield.

In corn or maize, this fungus infestation, also known as "Gibberella ear rot," ruins grain kernels, which reduces yield.

As a by-product of its metabolism, this fungus can sometimes produce the mycotoxins **deoxynivalenol** (also known as DON or "vomitoxin") and **zearalenone**.

See also FUNGUS, *FUSARIUM*, CORN, WHEAT, TOXIN, METABOLISM, MYCOTOXINS, DEOXYNIVALENOL, DON, VOMITOXIN, ZEARALENONE

Fusarium moniliforme One of the *Fusarium* fungi, therefore, it can produce one or more **fumonisins** (a group of mycotoxins) under certain environmental conditions when it grows in some grains.

When *Fusarium moniliforme* grows within growing plants of domesticated rice (*Oryza sativa*), it can cause the plant disease known as **Bakanae (also known as "foolish seedling" disease)**. Symptoms of Bakanae include rice plants that are much taller than normal rice plants and leaves that are much longer than normal.

That abnormal growth (of rice plant and leaves) is caused by a gibberellin compound that is excreted by the *Fusarium moniliforme* fungus. The fungus also excretes fusaric acids, which can stunt or kill rice plants.

See also *FUSARIUM*, MYCOTOXINS, FUMONISINS, FUNGUS, GIBBERELLINS

Fusion Inhibitors See CD4-PE40, SOLUBLE CD4

Fusion Protein A protein consisting of all or part of the amino acid sequences (known as the "domain") of two or more proteins. Fusion proteins are formed by the following:

- Some natural cellular processes. For example, a naturally occurring fusion protein results when the ubiquitin protein fuses with certain (degraded or misfolded) protein molecules inside cells to "mark" those degraded protein molecules for destruction by the cell's proteasomes. In some specific instances, the fusion of ubiquitin to certain protein molecules in cells causes that "partner protein" to be expressed in larger amounts than before.

- Scientists fusing the two protein-encoding genes (which causes the cell's ribosome to subsequently produce the desired fusion protein). This fusion is generally for the following reasons:
  - Put the expression of one of the (fused) genes under the control of the strong promoter for the first gene.
  - Allow the gene of interest (that is difficult to assay) to be more easily studied via substituting some of the (gene) protein with a more easily measured (assayed) function. For example, fusing a difficult-to-study gene with the β-galactosidase gene, the (protein) product of which can easily be measured (assayed) using chromatography. Another example is to fuse the gene of a fluorescent protein to that of a gene coding for a given protein being assayed regarding its folding inside a living cell (i.e., fluorescence then indicates that protein to have folded properly).
  - Create a pharmaceutical consisting of relevant domains of two different proteins. For example, the pharmaceutical Enbrel™ (etanercept) is a fusion protein consisting of the **extracellular (i.e., portion sticking out of cell's plasma membrane) sequence** of human TNFR (tumor necrosis factor receptor) and the **Fc sequence of the human antibody IgG1**. When injected, the TNFR segment of the etanercept fusion protein binds to a tumor necrosis factor molecule, and the Fc segment of the etanercept protein marks that molecule for removal by other immune system cells, thereby reducing the structural damage (to body joints) caused by excess tumor necrosis factor in the autoimmune disease rheumatoid arthritis.

F

See also PROTEIN, AMINO ACID, SEQUENCE (OF A PROTEIN MOLECULE), GENE, EXPRESS, CELL, RIBOSOMES, PROMOTER, ASSAY, CODING SEQUENCE, DOMAIN (OF A PROTEIN), UBIQUITIN, PROTEASOMES, PROTEIN FOLDING, GENE FUSION, FLUORESCENCE, VISIBLE FLUORESCENT PROTEINS, GREEN FLUORESCENT PROTEIN, TUMOR NECROSIS FACTOR (TNF), PLASMA MEMBRANE, RECEPTORS, ANTIBODY, SEQUENCE (OF A PROTEIN MOLECULE), RAPID PROTEIN FOLDING ASSAY, CD4-PE40, FUSION INHIBITORS

Fusion Toxin A fusion protein that consists of a toxic protein (domain) plus a cell receptor binding region (protein domain). The cell receptor portion (of the total fusion toxin molecule) delivers the toxin directly to the (diseased) cell, thus sparing other healthy tissues from the effect of the toxin.

See also FUSION PROTEIN, TOXIN, RICIN, PROTEIN, PROTEIN ENGINEERING, DOMAIN (OF A PROTEIN), RECEPTORS, ENDOCYTOSIS

Fusogenic Agent Any compound, virus, etc., that causes cells to fuse together. For example, one of the effects of the HIV (i.e., AIDS-causing) viruses is to cause the T cells of the human immune system to fuse (causing collapse of the immune system).

See also ACQUIRED IMMUNE DEFICIENCY SYNDROME (AIDS), HUMAN IMMUNODEFICIENCY VIRUS TYPE 1 (HIV-1), HUMAN IMMUNODEFICIENCY VIRUS TYPE 2 (HIV-2), HELPER T CELLS (T4 CELLS), ADHESION MOLECULE

Futile Cycle An enzyme-catalyzed set of cyclic reactions that results in release of thermal energy (heat) through the hydrolysis of ATP (adenosine triphosphate). The hydrolysis of ATP is normally coupled to other cycles and reactions in which the energy released is metabolically used. However, futile cycles would appear to waste the energy of ATP as heat — except when one is shivering to keep warm.

The production of heat by shivering is an example of the futile cycle.

See also ADENOSINE TRIPHOSPHATE (ATP), ENZYME, HYDROLYSIS

FXR Acronym for **Farnesoid X receptor**.

See FARNESOID X RECEPTOR (FXR)

G

G Proteins See G-PROTEINS

G-Proteins (Guanyl-Nucleotide Binding Proteins) Discovered by Rodbell and coworkers at National Institutes of Health (NIH), U.S. and Alfred G. Gilman and coworkers at the American University of Virginia-Charlottesville during the 1970s–1980s. These are proteins embedded in the surface membranes of cells. G-proteins "receive chemical signals" from outside the cell (e.g., hormones) and "pass the signal" into the cell so that it can "respond to the signal."

For example, a hormone, drug, neurotransmitter, or another "signal" binds to a receptor molecule on the surface of the cell's exterior membrane. That receptor then activates the G-protein. This causes an effector inside the cell to produce a second "signal" chemical inside the cell, which causes the cell (nucleus) to react to the original external chemical signal. G-proteins are called thus because they become GTP and GDP forms alternately as part of their reaction cycle (i.e., in "passing the signal").

G-protein-coupled receptors play crucial roles in many biological processes such as pain, vision, allergic responses, etc. In addition to **carrying to the cell nucleus** these signals, cytoplasmic G-proteins also regulate certain cellular processes.

Dysfunction of G-proteins in humans causes the salt and water losses inherent in cholera (the body's compromised immune defense inherent in pertussis), and is believed to be responsible for some symptoms of diabetes and alcoholism. Dysfunction of G-proteins in plants causes rapid water loss (wilting).

See also PROTEIN, PLASMA MEMBRANE, LIPID RAFTS, SIGNALING, SIGNAL TRANSDUCTION, MAPK, MITOGEN-ACTIVATED PROTEIN KINASE CASCADE, HORMONE, CELL, NUCLEUS, BETA CELLS, GTPases, GPA1, INSULIN, RECEPTORS, NUCLEAR RECEPTORS, NATIONAL INSTITUTES OF HEALTH (NIH), NEUROTRANSMITTERS, TRANSMEMBRANE PROTEINS, ION CHANNELS, CHOLERA TOXIN, PROSTAGLANDINS, LIGAND (IN BIOCHEMISTRY)

G-Protein-Coupled Receptors See G-PROTEINS

G+ See GRAM-POSITIVE (G+)

G See GRAM-NEGATIVE (G)

GA21 A naturally occurring gene (i.e., expressed at low levels in some plants) that confers resistance to glyphosate-containing herbicides. When the **GA21 gene** is inserted by man into crop plants (e.g., maize or corn) in a way that causes high expression, those crop plants are unaffected when glyphosate-containing herbicides are applied to fields to control weeds in those crops.

See also GENE, EXPRESS, EXPRESSIVITY, PROTEIN, GENETIC ENGINEERING, CORN, HERBICIDE-TOLERANT CROP, GLYPHOSATE

GAL4 See TWO-HYBRID SYSTEMS

Galactomannan See HIGH-MANNOGALACTAN SOYBEANS

Galactose (Gal) A monosaccharide occurring in both levo (L) and dextro (D) forms as a constituent of plant and animal oligosaccharides (lactose and raffinose) and polysaccharides (agar and pectin). Galactose is also known as cerebrose.

See also STEREOISOMERS, DEXTROROTARY (D) ISOMER, LEVOROTARY (L) ISOMER

Gall See Ti PLASMID

GalNAc *N*-acetyl-D-galactosamine.

GALT See GUT-ASSOCIATED LYMPHOID TISSUE (GALT)

Gamete A germ or reproductive cell. In animals (and humans) the functional, mature, male gamete is called spermatozoon; in plants it is called spermatozoid. In both animals and plants, the female gamete is called the ovum, or egg.

See also OOCYTES

Gamma Globulin A type of blood protein that plays a major role in the process of immunity (immune system response). Sometimes the term "gamma globulin" refers to a whole group of blood proteins that are known as antibodies or immunoglobulins (Ig). Most often, however, it applies to a particular immunoglobulin, designated as IgG, believed to be the most abundant type of antibody in the body.
See also ANTIBODY, GUT-ASSOCIATED LYMPHOID TISSUE (GALT), PROTEIN, IMMUNOGLOBULIN

Gamma Interferon Produced by T lymphocytes.
See INTERFERONS, T LYMPHOCYTES

GAP A double-stranded DNA is said to be "gapped" when one strand over a short region of the molecule is missing.
See also DEOXYRIBONUCLEIC ACID (DNA)

GAT Acronym for **glyphosate *N*-acetyltransferase**.
See GLYPHOSATE *N*-ACETYLTRANSFERASE

Gated Transport (of a protein) One of three means for a protein molecule to pass between compartments within eucaryotic cells. The compartment "wall" (membrane) possesses a "sensor" (receptor) that detects the presence of a correct protein (e.g., after that protein has been synthesized in the cell's ribosomes), then opens a "gate" (pore) in the membrane to allow that protein to pass from the first compartment to the second compartment.
See also PROTEIN, EUCARYOTE, CELL, RIBOSOMES, SIGNALING, VESICULAR TRANSPORT

GDH Gene See GLUTAMATE DEHYDROGENASE

GDNF See GLIAL-DERIVED NEUROTROPHIC FACTOR

GEAC India's Genetic Engineering Approval Committee. GEAC must approve an rDNA product (e.g., a genetically engineered crop plant that has earlier received its "bio safety clearance" from the Indian Department of Biotechnology) before it is allowed to be commercially planted in India.
See also GENETIC ENGINEERING, rDNA, INDIAN DEPARTMENT OF BIOTECHNOLOGY

Gel A colloid, where the dispersed phase is liquid and the dispersion medium is solid.

Gel Electrophoresis See TWO-DIMENSIONAL (2-D) GEL ELECTROPHORESIS, POLYACRYLAMIDE GEL ELECTROPHORESIS (PAGE), ELECTROPHORESIS, DENATURING GRADIENT GEL ELECTROPHORESIS

Gel Filtration Also known as **exclusion chromatography**. An effective technique for separating molecules (such as peptide mixtures) on the basis of size. This is accomplished by passing a solution of the molecules to be separated over a column of, for example, Sephadex®, which is a polymerized carbohydrate derivative that contains tiny holes. The holes are of such a size that some of the smaller molecules diffuse through them and are in this way retained (held back), while the larger molecules are not able to get through the holes and they pass through the solid phase (Sephadex®, in this example). This, simplistically, is how separation is effected.
See also ELECTROPHORESIS, CHROMATOGRAPHY, FIELD INVERSION GEL ELECTROPHORESIS

GEM This acronym stands for **Germplasm Enhancement for Maize**, a project conducted under the auspices of the United States Department of Agriculture, in concert with 16 U.S. universities and 20 corn (maize) seed companies. GEM's intent is to cross exotic (not in current use) germplasm with commercial maize lines in order to increase corn yield.
See also CORN, GERMPLASM, HYBRIDIZATION (PLANT GENETICS), PLEIOTROPIC

GEMP (Genetically Engineered Microbial Pesticide) See GENETICALLY ENGINEERED MICROBIAL PESTICIDE, INTEGRATED PEST MANAGEMENT (IPM)

Gene A natural unit of hereditary material, which is the physical basis for transmission of the characteristics of living organisms from one generation to another. The basic genetic material is fundamentally the same in all living organisms: it consists of chainlike molecules of nucleic acids — deoxyribonucleic acid (DNA) in most organisms and ribonucleic acid (RNA) in certain viruses — and is usually in a linear arrangement, constituting (in part) a chromosome.

A gene is also the segment of DNA that is involved in producing a polypeptide chain. It includes regions preceding and following the coding region (leader and trailer) as well as intervening sequences (introns) between individual coding segments (exons). More than one protein can be expressed (made) from a given gene, i.e., the particular protein expressed is determined by factors including the following:

- The cell's temperature or other environmental variable
- The presence of STATs (some of which **themselves** are proteins)

See also INFORMATIONAL MOLECULES, DEOXYRIBONUCLEIC ACID (DNA), RIBONUCLEIC ACID (RNA), GENE EXPRESSION, CHROMOSOMES, EXPRESS, MESSENGER RNA (mRNA), CODON, INTRON, EXON, CODING SEQUENCE, GENE EXPRESSION CASCADE, CENTRAL DOGMA (NEW), SIGNAL TRANSDUCERS AND ACTIVATORS OF TRANSCRIPTION (STATs)

Gene Amplification The copying of segments (e.g., genes) within the DNA or RNA molecule. This can be done by man (e.g., polymerase chain reaction), can be caused by certain chemical carcinogens (e.g., phorbol ester), or can occur naturally (e.g., in procaryotes and certain lower eucaryotes). The five primary techniques that are used to perform gene amplification are the following:

1. Polymerase chain reaction (PCR)
2. Ligase chain reaction (LCR)
3. Self-sustained sequence replication (SSR)
4. Q-beta replicase technique
5. Strand displacement amplification (SDA)

See also GENE, Q-BETA REPLICASE TECHNIQUE, POLYMERASE CHAIN REACTION (PCR), CARCINOGEN, PROCARYOTES, EUCARYOTE

Gene Array Systems See BIOCHIPS, PROTEOMICS, GENE EXPRESSION ANALYSIS

Gene Chips See BIOCHIPS, GENE EXPRESSION ANALYSIS, PROTEOMICS

Gene Correction See EDITING

Gene Delivery (Gene Therapy) The insertion of genes (e.g., via retroviral vectors) into selected cells in the body in order to achieve the following:

- Cause those cells to produce specific therapeutic agents (e.g., growth hormone in livestock, factor VIII in hemophiliacs, insulin in diabetics, etc.). A potential way of curing some genetic diseases, in that the inserted gene will produce the protein and/or enzyme that is missing in the body because of a defective gene (causing the genetic disease). Approximately 4000 genetic diseases are known to man. Examples of genetic diseases include cystic fibrosis, sickle cell anemia, Huntington's disease, phenylketonuria (PKU), Tay-Sachs disease, ADA deficiency (adenosine deaminase enzyme deficiency), and thalassemia.
- Cause those cells to produce a specific compound (e.g., interleukin-12) that will result in the body's immune system becoming more active against a specific disease (e.g., melanoma).
- Cause those cells to become (more) susceptible to a conventional therapeutic agent that previously was ineffective against that particular condition or disease (e.g., insertion of Hs-tk gene into brain tumor cells to make those tumor cells susceptible to the Syntex drug Ganciclovir®).
- Cause those cells to become less susceptible to a conventional therapeutic agent (e.g., insert genes into healthy tissue in order to enable that healthy tissue to resist the harmful effects of such conventional chemotherapy agents as vincristine).
- Counter the effects of abnormal (damaged) tumor suppressor genes

G

via insertion of normal tumor suppressor genes.

- Cause expression of ribozymes that cleave oncogenes (cancer-causing genes).
- Be used for other therapeutic applications of genes in cells.

See also GENE, TUMOR SUPPRESSOR GENES, ONCOGENES, CANCER, p53 GENE, TUMOR, MELANOMA, PROTO-ONCOGENES, RETROVIRAL VECTORS, RETROVIRUSES, HUNTINGTON'S DISEASE, GENETIC CODE, INFORMATIONAL MOLECULES, DEOXYRIBONUCLEIC ACID (DNA), CHROMOSOMES, HORMONE, ENZYME, PROTEIN, GENETIC TARGETING, POLYCATION CONJUGATE, ELECTROPORATION

Gene Expression Conversion of the **genetic information** within a gene into an actual protein (or cell process). Note that many genes are only expressed at specific times during the lifetime of a cell or organism. Some genes are expressed in a "cascade" of related expressions.

See also GENE, GENETIC CODE, INFORMATIONAL MOLECULES, EXPRESS, GENE EXPRESSION ANALYSIS, BIOCHIPS, GENE EXPRESSION CASCADE, MICRORNAs, CENTRAL DOGMA (NEW), CHO CELLS

Gene Expression Analysis Generally done via the use of two-dimensional gel electrophoresis, "biochips" (which have numerous detection or analysis devices fabricated on their silicon surface), or "microarrays" (e.g., with specific cDNA molecules attached to surface). In whole or in part, gene expression analysis involves evaluation of the expression (and expression **levels**) of numerous genes in a biological sample, to analyze or compare any differences between gene expression or products in the following:

- Normal cells vs. diseased cells
- Normal cells vs. those responding to a stimulus
- Cells from same organism, at different stages of development (e.g., embryo vs. adult)
- Normal (historic wild-type) cells vs. genetically engineered cells (e.g., those that have been engineered to cure a disease, resist a herbicide, etc.)
- Normal cells vs. those same cells treated with a given pharmaceutical or nutraceutical (candidate)

Analysis generally involves measurement of **gene expression markers** (i.e., molecules synthesized or cellular consequences such as apoptosis) to determine which genes are expressed (and when/**how much**, etc.). For example, during 2002, Yiwei Li utilized a cDNA-based microarray to show that genistein (an isoflavone obtained from soybeans) down-regulated the expression levels of eleven human genes (which have been shown to be involved in angiogenesis and/or cancer metastasis) and upregulated (i.e., increased the expression levels of) two human genes associated with connective tissue cell signaling.

See also GENE, GENE EXPRESSION, GENE EXPRESSION PROFILING, CAPILLARY ELECTROPHORESIS, MICROARRAY (TESTING), GENOMICS, FUNCTIONAL GENOMICS, EXPRESS, EXPRESSED SEQUENCE TAGS (EST), ZINC FINGER PROTEINS, BIOCHIPS, HIGH-THROUGHPUT SCREENING (HTS), MICROFLUIDICS, HERBICIDE-TOLERANT CROP, GENE DELIVERY (GENE THERAPY), HORMONE, PROTEOMICS, PROMOTER, GENE EXPRESSION MARKERS, GENE EXPRESSION CASCADE, APOPTOSIS, RT-PCR, DIFFERENTIAL DISPLAY, ISOELECTRIC FOCUSING (IEF), TWO-DIMENSIONAL (2-D) GEL ELECTROPHORESIS, GENISTEIN (GEN), NUTRACEUTICALS, ANGIOGENESIS, METASTASIS, ANTIANGIOGENESIS, SIGNALING, SERIAL ANALYSIS OF GENE EXPRESSION (SAGE)

Gene Expression Cascade A sequential series of **individual gene expressions** (i.e., each gene causing a separate or different protein to be "manufactured") that is initiated (i.e., "set off") by the first gene expression.

For example, a **gene expression cascade** is often initiated by the first gene, causing expression of a transcription factor (i.e., protein that **itself**

G

interacts with cell's DNA to either cause or speed up yet **another** gene expression). The protein resulting from that gene expression could be yet **another** transcription factor that triggers another (i.e., third) gene expression, and so on.

See also GENE, EXPRESS, GENE EXPRESSION, CASCADE, PROTEIN, CELL, DEOXYRIBONUCLEIC ACID (DNA), PROMOTER, TRANSCRIPTION FACTORS, APOPTOSIS

Gene Expression Markers Refers to molecules (e.g., synthesized because of a specific gene's expression) or consequences (e.g., cell apoptosis due to a specific gene's expression) that can be measured as **proof of a gene's expression** in gene expression analysis.

See also GENE EXPRESSION, GENE, GENE EXPRESSION ANALYSIS, EXPRESS, BIOCHIPS, PROTEIN, CELL, APOPTOSIS, GREEN FLUORESCENT PROTEIN, KUSABIRA ORANGE

Gene Expression Profiling Determination of specifically **which genes are "switched on" (e.g., in a cell)**, which thereby enables precise definition of the phenotypic condition of that cell (i.e., the phenotype of that cell at that moment).

Typical uses (i.e., comparison of such tissue phenotypes) include the following:

- Comparing **diseased** cell with **normal** cell
- Defining quantitatively the **"normal"** state
- Comparing a given drug's impact, i.e., **treated** cell vs. **untreated** cell
- Comparing the impact of a given **nutraceutical's consumption** (i.e., treated cell vs. untreated cell)
- Comparing **old** cells with **young** cells

In subsequent gene expression analysis, the quantitative **amounts of each protein being expressed** can be determined via use of such technologies as two-dimensional (2-D) gel electrophoresis, Southern blot analysis, fluorescence tagging, radiolabeling, RT-PCR, QPCR, fluorescence polarization (FP), plane polarimetry, etc.

See also GENE, GENE EXPRESSION, PROTEIN, CELL, PHENOTYPE, GENE EXPRESSION ANALYSIS, TWO-DIMENSIONAL (2-D) GEL ELECTROPHORESIS, SOUTHERN BLOT ANALYSIS, RADIOLABELED, RT-PCR, QPCR, GENE EXPRESSION MARKERS, MICROARRAY (TESTING), MULTIPLEXED ASSAY, FLUORESCENCE, FLUORESCENCE POLARIZATION (FP), NUTRACEUTICALS

Gene Function Analysis The determination of which protein is expressed (i.e., caused to be "manufactured") by each gene in an organism's genome/DNA. Typically, gene function analysis follows after discovery of gene sequences found via **structural genomics** study. Some methods utilized to determine which proteins result from which genes are the following:

- Site-directed mutagenesis (SDM): to compare two same-species organisms possessing two different genes at the same site (SNP) on the genome (i.e., on the organism's DNA)
- Antisense DNA sequences: to compare two same-species organisms, one of which has the gene at the same site "turned off" (silenced) via antisense DNA
- Reporter gene: to compare two same-species organisms (possessing two different genes at same site on genome or DNA) via a **reporter gene** adjacent to the gene or site, to detect the presence or absence of the desired trait or function
- Comparison of the same organism (e.g., crop plant) when one of the two is "challenged" by a specific plant disease
- Chemical genetics: To compare two same-species organisms (one of which has the gene at the specific site at least partially **inactivated by a specific chemical**)
- "Silencing" or "knocking out" a particular gene via **other methods than antisense or chemical genetics**: to compare

G

- Use of already-known "model organisms" (e.g., *Drosophila* for comparing insect genes, *Arabidopsis thaliana* for plant genes, *Caenorhabditis elegans* for animal genes)

See also GENE, GENE EXPRESSION, GENETIC CODE, INFORMATIONAL MOLECULES, EXPRESS, PROTEIN, GENOME, GENOMICS, STRUCTURAL GENOMICS, FUNCTIONAL GENOMICS, ZINC FINGER PROTEINS, TRAIT, DEOXYRIBONUCLEIC ACID (DNA), SEQUENCE (OF A DNA MOLECULE), POINT MUTATION, SITE-DIRECTED MUTAGENESIS (SDM), ANTISENSE (DNA SEQUENCE), GENE SILENCING, REPORTER GENE, METHYLATION, POSITIONAL CLONING, DNA METHYLATION, CHEMICAL GENETICS, MODEL ORGANISM, DROSOPHILA, *ARABIDOPSIS THALIANA*, *CAENORHABDITIS ELEGANS (C. ELEGANS)*, CENTRAL DOGMA (OLD), CENTRAL DOGMA (NEW), TRANSCRIPTION FACTORS, TRANSWITCH®, SINGLE-NUCLEOTIDE POLYMORPHISMS (SNPs)

Gene Fusion Refers to the technology or methods utilized to fuse two or more genes. When such a "fused gene" is then inserted into a genome (e.g., the DNA of a plant), it causes production (in plant's ribosomes) of proteins consisting of all or part of the amino acid sequences (known as the "domain") of the two proteins typically coded by those two genes. This fusion is often done in order to put expression of the "second" (fused) gene under the control of the (strong) promoter of the "first" gene.

During 2001, Rajbir Sangwan and colleagues inserted a fused gene into a potato plant (*Solanum tuberosum*), a major source of plant starch. That fused gene coded for the production of two proteins α-**amylase** and **glucose isomerase** (both are enzymes). α-amylase catalyzes the conversion of potato starch into glucose (a sugar), and glucose isomerase catalyzes conversion of glucose to fructose (a more valuable sugar).

See also GENE, GENOME, DEOXYRIBONUCLEIC ACID (DNA), GENETIC ENGINEERING, RIBOSOMES, CODING

SEQUENCE, PROTEIN, AMINO ACID, SEQUENCE (OF A PROTEIN MOLECULE), FUSION PROTEIN, RAPID PROTEIN FOLDING ASSAY, EXPRESS, PROMOTER, ENZYME, AMYLASE, GLUCOSE, ISOMERASE

Gene Imprinting See IMPRINTING

Gene Machine An instrument that when fed information on the amino acid sequence of a protein (usually via a protein sequencer), will automatically produce polynucleotide gene segments to code for that protein.

See also SEQUENCING (OF DNA MOLECULES), SYNTHESIZING (OF DNA MOLECULES), GENE, AMINO ACID, PROTEIN

Gene Manipulation See GENETIC ENGINEERING

Gene Map See LINKAGE MAP, GENETIC MAP, PHYSICAL MAP (OF GENOME)

Gene Mapping See SEQUENCING (OF DNA MOLECULES), GENETIC MAP, LINKAGE MAP, PHYSICAL MAP (OF GENOME)

Gene Probe See DNA PROBE

Gene Repair (natural) Refers to the natural processes via which all cells in an organism are continually repairing their DNA (which can be damaged by ultraviolet light, various chemicals, etc.). In these natural cell (gene repair) processes, the following take place:

- First, an enzyme complex detects the damaged DNA (e.g., on one of the two strands of the DNA molecule).
- Next, an enzyme cuts out the damaged portion of the DNA (on that one strand, leaving the good strand intact).
- Then, a DNA polymerase enzyme enters the gap and synthesizes (i.e., "manufactures") the new DNA (to replace the portion that was cut out), using the intact (good) DNA strand as a **template**.
- Finally, the new DNA is joined to the "old" DNA via the help of DNA ligase enzyme.

See also CELL, ENZYME, DEOXYRIBONUCLEIC ACID (DNA), DNA REPAIR, DNA POLYMERASE, DNA LIGASE, TEMPLATE, EDITING, ZINC FINGER PROTEINS

Gene Repair (synthetic) A term with several different meanings, as follows:

- One of the natural modes of **DNA repair**, when engendered by man.
- The "repair" of a **damaged gene (e.g., mutation)** or replacement of a given gene via a process invented by Eric Kmiec in 1993. The desired DNA (gene) is added to a cell, along with RNA, in a paired group known as a chimeraplast. The chimeraplast attaches itself to the cell's DNA at the site of the specific gene (i.e., the one that is to be changed), and "repairs" it using its (new) chimeraplast DNA as a "template."
- The gene therapy form of **editing**.

See also DNA REPAIR, GENE, CHIMERAPLASTY, MUTATION, DEOXYRIBONUCLEIC ACID (DNA), RIBONUCLEIC ACID (RNA), CELL, TEMPLATE, EDITING, GENE THERAPY

Gene Replacement Therapy See GENE DELIVERY

Gene Silencing The suppression of gene expression (e.g., of the gene for polygalacturonase, which causes fruit to ripen, of the gene for P34 protein in soybeans, etc.) via a variety of methods (e.g., via RNA interference (RNAi), chemical genetics, effect of certain viruses, "zinc finger proteins," sense or antisense genes, etc.). Also occurs with some genes in an organism as the organism matures (e.g., from an embryo to a seedling or juvenile).

See also GENE, EXPRESS, GENE EXPRESSION, TRANSCRIPTION, RNA INTERFERENCE (RNAi), KNOCKOUT, SHORT INTERFERING RNA (siRNA), GENETIC CODE, INFORMATIONAL MOLECULES, PROTEIN, CHEMICAL GENETICS, ZINC FINGER PROTEINS, VIRUS, GENE FUNCTION ANALYSIS, COSUPPRESSION, ANTISENSE (DNA SEQUENCE), TRANSWITCH®, SENSE, POLYGALACTURONASE (PG), GPA1, REDUCED-ALLERGEN SOYBEANS, POSTTRANSCRIPTIONAL GENE SILENCING (PTGS), EPIGENETIC, IMPRINTING, MICRORNAs

Gene Splicing The enzymatic attachment (joining) of one gene (or part of a gene) to another. Also the removal of introns and splicing of exons during mRNA synthesis.

Another category of gene splicing occurs when chromatin remodeling results in two **recombination signal sequences (RSS)** — which flank a relevant gene or sequence within the DNA that is looped around histones in the chromatin — becoming close enough or exposed so that cellular recombinase enzymes recognize them and catalyze their splicing together (along with relevant genes or sequences). For example, B lymphocyte cells are thereby able to splice together large numbers of gene segments that enable those B lymphocytes to collectively possess antigen receptors (Ig) specific to a huge number of antigens on innumerable pathogens.

See also SPLICING, CENTRAL DOGMA (NEW), MESSENGER RNA (mRNA), CELL, GENE, CHROMATIN, HISTONES, CHROMATIN REMODELING, B LYMPHOCYTES, ENZYME, RECOMBINASE, RECOMBINATION, SEQUENCE (OF A DNA MOLECULE), ANTIGEN, RECEPTORS, PATHOGEN

Gene "Stacking" See "STACKED" GENES

Gene Switching See GENE, GENETIC CODE, CODING SEQUENCE, DEOXYRIBONUCLEIC ACID (DNA), SEQUENCE (OF A DNA MOLECULE), REGULATORY SEQUENCE, TRANSCRIPTION FACTORS, CBF1, COLD HARDENING, CESSATION CASSETTE, SYSTEMIC ACQUIRED RESISTANCE (SAR)

Gene Targeting See GENETIC TARGETING, GENE SPLICING, GENE DELIVERY, GENETIC ENGINEERING

Gene Taxi A term used in some regions (e.g., Europe) to refer to a vector (e.g., *Agrobacterium tumefaciens*, etc.) that is utilized to carry a gene or cassette into an organism, and insert that gene or cassette into the organism's DNA.

See also VECTOR, *AGROBACTERIUM TUMEFACIENS, ORGANISM, GENE, CASSETTE, DEOXYRIBONUCLEIC ACID (DNA)*

Gene Technology Office An agency of the Australian government, established in 1997, to oversee and regulate all genetic engineering activities conducted in the country of Australia. Replaced or superceded by Australia's newly

G

formed Interim Office of the Gene Technology Regulator (IOGTR) in 1999.

See also IOGTR, GENE TECHNOLOGY REGULATOR (GTR), GENETIC ENGINEERING, RECOMBINANT DNA ADVISORY COMMITTEE (RAC), ZKBS (CENTRAL COMMITTEE ON BIOLOGICAL SAFETY), INDIAN DEPARTMENT OF BIOTECHNOLOGY, COMMISSION OF BIOMOLECULAR ENGINEERING

Gene Technology Regulator (GTR) The regulatory body of the Australian government that is responsible for approvals of new rDNA products (e.g., new genetically engineered crops) before they can be introduced into Australia. GTR replaced Australia's IOGTR (Interim Office of the Gene Technology Regulator) in this role on June 21, 2001.

See also INTERIM OFFICE OF THE GENE TECHNOLOGY REGULATOR (IOGTR), GENE TECHNOLOGY OFFICE, GENETIC MANIPULATION ADVISORY COMMITTEE (GMAC), rDNA, DEOXYRIBONUCLEIC ACID (DNA), GENETIC ENGINEERING, RECOMBINANT DNA ADVISORY COMMITTEE (RAC), COMMISSION OF BIOMOLECULAR ENGINEERING, INDIAN DEPARTMENT OF BIOTECHNOLOGY

Gene Therapy See GENE DELIVERY, EDITING

Gene Transcript See TRANSCRIPT

Generation Time The time required for a population of cells to double. The average time required for a round of cell division.

See also CELL, MITOSIS

Genestein See GENISTEIN (Gen)

Genetic Code The set of triplet code words in DNA, coding for all of the amino acids. There are more than 20 different amino acids and only four bases (adenine, thymine, cytosine, and guanine). The mRNA code is a triplet code, that is, each successive "frame" of three nucleotides (sometimes called a codon) of the mRNA corresponds to one amino acid of the protein. This rule of correspondence is the genetic code. The genetic code consists of 64 entries — the 64 triplets possible when there are four possible nucleotides, each of which can be at any of three places ($4 \times 4 \times 4 = 64$). A triplet code was required because a doublet code would have

only been able to code for ($4 \times 4 \times 16$) 16 amino acids. A triplet code allows for the coding of 64 theoretical amino acids. Because only a little over 20 exist, there is some redundancy in the system. Hence, certain amino acids are coded for by two or three different triplets.

See also MESSENGER RNA (mRNA), DEOXYRIBONUCLEIC ACID (DNA), INFORMATIONAL MOLECULES

Genetic Drift See ADAPTATION

Genetic Engineering The selective, deliberate alteration of genes (genetic material) by humans. This term has come to have a very broad meaning, including the manipulation and alteration of the genetic material (constitution) of an organism in such a way as to allow it to produce endogenous proteins with properties different from those of the traditional (historic or typical) or to produce entirely different (foreign) proteins altogether. Some other words often applicable to the same process are gene splicing, gene manipulation, or recombinant DNA technology (techniques).

See also GENE, INFORMATIONAL MOLECULES, CHROMOSOMES, GENE AMPLIFICATION, VECTOR, PLASMID, *AGROBACTERIUM TUMEFACIENS*, GENE SPLICING, DEOXYRIBONUCLEIC ACID (DNA), TRANSGENIC (ORGANISM), BIOLISTIC® GENE GUN, WHISKERS™, "SHOTGUN" METHOD, NUCLEAR TRANSFER, GMO, RECOMBINANT DNA (rDNA), RECOMBINATION, HETEROKARYON, HEREDITY, MESSENGER RNA (mRNA), HETERODUPLEX, POSITIVE AND NEGATIVE SELECTION (PNS), POLYMERASE CHAIN REACTION (PCR) TECHNIQUE, BIOTECHNOLOGY, METABOLIC ENGINEERING

Genetic Engineering Approval Committee See GEAC

Genetic Event See EVENT

Genetic Fingerprinting Another name for **DNA profiling**.

See DNA PROFILING

Genetic Linkage See LINKAGE, LINKAGE GROUP

Genetic Manipulation See GENETIC ENGINEERING

Genetic Manipulation Advisory Committee (GMAC) A body that advises the Australian government on matters pertaining to genetic engineering (e.g., new rDNA product approvals). GMAC is analogous to Germany's ZKBS (Central Commission on Biological Safety), Brazil's CTNBio (National Technical Biosafety Commission), and the Kenya Biosafety Council.

See also GMAC, ZKBS (CENTRAL COMMISSION ON BIOLOGICAL SAFETY), RECOMBINANT DNA ADVISORY COMMITTEE (RAC), GENETIC ENGINEERING, rDNA, DEOXYRIBONUCLEIC ACID (DNA), CTNBIO, KENYA BIOSAFETY COUNCIL, GENE TECHNOLOGY OFFICE, GENE TECHNOLOGY REGULATOR (GTR)

Genetic Map A diagram showing the relative sequence and position of specific genes along a chromosome (DNA) molecule. **Markers** utilized as "signposts" or guideposts in such maps include single-nucleotide polymorphisms (SNPs), restriction sites (i.e., the specific locations where each restriction endonuclease "cuts" a DNA strand), and microsatellites. Such **markers** located in or close to the **gene of interest** (e.g., a disease-causing gene within a chromosome) **to a researcher** are more likely to be inherited along with that gene.

See also POSITION EFFECT, GENE, GENOME, CHROMOSOMES, DEOXYRIBONUCLEIC ACID (DNA), PHYSICAL MAP (OF GENOME), SINGLE-NUCLEOTIDE POLYMORPHISMS (SNPs), RESTRICTION SITE, MICROSATELLITE DNA, MARKER-ASSISTED SELECTION

Genetic Marker Refers to a segment of DNA (e.g., gene) within an organism's overall DNA, which can be detected by man (e.g., via use of FISH) and is a reliable indicator that that particular organism possesses a specific trait of interest.

MARKER (DNA SEQUENCE), GENE, DEOXYRIBONUCLEIC ACID (DNA), FLUORESCENCE *IN SITU* HYBRIDIZATION (FISH), TRAIT, HER-2 GENE, GLEEVEC™, MARKER-ASSISTED SELECTION

Genetic Probe See DNA PROBE

Genetic Targeting The insertion of antisense DNA molecules *in vivo* into selected cells of the body in order to block the activity of undesirable genes. These genes might include oncogenes or genes crucial to the life cycle of parasites such as trypanosomes (cause sleeping sickness).

See also ANTISENSE (DNA SEQUENCE), GENE, GENE DELIVERY, ONCOGENES, DENDRIMERS

Genetic Use Restriction Technologies (GURTs) A general term utilized to refer to several different technologies intended to control the expression (or nonexpression) of the genes for specific (e.g., valuable) traits.

See also CESSATION CASSETTE, GENE, TRAIT, EXPRESS, VALUE-ENHANCED GRAINS

Genetically Engineered Microbial Pesticides (GEMP) One or more microbes that have been genetically engineered in such a way as to cause them to be effective in combating pests that attack crops or livestock. For example, a microbe that naturally attacks a crop pest could be genetically engineered to make the microbe more potent or more durable in the field environment when applied to the field via a selected method of microbe application.

See also MICROBE, GENETIC ENGINEERING, WHEAT TAKE-ALL DISEASE, BACULOVIRUS, *BACILLUS THURINGIENSIS (B.t.)*, FEDERAL INSECTICIDE FUNGICIDE AND RODENTICIDE ACT (FIFRA), TOXIC SUBSTANCES CONTROL ACT (TSCA)

Genetically Engineered Organism (GEO) See GEO

Genetically Manipulated Organism (GMO) See GMO

Genetically Modified Microorganism (GMM) See GMM

Genetically Modified Organism (GMO) See GMO

Genetically Modified Pest Protected (GMPP) Plants Plants that have been genetically engineered so that they resist (or are more tolerant to) attacks by pests (e.g., insects).

See also GENETIC ENGINEERING, *BACILLUS THURINGIENSIS (B.t.)*, COWPEA TRYPSIN INHIBITOR (CpTI), CRY PROTEINS, CRY1A (b) PROTEIN, CRY1A (c) PROTEIN, CRY9C PROTEIN, *B.t. KURSTAKI*, *B.t. TENEBRIONIS*,

G

B.t. ISRAELENSIS, PATHOGENESIS-RELATED PROTEINS, *PHOTORHABDUS LUMINESCENS*

Genetics The branch of biology concerned with heredity. It was invented by Gregor Mendel in the 19th century. It is a study of the manner in which genes operate and are transmitted from parents to offspring. In 1865, Mendel defined what gene (alleles) are and showed that they can be **dominant** or **recessive** (within the offspring's genome or DNA, which has two "copies" of each gene).

For example, if a given trait (e.g., black hair) is **dominant**, and that gene is inherited from only one of the parents (e.g., the father), the offspring will have that trait (i.e., black hair). But if a given trait (e.g., red hair) is **recessive**, the offspring will not have that trait (i.e., red hair) unless the "red hair gene" is inherited from **both** parents.

Similarly, **dominantly inherited diseases,** such as Huntington's disease, result even if only one copy of the damaged or mutant gene (i.e., **HD gene** in this example) is inherited.

Genetics also involves the study of the mechanism of gene action — the manner in which the genetic material (DNA) affects physiological reactions within the cell.

See also GENE, DEOXYRIBONUCLEIC ACID (DNA), HYBRIDIZATION (PLANT GENETICS), HEREDITY, DOMINANT ALLELE, RECESSIVE ALLELE, CELL, GENE EXPRESSION ANALYSIS, DYNAMICS, HUNTINGTON'S DISEASE, HD GENE

Genistein (Gen) One of several phytochemicals produced by the soybean plant as a defense against certain plant diseases and to signal the *Rhizobium japonicum* bacteria to produce nitrogen for the soybean plant via colonization of its roots, followed by nitrogen fixation from the air. Genistein can also be produced as a by-product of mycobacterium fermentation (a process used to produce commercial amounts of certain antibiotics). Genistein is an isoflavone, a steroid-like compound that can be lethal to certain animal cells via its kinase-inhibiting and other properties. Genistein fights cancer (tumor cells) by inhibiting protein tyrosine kinase and topoisomerase II. Genistein also exhibits the property of antiangiogenesis (i.e., inhibition of tumor growth via prevention of the formation or development of new blood vessels in tumors).

Attached to a pharmaceutical "guided missile" such as a monoclonal antibody or the CD4 protein, genistein is potentially useful for treatment against some tumors and has been investigated as a possible treatment against B cell precursor leukemia. A human diet containing a large amount of genistein has been shown to increase bone density and to decrease total serum (blood) cholesterol, thereby lowering the risk of osteoporosis and coronary heart disease.

Research indicates that consumption of genistein by humans can help to prevent breast cancer, prostate cancer or metastasis, and adverse increases in blood platelet aggregation, and inhibit the proliferation of **smooth-muscle cells** in plaque deposits (inside blood vessels).

Research also indicates that consumption of genistein can enhance the effectiveness of both radiation and of chemotherapy drugs (e.g., Cisplatin) used in the treatment of cancer in humans.

See also IMMUNOTOXIN, MONOCLONAL ANTIBODIES (MAb), CD4 PROTEIN, GENETIC ENGINEERING, NITROGEN FIXATION, NODULATION, PHYTOCHEMICALS, FUSION PROTEIN, FUSION TOXIN, SOLUBLE CD4, ISOFLAVONES, SOYBEAN PLANT, RICIN, TYROSINE (Tyr), STEROID, CANCER, INHIBITION, STRESS PROTEINS, "MAGIC BULLET," TYROSINE KINASE, CORONARY HEART DISEASE (CHD), CHOLESTEROL, OSTEOPOROSIS, SELECTIVE ESTROGEN EFFECT, ANTIANGIOGENESIS, PROTEIN TYROSINE KINASE INHIBITOR, GENE EXPRESSION ANALYSIS, PLAQUE, METASTASIS

Genistin The β-glycoside form (isomer in which glucose is attached to the molecule at the 7 position of the A ring) of the isoflavone known as genistein (aglycone form).

See also GENISTEIN (Gen), ISOFLAVONES, ISOMER

Genome The entire hereditary material (which was proven by Oswald Avery in 1944 to be DNA) in a cell. In addition to the DNA contained in cell nuclei (known as nuclear DNA), an organism's cells contain DNA in other locations within those cells, as given in the following text:

- Bacteria also contain some DNA in PLASMIDS.
- Plants also contain some DNA in PLASTIDS.
- Animals also contain some DNA in MITOCHONDRIA.

An organism's nuclear DNA is composed of one or more chromosomes, depending on the complexity of the organism.

See also DEOXYRIBONUCLEIC ACID (DNA), CHROMOSOMES, PLASTID, PLASMID, MITOCHONDRIA, MITOCHONDRIAL DNA

Genomic Sciences An encompassing term utilized to refer to all knowledge of, and attempts to decipher or understand the structure and function of, the genomes of organisms.

See also GENOMICS, GENOME, STRUCTURAL GENOMICS, FUNCTIONAL GENOMICS, GENOTYPE, GENE, GENETICS, GENETIC MAP, GENETIC TARGETING, GENETIC CODE, SEQUENCING (OF DNA MOLECULES), INFORMATIONAL MOLECULES, DEOXYRIBONUCLEIC ACID (DNA), GENE AMPLIFICATIONS, CODING SEQUENCE, CHEMICAL GENETICS

Genomics The scientific study of genes and their role in an organism's structure, growth, health, and disease (and/or resistance to disease, etc.). For example, how the (approximately) 3000 genes in a given strain of bacteria or the (approximately) 6000 genes in a given strain of yeast contribute to the shape, function, and development of those whole organisms.

Some tools or methods utilized in genomics include the following:

- Structural Genomics—The study or discovery of what particular gene sequences are present, and where they are located within an organism's DNA.
- Gene Function Analysis—The determination of which protein is expressed (i.e., caused to be "manufactured") by

each gene in an organism's genome. Typically, gene function analysis follows a structural genomics study.

- Functional Genomics—The study or discovery of what traits or functions are conferred on an organism by given gene sequences.
- Chemical Genetics—Used to compare two same-species organisms (one of which has a given gene, or genes, inactivated by a specific chemical or site mutation).
- Gene Expression Analysis—Used to determine products produced (such as an enzyme or other critical protein) when a given gene is "switched on," by measuring fluorescence of individual messenger RNA (mRNA) molecules (specific to which particular gene is "switched on" at the time) when that mRNA hybridizes (with DNA pieces corresponding to proteins produced and analyzed that were attached to hybridization surface on biochip).

See also GENOTYPE, GENE, GENETIC MAP, GENETIC TARGETING, GENETICS, GENETIC CODE, SEQUENCING (OF DNA MOLECULES), INFORMATIONAL MOLECULES, DEOXYRIBONUCLEIC ACID (DNA), FUNCTIONAL GENOMICS, GENE AMPLIFICATION, CODING SEQUENCE, STRUCTURAL GENOMICS, GENOMIC SCIENCES, BACTERIA, YEAST, STRAIN, CHEMICAL GENETICS, FLUORESCENCE, ENZYME, PROTEIN, MESSENGER RNA (mRNA), BIOCHIPS, EXPRESS, EXPRESSED SEQUENCE TAGS (EST), HYBRIDIZATION SURFACES, GENE EXPRESSION, GENE EXPRESSION ANALYSIS, GENE FUNCTION ANALYSIS

Genosensors Biosensors (electronic) that can detect the individual nucleotides that comprise a genome (DNA) molecule. Automated genosensors enable rapid, nondestructive sequencing of DNA molecules.

See also GENOME, NUCLEOTIDE, DEOXYRIBONUCLEIC ACID (DNA), SEQUENCING (OF DNA MOLECULES),

G

TEMPLATE, BIOSENSORS (ELEC-TRONIC), FOOTPRINTING, NANOTECH-NOLOGY, BIOCHIPS

Genotoxic Refers to compounds that interfere with normal functioning of genetic material (i.e., DNA). For example, the antitumor antibiotic family of duocarmycin drugs.

See also DEOXYRIBONUCLEIC ACID (DNA), GENOTOXIC CARCINOGENS, FOOTPRINTING

Genotoxic Carcinogens Compounds that act directly on the genetic material (i.e., DNA) of an organism, thus causing cancer in that organism. Of the numerous chemicals that have been documented to be human carcinogens, the majority of them are genotoxic.

See also CARCINOGEN, CANCER, GENE, DEOXYRIBONUCLEIC ACID (DNA)

Genotype The total genetic, or hereditary, constitution that an individual receives from its parents. An individual organism's genotype is distinct from its phenotype, which is its appearance or observable character.

See also TRAIT, PHENOTYPE, WILD TYPE

Gentechnik Gesetz (Gene Technology Law) The 1990 law that governs recombinant DNA research and development in the country of Germany. It was amended January 1, 1994, to make it somewhat less restrictive.

See also ZKBS (CENTRAL COMMISSION ON BIOLOGICAL SAFETY), RECOMBINANT DNA ADVISORY COMMITTEE (RAC), GENETIC ENGINEERING, RECOMBINANT DNA (rDNA), RECOMBINATION, BIOTECHNOLOGY, BUNDESGESUNDHEITSAMT (BGA), INDIAN DEPARTMENT OF BIOTECHNOLOGY

Genus A group of closely related species.

See also SPECIES, CLADES

GEO Genetically engineered organism.

See also GENETIC ENGINEERING, GMO, GENE, GENE SPLICING, GMM

Geomicrobiology Applications of microbiological knowledge to an understanding of geological phenomena.

See also FERROBACTERIA

GEP Acronym for **gel electrophoresis**.

See GEL ELECTROPHORESIS

Germ Cell The sex cell (sperm or egg). It differs from other cells in that it contains only half (haploid) the usual number of chromosomes.

See also GAMETE, HAPLOID

German Gene Law See GENTECHNIK GESETZ (GENE TECHNOLOGY LAW)

Germplasm The total genetic variability to an organism represented by the total available pool of germ cells or seed.

See also ORGANISM, CELL, GERM CELL, GEM

GFP Acronym for **Green Fluorescent Protein**.

See GREEN FLUORESCENT PROTEIN

GH See GROWTH HORMONE

Gibberella Ear Rot See *FUSARIUM GRAMINEARUM*

Gibberella zeae See *FUSARIUM GRAMINEARUM*

Gibberellins Plant hormones that, among other functions, regulate the growth of grass species, including rice (after the relevant gibberellin is activated by an enzyme). A gene known as **sd1** controls the amount of that enzyme produced (e.g., less of the enzyme = less gibberellin = shorter plant stalk).

In 1996, Lew Mander and Richard Pharis discovered an analogue (i.e., a chemical that is similar) to grass gibberellin that does *not* cause grass to grow. When this analogue is sprayed onto grass, it mixes with the naturally occurring grass gibberellin and significantly slows grass growth (thus potentially reducing the amount of mowing required for lawns, golf courses, etc.).

See also PLANT HORMONE, ENZYME, ANALOGUE, *FUSARIUM MONILIFORME*

GIST See GLEEVEC™

Gleevac™ See GLEEVEC™

Gleevec™ A pharmaceutical (imatinib mesylate, also known as STI571), developed and trademarked by Novartis AG, that is used to treat the blood cancer known as **chronic myelogenous leukemia** or **chronic myeloid leukemia** or **chronic myelocytic leukemia (CML)**. CML results from a genetic defect (single-nucleotide polymorphism) that causes excessive production of white blood cells in the (human) body of the affected. That excessive production of white blood cells results when the defective gene (i.e., SNP) causes excessive production of the enzyme **Bcr-Abl tyrosine kinase**.

Because Gleevec™ is a protein tyrosine kinase **inhibitor**, it inhibits excessive production of white blood cells (and induces apoptosis — cell death — in the cells that have the Bcr-Abl gene/SNP). Gleevec™ can also be utilized to treat GIST (gastrointestinal stromal tumors); where it targets the receptor tyrosine kinase known as KIT.

See also CANCER, WHITE BLOOD CELLS, GENE, MUTATION, SINGLE-NUCLEOTIDE POLYMORPHISMS (SNPs), ENZYME, APOPTOSIS, PROTEIN TYROSINE KINASE INHIBITOR, FLUORESCENCE *IN SITU* HYBRIDIZATION (FISH), KINASE ASSAYS, RECEPTORS, RECEPTOR TYROSINE KINASE

Glial-Derived Neurotrophic Factor (GDNF) A neurotrophic factor that assists the survival and functional activity of the brain's dopaminergic neurons. Because dopaminergic neurons in the brains of the victims of Parkinson's disease typically deteriorate and die, it is possible that GDNF may someday be used in treatment of Parkinson's disease.

See also NEUROTRANSMITTER, PARKINSON'S DISEASE

Globular Protein A soluble protein in which the polypeptide chain is tightly folded in three dimensions to yield a globular (roughly oval, circular) shape.

See also PROTEIN FOLDING, POLYPEPTIDE (PROTEIN), CONFORMATION, TERTIARY STRUCTURE

Glomalin A "sticky" protein molecule naturally produced by certain fungi that grow on most plant roots (in the soil). It was discovered and named by Sara F. Wright in 1996. As plant roots grow, glomalin is sloughed into the surrounding soil.

Glomalin acts as a sort of glue, thereby improving soil stability by "gluing" soil into clumps. Proper soil "clumping" (i.e., glomming together) allows air and water to pass through the soil more easily, increases the amount of carbon contained within the soil (thereby removing that "greenhouse gas" carbon dioxide from the atmosphere), increases the number of ("healthy") bacteria in the soil, and improves the soil's overall fertility (i.e., its ability to produce high-yield crops or a large amount of biomass per hectare or acre). The glomalin (and thus carbon) content of soil in

a field is increased by farmer utilization of low-tillage or "no-tillage" methods of crop production.

See also PROTEIN, FUNGUS, MYCORRHIZAE, BACTERIA, BIOMASS, CONSERVATION TILLAGE, LOW-TILLAGE CROP PRODUCTION, NO-TILLAGE CROP PRODUCTION

GLP See GOOD LABORATORY PRACTICES (GLP)

GLQ223 See TRICHOSANTHIN

GLS Abbreviation for **glucosinolates**.
See GLUCOSINOLATES

Glucagon A hormone produced by the pancreas that causes the breakdown of glycogen in the liver.

Glycogen is a form of storage sugar, and its breakdown releases glucose for energy production.

See also GLYCOGEN, HORMONE, GLUCOSE, PANCREAS

Glucagon See WATER-SOLUBLE FIBER, POLYPHENOLS

Glucocerebrosidase (Trade Name is Ceredase) An enzyme used in treatment of inherited Gaucher's disease, in which there is abnormal deposition of glucocerebrosides (hydrophobic lipid molecules that contain a hydrophilic sugar head group). Gaucher's disease is an enzyme deficiency disease that may be amenable to cure by incorporation via gene delivery techniques of the gene that codes for glucocerebrosidase into the patient's genome.

See also ENZYME, GENE DELIVERY

Glucogenic Amino Acid Amino acids whose carbon chains can be metabolically converted by cells into glucose or glycogen.

See also GLUCONEOGENESIS, CELL, AMINO ACID, METABOLISM

Gluconeogenesis The net biosynthesis (formation) of new glucose from noncarbohydrate precursors such as pyruvate, lactate, glycerol, acetyl-CoA (in plants), certain amino acids, and intermediates of the citric acid cycle.

See also CARBOHYDRATES, GLUCOSE (GLc), CITRIC ACID CYCLE, AcCoA, BIOTIN

Glucose (GLc) A prime fuel for the generation of energy by organisms. It is broken down (to obtain energy) via a metabolic process called glycolysis. Glucose is a hexose, a sugar

G

possessing six carbon atoms in its molecule. The six carbon atoms are connected to each other to form a closed ring structure known as a hexose (6) ring.

Animal cells store glucose in the form of glycogen (sometimes called animal starch), a large branched polymer of glucose units. Plant cells store glucose in the form of starch, a large polymer of glucose units.

Yeasts and bacteria store glucose in the form of dextran, a polymer of glucose units. The difference between the forms of storage glucose is (1) in the size (molecular weight) of the final polymer formed, (2) in the type of linkages that connect the single glucose units together in the branched molecule, and (3) in the degree of branching that occurs in the polymer. Note that a glucose polymer does not consist of just a single long straight chain. The backbone chain has other polymer chains branches. The whole molecule may be visualized as a tree without the trunk. The other very abundant polymer formed by glucose units is structural in nature and is called cellulose. It is the most abundant cell wall and structural polysaccharide in the plant world. Hence, glucose is used not only as an energy source but also as a structural material.

See also AMYLOSE, AMYLOPECTIN, GLYCOLYSIS, GLUCONEOGENESIS, GLYCOGEN, STARCH, DEXTRAN, CELLULOSE

Glucose Isomerase An enzyme that catalyzes the conversion of glucose to fructose. A molecule of fructose contains the same atoms as a molecule of glucose (but in a different arrangement).

See also ENZYME, GLUCOSE, GENE FUSION

Glucose Oxidase An enzyme that breaks down sugar molecules (causing oxygen consumption in an organism). Industrial uses include removal of dissolved oxygen from certain food products (e.g., sugar-containing drink).

See also ENZYME, GLUCOSE (GLc), GLYCOLYSIS, SUGAR MOLECULES, ORGANISM

Glucosinolates Toxins (neurotoxic phytotoxins) that are naturally produced in the seeds of some plants, for example, rapeseed, wild mustard (*Brassica juncea/Brassica rapa,* and

Sinapis arvensis), grass pea (*Lathyrus sativus*), etc., in order to dissuade wild animals from eating the seeds.

For example, when large amounts of grass pea (*Lathyrus sativus*) are consumed by humans, glucosinolates build up in the body and can cause Lathyrism (i.e., an irreversible spastic paralysis of the legs). The glucosinolates in rapeseed (high-erucic-acid) oil have been linked to heart damage in humans; these can also impart a bitter taste to such plant oils.

The rapeseed glucosinolate 5-vinyl oxazolidine I cyano-2-hydroxy-3-butene causes poultry liver to hemorrhage (bleed internally) if poultry are fed rapeseed meal or rapeseed oil for several weeks (at 20% of total diet). Such feeding of rapeseed meal or oil to poultry also predispose those poultry to develop fatty liver syndrome (FLS), a metabolic disease.

When glucosinolates from seeds of the wild mustard weed (*Sinapis arvensis*) family are mixed into canola meal (e.g., when those weeds grew in a canola field and that resultant canola is processed into canola meal), the meal must first be diluted (e.g., via mixing some soybean meal) in order to reduce glucosinolate concentration (below the legal maximum allowance in Canada) before it is fed to livestock.

See also CANOLA, *BRASSICA*, TOXIN, PHYTOTOXINS, METABOLISM, SOYBEAN MEAL

Glufosinate See PAT GENE, BAR GENE, HERBICIDE-TOLERANT CROP, GENE, GLUTAMINE SYNTHETASE

Gluphosinate See PAT GENE, BAR GENE, HERBICIDE-TOLERANT CROP, GENE, GLUTAMINE SYNTHETASE

Glutamate Dehydrogenase An enzyme found naturally in certain soil bacteria that helps them to utilize soilborne nitrogen. When its gene (GDH gene) is inserted into corn plant via genetic engineering, the resultant plant production of glutamate dehydrogenase enables the corn plant to better utilize soilborne nitrogen. As a result, such genetically engineered corn (*Zea mays* L.) has a protein-yield increase of approximately 10%, according to research begun in 1991 by David Lightfoot.

See also ENZYME, BACTERIA, GENE, CORN, NITROGEN CYCLE, DEHYDRO-

GENASES, PROTEIN, GENETIC ENGI-
NEERING

Glutamic Acid A dicarboxylic amino acid of
the α-ketoglutaric acid family.

See also AMINO ACID

Glutamic Acid Decarboxylase (GAD)
Refers to a type of enzyme present in the insulin-producing cells of mammalian pancreas.

During 2003, Anthony Jevnikav discovered that
feeding mice (of laboratory strain predisposed
to developing Type 1 diabetes) a diet containing some GAD helped to make their immune
systems less likely to be attacked by their own
pancreatic insulin-producing cells (i.e., a
cause of type 1 diabetes).

The result of such feeding (small amounts of a
particular protein, to cause a mammal's
immune system to tolerate and not "attack"
that protein) is known as **oral tolerance**.

See also ENZYME, TYPE I DIABETES,
INSULIN, BETA CELLS, AUTOIMMUNE
DISEASE, PROTEIN, STRAIN

Glutamine An amino acid, the monamide
molecular form of glutamic acid. Glutamine
is of fundamental importance for amino acid
biosynthesis in all forms of life.

See also GLUTAMINE SYNTHETASE,
AMINO ACID, PAT GENE, BAR GENE

Glutamine Synthetase An enzyme that catalyzes the synthesis of glutamine (which is crucial for amino acid biosynthesis).

See also GLUTAMINE, ENZYME, PAT
GENE, BAR GENE, AMINO ACID

Glutathione A tripeptide that is found in all
cells of higher animals, that acts to help protect against oxidative stress. Composed of the
amino acids glutamic acid, cysteine, and glycine. Cysteine possesses a sulfhydryl group
that makes glutathione a weak reducing agent.

See also OXIDATIVE STRESS, REDUCTION
(IN A CHEMICAL REACTION)

Gluten A term that refers to a naturally occurring mixture of two different proteins —
glutenin and gliadin — in the seeds of bread
wheat (*Triticum aestivum*). In flour made from
traditional varieties of wheat, glutenin proteins constitute approximately 50% of the
total gluten. The relative content of those two
proteins determines one of the most commercially important properties of the wheat, i.e.,
the strength and elasticity of flour made from

that particular wheat. For example, more of
the high molecular weight glutenin (which is
"stretchy" and imparts physical strength to a
dough made from such flour so that dough
holds together while rising) results in a flour
that is better suited to manufacture higher-
quality yeast-raised bread products.

See also WHEAT, PROTEIN, GLUTENIN,
HIGH-GLUTENIN WHEAT, YEAST,
MOLECULAR WEIGHT, POLYMER

Glutenin A protein that is naturally present in
the gluten within seeds of wheat (*Triticum
aestivum*).

See also GLUTEN, WHEAT, PROTEIN

GLV Acronym for **Green Leafy Volatiles**.

See VOLICITIN

Glyceraldehyde (D- and L-) One of the
smallest monosaccharides. It is called an
aldose because it contains an aldehyde group.
Glyceraldehyde has a single asymmetric carbon atom; thus there are two stereoisomers
(D-glyceraldehyde and L-glyceraldehyde).

See also MONOSACCHARIDES, STEREOI-
SOMERS

Glycetein See ISOFLAVONES

Glycine (Gly) The simplest (and smallest) of
the amino acids found in proteins. It is the
only amino acid that does not have an asymmetric carbon atom within its molecule. Thus,
it is not optically active.

See also AMINO ACID, PROTEIN, STEREOI-
SOMERS, OPTICAL ACTIVITY

Glycine max See SOYBEAN PLANT

Glycinin One of the (structural) categories of
proteins that are produced within seeds of
legumes. In general, glycinins contain 3 to 4
times more cysteine (Cys) and methionine (Met)
per unit of protein than does β-conglycinin.

Glycinin tends to promote gelling (in water), so
soybeans containing a greater proportion of
glycinin would tend to enable the manufacture
of a firmer tofu.

See also PROTEIN, CYSTEINE (Cys),
METHIONINE (Met)

Glycitein See ISOFLAVONES

Glycitin The β-glycoside form (isomer in
which glucose is attached to molecule at the
7 position of the A ring) of the isoflavone
known as glycitein (aglycone form).

See also ISOFLAVONES, ISOMER, GLY-
CITEIN

G

Glycoalkaloids See ALKALOIDS

Glycobiology The study of the involvement (function) of sugars in biological processes.

See also GLUCOSE (GLc), GLUCOSE OXIDASE, GLYCOGEN, GLYCOLIPID, GLYCOLYSIS, GLYCOPROTEIN, GLYCOSIDASES, GLYCOSIDE, GLYCOSYLATION

Glycocalyx A polysaccharide matrix that is involved (in some microorganisms) in the firm attachment of the organism to a solid surface.

Glycoform One of several molecular arrangements that a given glycoprotein can possess (varieties are determined by the attachment of various oligosaccharides). Some glycoforms of a given glycoprotein may exhibit greater or lesser biological activity (e.g., pharmaceutical effectiveness for biotherapeutic glycoproteins) because the oligosaccharide units of the glycoprotein molecule mediate interactions of the glycoprotein with the cells of the body.

See also GLYCOPROTEIN, OLIGOSACCHARIDES

Glycogen A polymer of glucose with a branching, tree-like molecular structure. It is the chief storage form of carbohydrates in animals. In mammals, glycogen is stored mainly in the liver and muscles. Its molecular weight may be on the order of several million.

See also GLUCOSE (GLc), GLUCAGON, MOLECULAR WEIGHT

Glycolipid A lipid containing at least one carbohydrate group within its molecule.

See also LIPIDS, GLYCOPROTEIN, GLYCOSYLATION, GLYCOLYSIS

Glycolysis A metabolic process in which sugars are broken down into smaller compounds with the release of energy. This series of chemical reactions is found in plant and animal cells as well as in many microorganisms. Except for the final reaction in the series, the chemical reaction pathway of glycolysis is the same as that for fermentation.

See also GLUCOSE (GLc), METABOLISM, FERMENTATION

Glycoprotein A conjugated protein containing at least one carbohydrate (oligosaccharide) group within its molecule. A commonly occurring category of glycoproteins found in nature is called mucoproteins. These are protein–polysaccharide compounds that occur in tissues, particularly in mucous secretions.

Other glycoproteins include lymphokines (e.g., interleukins), hormones (e.g., somatotropins), receptors (e.g., GP120), enzymes (e.g., tissue plasminogen activator), and some therapeutics (e.g., CD4-PE40).

See also GLYCOFORM, CONJUGATED PROTEIN, GP120 PROTEIN, CONJUGATE, PROTEIN, OLIGOSACCHARIDES, POLYSACCHARIDES, SIALIC ACID

Glycoprotein C A blood-clot-regulating glycoprotein.

See also PROTEIN C, GLYCOPROTEIN

Glycoprotein Remodeling The use of restriction endoglycosidases to (enzymatically) remove sugar (i.e., oligosaccharide) "branches" from glycoprotein (i.e., part protein, part oligosaccharide) molecules.

One reason for such glycoprotein remodeling done by scientists would be to remove one or more oligosaccharide branches so that the glycoprotein is less or no longer antigenic (i.e., triggers an immune response). This allows the glycoprotein to be injected into the body (e.g., for pharmaceutical purposes) without incurring an unwanted immune response.

Glycoprotein remodeling by bacteria (e.g., certain pathogenic bacteria) can enable them to become resistant to some antibiotics.

See also GLYCOPROTEIN, RESTRICTION ENDOGLYCOSIDASES, ENZYME, OLIGOSACCHARIDES, ANTIGEN, CELLULAR IMMUNE RESPONSE, HUMORAL IMMUNITY, ANTIBODY, EPITOPE, HAPTEN, BACTERIA, PATHOGEN, PATHOGENIC, ANTIBIOTIC, ANTIBIOTIC RESISTANCE

Glycosidases Enzymes that catalyze the cleavage (hydrolysis) of glycosidic molecular bonds. For example, lysozyme (an enzyme found in human tears) lyses (cuts up) certain bacteria by cleaving the (β configuration) glycosidic linkages (bonds) between the monosaccharide units that (when linked) comprise the polysaccharide component of the bacterial cell walls. A bacterial cell devoid of a cell wall usually bursts.

See also ENDOGLYCOSIDASE, EXOGLYCOSIDASE, RESTRICTION ENDOGLYCOSIDASES

Glycoside A member of a group of compounds that yield sugar molecules on hydrolysis. All parts of a glycoside compound may be sugar molecules so that sucrose, raffinose, starch, and cellulose — all of which hydrolyze into sugar molecules — may all be considered to be glycosides. However, the name glycoside is usually applied to a compound in which part of the molecule is not a sugar. This nonsugar component is called the aglycon.

See also HYDROLYSIS, FRUCTAN

Glycosinolates See GLUCOSINOLATES

Glycosylation (to glycosylate) Addition of oligosaccharide units (e.g., to protein molecules). The oligosaccharide units are linked to either asparagine side chains by *N*-glycosidic bonds or to serine and threonine side chains by O-glycosidic bonds.

See also OLIGOSACCHARIDES, PROTEIN, GOLGI BODIES, PLANTIBODIES™, BACULOVIRUS

Glycosyltransferases A class of enzymes (transferases) that catalyze the addition (chemical reaction) of specific sugars (molecular groups) to oligosaccharides, glycoproteins, or glycosides.

See also OLIGOSACCHARIDES, MONOSACCHARIDES, ENZYME, GLYCOPROTEIN, GLYCOSIDE, TRANSFERASES

Glyphosate An active ingredient in some herbicides, it kills plants (e.g., weeds) by inhibiting the crucial plant enzyme EPSP synthase.

See also ENZYME, EPSP SYNTHASE, CP4 EPSPS, GLYPHOSATE OXIDASE, GLYPHOSATE-TRIMESIUM, GLYPHOSATE ISOPROPYLAMINE SALT, GA21

Glyphosate Isopropylamine Salt One of several forms of active ingredients utilized in some glyphosate-based herbicides.

See also GLYPHOSATE, EPSP SYNTHASE, CP4 EPSPS, GLYPHOSATE OXIDASE, GLYPHOSATE-TRIMESIUM

Glyphosate *N*-acetyltransferase An enzyme that is naturally produced in the soil-dwelling bacteria *Bacillus licheniformis*. It catalyzes the **acetylation (i.e., the "attaching" of an acetyl group to a molecule)** of glyphosate, the active ingredient in some herbicides. Such acetylation prevents glyphosate molecules from killing plants.

If the genes that code for the production of glyphosate *N*-acetyltransferase (GAT) are inserted via genetic engineering into crop plants, it could help such plants to survive postemergence applications of glyphosate-containing herbicides.

See also ENZYME, BACTERIA, GENE, GENETIC ENGINEERING, CODING SEQUENCE, GLYPHOSATE

Glyphosate Oxidase An enzyme that (via catalysis) chemically breaks down glyphosate (i.e., the active ingredient in some herbicides). Glyphosate oxidase is produced in nature by acclimated microorganisms.

In 1988, Michael Heitkamp discovered a strain of *pseudomonas* bacteria that possessed a gene (GO) that caused those bacteria to produce unusually large amounts of glyphosate oxidase. The gene can be incorporated into a variety of crop plants (e.g., soybean, cotton, etc.) in order to enable those plants to survive postemergence applications of glyphosate-containing herbicides.

Additionally, a plant can be genetically engineered to survive postemergence applications of glyphosate-containing and/or sulfosate-containing herbicides via insertion of gene (cassette) for plant production of the enzyme CP4 EPSPS.

See also ENZYME, ACCLIMATIZATION, STRAIN, *PSEUDOMONAS FLUORESCENS*, GENE, GENETIC ENGINEERING, BACTERIA, MICROORGANISM, SOYBEAN PLANT, EPSP SYNTHASE, CP4 EPSPS, CASSETTE, GLYPHOSATE, SULFOSATE, GA21

Glyphosate Oxidoreductase An enzyme that is naturally produced in one strain of the microorganism *Ochrobactrum anthropi*. It chemically breaks down (by catalysis) glyphosate (i.e., the active ingredient in some herbicides).

If the gene (called **goxv247**) that codes for the production of glyphosate oxidoreductase is inserted via genetic engineering into crop plants, it would help enable such plants to survive postemergence applications of glyphosate- and/or sulfosate-containing herbicides.

Additionally, a plant can be genetically engineered to survive postemergence applications of glyphosate- and/or sulfosate-containing herbicides via insertion of gene (cassette) for plant production of the enzyme CP4 EPSPS.

G

See also ENZYME, STRAIN, MICROOR-GANISM, GENE, GENETIC ENGINEER-ING, EPSP SYNTHASE, CP4 EPSPS, CAS-SETTE, GLYPHOSATE, SULFOSATE

Glyphosate-Trimesium One of several forms of active ingredient utilized in some glyphosate-based herbicides.

See also GLYPHOSATE, EPSP SYNTHASE, CP4 EPSPS, GLYPHOSATE OXIDASE, GLY-PHOSATE ISOPROPYLAMINE SALT, GA21

Gm Fad2-1 A (plant) gene that codes for delta 12 desaturase (Δ 12).

See also GENE, DELTA 12 DESATURASE, COSUPPRESSION

GMAC Acronym for the **Genetic Manipulation Advisory Committee of Australia**, which advises the Australian government on matters pertaining to genetic engineering (e.g., new rDNA product approvals).

The GMAC is analogous to Germany's ZKBS (Central Commission on Biological Safety), Brazil's CTNBio (National Technical Biosafety Commission), and the Kenya Biosafety Council.

See also GENE TECHNOLOGY REGULA-TOR (GTR), ZKBS (CENTRAL COMMIS-SION ON BIOLOGICAL SAFETY), RECOMBINANT DNA ADVISORY COM-MITTEE (RAC), GENETIC ENGINEER-ING, rDNA, DEOXYRIBONUCLEIC ACID (DNA), CTNBIO, KENYA BIOSAFETY COUNCIL, GENE TECHNOLOGY OFFICE, INTERIM OFFICE OF THE GENE TECHNOLOGY REGULATOR (IOGTR)

GMO Genetically manipulated organism or genetically modified organism.

See also GENE, GENE SPLICING, GENETIC ENGINEERING

GMP See GOOD MANUFACTURING PRACTICES (GMP)

GMP Guanylate See G-PROTEINS

GMPP See GENETICALLY MODIFIED PEST PROTECTED (GMPP) PLANTS

GMS Genetically modified soya.

See also GMO, SOYBEAN PLANT

GNE Group of National Experts on Safety in Biotechnology. The group of people within the OECD that developed OECD's guidelines for nations to utilize in their safety evaluations of foods derived from biotechnology.

See also ORGANIZATION FOR ECONOMIC COOPERATION AND DEVELOPMENT (OECD), BIOTECHNOLOGY, GENETIC ENGINEERING

GO Gene See GLYPHOSATE OXIDASE

Golden Rice A biotechnology-derived rice (*Oryza sativa*) created in the 1990s by Ingo Potrykus and Peter Beyer, which contains large amounts of beta-carotene (precursor of vitamin A) in its seeds. The human body converts beta-carotene into vitamin A.

Potrykus and Beyer utilized *Agrobacterium tumefaciens* bacteria to genetically engineer rice plant by inserting the following genes from daffodil and from the bacterium *Erwinia uredovora*:

- Phytoene synthase from daffodil (narcissus), which converts geranylgeranyl-diphosphate into phytoene.
- "CRTL" gene from *Erwinia uredovora*, which codes for phytoene desaturase and causes the rice plant to convert phytoene (a "light harvesting" carotenoid involved in photosynthesis) into lycopene (a carotenoid that is then utilized by the rice plant in the production of beta-carotene). See the following item.
- Lycopene beta-cyclase from daffodil, which converts lycopene into beta-carotene.

The United Nations (UNICEF) estimates that 1 to 2 million deaths of children aged 1 to 4 yr could be prevented annually around the world if they received a little more vitamin A daily in their diet (e.g., via such a rice).

Some of the diseases caused by lack of vitamin A include:

- Childhood blindness (estimated to afflict 350,000 to 500,000 children per year)
- Coronary heart disease
- Certain cancers (e.g., cancer of the lungs, prostate, etc.)
- Macular degeneration, a leading cause of blindness in older people
- Various childhood diseases that result in death (e.g., due to a weakened immune system)

Research indicates that, when commercialized in the future, "golden rice" will also contribute more iron (bioavailable) to the human diet. That will be due to inserted genes for ferritin (an iron-rich storage protein) and phytase. Because iron deficiency anemia (IDA) is a major cause of maternal and childhood illnesses in developing countries, such a reduction in IDA via consumption of this rice could confer major health benefits.

See also BIOTECHNOLOGY, BETA-CARO-TENE, VITAMIN, PHYTOCHEMICALS, NUTRACEUTICALS, CAROTENOIDS, GENE, GENETIC ENGINEERING, BAC-TERIA, *AGROBACTERIUM TUMEFA-CIENS*, PHOTOSYNTHESIS, LYCOPENE, CORONARY HEART DISEASE (CHD), IRON DEFICIENCY ANEMIA (IDA), PRO-TEIN, PHYTASE, PATHWAY, METABOLIC PATHWAY, METABOLIC ENGINEERING

GoldenRice™ A registered trademark now owned by the company Syngenta AG.

See also GOLDEN RICE

Golgi Apparatus See GOLGI BODIES

Golgi Bodies (also known as Golgi complexes) First described by Camillo Golgi in 1898, these are the primary locations of the "sorting centers" of cells and of the mechanism for glycosylation of (i.e., adding oligosaccharide and polysaccharide branches onto) proteins, before those proteins are subsequently transported by transfer vesicles to lysosomes, secretory vesicles, or the plasma membrane.

In plant cells, Golgi complexes are where complex polysaccharides are "sorted" and assembled in preparation for making the cell wall (located just outside the cell's plasma membrane).

A Golgi complex is a stack of flattened membranous sacs (usually 6 sacs in mammal cells and 20 sacs in plant cells).

See also GLYCOSYLATION, CELL, OLI-GOSACCHARIDES, POLYSACCHA-RIDES, PROTEIN, LYSOSOME, VESI-CLES, PLASMA MEMBRANE

Golgi Complexes See GOLGI BODIES

Good Laboratory Practice for Nonclinical Studies (GLPNC) The Good Laboratory Practice (GLP) that is required by the U.S. Food and Drug Administration (FDA) for studies of the safety and toxicological effects of new drugs for livestock.

See also GOOD LABORATORY PRACTICES (GLP), NADA

Good Laboratory Practices (GLP) A set of rules and regulations issued by the Food and Drug Administration (FDA) that establishes broad methodological guidelines for procedures and record keeping. They are to be followed in laboratories involved in the testing and/or preparation of pharmaceuticals. GLPs also apply to the Environmental Protection Agency (EPA) (e.g., toxicity testing of new herbicides).

Good Manufacturing Practices (GMP) The set of general methodologies, practices, and procedures mandated by the Food and Drug Administration (FDA) that is to be followed in the testing and manufacture of pharmaceuticals. The purpose of GMPs is essentially to provide for record keeping and, in a wider context, to protect the public. GMP guidelines exist instead of specific regulations because of the newness of the technology, and may later be superceded (modified) because of further advances in technology and understanding.

See also cGMP

Gossypol A yellow pigment produced in glands and seeds of the cotton plant (*Gossypium* spp.) and some other plants.

When consumed by monogastric animals (e.g., swine, poultry, etc.), gossypol is somewhat toxic to those animals. Recent research indicates that, when administered (in the form of a purified pharmaceutical compound) to humans, gossypol is active against certain forms of cancer.

See also COTTON, PHYTOTOXIN, CANCER

GP120 Protein An adhesion molecule (glycoprotein) on the envelope (surface membrane) of HIV (i.e., AIDS-causing) viruses that directly interacts with the CD4 protein on helper T cells, enabling the HIV viruses to bind to and infect helper T cells. In 1994, a group at America's Scripps Research Institute led by Dennis Burton and Carlos Barbas III announced that they had generated a recombinant human antibody to the GP120 protein that neutralized more than 75% of HIV isolates that it was tested against. This advance

G

holds the potential to someday lead to a vaccine against AIDS.

See also MONOCLONAL ANTIBODIES (MAb), HUMAN IMMUNODEFICIENCY VIRUS TYPE 1 (HIV-1), HUMAN IMMUNODEFICIENCY VIRUS TYPE 2 (HIV-2), ACQUIRED IMMUNE DEFICIENCY SYNDROME (AIDS), SOLUBLE CD4, CD4 PROTEIN, HELPER T CELLS (T4 CELLS), CD44 PROTEIN, ADHESION MOLECULE, CONSERVED, GLYCOPROTEIN, SELECTINS, LECTINS, PROTEIN

GPA1 A gene, found in most plants, that is responsible for controlling water retention and cell division in those plants. The GPA1 gene codes for a G-protein, which transmits or regulates signals (e.g., light, temperature, phytohormones, nutrients, etc.) controlling the plant's development.

During 2001, Alan Jones and colleagues discovered that "knocking out" (i.e., silencing) the GPA1 gene caused the (then-resultant) G-protein to be insensitive to abscisic acid. Because abscisic acid is a phytohormone (i.e., plant hormone) utilized by plants to control the size of stomatal pores, i.e., the openings in leaves through which plants exchange oxygen and carbon dioxide (and also water inadvertently) with the atmosphere, the "knocked out GPA1" plants wilted because of uncontrolled water loss to the atmosphere.

See also GENE, CELL, MITOSIS, G-PROTEINS, PLANT HORMONE, ABSCISIC ACID, KNOCKOUT (GENE)

GPCRs Acronym for **G-protein-coupled receptors**.

See G-PROTEIN-COUPLED RECEPTORS

Graft-Versus-Host Disease (GVHD) The rejection of transplanted organs by the recipient's immune system. Also known as hyperacute rejection. It is caused by the attack of the recipient's T lymphocytes (i.e., T cells, a certain class of white blood cells) on the transplanted organ. The recipient's T cells are able to distinguish between self and foreign cells and are hence able to recognize the foreign (nonself) cells of the transplanted organ. They then, naturally, try to destroy the "foreign invaders" in the body. This then constitutes rejection of the transplanted organ. From this it should be understood that there is nothing wrong with the body, but that it is behaving exactly as it should.

See also CELLULAR IMMUNE RESPONSE, HUMORAL IMMUNITY, XENOGENEIC ORGANS, FIBROBLASTS, CYCLOSPORIN

Gram Molecular Weight The weight in grams of a compound that is numerically equal to its molecular weight; the weight of one mole ($6.022141527 \times 10^{23}$ molecules).

See also MOLECULAR WEIGHT, MOLE

Gram Negative (G) Pertaining to one of the most important ways of classifying bacteria by means of the differences in the way they stain. The set of bacteria that cannot be stained (blue) when treated with the Gram staining procedure. Gram negativity (and Gram positivity) is conferred not by the chemical constituents of the bacteria, but rather by the physical structure of the bacteria cell wall. The staining procedure involves the staining of all cells in a sample with a blue dye. Gram-negative bacteria have a very thin peptidoglycan cell wall (capsule). Hence, the washing procedure, which is an integral part of the overall staining procedure, washes out the blue dye (known as crystal violet). This leaves the Gram-negative bacteria colorless. The cells are then stained with a red acidic counterstain (dye) such as acid fuchsin or safranine. After treatment with counterstain, the Gram-negative cells are red and the gram-positive cells are blue.

See also GRAM POSITIVE (G+), BACTERIA, CELL, GRAM STAIN

Gram Positive (G+) Pertaining to bacteria, this refers to them holding the color of the primary stain (blue) when treated with Gram's stain (a commercial staining agent) or Gentian violet solution.

In contrast to the Gram-negative bacteria, Gram-positive bacteria possess a much thicker peptidoglycan cell wall (capsule). Because of this, the blue crystal violet dye (with which the bacteria were stained) does not wash out of the cell and the bacteria appear blue under the microscope.

Most Gram-positive species of bacteria (e.g., *enterococci*) utilize peptides for quorum sensing. The human pathogen *Enterococcus faecalis* utilizes the peptide **cytolysin** for both the following:

G

- Quorum sensing
- Lysing of **target cells (i.e., of the host organism)** at a distance from the bacteria cell.

See also GRAM NEGATIVE (G), BACTERIA, CELL, GRAM STAIN, CAPSULE, PATHOGEN, PEPTIDE, QUORUM SENSING, LYSE

Gram Stain Devised by Hans Christian Joachim Gram in 1884, this is a test that illuminates the composition or makeup of the physical structure of the cell wall of bacteria being tested. It is utilized to judge the effectiveness of a given chemical compound (e.g., an antibiotic) against bacteria types.

The test consists of a differential staining procedure, which allows most bacteria to be visually separated into two groups — Gram positive (G+) and Gram negative (G). An antibiotic is defined in terms of the group of (pathogenic) bacteria that it is effective against, which is known as that antibiotic's "spectrum of activity." An antibiotic is said to have a spectrum of activity against gram-positive bacteria, gram-negative bacteria, or the bacteria of *both* groups. An antibiotic that is effective against both groups of bacteria is termed "broad spectrum" or "wide spectrum."

See also BACTERIA, GRAM POSITIVE (G+), GRAM NEGATIVE (G), PATHOGENIC, CELL, ANTIBIOTIC

Granulation Tissue A mixture of proteins and cells produced by the fibroblast growth that results from a wound.

See also FIBROBLASTS, PROTEIN

Granulocidin A protein produced by white blood cells, which has demonstrated (in the laboratory) the ability to kill a broad spectrum of pathogens.

See also PATHOGEN, PROTEIN

Granulocyte Colony-Stimulating Factor (G-CSF) A colony-stimulating factor (CSF, a protein) that stimulates production of granulocytes, particularly neutrophils.

See also COLONY-STIMULATING FACTORS, GRANULOCYTES, NEUTROPHILS

Granulocyte-Macrophage Colony-Stimulating Factor (GM-CSF) (or granulocyte-monocyte colony-stimulating factor). A colony-stimulating factor (CSF, a protein) that stimulates production of granulocytes or macrophages or monocytes.

Research indicates that injection of GM-CSF into the human body will also stimulate the growth of new blood vessels around the heart in those people whose heart arteries are clogged, e.g., via arteriosclerosis.

See also COLONY-STIMULATING FACTORS (CSFs), MACROPHAGE, MONOCYTES, ANGIOGENESIS, ARTERIOSCLEROSIS

Granulocytes (Polymorphonuclear Granulocytes) Phagocytic (scavenging and ingesting) cells that are part of the immune system. When their cell nucleus is segmented into lobes and they have granule-like inclusions within their cytoplasm (the neutrophils, eosinophils, and basophils), they are collectively known as polymorphonuclear granulocytes.

See also PHAGOCYTE

GRAS List A list of food additives or ingredients considered to be Generally Recognized as Safe by the U.S. government's Food and Drug Administration (FDA). This list of additives is judged to be safe by a panel of FDA pharmacologists and toxicologists, who base their judgment upon data that is available for each ingredient. In practice, additives for which extensive experience of common use in foods (without known ill effects) has been accumulated over time (e.g., common table salt) are often approved by the FDA more because of the "common use factor" than any toxicology data *per se*.

See also FOOD AND DRUG ADMINISTRATION (FDA), DELANEY CLAUSE, PHARMACOLOGY, CANOLA

Grass Pea See GLUCOSINOLATES

Green Biotechnology Term utilized in some countries to refer to **agricultural** applications of genetic engineering. One example would be herbicide-tolerant crops.

See also GENETIC ENGINEERING, HERBICIDE-TOLERANT CROPS

Green Fluorescent Protein A protein that is naturally present within the jellyfish *Aequorea victoria*. Green fluorescent protein (GFP) is utilized by scientists to do the following:

- "Label" certain protein molecules that are of interest to scientists (e.g., in cell samples).

G

- Help visualize thin layers of biological tissue in fluorescence microscopy.
- "Mark" certain end points in experiments (at which point the green light signals that the end point was reached).

When GFP binds to double-stranded DNA, its fluorescence is greatly enhanced (i.e., also "marking" end point). GFP's gene (which codes for production of the protein) can be utilized as a "reporter gene" for monitoring gene expression (i.e., of another protein that is of interest to a researcher) in a variety of living systems; for example, inside transparent tissues of the zebra fish (*Danio rerio*), the roundworm *Caenorhabditis elegans*, in tissues that are being grown via cell culture, etc.

See also FLUORESCENCE, PROTEIN, GENE, TRANSFECTION, GENE EXPRESSION MARKERS, CELL, CELL ARRAY, CELL CULTURE, REPORTER GENE, LABEL (FLUORESCENT), DEOXYRIBONUCLEIC ACID (DNA), DOUBLE HELIX, CODING SEQUENCE, *CAENORHABDITIS ELEGANS (C. elegans)*, FLUORESCENCE-ACTIVATED CELL SORTER (FACS), TIRF MICROSCOPY, RAPID PROTEIN FOLDING ASSAY

Green Leafy Volatiles See VOLICITIN

GRF See GROWTH-HORMONE-RELEASING FACTOR

GRH See GROWTH-HORMONE-RELEASING FACTOR

Group of National Experts on Safety in Biotechnology See GNE

Growth (Microbial) An increase in the number of cells.

See also GENERATION TIME

Growth Curve The change in the number of cells in a growing culture as a function of time.

See also GENERATION TIME

Growth Factor A specific substance that must be present in the organism's tissues (when *in vivo*) or growth medium (when *in vitro*) so that the growth-factor-specific cells grow or multiply.

See also FIBROBLAST GROWTH FACTOR (FGF), NERVE GROWTH FACTOR (NGF), EPIDERMAL GROWTH FACTOR (EGF), VASCULAR ENDOTHELIAL GROWTH FACTOR (VEGF), ANGIOGENIC GROWTH FACTORS, ANGIOGENIN, BONE MORPHOGENETIC PROTEINS (BMP), PRE-B CELL COLONY-ENHANCING FACTOR, INSULIN-LIKE GROWTH FACTOR-2 (IGF-2)

Growth Hormone (GH) A hormone produced by the anterior pituitary gland. This hormone is a protein (somatotropin) and can be obtained from the bodies of animals or produced by genetically engineered microorganisms. Its major action in humans (human growth hormone) is a generalized stimulation of skeletal growth. However, the human growth hormone (HGH) is also known to affect the growth of other tissues, to be important in fat, protein, and carbohydrate metabolism, and to enhance the effects of various other hormones.

See also BOVINE SOMATOTROPIN (BST), PORCINE SOMATOTROPIN (PST), PITUITARY GLAND

Growth-Hormone-Releasing Factor (GRF or GHRF) Also termed growth-hormone-releasing hormone (GRH). A factor that causes the release of growth hormone. It is 44 amino acids in length.

See also GROWTH HORMONE (GH), GROWTH FACTOR, AMINO ACID, HORMONE

GT-AG Rule Describes the presence of these constant dinucleotides at the first two and last two positions of introns of nuclear genes.

See also INTRON, GENE

GT/PT Correlation Abbreviation for **genotype/phenotype correlation**.

See also GENOTYPE, PHENOTYPE

GTO Abbreviation for **Gene Technology Office**.

See also GENE TECHNOLOGY OFFICE

GTP See GMP

GTPases Guanosine triphosphatases. These are G-proteins (enzymes) that are crucial for growth, movement, and maintenance of the cell's shape. When active, GTPases are bound to cell membranes (surfaces) by an isoprene molecule (receptor).

See also G-PROTEINS, ENZYME, CELL, PHOSPHORYLATION, RECEPTORS, PROTEIN

GTR See GENE TECHNOLOGY REGULATOR (GTR)

GTS Glufosinate-ammonium-tolerant soybean.

See also HERBICIDE-TOLERANT CROP, SOYBEAN PLANT, PAT GENE, GLUFOSINATE

GTS Glyphosate-tolerant soybean.

See also HERBICIDE-TOLERANT CROP, SOYBEAN PLANT, CP4 EPSPS, GLYPHOSATE

Guanine A purine base. It occurs naturally as a fundamental component of nucleic acids.

See also PURINE, NUCLEIC ACIDS

GURTs See GENETIC USE RESTRICTION TECHNOLOGIES

GUS See GUS GENE

GUS Gene A gene that codes for production of B-glucuronidase (i.e., GUS protein) in certain organisms (e.g., *Escherichia coli* bacteria).

The GUS gene is commonly utilized as a "marker gene" for genetically engineered plants. B-glucuronidase causes a color change, in the presence of the chemical 5-bromo-4-chloro-3-indoyl-beta-D-glucuronic acid, by cleaving (i.e., "cutting") a glucuronic acid molecule off the 5-bromo-4-chloro-3-indoyl-beta-D-glucuronic acid. The (remaining) molecule is an insoluble blue dye.

See also GENE, CODING SEQUENCE, *ESCHERICHIA COLIFORM (E. COLI)*, MARKER (GENETIC MARKER), GENETIC ENGINEERING, ENZYME

Gut-Associated Lymphoid Tissues (GALT) A variety of specialized lymph-reticular tissues that line the inside of an animal's digestive system. GALT include Peyer's patches, the appendix, and small solitary lymphoid tissues in the gut. They constitute the intestinal immune system (response to antigens).

See also LYMPHOCYTE, PEYER'S PATCHES, ANTIGEN, HUMORAL IMMUNITY, CELLULAR IMMUNE RESPONSE, EDIBLE VACCINES, PLANTIGENS

Gyrase See HELICASE

G

H

HA Abbreviation for the word **hemagglutinin**. See HEMAGGLUTININ

Habitat The natural environment of an organism within an ecosystem. The place, in an ecosystem, where an organism lives.
See also ECOLOGY

HAC See HUMAN ARTIFICIAL CHROMOSOMES (HAC)

HACCP See HAZARD ANALYSIS AND CRITICAL CONTROL POINTS (HACCP)

Hairpin Loop A section of highly curving, single-stranded DNA or RNA formed when a long piece (string) of the DNA or RNA bends back on itself and hydrogen-bonds (is able to base pair) in some regions to form double-stranded regions. The structure can be visualized by taking a human hair, bending it back on itself and holding it in such a way as to halve its original length. The section where the two ends of hair lie next to each other represents the section of double-stranded DNA or RNA. At one end the hair will have to make a sharp turn and will form a loop. This loop represents the single-stranded hairpin loop.

Hairpin loops can also form in peptide (molecules). For example, during 2002, Joel P. Schneider and Darrin J. Pochan designed a 20-residue peptide that spontaneously assembles (by the millions) into a *hydrogel*, when a solution containing those peptides is caused to have a pH of 9.
See also RIBONUCLEIC ACID (RNA), DEOXYRIBONUCLEIC ACID (DNA), SELF-ASSEMBLY (OF A LARGE MOLECULAR STRUCTURE), MOLECULAR BEACON

Halophile Microorganisms that require NaCl (salt) for growth (they are called obligate halophiles). Those that do not require salt, but can grow in the presence of high NaCl concentrations, are called facultative halophiles. Natural habitats containing high salt concentrations are, for example, the Great Salt Lake in Utah, the Dead Sea in Israel, and the Caspian Sea in Russia.
See also HABITAT

HAP Gene See LOW-PHYTATE CORN

Haploid A cell with one set of chromosomes, i.e., half as many chromosomes as the normal somatic body cells contain. A characteristic of sex cells.
See also GAMETE

Haplophase A phase in the life cycle of an organism in which it has only one copy of each gene. The organism is then said to be haploid. Yeast can exist as true haploids. Humans are haploid for only a few genes and cannot exist as true haploids.
See also HAPLOID

Haplotype A subgroup (e.g., an ethnic minority, all members of a genetically related family group, etc.) of organisms (e.g., humans) whose phenotype results in their body responding in the same way to a physical agent (e.g., a certain pharmaceutical, a toxin, a food, etc.), or are predisposed to particular diseases. For example, more than 70% of black people in North America are lactose intolerant (e.g., their bodies cannot metabolize the lactose sugar in cow's milk), but fewer than 19% of Caucasian people in North America are lactose intolerant.

Analogous to that, the drugs acetaminophen, aspirin, and Valium remain in the bodies of women (who constitute a haplotype) longer than in the bodies of men. Haplotypes for the β_2-adrenergic gene are predictive of asthma patients' response to the pharmaceutical **albuterol**.

Haplotypes of women possessing the BRCA 1 gene or the BRCA 2 gene have a higher-than-average chance of developing ovarian cancer or breast cancer. Haplotypes of people possessing the APOE4 gene or the CYP46 gene have a higher-than-average chance of developing Alzheimer's disease.

In terms of molecular biology, haplotypes consist of individuals whose DNA contains

H

165

"grouped **SNPs**" **(single-nucleotide poly-morphisms),** which **collectively** confer the particular aspect (e.g., sensitivity to certain pharmaceuticals, susceptibility to certain diseases, etc.) when they are inherited.

For example, during 2002, a haplotype consisting of people possessing **70 genes inherited together** was found to be predictive of breast cancer metastasis.

During 2003, Jeffrey Mogil discovered that a haplotype consisting of red-haired women possessing certain versions of the ***MC1R*** **(melanocortin 1 receptor)** gene was predictive of a heightened response to the opioid pharmaceutical pentazocine in those women.

See also PHARMACOGENOMICS, HERITABILITY, HEREDITY, TRAIT, GENE, GENETICS, PHENOTYPE, TOXIN, INSULIN, METABOLISM, SINGLE-NUCLEOTIDE POLYMORPHISMS (SNPs), CANCER, BRCA GENES, LINKAGE, APOE4, CYTOCHROME P450 (CYP), CYP46 GENE, ALZHEIMER'S DISEASE, METASTASIS, FLUORESCENCE *IN SITU* HYBRIDIZATION (FISH), ALLELE

Haplotype Map See SINGLE-NUCLEOTIDE POLYMORPHISMS (SNPs)

HapMap Acronym for **Haplotype Map**.
See also HAPLOTYPE MAP

Hapten A small foreign molecule that will stimulate an immune system response (e.g., antibody production) if the small molecule (now called a haptenic determinant) is attached to a macromolecule (carrier) to make it large enough to be recognized by the immune system.

See also EPITOPE, CELLULAR IMMUNE RESPONSE, HUMORAL IMMUNITY, CARRIER PROTEIN

Haptoglobin A protein that is a component of human blood; it can occur in one of two different molecular forms (i.e., a "large" or a "small" version of the molecule).

The "small" version of haptoglobin is very effective in "capturing" and removing free radicals (high-energy oxygen atoms that bear an "extra" electron) **from the bloodstream** before they damage tissues (e.g., in the eyes, kidneys, or arteries).

The "large" version of haptoglobin, which is the only haptoglobin molecule in the bloodstream of one particular haplotype (genetic

subgroup) of people, is not effective in the capture and removal of those free radicals (e.g., generated at a high rate in people with diabetes disease), and therefore diabetics within that particular haplotype tend to suffer extreme damage to eyes, kidneys, nerves, and arteries (sometimes necessitating limb amputation).

See also FREE RADICAL, HAPLOTYPE, INSULIN, OXIDATIVE STRESS, DIABETES

Hardening See COLD HARDENING, HYDROGENATION

Harpin A protein that is naturally produced by the *Erwinia amylovora* bacteria (which usually causes the plant disease known as **fire blight** in apple trees, pear trees, and some ornamental plants of the rose family).

Discovered in 1992 by Zhong-Min Wei and colleagues, harpin causes numerous species of plants to initiate a protective or defensive response (cascade) against bacteria, viruses, fungi, and some insects and nematodes. Harpin also causes plants (that it is sprayed on to) to increase their photosynthesis and to have increased root growth and proliferation, which can lead to greater crop yields.

See also PROTEIN, BACTERIA, PHYTOALEXINS, PATHOGENESIS-RELATED PROTEINS, SIGNALING, SIGNALING MOLECULE, SIGNAL TRANSDUCERS AND ACTIVATORS OF TRANSCRIPTION (STATs), SALICYLIC ACID (SA), JASMONIC ACID, SYSTEMIC ACQUIRED RESISTANCE (SAR), CASCADE, R GENES, NEMATODES

Harvesting A term used to describe the recovery of microorganisms from a liquid culture (in which they have been grown by man). This is usually accomplished by means of filtration or centrifugation.

See also MICROORGANISM, CULTURE MEDIUM, ULTRACENTRIFUGE, DIALYSIS

Harvesting Enzymes Enzymes that are used to gently dissociate (i.e., break apart) cells in living tissues in order to produce single, separate cells that can then be established and propagated in a cell culture reactor. Harvesting enzymes are also used to dissociate cells that have been grown for some time in a cell culture reactor.

See also CELL CULTURE, MAMMALIAN CELL CULTURE, ENZYME, CULTURE MEDIUM

Hazard Analysis and Critical Control Points (HACCP) A quality control program (for food processing) to systematically prevent hazards (e.g., pathogens) from entering the production process. HACCP was initially developed in the 1950s by the Pillsbury Company to supply food products for astronauts in the U.S. space program. Under HACCP, food processors and handlers must analyze and identify in advance the points where hazards are most likely to occur, and eliminate them. For example, because melons lie in pathogen-contaminated dirt while growing, a "critical control point" for restaurants serving sliced melon is cleansing of the knife after each melon is cut (to prevent the knife from carrying pathogens from one infected melon to other melons).

See also PATHOGEN, RAPID MICROBIAL DETECTION (RMD)

HCC See ANGIOGENESIS

HCS Acronym for **high-content screening**. See HIGH-CONTENT SCREENING

HD Gene Refers to the damaged (mutant) allele that causes Huntington's disease, when present in a human's genome.

See also GENE, DOMINANT ALLELE, GENOME, HUNTINGTON'S DISEASE, GENETICS, MUTATION

HDL See HIGH-DENSITY LIPOPROTEINS (HDLPs)

Heat-Shock Proteins See STRESS PROTEINS

Heavy-Chain Variable (VH) Domains The regions (domains) of the antibody molecule's "heavy chain" that vary in their amino acid sequence. The "chains" (of atoms) comprising the antibody (immunoglobulin) molecule consist of a region of variable (V) amino acid sequence and another region in which the amino acid sequence remains constant (C). An antibody molecule possesses two antigen-binding sites, and it is the variable domains of the light (VL) and heavy (VH) chains which contribute to this (antigen-binding ability).

See also ANTIBODY, PROTEIN, IMMUNO-GLOBULIN, SEQUENCE (OF A PROTEIN MOLECULE), ANTIGEN, AMINO ACID, COMBINING SITE, DOMAIN (OF A PROTEIN), LIGHT-CHAIN VARIABLE (VL) DOMAINS

Hedgehog Proteins A "family" of related signaling molecules (consisting of "signaling protein" with a cholesterol molecule attached to it), which direct or control tissue differentiation during animal and insect embryo development (into various organs, limbs, etc.). They also control left–right asymmetry of the developing body. Some of the hedgehog proteins are **Sonic Hedgehog (Shh), Indian Hedgehog (Ihh), Desert Hedgehog (Dhh)**. The applicable hedgehog protein (within an embryo cell) cleaves itself into two peptides, one of which then acts as a transferase (i.e., enzyme that catalyzes the addition of a functional group to a given molecule — in this case to the other "hedgehog peptide").

When the cell then secretes the cholesterol or peptide molecule, the cholesterol (functional group) "anchors" it to the cell surface, whereas the "signaling protein" end of the cholesterol or peptide directs differentiation of nearby cells.

See also PROTEIN, SIGNALING MOLE-CULES, SIGNALING, CHOLESTEROL, SIGNAL TRANSDUCTION, PEPTIDE, CELL, TRANSFERASES, ENZYME, FUNCTIONAL GROUP, DIFFERENTIA-TION, CELL DIFFERENTIATION

Hedgehog Signaling Pathway A signaling pathway that is critical to development of many embryonic organisms into adult organisms. Via this pathway, hedgehog proteins direct or control tissue differentiation (into various organs, limbs, etc.) as the embryo develops into an adult body. Hedgehog proteins also control left–right asymmetry of the developing body. When the body reaches adult form, the hedgehog signaling pathway shuts down (epigenetically).

Research indicates that if the hedgehog signaling pathway is (wrongly) "turned on" in an adult body, it can promote development of some cancers.

See also PATHWAY, SIGNALING, PRO-TEIN, SIGNALING PROTEIN, SIGNAL TRANSDUCTION, HEDGEHOG PRO-TEINS, DIFFERENTIATION, CELL, CELL

H

DIFFERENTIATION, CELL MOTILITY, EPIGENETIC, CANCER

HeLa Cells A cell line (i.e., cells propagated in cell culture) utilized by researchers studying human physiology or malignancy. Named after **Henrietta La**cks, who donated it to science (from a tumor in her body) in 1951.

See also CELL, CELL CULTURE, CANCER, TUMOR, MONOCLONAL ANTIBODIES (MAb)

Helicase An enzyme that "unwinds" the DNA molecule's **double helix structure** during DNA replication.

See also ENZYME, DEOXYRIBONUCLEIC ACID (DNA), DOUBLE HELIX, REPLICATION (OF DNA)

Helicobacter pylori Bacteria.

See *H. PYLORI*

Helicoverpa armigera See *HELICOVERPA ZEA* (*H. zea*)

Helicoverpa zea (*H. zea*) Known as the corn earworm (when it is on corn plants) and as the tomato fruitworm (when it is on tomato plants), this is one of three insect species that is called "bollworms" (when on cotton plants). *H. zea* chews on these crop plants, and is one of the insects that can act as a vector (carrier) of *Aspergillus flavus* fungus. In India, the "cotton bollworm" is *Helicoverpa armigera*. In 1997, scientists at the U.S. Department of Agriculture created and optimized a monoclonal antibody against *Helicoverpa zea* **vitellin**, which thus holds potential to be used as a means to control that insect.

See also *B.t. KURSTAKI, HELIOTHIS VIRESCENS* (*H. VIRESCENS*), HIGH-MAYSIN CORN, FUNGUS, *PECTINOPHORA GOSSYPIELLA, ASPERGILLUS FLAVUS*, CORN, MONOCLONAL ANTIODIES (MAb)

Heliothis virescens (*H. virescens*) Known as the tobacco budworm (when it is on tobacco plants), this is one of three insect species that is called "bollworms" (when they are on cotton plants). As part of Integrated Pest Management (IPM), farmers can utilize the parasitic *Euplectrus comstockki* wasp to help control the tobacco budworm and cotton bollworm. When the wasp's venom is injected into *Heliothis* larva, it stops the larva from molting (and thus maturing).

See also *B.T. KURSTAKI, HELICOVERPA ZEA* (*H. ZEA*), *PECTINOPHORA GOSSYPIELLA*, INTEGRATED PEST MANAGEMENT (IPM)

Helix A spiral, staircase-like structure with a repeating pattern described by two simultaneous operations (rotation and translation). It is one of the natural conformations exhibited by biological polymers.

See also BIOMIMETIC MATERIALS, ANALOGUE

Helper T Cells (T4 Cells) T cells (lymphocytes) that bind B cells (upon recognizing a foreign epitope on B cell surface). The binding stimulates B cell proliferation by secreting B cell growth factor.

See also B CELLS, CYTOKINES, T CELL, T CELL RECEPTORS, SUPPRESSOR T CELLS

Hemagglutinin (HA) A special protein that some viruses utilize to gain entry into the cells they have "targeted." The HA protein helps the virus to **adhere** to the cell that it "targets."

Hemaglutinin is also used to refer to specific plant cell proteins (lectins) that are naturally produced by certain plants such as the soybean plant (*Glycine max* (L) Merrill). The presence of those lectin molecules (e.g., on surfaces of root cells of the soybean plant) help nitrogen-fixing *Rhizobium japonicum* bacteria to adhere to soybean plant roots, where they begin to "fix nitrogen" (i.e., create natural nitrate fertilizer, which improves the soil and helps plants to grow).

See also PROTEIN, VIRUS, CELL, LECTINS, SOYBEAN PLANT, NITROGEN FIXATION, BACTERIA, *RHIZOBIUM* (BACTERIA), NITRATES, NODULATION

Hematologic Growth Factors (HGF) A class of colony-stimulating factors (proteins) that stimulates bone marrow cells to produce certain types of red and white blood cells. Some colony-stimulating factors are (1) granulocyte-macrophage colony-stimulating factor (GM-CSF), (2) granulocyte-monocyte colony-stimulating factor, (3) granulocyte colony-stimulating factor (GM-CSF), (4) erythropoietin (EPO), (5) interleukin-3 (IL-3), and (6) macrophage colony-stimulating factor (M-CSF).

Hematopoietic Growth Factors Growth factors that stimulate the body to produce blood cells.

H

See also GROWTH FACTOR, INTERLEU-KIN-6 (IL-6)

Hematopoietic Stem Cells Certain stem cells present (e.g., in infants' bodies and in the umbilical cords of newborn infants) that can be differentiated (via chemical signals in the growing body) to give rise to red blood cells and the infection-fighting cells of the immune system.

See also STEM CELLS, MULTIPOTENT ADULT STEM CELLS, MESODERMAL ADULT STEM CELLS, CELL, ORGAN-ISM, SIGNALING

Heme The iron porphyrin prosthetic group of a class of proteins called "heme proteins."

See also PROSTHETIC GROUP, CHELAT-ING AGENT, PROTEIN, TRANSFERRIN

Hemoglobin An oxygen-transporting respiratory pigment; it is present in humans, animals, and some plants (e.g., land plants that withstand occasional immersion and flooding).

In humans, hemoglobin is carried in the red blood cells (erythrocytes) and is responsible for the red color of the blood. It is composed of two pairs of identical polypeptide chains and iron-containing heme groups, comprising the (total) hemoglobin molecule. The molecular structure of hemoglobin was determined by Max Perutz in 1959. A human disease known as sickle cell anemia is caused by a (genetically-induced) small change (i.e., due to SNP) in the hemoglobin molecule's structure (in victims of that disease).

See also HEME, POLYPEPTIDE (PROTEIN), GENETICS, BILIRUBIN, HEREDITY, ERYTHROCYTES, PROTEIN STRUC-TURE, SINGLE-NUCLEOTIDE POLY-MORPHISMS (SNPs)

Hemostasis See FIBRIN

Heparin A polysaccharide sulfuric acid ester found in liver, lung, and other tissues that prolongs the clotting time of blood by preventing the formation of fibrin. Used in vascular surgery and in treatment of postoperative thrombosis and embolism.

See also FIBRIN, THROMBOSIS

HER-2 Gene Abbreviation often utilized for **human epidermal growth factor receptor-2 gene/neu**, which is an oncogene that is responsible for approximately 30% of breast cancers (i.e., in those women whose body **overexpresses** that particular oncogene), and it spreads via metastatis.

In addition to conventional treatment (e.g., mastectomy, chemotherapy, etc.), the U.S. Food and Drug Administration (FDA) in 1998 approved use of a humanized monoclonal antibody (trastuzumab) to be utilized alone, or in combination with certain chemotherapy agents (e.g., paclitaxel) against such metastatic breast cancers. That monoclonal antibody attaches to the **extracellular domain** (i.e., portion of the Her-2 receptor sticking out of surface of breast tissue cells) and **downregulates** the Her-2 gene (i.e., resulting in fewer Her-2 receptors being produced on the plasma membrane surfaces of those breast tissue cells).

See also GENE, RECEPTORS, HER-2 RECEPTOR, *ras* GENE, EGF RECEPTOR, ONCOGENES, CANCER, EXPRESS, EXPRESSIVITY, METASTASIS, MONO-CLONAL ANTIBODIES (MAb), BRCA GENES, PACLITAXEL, FOOD AND DRUG ADMINISTRATION (FDA), PLASMA MEMBRANE, FLUORESCENCE *IN SITU* HYBRIDIZATION (FISH), PHARMACO-GENOMICS, PHARMACOGENETICS, TRASTUZUMAB, NUTRITIONAL GENOMICS

HER-2 Protein See HER-2 RECEPTOR

HER-2 Receptor An epidermal growth factor receptor (protein molecule embedded in the surface of cells) that is present in abundance in the plasma membrane surface of breast tissue cells in humans possessing the **HER-2 gene**.

See also RECEPTORS, EPIDERMAL GROWTH FACTOR RECEPTOR, PLASMA MEMBRANE, HER-2 GENE

HER-2/neu Gene See HER-2 GENE

Herbicide Resistance See HERBICIDE-TOLERANT CROP

Herbicide-Resistant Crop See HERBICIDE-TOLERANT CROP

Herbicide-Tolerant Crop Crop plants, cultivated by humans, that have been altered to be able to survive applications of one or more herbicides by the incorporation of certain genes by either genetic engineering, natural mutation, or mutation breeding (i.e., soaking seeds in mutation-causing chemicals, or bombardment of seeds with ionizing radiation, to cause random genetic mutations, followed by selection of the **particular mutation in which herbicide-tolerance occurs**).

Because it has been utilized for decades, most relevant national laws consider mutation breeding to be one of the so-called "traditional plant breeding" techniques.

For example, European laws that require special labeling of food products containing genetically engineered (via rDNA) crops do not require such special labeling for food products that contain **crops that were created via mutation breeding**.

Several crops (e.g., soybean, canola, cotton, etc.) are made tolerant to glyphosate- or sulfosate-containing herbicides by the insertion (via genetic engineering techniques) of the aroA transgene (cassette) for CP4 EPSPS. Corn (maize) is made tolerant to glyphosate-containing herbicides by insertion (via genetic engineering techniques) of the mEPSPS or GA21 transgene (cassette).

Some soybean varieties are made tolerant to sulfonylurea-based herbicides by adding (via traditional breeding methods) the **ALS gene** (which confers the sulfonylurea-tolerance trait).

Corn (maize) and rice (*Oryza sativa*) are made tolerant to imidazolinone-containing herbicides by adding (via traditional breeding techniques) the imidazolinone tolerance trait. That trait is imparted by the T-Gene, IT-Gene, or IR-Gene.

See also GENE, GENETIC ENGINEERING, CASSETTE, TRANSGENIC, DEOXYRIBONUCLEIC ACID (DNA), rDNA, EPSP SYNTHASE, GLYPHOSATE OXIDASE, PAT GENE, BAR GENE, GENETICS, GLYPHOSATE, GA21, SULFOSATE, ALS GENE, CP4 EPSPS, CHLOROPLAST TRANSIT PEPTIDE (CTP), ACURON™ GENE, TRANSGENE, TRAIT, CANOLA, SOYBEAN PLANT, CORN, MUTATION BREEDING, TRADITIONAL BREEDING METHODS, IMIDAZOLINONE-TOLERANT SOYBEANS, DROUGHT TOLERANCE

Heredity Transfer of genetic information from parent cells to progeny.

See also INFORMATIONAL MOLECULES, GENE, GENETIC CODE, GENOME, GENETICS, GENOTYPE, DEOXYRIBONUCLEIC ACID (DNA), HERITABILITY, QUANTITATIVE TRAIT LOCI (QTL)

Heritability The fraction of variation (of an individual's given trait) that is due to genetics. For example, if a pig's trait (e.g., weight at birth) is 30% heritable, it means that 30% of the (birth weight) difference between that individual pig and its (statistically representative) group of contemporaries (pigs) is due to genetics. The other 70% would be due to factors such as nutrition of the mother during pregnancy, etc.

See also HEREDITY, TRAIT, GENETICS, INFORMATIONAL MOLECULES, GENE, GENETIC CODE, GENOME, GENOTYPE, DEOXYRIBONUCLEIC ACID (DNA), QUANTITATIVE TRAIT LOCI (QTL)

Hetero A chemical nomenclature prefix meaning "different." For example, a **heterocyclic** compound is one with a (ring) structure made up of **more than one kind** of atom. A **heterokaryon** refers to a cell containing nuclei of **different species.**

See also HETEROCYCLIC, HETERODUPLEX, HETEROGENEOUS (CATALYSIS), HETEROGENEOUS (CHEMICAL REACTION), HETEROGENEOUS (MIXTURE), HETEROKARYON, HETEROLOGOUS PROTEINS, HETEROLOGOUS DNA, HETEROLOGY, HETEROSIS, HETEROTROPH, HETEROZYGOTE

Heterocyclic See HETERO

Heteroduplex A DNA molecule, the two strands of which come from different individuals so that there may be some base pairs or blocks of base pairs that do not match. Can arise from mutation, recombination, or by annealing DNA single strands *in vitro*.

See also DEOXYRIBONUCLEIC ACID (DNA)

Heterogeneous (catalysis) Catalysis occurring at a phase boundary, usually a solid–fluid interface.

See also HETERO, HETEROGENEOUS (MIXTURE), CATALYST

Heterogeneous (chemical reaction) A chemical reaction in which the reactants are of different phases; for example, gas with liquid, liquid with solid, or a solid catalyst with liquid or gaseous reactants.

H

See also HETERO, HETEROGENEOUS (CATALYSIS), CATALYST

Heterogeneous (mixture) One that consists of two or more phases such as liquid–vapor, or liquid–vapor–solid.

See also HETERO

Heterokaryon A fused cell containing nuclei of different species.

See also NUCLEOID

Heterologous DNA Refers to a DNA molecule in which each of the (double) strands is from different sources (e.g., different species).

See also DEOXYRIBONUCLEIC ACID (DNA), HETERO, SPECIES

Heterologous Proteins Those proteins produced by an organism that is not the wild-type source of those proteins. For example, bacteria have been genetically engineered to produce human growth hormone and bovine (i.e., cow) somatotropin.

See also PROTEIN, WILD TYPE, GROWTH HORMONE (GH), BOVINE SOMATOTROPIN (BST), HOMOLOGOUS PROTEIN

Heterology A sequence of amino acids in two or more proteins that are not identical to each other.

See also AMINO ACID, PROTEIN, HOMOLOGY

Heterosis Also known as "hybrid vigor."

See F1 HYBRIDS

Heterotroph An organism that obtains nourishment from the ingestion and breakdown of organic matter.

Heterozygote An individual organism with different alleles at one or more particular loci.

See also ALLELE

Hexadecyltrimethylammonium Bromide (CTAB) A solvent that is widely utilized to dissolve plant DNA samples (e.g., when a scientist wants to sequence that sample of plant DNA). CTAB solvent helps the scientist to separate out contaminants that are commonly present in samples from plant tissues (i.e., polysaccharides, quinones, etc.) because DNA molecules are much more soluble in CTAB than are the contaminant molecules.

See also DEOXYRIBONUCLEIC ACID (DNA), POLYSACCHARIDES, SEQUENCING (OF DNA MOLECULES), SDS

Hexose See GLUCOSE (GLc)

HF Cleavage A research process in which hydrofluoric acid is used to sequentially remove side-chain protective groups from peptide chains. Also used to remove the resin support from peptides that have been prepared via solid-phase peptide synthesis. The HF cleavage reaction is a temperature-dependent process.

See also PROSTHETIC GROUP, SYNTHESIZING (OF PROTEINS)

HGT Acronym for **horizontal gene transfer**. See INTROGRESSION

Hh Abbreviation for **hedgehog proteins** or **hedgehog signaling pathway**.

See HEDGEHOG PROTEINS, HEDGEHOG SIGNALING PATHWAY

High-Amylose Corn Refers to those corn (maize) hybrids that produce kernels in which the starch that is contained within those kernels is at least 50% amylose, as against the average of 24 to 28% amylose in traditional cornstarch.

See also CORN, STARCH, AMYLOSE

High-Content Screening Refers to any analytical methodology or technology by which **multiple** parameters (e.g., secretion of **specific** proteins, the **amounts** of each protein secreted, etc.) of complex systems (e.g., living cells, living multicell organisms, etc.) are simultaneously analyzed.

See also CELL, HIGH-THROUGHPUT IDENTIFICATION, HIGH-THROUGHPUT SCREENING (HTS), TARGET–LIGAND INTERACTION SCREENING, GENE EXPRESSION PROFILING, MULTIPLEX ASSAY, CONFOCAL MICROSCOPY, MULTIPLEXED (ASSAY)

High-Density Lipoproteins (HDLPs) The so-called good cholesterol, it consists of lipoproteins that can help move excess low-density lipoproteins (i.e., "bad" cholesterol, which can clog arteries) from the human body by binding to the low-density lipoproteins (also known as LDL cholesterol) in the blood and then attaching to special LDLP receptor molecules in the liver. The liver then clears those (bound) low-density lipoproteins from the body as a part of regular liver functions.

Studies have shown that humans having high bloodstream levels of HDLPs will offset high levels of LDLPs (e.g., the HDLPs can still

H

help lower the risk of developing coronary heart disease).

Because cholesterol does not dissolve in water (which constitutes most of the volume of blood), the body makes HDL cholesterol into little "packages" surrounded by a hydrophilic (i.e., "water-loving") protein. This protein "wrapper" is known as apolipoprotein A-1, or apo A-1, and it enables HDL cholesterol to be transported in the bloodstream because the apolipoprotein A-1 is attracted to water molecules in the blood.

See also LOW-DENSITY LIPOPROTEINS (LDLP), RECEPTORS, APOLIPOPROTEINS, WATER-SOLUBLE FIBER, CHOLESTEROL, CORONARY HEART DISEASE (CHD)

High-Galactomannan Soybeans See HIGH-MANNOGALACTAN SOYBEANS

High-Glutenin Wheat See GLUTEN

High-Isoflavone Soybeans Developed in the U.S. in the 1990s, these are soybean varieties that contain greater content of isoflavones than do traditional soybean varieties (i.e., isoflavones constitute 0.15 to 0.3% of a traditional variety soybean's dry weight).

Consumption of isoflavones helps to reduce the level of low-density lipoproteins (i.e., "bad cholesterol") in the blood of humans.

A human diet containing a large amount of isoflavones helps prevent osteoporosis, causes reduced risk of certain cancers (e.g., breast cancer, prostate cancer, endometrial cancer, etc.), and decreases risk of prostate enlargement.

See also ISOFLAVONES, SOYBEAN PLANT, CHOLESTEROL, CANCER, PROSTATE-SPECIFIC ANTIGEN (PSA), LOW-DENSITY LIPOPROTEINS (LDLP), OSTEOPOROSIS

High-Lactoferrin Rice Refers to rice plants (*Oryza sativa*) that have been genetically engineered to produce substantial amounts of lactoferrin in the grain they yield. Lactoferrin is a compound that is naturally produced in human breast milk. Consumption of lactoferrin by infants helps to strengthen their immune system.

Consumption of lactoferrin (e.g., from genetically engineered rice) by older humans helps their immune systems to resist some infectious diseases. Lactoferrin "binds" free iron (e.g., in body fluids), thereby **denying that iron** to pathogenic bacteria (which need free iron to grow and infect). Lactoferrin also promotes intestinal cell growth in humans.

See also GENETIC ENGINEERING, PATHOGEN, BACTERIA, VALUE-ENHANCED GRAINS, GROWTH (MICROBIAL), CELL

High-Laurate Canola Refers to canola (*Brassica napus/campesris*) varieties that have been genetically engineered (e.g., via insertion of gene for **lauroyl-ACP thioesterase**) to produce at least 40% laurate (lauric acid) in their oil (in seed).

See also LAURATE, CANOLA, GENETIC ENGINEERING, FATTY ACID, LAUROYL-ACP THIOESTERASE, VALUE-ENHANCED GRAINS

High-Linolenic-Oil Soybeans Soybeans from soybean plants that have been genetically engineered to produce soybeans bearing oil that contains more than 40% linolenic acid, instead of the typical 8% in oil produced from traditional varieties of soybeans. Scientists accomplish that via upregulation (i.e., increased expression) of the *Fad3* gene within the soybean plant's oil synthesis pathway.

See also SOYBEAN PLANT, SOYBEAN OIL, FATTY ACID, LINOLENIC ACID, POLYUNSATURATED FATTY ACIDS (PUFA), GENE, FAD3 GENE, GENETIC ENGINEERING, EXPRESS, UPREGULATION, PATHWAY

High-Lysine Corn Developed in the U.S. in the mid-1960s, these were initially corn (maize) varieties possessing the **opague-2** gene. The opague-2 gene causes such corn to contain 0.30 to 0.55% lysine (i.e., 50 to 80% more than traditional No. 2 yellow corn).

Other genes have subsequently been discovered that, when inserted into corn or maize genome (e.g., via genetic engineering techniques), cause production of larger amounts of lysine than in traditional corn or maize varieties.

High-lysine corn is particularly useful for feeding of swine, because traditional No. 2 yellow corn does not contain enough lysine for optimal swine growth.

See also CORN, LYSINE (Lys), GENE, OPAGUE-2, GENETIC ENGINEERING, GENOME, VALUE-ENHANCED GRAINS,

H

"IDEAL PROTEIN" CONCEPT, MAL (MULTIPLE ALEURONE LAYER) GENE

High-Mannogalactan Soybeans Developed in the U.S. following the 2003 discovery by Kanwarpal S. Dhugga and coworkers that the soybean plant (*Glycine max* (L.)) produces guar gum mannogalactan (i.e., a copolymer of galactose and mannose) when the **CtManS** gene from guar plant (*Cyanmopsis tetragonoloba*) is inserted via genetic engineering; these will be soybean varieties that contain significant amounts of the food-thickening agent currently known as guar gum.

See also SOYBEAN PLANT, GENE, GENETIC ENGINEERING, GALACTOSE (Gal), WATER-SOLUBLE FIBER

High-Maysin Corn Developed in the U.S. during the 1980s and 1990s, these are corn (maize) varieties possessing at least ten times the typical amount of maysin found in traditional corn (maize) varieties.

Maysin is a chemical compound that "binds up" essential amino acids within the gut of certain pest insects, so those insects starve in spite of eating these corns (but humans, animals, and nonpest insects are unharmed). Maysin primarily acts against the corn earworm (*Helicoverpa zea*).

See also CORN, MAYSIN, AMINO ACID, ESSENTIAL AMINO ACIDS, *HELICOVERPA ZEA (H. ZEA)*

High-Methionine Corn Developed in the U.S. in the mid-1960s, these were initially corn (maize) varieties possessing the **floury-2** gene. The floury-2 gene causes such corn to contain slightly higher levels of methionine than traditional No. 2 yellow corn.

Other genes have subsequently been discovered that, when inserted into corn or maize genome (e.g., via genetic engineering techniques), cause production of larger amounts of methionine than in traditional corn or maize varieties.

High-methionine corn is particularly useful for feeding of poultry, because traditional No. 2 yellow corn does not contain enough methionine for optimal poultry (especially feather) growth.

See also METHIONINE (Met), CORN, FLOURY-2, GENE, GENOME, GENETIC ENGINEERING, VALUE-ENHANCED

GRAINS, OPAGUE-2, "IDEAL PROTEIN" CONCEPT, MAL (MULTIPLE ALEURONE LAYER) GENE

High-Oil Corn Conceived in 1896 at the University of Illinois, high-oil corn (HOC) is defined to be corn (maize) possessing a kernel oil content of 5.8% or greater. Traditional No. 2 yellow corn varieties tend to contain 4.5% or less oil content.

See also VALUE-ENHANCED GRAINS, CORN, CHEMOMETRICS

High-Oleic-Oil Corn Conceived in 2002 at Iowa State University, high-oleic-oil corn is defined to be corn (maize) whose kernels possess oil containing more than 40% oleic acid, instead of the 20 to 30% present in kernel oil from traditional varieties of corn.

High-oleic-oil corn varieties were created via the incorporation of certain genes from **eastern gamagrass** (*Tripsacum dactyloides*), which causes the higher-than-traditional amount of oleic acid in the corn oil.

See also VALUE-ENHANCED GRAINS, CORN, FATTY ACID, OLEIC ACID, MONOUNSATURATED FATS

High-Oleic-Oil Soybeans Soybeans from soybean plants that have been genetically engineered to produce soybeans bearing oil that contains more than 70% oleic acid, instead of the typical 24% in the oil produced from traditional varieties of soybeans. Cosuppression, via inserted gene for Δ 12 desaturase (i.e., enzyme that normally converts oleic acid to linoleic acid as part of the oil creation process in traditional varieties of soybean plants), causes the **higher than the traditional** amount of oleic acid in the soybean oil.

High-oleic soybean oil would tend to have greater oxidative stability (especially at elevated temperatures) than soybean oil from traditional varieties of soybeans. Because of this property, nuts that were fried in **high-oleic oil** have been shown to possess a longer shelf life than nuts fried in traditional vegetable oils.

A human diet containing a large amount of oleic acid causes lower blood cholesterol level and, thus, lower risk of coronary heart disease (CHD).

See also SOYBEAN PLANT, SOYBEAN OIL, FATTY ACID, OLEIC ACID, MONOUN-

H

SATURATED FATS, GENETIC ENGI-
NEERING, DELTA 12 DESATURASE,
CHOLESTEROL, CORONARY HEART
DISEASE (CHD), PALMITIC ACID,
COSUPPRESSION, ENZYME, LINOLEIC
ACID, FAD GENES, FAD3 GENE

High-Oleic Sunflowers Refers to sunflower
(*Helianthus annus* L.) plant varieties that have
been bred so their seeds contain 80 to 90% oleic
acid within the oil in those seeds as against the
historical average of 20% in the oil of traditional sunflower (crop) plant varieties.

To create the high-oleic sunflowers, a mutation
known as "**Pervenet**" was obtained via chemical mutagenesis that acts via Δ-12 desaturase
and Δ-9 desaturase enzymes.

See also FATTY ACID, OLEIC ACID, MID-
OLEIC SUNFLOWERS, MUTATION
BREEDING, TRADITIONAL BREEDING
METHODS, ENZYME, DESATURASE,
DELTA 12 DESATURASE, HIGH-OLEIC-
OIL SOYBEANS

High-Phytase Corn and Soybeans Crop plants
that have been genetically engineered to contain in their grain or seed higher levels of the
enzyme phytase (which aids digestion and
absorption of phosphate in that grain or seed).
High-phytase grains or oilseeds are particularly useful for the feeding of swine and poultry, because traditional No. 2 yellow corn
(maize) or traditional soybean varieties do not
contain phytase in amounts needed for complete digestion and absorption of phosphate
naturally contained in those traditional soybeans and corn (maize) in the form of phytate.

See also PHYTASE, ENZYME, PHYTATE,
VALUE-ENHANCED GRAINS, LOW-
PHYTATE CORN, LOW-PHYTATE SOY-
BEANS

High-Protein Rice Developed during 2002,
these are varieties of rice (*Oryza sativa*)
whose grain contains at least 12% protein, in
contrast to traditional varieties of rice, which
average 8% protein content.

See also PROTEIN

High-Stearate Canola Canola varieties that
have been genetically engineered so that their
seeds contain a higher percentage of stearate
(also called stearic acid) in the canola oil than
the typical stearate content in canola oil produced from traditional canola varieties.

Cosuppression, via inserted gene for Δ-
stearoyl-ACP desaturase (i.e., enzyme that
normally converts stearic acid to oleic acid in
the oil creation process in traditional varieties
of canola), causes the **higher-than-traditional** amount of stearic acid in the canola oil.

See also CANOLA, STEARATE, SATU-
RATED FATTY ACIDS (SAFA), GENE,
GENETIC ENGINEERING, VALUE-
ENHANCED GRAINS, FATTY ACID,
COSUPPRESSION, ENZYME, OLEIC
ACID, STEAROYL-ACP DESATURASE,
CHOLESTEROL, CORONARY HEART
DISEASE (CHD)

High-Stearate Soybeans Soybean plant varieties that have been bred or genetically engineered so that their beans contain at least
12% stearate (also known as stearic acid)
within their soybean oil (i.e., more than four
times the typical 3% stearic acid content in
the soybean oil produced from traditional
soybean varieties). Some high-stearate soybeans contain more than 20% stearate.
Cosuppression, e.g., via inserted gene for Δ-
stearoyl-ACP desaturase (i.e., enzyme that
normally converts stearic acid to oleic acid
in the oil creation process in traditional varieties of soybeans), is the primary way to
cause **higher-than-traditional** amount of
stearic acid in the resultant soybean oil.

A human diet containing stearate instead of
alternative saturated fatty acids does not cause
an increase in blood cholesterol levels
(whereas human consumption of the **other**
saturated fatty acids causes bloodstream cholesterol levels to increase, which increases risk
of coronary heart disease).

See also STEARATE, VALUE-ENHANCED
GRAINS, SOYBEAN PLANT, SOYBEAN
OIL, GENE, GENETIC ENGINEERING,
FATTY ACID, COSUPPRESSION,
ENZYME, OLEIC ACID, CHOLESTEROL,
SATURATED FATTY ACIDS (SAFA), COR-
ONARY HEART DISEASE (CHD),
STEAROYL-ACP DESATURASE

High-Sucrose Soybeans Another name for
low-stachyose soybeans because the soybeans
replace the (reduced) stachyose with (additional) sucrose.

See also LOW-STACHYOSE SOYBEANS,
STACHYOSE, VALUE-ENHANCED

GRAINS, SOYBEAN PLANT, SUGAR MOLECULES

High-Throughput Identification Determination of the identification of a given **chemical compound** (e.g., within a mixture), the desired **impact** (e.g., cell apoptosis, etc.), a specific **segment (sequence) of DNA (i.e., a specific gene),** a specific **ligand or receptor (e.g., "attaching" itself to a given molecule),** etc., within the overall process known as high-throughput screening.

See also HIGH-THROUGHPUT SCREENING (HTS), COMBINATORIAL CHEMISTRY, BIOCHIPS, CELL, APOPTOSIS, GENE, DEOXYRIBONUCLEIC ACID (DNA), GENE EXPRESSION, TARGET–LIGAND INTERACTION SCREENING, RECEPTORS, CHARACTERIZATION ASSAY, SEQUENCE (OF A DNA MOLECULE), GENE EXPRESSION ANALYSIS, *CAENORHABDITIS ELEGANS (C. ELEGANS)*, MOLECULAR BEACON

High-Throughput Screening (HTS) A methodology utilized to quickly screen large numbers of compounds for use as pharmaceuticals or agrochemicals (e.g., herbicides).

For example, when screening chemical compounds for potential use as a pharmaceutical, the goal often is to assess differences between diseased and (treated) cells, enabling identification of a pharmaceutical candidate that favorably impacts change in protein level (i.e., gene expression) that characterizes a diseased state or some other gene expression marker (e.g., apoptosis).

When screening compounds for potential use as herbicide active ingredients, the goal is to assess differences between normal and (treated) weed plant cells, enabling identification of a potential herbicide candidate that imparts desired (fatal) change.

Although whole living cells or whole microscopic animals such as nematodes could be utilized in HTS, it is more common to use a proxy (e.g., receptors, enzymes, or STATs from applicable cells) whose interaction with candidate compounds can be inferred to cell (or organism) effects.

See also COMBINATORIAL CHEMISTRY, BIOCHIP, TARGET–LIGAND INTERACTION SCREENING, CELL, ORGANISM, CHARACTERIZATION ASSAY, PROTEIN, GENE, GENE EXPRESSION, CELL ARRAY, HIGH-THROUGHPUT IDENTIFICATION, RECEPTORS, GENE EXPRESSION ANALYSIS, BIOASSAY, GENE EXPRESSION MARKERS, SIGNAL TRANSDUCERS AND ACTIVATORS OF TRANSCRIPTION (STATs), APOPTOSIS, *IN SILICO* SCREENING, NEMATODES, *CAENORHABDITIS ELEGANS (C. ELEGANS)*, ENZYME, NORTHERN BLOT ANALYSIS, FLUORESCENCE, MOLECULAR BEACON, FLUORESCENCE POLARIZATION (FP), LIVE CELL ARRAY, MICROARRAY (TESTING), TOXICOGENOMICS, LABEL (RADIOACTIVE), WHOLE-CELL PATCH-CLAMP RECORDING

Highly Available Phosphate Corn (Maize)
See LOW-PHYTATE CORN

Highly Available Phosphorous (HAP) Gene
See LOW-PHYTATE CORN

Highly Unsaturated Fatty Acids (HUFA)
Refers to a number of unsaturated fatty acids (e.g., that the human body forms from polyunsaturated fatty acids it consumes in diet) containing four or more **double** (molecular) **bonds.** Examples include arachidonic acid, docosahexanoic acid, and eicosapentanoic acid.

These HUFAs are utilized (by the human body) to make prostaglandins and other eicosanoids.

See also POLYUNSATURATED FATTY ACIDS (PUFA), UNSATURATED FATTY ACIDS, ESSENTIAL FATTY ACIDS, CORONARY HEART DISEASE (CHD), n-3 FATTY ACIDS, n-6 FATTY ACIDS, DOCOSAHEXANOIC ACID (DHA), EICOSAPENTANOIC ACID (EPA), ARACHIDONIC ACID (AA), PROSTAGLANDIN ENDOPEROXIDE SYNTHASE

Hirudin A compound, naturally produced by leeches (e.g., *Hirudo medininalis*), which, in humans, prolongs the clotting time of blood (i.e., hirudin acts as an anticoagulant). The U.S. Food and Drug Administration approved the use of hirudin as an anticoagulant pharmaceutical in 1998.

Used in vascular surgery and in postoperative treatment of thrombosis.

See also THROMBOSIS, FOOD AND DRUG ADMINISTRATION (FDA)

Histamine A base that is naturally present in ergot (a fungus) and plants; it is also naturally produced by basophils (basophilic leukocytes) in the human body. It is formed from histidine by decarboxylation, and is held responsible for the dilation and increased permeability of blood vessels, which play a major role in allergic reactions.

See also BASE (GENERAL), HISTIDINE (His), BASOPHILS

Histidine (His) A basic amino acid that is essential in the nutrition of the rat. It is formed by the decomposition of most proteins (as globin).

See also PROTEIN

Histiocyte See MACROPHAGE

Histoblasts See B LYMPHOCYTES

Histone Modification See CHROMATIN REMODELING

Histones Proteins rich in basic amino acids (e.g., lysine) that are found complexed with DNA in the chromosomes of all eucaryotic cells except sperm.

Histones play a significant role in the regulation of gene expression. Examples include the following:

- ACETYLATION (i.e., addition of acetyl molecular group) of histones results in some genes within the DNA looped around that histone to become (more) accessible to the cell's transcriptional "machinery," thereby turning on those genes.
- METHYLATION (i.e., addition of methyl molecular group) of a protruding amino acid (e.g., lysine) in a histone, thereby "turning on" or upregulating those genes.

See also CHROMOSOMES, CHROMATIDS, CHROMATIN, CELL, PROTEIN, DEOXYRIBONUCLEIC ACID (DNA), GENE, GENE EXPRESSION, TRANSCRIPTION, EXPRESSIVITY, METHYLATED, AMINO ACID, LYSINE (Lys), UPREGULATING, CHROMATIN REMODELING

Histopathologic Refers to changes in tissue caused by a disease. For example, certain diseases (such as jaundice) cause the skin to turn yellow.

See also PATHOGENIC, VIRUS, CANCER, ADHESION MOLECULE

HIV-1 and HIV-2 See HUMAN IMMUNODEFICIENCY VIRUS TYPE 1 (HIV-1), HUMAN IMMUNODEFICIENCY VIRUS TYPE 2 (HIV-2)

HLA See HUMAN LEUKOCYTE ANTIGENS

HNE The common chemical by-product of lipid oxidation, known as 4-hydroxy-2-nonenal, that is an aldehyde.

See OXIDATIVE STRESS, OXIDATION, PLASMA MEMBRANE, LIPIDS

HNGF Human nerve growth factor.

See also NERVE GROWTH FACTOR (NGF)

HOC See HIGH-OIL CORN

Holins Small proteins that are produced by bacteriophages during infection of bacteria. Holins "punch" holes into the bacterial cell membranes, thereby allowing the cell contents to leak out, and thus killing the bacteria.

See also BACTERIA, BACTERIOPHAGE, PROTEIN, LYTIC INFECTION

Hollow Fiber Separation (of proteins) The separation of proteins from a mixture by means of "straining" the mixture through hollow, semipermeable fibers (e.g., polysulfone fibers) under pressure. The hollow fibers are constructed in such a way that they have very tiny (molecular size) holes in them. In this way large molecules are retained in the original liquid, whereas smaller molecules that are able to pass through the holes are filtered out.

See also DIALYSIS, PROTEIN, ULTRAFILTRATION

Holoenzyme The entire, functionally complete enzyme. The term is used to designate an enzyme that requires a coenzyme in order for it to function (possess catalytic abilities). The holoenzyme consists of the protein part (apoenzyme) plus a dialyzable, nonprotein, coenzyme part that is bound to the apoenzyme protein.

See also COENZYME, APOENZYME, DIALYSIS

Homeobox A short sequence of DNA that is 180 base pairs long and located in the 3′ exon of certain genes of the *Drosophila* fly (where they were discovered by Walter Gehring during the 1970s). In the 1980s, Jani Christian Nusslein-Volhard discovered that one

H

homeobox was attached (in adjacent exon) to each of the genes that are responsible for embryonic development (i.e., "switched on" only in an embryo that is developing into an adult) in a wide variety of species, including invertebrates, birds, and mammals. Thus, it is now possible to locate many embryonic-development genes in many species by using a DNA probe (made via a *Drosophila* homeobox DNA sequence) to find homeobox sequences attached to those embryonic-development genes. In such a role, the respective homeobox sequences attached to each gene are known as DNA markers.

See also GENE, DEOXYRIBONUCLEIC ACID (DNA), DNA PROBE, DNA MARKER, SEQUENCE (OF A DNA MOLECULE), BASE PAIR (bp), DROSOPHILA, EXON, SPECIES

Homeostasis A tendency toward maintenance of a relatively stable internal environment in the bodies of higher animals through a series of interacting physiological processes. An example is the mammal's maintenance of a constant body temperature despite extremes in ambient (weather) temperature.

See also SELECTINS, LECTINS, ADHESION MOLECULE, CORTISOL

Homing Receptor Also known as L-selectin.

See also SELECTINS, LECTINS, ADHESION MOLECULES

Homocysteine A metabolite compound (i.e., amino acid derived via metabolism from methionine) that, when present in the bloodstream in elevated amounts, increases the risk of stroke and the likelihood for a person's developing arteriosclerosis and/or coronary heart disease (CHD).

Folic acid, vitamin B_{12}, and vitamin B_6 act as cofactors in the conversion of homocysteine back to methionine or cysteine.

Consumption of choline or folic acid has been shown to reduce bloodstream levels of homocysteine. Research also has shown that moderate consumption of beer and B vitamins will reduce bloodstream levels of homocysteine.

See also METABOLISM, ARTERIOSCLEROSIS, CORONARY HEART DISEASE (CHD), METHIONINE, AMINO ACID, COFACTOR, CYSTEINE (Cys), CHOLINE, VITAMIN

Homologous (chemically) See HOMOLOGY

Homologous (chromosomes or genes) Chromosomes or chromosome segments that are identical with respect to their constituent sequence, genetic loci, or their visible structure (in the case of chromosomes).

So, for example, a gene of "unknown" function in humans could be compared (in a database) with genes of a simpler organization (e.g., *Caenorhabditus elegans*). If the human gene is homologous and the function of the *Caenorhabditus elegans* gene is known, the function of the human gene could be inferred by comparison.

See also CHROMOSOMES, GENE, SEQUENCE (OF A DNA MOLECULE), LOCUS, *CAENORHABDITUS ELEGANS*, MODEL ORGANISM

Homologous Protein A protein having identical functions and similar properties in different species. For example, the hemoglobins that perform identical functions in the blood of different species.

See also PROTEIN, SPECIES

Homologous Recombination Refers to the fact that insertion (into living cells or organism) of the DNA sequence of a given gene can (under certain conditions) "knock out" or silence that particular gene in that cell.

See also GENE, CELL, ORGANISM, DEOXYRIBONUCLEIC ACID (DNA), KNOCKOUT, GENE SILENCING, COSUPPRESSION

Homology A sequence of amino acids in two or more proteins that are identical to each other. **Nucleic acids homology** refers to complementary strands that can hybridize with each other.

See also TATA HOMOLOGY, PROTEIN, HYBRIDIZATION (MOLECULAR GENETICS)

Homology Modeling Refers to the use (e.g., in computerized molecule models) of **known** proteins' structural and functional properties as a "predictive template" for computer-generated **hypothetical proteins** (whose structure is not known).

Such predictive structural modeling of hypothetical proteins becomes more accurate as more and more of the known structures (i.e., **parts** comprising the large protein molecule) are added to the computer model.

See also PROTEIN, CONFORMATION, PRO-
TEIN FOLDING, PROTEIN STRUCTURE,
PROTEIN ENGINEERING, ABSOLUTE
CONFIGURATION

Homotropic Enzyme An allosteric enzyme
whose own substrate functions as an activity
modulator.
See also ENZYME

Homozygote An organism in which the corresponding genes (alleles) on the two genomes
are identical. An organism that possesses an
identical pair of alleles in regard to a given
(genetic) characteristic.
See also GENE, ALLELE, GENOME, GENO-
TYPE, PHENOTYPE, HOMOZYGOUS,
HETEROZYGOTE

Homozygous In a diploid organism, a state in
which both alleles of a given gene are the
same.
See also HETEROZYGOTE, ALLELE, DIP-
LOID, DIPLOPHASE, HOMOZYGOTE

Hormone Coined in 1905, the term hormone
refers to a type of chemical messenger (peptide), occurring in both plants and animals,
that acts to inhibit or excite metabolic activities (in that plant or animal) by binding to
receptors on specific cells to deliver its
"message." A hormone's site of production is
distant from the site of biological activity (i.e.,
where the message is delivered).
See also PEPTIDE, MINIMIZED PROTEINS,
SIGNALING, SIGNALING MOLECULE,
NUCLEAR HORMONE RECEPTORS,
ALBUMIN

Hormone Response Elements See NUCLEAR
RECEPTORS

Hormone-Sensitive Lipase (HSL) See LIPASE

Host Cell A cell whose metabolism is used by
a virus for growth and reproduction. Also, the
cell into which a plasmid is introduced (in
recombinant DNA experiments).

Host Vector (HV) System The host is the
organism into which a gene from another
organism is transplanted. The guest gene is
carried by a vector (i.e., a larger DNA molecule, such as a plasmid, or a virus into which
that gene is inserted) that then propagates in
the host.

Hot Spots Sites in genes where events such
as mutations occur with unusually high
frequency.

See also GENE, JUMPING GENES, MUTA-
TION, TRANSLOCATION

HPLC Initially known as **high-performance
liquid chromatography** when developed during the 1970s, this separation and analysis
technology was later renamed **high-pressure
liquid chromatography**.
See CHROMATOGRAPHY

H. pylori A bacteria that has been linked (possibly as a cause) to gastric ulcers, stomach cancers, and other gastric problems in humans. The
link was first announced by Barry Marshall in
the early 1990s.
See also BACTERIA, *HELICOBACTER
PYLORI*, CANCER, SULFORAPHANE

hSOD See HUMAN SUPEROXIDE DISMU-
TASE (hSOD)

HSP Acronym for **heat-shock protein**.
See HEAT-SHOCK PROTEINS

HTC See HERBICIDE-TOLERANT CROP,
STS, PAT GENE, EPSP SYNTHASE, ALS
GENE, BAR GENE, CP4 EPSPS, GLYPHO-
SATE OXIDASE

HTMS Acronym for **High-throughput Mass
Spectrometry**.
See HIGH-THROUGHPUT SCREENING
(HTS), MASS SPECTROMETER, MALDI-
TOF-MS

HTS Herbicide-tolerant soybeans.
See SOYBEAN PLANT, GLYPHOSATE, CP4
EPSPS, EPSP SYNTHASE, GLYPHOSATE
OXIDASE, HERBICIDE-TOLERANT CROP,
STS, GLUFOSINATE, PAT GENE, BAR
GENE

HTS See HIGH-THROUGHPUT SCREEN-
ING (HTS)

Human Artificial Chromosomes (HAC)
Chromosomes that have been synthesized
(made) from chemicals, and are identical to
chromosomes within human cells.
See also YEAST ARTIFICIAL CHROMO-
SOMES (YAC), BACTERIAL ARTIFICIAL
CHROMOSOMES (BAC), CHROMO-
SOMES, *ARABIDOPSIS THALIANA*, SYN-
THESIZING (OF DNA MOLECULES)

Human Chorionic Gonadotropin A human
hormone. In 1986, Mark Bogart discovered that
elevated levels of human chorionic gonadotropin in pregnant women are correlated with
babies (later) born with Down's Syndrome.
See also HORMONE

H

Human Colon Fibroblast Tissue Plasminogen Activator A second generation tissue plasminogen activator (tPA), which has the clot-sensitive activation of plasminogen with potentially greater selectivity and (clot) specificity.

See also TISSUE PLASMINOGEN ACTIVATOR (tPA)

Human EGF-Receptor-Related Receptor (HER-2) A gene that appears to be directly related to human breast cancer mortality. More the copies of the HER-2 gene in a patient's breast tumor cells, the more dismal the prospects for survival.

Human Embryonic Stem Cells Those cells (in the early embryo's inner cell mass) from which each of the human body's 210 different types of tissues arise via differentiaion, proliferation, and growth processes.

See also STEM CELLS, PLURIPOTENT, STEM CELL GROWTH FACTOR (SCF), DIFFERENTIATION, ADULT STEM CELL

Human Gamma-Glutamyl Transpeptidase A glycoprotein that is thought to possess a different oligosaccharide when it is produced by a (liver) tumor cell instead of a healthy cell. Thus, it is a possible early warning marker for liver cancer.

See also GLYCOPROTEIN, OLIGOSACCHARIDES

Human Growth Hormone (HGH) See GROWTH HORMONE (GH)

Human Immunodeficiency Virus Type 1 (HIV-1) One of the two "families" of the viruses identified (so far) that cause acquired immune deficiency syndrome (AIDS), although not all strains of HIV-2 cause AIDS. HIV-1 and HIV-2 show a preferential tropism (affinity) toward the helper T cells, although other immune system (and nervous system) cells are also infected. The GP120 envelope (surface) protein of HIV-1 and HIV-2 directly interacts (binds) with the CD4 proteins (receptors) on the surface of helper T cells, enabling the viruses to bind (attach to) and infect the helper T cells. In order to successfully enter and infect cells, HIV must also bind with CKR-5 proteins (receptors) located on the surface of cells of most humans. In 1996, Nathaniel Landau and Richard Koup discovered that approximately 1% of humans carry a gene for a version of CKR-5 receptor that resists entry to cells by HIV. As of 1996, a total of nine separate strains (serotypes) of human immunodeficiency virus were known and were identified by the letters A, B, C, D, E, F, G, H, and I.

See also CD4 PROTEIN, TAT, TATA HOMOLOGY, ADHESION MOLECULE, GP120 PROTEIN, ACQUIRED IMMUNE DEFICIENCY SYNDROME (AIDS), RECEPTORS, TROPISM, HELPER T CELLS (T4 CELLS), STRAIN, T CELL RECEPTORS, VIRUS, SEROTYPES, HUMAN IMMUNODEFICIENCY VIRUS TYPE 2 (HIV-2)

Human Immunodeficiency Virus Type 2 (HIV-2) See HUMAN IMMUNODEFICIENCY VIRUS TYPE 1 (HIV-1)

Human Leukocyte Antigens (HLA) A very complex array of six proteins that cover the surface of leukocytes (and the bone marrow cells that produce leukocytes). These HLA are usually different (i.e., a nonmatch) for individuals that are not genetically related to each other (e.g., a father and son or a father and daughter), so they have been used in the past to prove paternity. HLA must also be matched (as nearly as possible) for successful bone marrow transplants to prevent the donated bone marrow and the marrow recipient from "rejecting" each other.

See also LEUKOCYTES, ANTIGEN, MAJOR HISTOCOMPATIBILITY COMPLEX (MHC), PROTEIN, GRAFT-VERSUS-HOST DISEASE (GVHD)

Human Protein Kinase C An enzyme that is involved in the control of blood coagulation and fibrinolysis.

See also FIBRIN

Human Superoxide Dismutase (hSOD) An enzyme that "captures" **oxygen free radicals (oxygen atoms bearing an extra electron and thus high in energy** — e.g., those that are sometimes generated in a biological system such as within the body of an organism). Oxygen free radicals are generated within occluded blood vessels when a blood clot blocks arteries in the heart, causing a heart attack. These oxygen free radicals are highly energized and can cause damage to blood vessel walls after the clot is dissolved (e.g., with

H

tissue plasminogen activator); therefore, hSOD may profitably be administered in conjunction with clot-dissolving pharmaceuticals to minimize damage when occluded arteries are reopened.

Research indicates that hSOD may help protect elderly patients from the lethal effects of influenza (i.e., the flu), because influenza often causes overproduction of free radicals in the victim's body.

Research indicates that administration of hSOD can help to relieve some pain and inflammation caused by certain clinical procedures (e.g., dental surgery), because overproduction of free radicals can result from those particular procedures.

See also FREE RADICAL, PEG-SOD (POLYETHYLENE GLYCOL SUPEROXIDE DISMUTASE), CATALASE, XANTHINE OXIDASE, TISSUE PLASMINOGEN ACTIVATOR (tPA), ANTIOXIDANTS

Human Thyroid-Stimulating Hormone (hTSH) A naturally occurring hormone that causes the thyroid gland to develop.

See also HORMONE

Humanized Antibody Refers to an (genetically engineered) antibody in which the complementarity-determining (i.e., antigen-binding) portion of an (animal source) antibody is imparted to a human antibody molecule via splicing the (sequence of) DNA responsible for that animal antibody's **complementarity (to a specific antigen)** into a cell line producing human monoclonal antibodies.

See also ANTIBODY, CHIMERIC ANTIBODY, ANTIGEN, AVIDITY, CHIMERIC PROTEINS, SEQUENCE (OF A DNA MOLECULE), MONOCLONAL ANTIBODIES (MAb), GENETIC ENGINEERING, TRASTUZUMAB, FLUORESCENCE *IN SITU* HYBRIDIZATION (FISH)

Humoral Immune Response Refers to the rapid manufacture and secretion, by the body, of the soluble blood serum components in response to an infection. Examples of the components are the following:

- Antibodies (by B cells)
- Complement proteins
- Lymphokines
- Cecrophins

See also ANTIBODY, COMPLEMENT, COMPLEMENT CASCADE, CECROPHINS, HUMORAL IMMUNITY, LYMPHOKINES, GAMMA INTERFERON

Humoral Immunity The immune system response consisting of the soluble blood serum components that fight an infection (e.g., antibodies, complement proteins, cecrophins, etc.).

See also ANTIBODY, COMPLEMENT, COMPLEMENT CASCADE, CECROPHINS, CELLULAR IMMUNE RESPONSE, IMMUNOGLOBULIN

Huntington's Disease A neurodegenerative disease that is dominantly inherited (i.e., disease results even if there is only one copy of the damaged gene in the genome).

The gene for Huntington's disease was discovered by Nancy Wexler.

See also GENE, DOMINANT ALLELE, HD GENE, GENOME, GENETICS, MUTATION

HuSNPs Abbreviation for **Human SNPs** (single-nucleotide polymorphisms).

See SINGLE-NUCLEOTIDE POLYMORPHISMS (SNPs)

H. virescens See *HELIOTHIS VIRESCENS (H. VIRESCENS)*

Hybrid Vigor See F1 HYBRIDS, HYBRIDIZATION (PLANT GENETICS)

Hybridization (molecular genetics) The pairing (tight physical bonding) of two complementary single strands of RNA and/or DNA to give a double-stranded molecule.

See also ANNEAL, STICKY ENDS, RIBONUCLEIC ACID (RNA), MESSENGER RNA (mRNA), BIOSENSORS (ELECTRONIC), BIOSENSORS (CHEMICAL), HYBRIDIZATION SURFACES, DNA PROBE, DEOXYRIBONUCLEIC ACID (DNA), ANTISENSE (DNA SEQUENCE), BIOMOTORS

Hybridization (plant genetics) The mating of two plants from different species or from *genetically very different* members of the same species to yield hybrids (first filial hybrids) possessing some of the characteristics of each parent. Those (hybrid) offspring tend to be more healthy, productive, and uniform than their parents — a phenomenon known as "hybrid vigor." Hybrids can also arise from more than two ("parent") species.

Hybrid corn or maize seed was first commercialized (in the U.S.) in 1922. Other recently created crop hybrids include tangelos (produced by crossing grapefruit with tangerines), nectarines (bred from peaches), brocciflower (produced by crossing broccoli with cauliflower), etc.

Some hybrids have occurred spontaneously in nature. For example, wheat (*Triticum aestivum*) arose centuries ago from a naturally occurring interbreeding of three Middle East grasses. In the 1980s, sugar beet (*Beta vulgaris* ssp. *vulgaris*) naturally interbred with the wild native weed known as sea beet (*Beta vulgaris* ssp. *maritima*) in Europe, resulting in an annual weed (in contrast to sugar beet, which is a biannual). Because that (new hybrid weed) is closely related to sugar beet, any herbicide that kills the (new hybrid weed) is likely to harm the sugar beet crop (unless the sugar beet crop is made herbicide tolerant).

See also F1 HYBRIDS, SPECIES, TRANSGRESSIVE SEGREGATION, GENETICS, CORN, WHEAT, GEM, EXOTIC GERMPLASM, BARNASE, HERBICIDE-TOLERANT CROP

Hybridization Surfaces Various physical substrates (surfaces) onto which genetic materials has been "attached" (DNA, RNA, oligonucleotides, etc.). Relevant complementary genetic material (e.g., DNA, RNA, oligonucleotides, etc.) are then hybridized onto those attached-to-surface genetic material for various specific purposes (e.g., detection of the presence of those unattached genetic material, in the case of biosensor's hybridization surface). One of the technologies that can be utilized to assay (evaluate) DNA from hybridization surfaces is matrix-assisted laser desorption ionization time-of-flight mass spectrometry (MALDI-TOF-MS).

See also SUBSTRATE (STRUCTURAL), HYBRIDIZATION (MOLECULAR GENETICS), COMPLEMENTARY DNA (c-DNA), DEOXYRIBONUCLEIC ACID (DNA), RIBONUCLEIC ACID (RNA), NANOCRYSTAL MOLECULES, DOUBLE HELIX, BIOSENSORS (ELECTRONIC), BIOSENSORS (CHEMICAL), BIOCHIPS, OLIGONUCLEOTIDE, OLIGONUCLEOTIDE PROBES, MALDI-TOF-MS, ASSAY, MICROARRAY (TESTING), DIRECTED SELF-ASSEMBLY, MASSIVELY PARALLEL SIGNATURE SEQUENCING

Hybridoma The cell line produced by fusing a myeloma (tumor cell) with a lymphocyte (which makes antibodies); it continues indefinitely to express the immunoglobulins (antibodies) of both parent cells.

See also MONOCLONAL ANTIBODIES (MAb), AGING

Hydrazine A chemical with formula N_2H_4. Used as a rocket fuel and in the hydrazinolysis of glycoproteins. Some hydrazine compounds are also naturally produced in certain mushrooms (*Agaricus bisporus, Gyomitra esculenta*, etc.).

See also HYDRAZINOLYSIS, GLYCOPROTEIN, REDUCTION (IN A CHEMICAL REACTION).

Hydrazinolysis (of glycoproteins to isolate unreduced oligosaccharide side chains) A technique that used the chemical hydrazine to separate and isolate the oligosaccharide portion from the protein portion of a glycoprotein. The hydrazine chemically "chews up" the polypeptide (i.e., protein) portion of a glycoprotein molecule, leaving the intact oligosaccharides behind. It can subsequently be analyzed (after chromatographic separation from the peptide pieces and other chemical components).

See also REDUCTION (IN A CHEMICAL REACTION), HF CLEAVAGE, POLYPEPTIDE (PROTEIN), GLYCOPROTEIN, SEQUENCING (OF OLIGOSACCHARIDES), HYDRAZINE, CHROMATOGRAPHY

Hydrofluoric Acid Cleavage See HF CLEAVAGE

Hydrogenation Invented by Wilhelm Normann in 1901, it is a chemical reaction or process in which hydrogen atoms are added to certain molecules (e.g., of unsaturated fatty acids) in edible oils. In the case of fatty acids, the fraction of each isomeric form (*trans* vs. *cis* fatty acids) and the molecular chain length (of the fatty acids present) have a large impact on the melting characteristics of each (fat or oil), with shorter-chain fats melting at lower temperatures.

Hydrogenation is the most common chemical reaction utilized in the edible oil (processing) industry. Hydrogenation increases the solids (i.e., crystalline fat) content of edible fats or oils, and improves their resistance to thermal and atmospheric oxidation (e.g., as in frying

H

of foods). Those increases in solids and resistance to oxidation result from the reduction in the fat or oil relative unsaturation plus the increased geometric and positional isomerization of the fat or oil molecules.

The edible oil or fat hydrogenation reaction is accomplished by treating fats or oils with pressurized hydrogen gas in the presence of a catalyst. As a result, the (usually) liquid oils are converted to more-saturated fats, which are semisolids at an ambient temperature of 72°F (22°C). The presence of *trans* fatty acids in hydrogenated edible oils can be reduced significantly via changes in catalyst, temperature, pressure, etc., utilized in the hydrogenation reaction. In general, natural oils and fats with melting points lower than 121°F (50°C) are nearly completely absorbed in the digestive system of typical humans.

See also FATTY ACID, MONOUNSATURATED FATS, SATURATED FATTY ACIDS (SAFA), DEHYDROGENATION, ESSENTIAL FATTY ACIDS, LAURATE, LECITHIN, TRIGLYCERIDES, UNSATURATED FATTY ACID, SOYBEAN OIL, CONJUGATED LINOLEIC ACID (CLA), OXIDATION, ISOMER, STEREOISOMERS, CATALYST, SUBSTRATE (CHEMICAL), *TRANS* FATTY ACIDS

Hydrolysis Literally means "cleaved by water." It is used for a chemical reaction in which the chemical bond attaching an atom, or a group of atoms, to the (rest of the) molecule is cleaved, followed by attachment of a hydrogen atom at the same chemical bond.

Hydrolytic Cleavage A chemical reaction in which a portion (e.g., an atom or a group of atoms) of a molecule is "cut" off via hydrolysis.

See also HYDROLYSIS

Hydrolyze To "cut" a chemical bond (i.e., with a molecule) via hydrolysis.

See also HYDROLYSIS

Hydrophilic This term means water-loving or having a great affinity for water. It is used to describe molecules or portions of molecules that have an affinity for water. For example, ordinary sugar that dissolves readily in water is said to be hydrophilic.

It is also the property of having an affinity for water in an oil–water interface.

See also AMPHIPHILIC MOLECULES

Hydrophobic This term means water hating or having a great dislike for water. It is used to describe molecules or portions of molecules that have very little or no affinity for water. The property of having an affinity for oil (nonpolar environments) in an oil–water interface. For example, a nonpolar hydrocarbon such as butane (as used in lighters) that does not dissolve in water but dissolves (be miscible) in oil is said to be hydrophobic.

See also AMPHIPHILIC MOLECULES

Hydroxylation Reaction A chemical reaction in which one or more hydroxyl groups (i.e., the OH group) is introduced (i.e., is chemically attached) to a molecule.

Hyperacute Rejection See GRAFT-VERSUS-HOST DISEASE (GVHD)

Hyperchromicity The increase in optical density that occurs when DNA is denatured.

See also DEOXYRIBONUCLEIC ACID (DNA), DENATURED DNA, OPTICAL DENSITY (OD)

Hypersensitive Response A protective or defensive response of certain plants to "infection" by plant pathogens (e.g., bacteria, fungi, and viruses), in which those plant cells that are immediately adjacent (to the infected area of plant) are "instructed" to self-destruct via apoptosis in order to cordon off the infected area (to prevent further spread of the infection).

The initiation of the hypersensitive response is often triggered by **signaling molecules** that are produced by the pathogens themselves. For example, one particular protein produced by the soil fungus *Fusarium oxysporum* triggers a hypersensitive response that often is so severe that the entire plant dies.

See also PATHOGENESIS-RELATED PROTEINS, PROTEIN, PATHOGEN, BACTERIA, FUNGUS, VIRUS, CELL, APOPTOSIS, SIGNALING, SIGNALING MOLECULE

Hyperthermophilic (organisms) See THERMOPHILE, THERMOPHILIC BACTERIA

Hypostasis Interaction between nonallelic genes in which one gene will not be expressed in the presence of a second.

See also EPISTASIS, GENE, EXPRESS, ALLELE

Hypothalamus A part of the brain structure, lying near the base of the brain, that regulates a number of hormones. As a part of the brain, it constantly receives (neurochemical) signals from nerve cells (neurons). The hypothalamus monitors those signals and converts them into hormonal "signals" (e.g., it generates a "burst" of hormones in response to certain visual stimuli, certain physical [e.g., sexual] stimuli, etc.). Also, the hypothalamus is able to monitor and detect changes in the blood levels of hormones coming from endocrine glands. For example, the metabolic hormone insulin (from the pancreas) and the reproductive hormone estrogen (from the ovaries) both trigger changes in function of the hypothalamus. The hypothalamus regulates biological processes (e.g., metabolic rate, appetite, etc.). A major function of the hypothalamus is to control reproduction, via secretion of gonadotropin-releasing hormone (GnRH) from the tips of hypothalamic nerve fibers that extend downward toward (into) the pituitary gland. Similarly, the hypothalamus also helps to control the body's growth (from birth until the end of puberty) via secretion of growth-hormone-releasing factor (GHRF) to the pituitary gland.

See also HORMONE, ENDOCRINE HORMONES, ENDOCRINE GLANDS, ENDOCRINOLOGY, PITUITARY GLAND, GROWTH HORMONE (GH), NEUROTRANSMITTER, GROWTH-HORMONE-RELEASING FACTOR (GHRF)

Hypoxia Used to refer to a state (e.g., of cells within a specific tissue in an organism) in which the media lacks enough oxygen (e.g., to sustain growth, etc.). Hypoxia can lead to epigenetic events in some organisms.

See also CELL, ORGANISM, EPIGENETIC

H. zea See *HELICOVERPA ZEA (H. zea)*

H

I

IBA See INDUSTRIAL BIOTECHNOLOGY ASSOCIATION

IBG See INTERNATIONAL BIOTECHNOLOGY GROUP

ICAM Intercellular adhesion molecule.

See also ADHESION MOLECULE

ICM Acronym for **intact-cell MALDI-TOF-MS**. Beginning in 1975, Catherine Fenselau and John Anhalt extended the use of MALDI-TOF-MS (previously utilized to identify only **molecules**) to encompass identification of certain intact cells (e.g., Gram-positive bacteria, after they were gently heated and dislodged via laser from a "soft" matrix or substrate that Fenselau–Anhalt had adhered them to).

See also MALDI-TOF-MS, CELL, BACTERIA, GRAM POSITIVE

IDA Acronym for **iron deficiency anemia**.

See IRON DEFICIENCY ANEMIA (IDA)

IDE "Investigational Device Exemption" application to the Food and Drug Administration (FDA) seeking approval to begin clinical studies of a new medical device.

Ideal Protein Concept Refers to the protein content in the feed ration (food) of livestock, poultry (and humans). Feed that contains **ideal protein** has proteins that, when digested by an animal, yield all of the essential amino acids, in proper proportions, for the growth and maintenance needs of that animal.

"Ideal protein" varies for different species (e.g., pigs require different amino acids or rations than chickens). Ideal protein varies for different stages in the life of a given animal (e.g., poultry require more sulfur-containing amino acids such as methionine during life stages when feather growth is at a comparatively high rate).

The animal's requirement for one essential amino acid is proportionally linked to its requirements for another. Increasing the supply (when deficient) of one essential amino acid in the animal's diet would improve its (growth) performance if no other amino acids were limiting.

Feed rations formulated to contain ideal protein have been shown to reduce the amount of nitrogen (nitrates) excreted by livestock and poultry by as much as 50%.

See also AMINO ACID, PROTEIN, ESSENTIAL AMINO ACIDS, ESSENTIAL NUTRIENTS, METHIONINE (Met), DIGESTION (WITHIN ORGANISMS), SOY PROTEIN, HIGH-LYSINE CORN, HIGH-METHIONINE CORN

Idiotope An antigenic determinant within the variable region of an antibody.

See also ANTIGENIC DETERMINANT, ANTIBODY

Idiotype The region of the antibody molecule (i.e., antigen-combining site) that enables each antibody to recognize a specific foreign structure (i.e., epitope or hapten) is said to have an idiotype (for that epitope or hapten). An identifying characteristic (or property) of an epitope or hapten.

See also EPITOPE, HAPTEN, ANTIGEN, ANTIBODY, CATALYTIC ANTIBODY

IDM See INTEGRATED DISEASE MANAGEMENT

IFBC See INTERNATIONAL FOOD BIOTECHNOLOGY COUNCIL

IFN-Alpha Alpha interferon.

See INTERFERONS

IFN-Beta Beta interferon.

See INTERFERONS

IGF-1 See INSULIN-LIKE GROWTH FACTOR-1

IGF-2 See INSULIN-LIKE GROWTH FACTOR-2

IGF-I See INSULIN-LIKE GROWTH FACTOR-1

IGF-II See INSULIN-LIKE GROWTH FACTOR-2

IGR Acronym for **intergenic region** (of an organism's DNA).

See GENE, DEOXYRIBONUCLEIC ACID (DNA), INTRON

IL-1 See INTERLEUKIN-1

IL-Ira See INTERLEUKIN-1 RECEPTOR ANTAGONIST

Imidazilinone-Tolerant Soybeans See IMIDAZOLINONE-TOLERANT SOYBEANS

Imidazolinone-Tolerant Soybeans Refers to soybeans (*Glycine max* (L.) Merrill) that are able to resist the (weed-killing) effects of imidazolinone-based herbicides (including imazethapyr and imazaquin). During 2003, Brazilian researchers developed such soybeans via genetic engineering.

See also HERBICIDE-TOLERANT CROP, SOYBEAN PLANT, STS SULFONYLUREA (HERBICIDE)-TOLERANT SOYBEANS, GENETIC ENGINEERING

Immobilization Refers to the process of "attaching" the molecular capture agents, biosensors or probes (e.g., fluorophore-labeled DNA segment or antibody, etc.) to the glass/silicon/plastic/gold surface of a **microarray** (e.g., DNA chip, SNP chip, protein microarray, proteome chip, cell array, etc.), **magnetic particle**, **surface plasmon resonance chip**, or other hybridization surface.

The particular immobilization that is utilized is dependent on the physical properties of the chip surface and the capture agent/probe molecule. Immobilization can be accomplished via a (covalent) chemical reaction between capture agent/probe and surface or via a noncovalent means such as physical adsorption-onto-surface, van der Waals forces, hydrogen bonding, electrostatic forces, etc.

See also BIOSENSORS (CHEMICAL), PROBE, DNA PROBE, DEOXYRIBONUCLEIC ACID (DNA), LABEL (FLUORESCENT), FLUOROPHORE, MICROARRAY (TESTING), DNA CHIP, BIOCHIP, CELL ARRAY, PROTEIN MICROARRAYS, PROTEOME CHIP, TARGET–LIGAND INTERACTION SCREENING, MULTIPLEXED ASSAY, IMMUNOSENSOR, SNP CHIP, SURFACE PLASMON RESONANCE (SPR), MAGNETIC PARTICLES, HYBRIDIZATION SURFACES, CAPTURE AGENT

Immune Effector Sites See PEYER'S PATCHES

Immune Response See CELLULAR IMMUNE RESPONSE, ANTIBODY, HUMORAL IMMUNITY, INNATE IMMUNE RESPONSE

Immunoadhesins See ADHESION MOLECULE

Immunoassay The use of antibodies to identify and quantify (measure) substances by a variety of methods. The binding of antibodies to antigen (substance being measured) is often followed by tracers such as fluorescence or (radioactive) radioisotopes to enable measurement of the substance.

See also ANTIBODY, TRACER (RADIOACTIVE ISOTOPIC METHOD), ANTIGEN, ELISA, RADIOIMMUNOASSAY, ASSAY, EIA, FLUORESCENCE, NEAR-INFRARED SPECTROSCOPY (NIR), CHEMILUMINESCENT IMMUNOASSAY (CLIA)

Immunoconjugate A molecule that has been formed by attachment to each of two originally different molecules. One of these is generally an antibody and hence the word "immunoconjugate." Classic organic drug molecules such as methotrexate, adriamycin chlorambucil, etc.; radionuclides; enzymes; toxins; and ribosome-inhibiting proteins may be conjugated to antibodies. The salient point is that the antibody portion of the conjugate exists to "steer" the biologically active molecule to its target.

See also CONJUGATE, "MAGIC BULLET," ANTIBODY, MAGNETIC PARTICLES

Immunocontraception Any process or procedure in which an organism's immune system is utilized to attack or inactivate the reproductive cells (e.g., sperm) within the organism.

See also CELLULAR IMMUNE RESPONSE, ANTIBODY, HUMORAL IMMUNITY, GERM CELL

Immunodominant Term utilized to refer to a compound (e.g., a food allergen) that causes an organism's immune system to respond so strongly that it causes harm to the organism.

See also ALLERGIES (FOODBORNE), ANTIGEN, IMMUNE RESPONSE

Immunogen A molecule or an organism (e.g., pathogenic bacteria) that is specifically "recognized" by the immune system (e.g., of humans it has entered) and triggers an immune response.

See also ANTIGEN, PATHOGENIC, HUMORAL IMMUNITY, CELLULAR IMMUNE RESPONSE

Immunoglobulin (IgA, IgE, IgG, and IgM) A class of (blood) serum proteins representing antibodies. Often used, along with the more specific monoclonal antibodies, in health diagnostic reagents. In certain people who are genetically predisposed to foodborne allergies, immunoglobulin-E (IgE) initiates an immune system response to antigens present on protein molecules in the particular food that the person is allergic to. Severe allergic reactions to foods may lead to death.

See also PROTEIN, ANTIGEN, ALLERGIES (FOODBORNE), ANTIBODY, IMMUNOASSAY, B LYMPHOCYTES

Immunomagnetic Refers to the usage of antibody molecules linked to magnetic particles (e.g., as part of an immunoassay).

See also ANTIBODY, MAGNETIC PARTICLES, IMMUNOCONJUGATE, IMMUNOASSAY, CELL SORTING

Immunosensor A biosensor with a selected antibody attached, which can sense when a given molecule (from sample) binds (i.e., "attaches to") that antibody.

For example, the selected antibody binding can be made to cause (simultaneous) fluorescence. If the biosensor (that the antibody is attached to) incorporates a fiber optic and light detector (e.g., CCD detector), the binding can be detected automatically and at a distance (e.g., from outside a reactor or outside the body in the case of an implanted-in-body sensor).

See also BIOSENSORS (ELECTRONIC), ANTIBODY, FLUORESCENCE, BIOSENSORS (CHEMICAL), CATALYTIC ANTIBODY

Immunosuppressive That which suppresses the immune system response (e.g., certain chemicals).

See also CELLULAR IMMUNE RESPONSE, HUMORAL IMMUNITY

Immunotoxin A conjugate formed by attaching a toxic molecule (e.g., ricin) to an agent of the immune system (e.g., a monoclonal antibody) that is specific for the pathogen or tumor to be killed. The immune system agent portion (of the conjugate) delivers the toxic chemical directly to the specified (disease) site, thus sparing other healthy tissues from the effect of the toxin.

See also RICIN, MONOCLONAL ANTIBODIES (MAb), "MAGIC BULLET"

Imprinting A cellular epigenetic process in which certain genes within an organism's cells

are "disabled" (e.g., via methylation) during the earliest stages of the organism's development. For example, the embryo of a female mammal (which receives two copies of the X chromosome — one from each parent) disables one of those copies, at random, in each of its cells, so the female becomes a **genetic mixture** of its two parents. Loss of imprinting (LOI) can sometimes occur in an adult organism. For example:

- In mice, LOI of the gene that codes for insulin-like growth factor-2 (IGF-2) results in the intestine's epithelial cells reverting to a less-developed state and also in development of significantly more intestinal tumors.
- In humans, LOI of the gene that codes for IGF-2 is correlated with development of colorectal cancer.

See also CELL, EPIGENETIC, GENE, GENETIC CODE, CHROMOSOMES, X CHROMOSOME, METHYLATED, DNA METHYLATION, EMBRYOLOGY, TUMOR, CANCER, INSULIN-LIKE GROWTH FACTOR-2

Inclusion Bodies See REFRACTILE BODIES (RB)

IND "Investigational New Drug" application to the Food and Drug Administration (FDA) seeking approval to begin clinical studies of a new pharmaceutical.

See also "TREATMENT" IND, IND EXEMPTION, PHASE I CLINICAL TESTING, FOOD AND DRUG ADMINISTRATION (FDA)

IND Exemption A permit by the Food and Drug Administration (FDA) to begin clinical trials on humans (of a new pharmaceutical) after toxicity data has been reviewed and approved by the FDA.

See also KEFAUVER RULE, IND, PHASE I CLINICAL TESTING

Indel See COLINEARITY

Indian Department of Biotechnology The governmental body in India that regulates all recombinant DNA research. It is the Indian counterpart of the American Government's Recombinant DNA Advisory Committee (RAC), the Australian government's Gene

Technology Regulator (GTR), and the French government's Commission of Biomolecular Engineering.

See also RECOMBINANT DNA ADVISORY COMMITTEE (RAC), ZKBS (CENTRAL COMMISSION ON BIOLOGICAL SAFETY), GENETIC ENGINEERING, RECOMBINANT DNA (rDNA), RECOMBINATION, BIOTECHNOLOGY, GENE TECHNOLOGY OFFICE, COMMISSION OF BIOMOLECULAR ENGINEERING, GENE TECHNOLOGY REGULATOR (GTR)

Indian Hedgehog Protein (Ihh) See HEDGEHOG PROTEINS

Induced Fit A substrate-induced change in the shape of an enzyme molecule that causes the catalytically functional groups of the enzyme to assume positions that are optimal for catalytic activity to occur.

See also ENZYME

Inducers Molecules that cause the production of larger amounts of the enzymes that are involved in the uptake and metabolism of the inducer (such as galactose). Inducers may be enzyme substrates.

See also ENZYME, INDUCIBLE ENZYMES, SUBSTRATE (CHEMICAL)

Inducible Enzymes Enzymes whose rate of production can be increased by the presence of certain chemical molecules. For example, **Paneth cells,** which line the human small intestine are induced by the presence of plant "natural pesticidal compounds" to excrete into passing food or plant materials large amounts of nucleases that degrade those plant natural pesticidal compounds (e.g., psoralene, caffeine, etc.), thereby protecting the human body. Other inducible enzymes include the **Phase I and Phase II detoxification enzymes** that work in tandem to eliminate some toxins from the body. The Phase I enzymes metabolize certain food compounds (sometimes into chemicals that happen to themselves be carcinogens), which are then transformed into harmless compounds by Phase II enzymes.

Research published during 2004 indicates that the presence of lycopene or sulforaphane in the human digestive tract induces excretion of some cancer-inhibiting Phase II detoxification enzymes.

Some diseases result in the production of certain chemicals that also thereby induce Phase I/II enzymes.

See also ENZYME, NUCLEASE, CAFFEINE, TOXIN, PSORALENE, LYCOPENE, SULFORAPHANE, CANCER, CARCINOGEN

Inducible Promoter Refers to a particular promoter, in which start or increase of promotion is caused (to initiate "defense" of the organism) by the presence of a disease, pathogen, or a toxin.

See also PROMOTER

Industrial Biotechnology Association (IBA) An American trade association of companies involved in biotechnology. Formed in 1981, the IBA tended to consist of the larger firms involved in biotechnology. In 1993, the Industrial Biotechnology Association (IBA) was merged with the Association of Biotechnology Companies (ABC) to form the Biotechnology Industry Organization (BIO).

See also ASSOCIATION OF BIOTECHNOLOGY COMPANIES (ABC), BIOTECHNOLOGY INDUSTRY ORGANIZATION (BIO), BIOTECHNOLOGY

Infliximab See TUMOR NECROSIS FACTOR (TNF)

Information RNA (iRNA) Refers to an RNA molecule (within cell) that does not code for production of a protein but only provides some "information" to **regulate** one or more cell functions (e.g., protein synthesis).

See also RIBONUCLEIC ACID (RNA), CELL, GENETIC CODE, PROTEIN, GENE, TRANSLATION, SYNTHESIZING (OF PROTEINS)

Informational Molecules Molecules containing information in the form of specific sequences of different building blocks. They include proteins and nucleic acids.

See also HEREDITY, GENE, GENETIC CODE, GENOME, GENOTYPE, NUCLEIC ACIDS, MESSENGER RNA (mRNA), DEOXYRIBONUCLEIC ACID (DNA), RIBONUCLEIC ACID (RNA), EDITOSOME

Ingestion Taking a substance into the body. For example, the amoeba surrounds a food particle and then ingests the particle.

Inhibition The suppression of the biological function of an enzyme or system by chemical or physical means.

See also APTAMERS, ENZYME, PROTEIN TYROSINE KINASE INHIBITOR, SOLANINE

Initiation Factors Refers to either:

- Specific proteins required to initiate synthesis of a polypeptide on ribosomes
- Specific proteins (e.g., C-reactive protein) that initiate an immune system response

See also RIBOSOMES, PROTEIN, POLYPEP-TIDE (PROTEIN), C-REACTIVE PROTEIN (CRP), IMMUNE RESPONSE, COMPLE-MENT FACTOR H GENE

Innate Immune Response Refers collectively to the inherent "first lines of immune defense" in the body (e.g., complement cascade), which are initiated by TLR (i.e., **toll-like receptors**), a category of cellular transmembrane proteins that "recognize" certain features (e.g., antigens) present on the exterior of invading pathogens.

For example, the **TLR 11** class of TLRs specifically sense the presence of pathogenic bacteria that infect the urinary tract. The **TLR 7** and **TLR 8** collectively specifically sense the single-stranded RNAs (ssRNA) which are present within some pathogenic viruses. Each of the TLRs thereby initiates the appropriate immune system response (e.g., against *bacteria* in the former case, and against *viruses* in the latter).

See also INNATE IMMUNE SYSTEM, HUMORAL IMMUNE RESPONSE, COM-PLEMENT, COMPLEMENT CASCADE, RECEPTORS, CELL, TRANSMEMBRANE PROTEINS, ANTIGEN, PATHOGEN, BAC-TERIA, VIRUS, RIBONUCLEIC ACID (RNA)

Innate Immune System Refers to an organism's "first line of defense" against pathogens. Typically consists of:

- Physical barriers (e.g., skin, epithelium, etc.)
- Chemical barriers (e.g., digestive enzymes and acids)
- Receptors (located on the surface of certain cells) that initiate the **innate immune response**
- Certain cells (e.g., neutrophils) that ingest or envelop pathogens as a part of the immune response
- Cytokines and other relevant signaling molecules that help regulate immunologic and inflammatory processes

See also ORGANISM, CELL, PATHOGEN, EPITHELIUM, ENZYME, DIGESTION (WITHIN ORGANISMS), RECEPTORS, INNATE IMMUNE RESPONSE, CYTO-KINES, SIGNALING MOLECULE

Inositol A cyclic (i.e., ring-shaped molecule) alcohol, initially characterized as a vitamin in 1941, which imparts certain (nutritional and other) benefits to animals and humans that consume it. Because it is critically important (nutritionally) during periods of rapid growth, the U.S. Food and Drug Administration (FDA) has mandated the inclusion of inositol in nonmilk infant formula products.

Research indicates that inositol and inositol-containing metabolites may also help to prevent type II diabetes, reduce or avoid several mental illnesses, and certain cancers.

See also VITAMIN, METABOLITE, TYPE II DIABETES, CANCER, PHYTATE, FOOD AND DRUG ADMINISTRATION (FDA)

Inositol Hexaphosphate (IP-6) See PHYTATE

Insect Cell Culture The propagation *in vitro* (e.g., in a vat or other container) of a population of living cells isolated from insects. Two insect species commonly utilized are fall armyworm (*Spodoptera frugiperda*) and cabbage looper (*Trichoplusia ni*).

Glycosylation of protein molecules produced in these (insect-source) cells is not identical to the glycosylation of rel. protein molecules produced by mammalian cells. That is because insect cells cannot put the sialic acid or galactose units onto the "ends" of the glycosylation molecular chains/branches). However, the glycoproteins (i.e., glycosylated protein molecules) produced by insect cells are **similar enough to mammalian-source glycoproteins** to possess a similar biological activity.

See also CELL, CELL CULTURE, *IN VITRO*, PROTEIN, BACULOVIRUS EXPRESSION VECTOR SYSTEM (BEVS), GLYCOSY-LATION, SIALIC ACID, GALACTOSE (Gal), BIOLOGICAL ACTIVITY, MAM-MALIAN CELL CULTURE, FALL ARMY-WORM

Insertional Knockout Systems See GENE SILENCING

In Silico See *IN SILICO* BIOLOGY

***In Silico* Biology** A set of computer-modeling technologies, using which researchers can do the following:

- Create computer models of specific cells, how a given disease impacts that cell, how a given pharmaceutical impacts that cell (e.g., by "docking" to it), or fails to impact that cell, etc.
- Create computer models of specific organs, how a given disease impacts that organ, how a given pharmaceutical impacts that organ, etc.
- Create computer models of specific organisms, how a given disease impacts that organism, how a given pharmaceutical then impacts that disease within that organism, etc.
- Create computer models of specific organisms that possess a given genome, how a given disease impacts that specific organism or phenotype, how a given pharmaceutical then impacts that disease within that organism or phenotype, etc.
- Create computer models of protein "digestion" (i.e., breaking apart into constituent peptides) for comparison with the **actual** peptides (fragments) that are determined (e.g., via MALDI-TOF-MS) to have resulted from **chemical digestion** of those protein molecules (e.g., via immersion in trypsin).

See also RATIONAL DRUG DESIGN, RECEPTOR MAPPING, CELL, BIOCHIPS, GENOME, GENOMICS, PHARMACOGE-NOMICS, PROTEIN, PROTEOMICS, PHE-NOTYPE, MALDI-TOF-MS, PEPTIDE, TRYPSIN, DOCKING (IN COMPUTA-TIONAL BIOLOGY), SYNTHETIC BIOL-OGY

***In Silico* Screening** A set of computer-model-ing technologies using which researchers can (vicariously) screen chemical compounds for their potential as pharmaceutical candidate compounds, pesticide candidate compounds, etc.

The chemical compounds are "generated" (e.g., from data available about compounds actually **created** in a laboratory in the past) and then computer modeling is utilized to do the fol-lowing:

- Assess their impact on "generated" specific cells, tissues, etc., via "dock-ing" (e.g., from data available about that **chemical-type** of molecule's impact on that **type of cell/tissue** when actually tested on it in a labo-ratory or clinic in the past).
- Generate an analogous chemical compound, that is likely to be more efficacious or have fewer undesirable side effects.
- Repeat the process.

For example, when **screening compounds** for potential usefulness as a pharmaceutical, the goal is to assess (modeled/predicted) differ-ences between **diseased** (untreated) and **treated** cells, thus enabling prediction of (bet-ter) pharmaceutuical candidate compounds for eventual actual testing on **real** cells/tissues.

Some of the more sophisticated *in silico* screen-ing software can even model ADME proper-ties for selected pharmaceutical candidate compounds.

See also RATIONAL DRUG DESIGN, *IN SIL-ICO* BIOLOGY, RECEPTOR MAPPING, CELL, BIOCHIPS, HIGH-THROUGHPUT SCREENING (HTS), COMBINATORIAL CHEMISTRY, PHARMACOGENOMICS, PROTEOMICS, QUANTITATIVE STRUC-TURE–ACTIVITY RELATIONSHIP (QSAR), ADME TESTS, TARGET (OF A THERAPEUTIC AGENT), TARGET (OF A HERBICIDE OR INSECTICIDE), DOCK-ING (IN COMPUTATIONAL BIOLOGY)

In Situ In the natural or original position (e.g., inside the body).

Insulin A protein hormone normally secreted by the beta (β) cells of the pancreas (when stimulated by glucose and the parasympa-thetic nervous system). Insulin and glucagon are the most important regulators of fuel (food) metabolism. In essence, insulin signals the "fed" state to the body's cells, which stim-ulates the storage of energy (fuel) in the form of fat and the synthesis of proteins (i.e., tissue building and repair) in a variety of ways.

Other impacts of insulin are to stimulate the uptake of amino acids by tissues, increase the permeability of cells to some ions (e.g., potassium), cause secretion of the hormone **angiotensin II,** which constricts arteries, promote synthesis of free fatty acids in the liver, inhibit the breakdown of fat in adipose tissue, etc. The disease known as **diabetes** results from a body's inability to produce insulin or its insensitivity to the insulin that is produced. That inability or insensitivity, and thus the disease, can result from several different causes:

- TYPE I (also known as **childhood** or **juvenile** or **early-onset**) DIABETES results when the body's insulin-making tissue is destroyed by autoimmune disease. See also the entry for INSULIN-DEPENDENT DIABETES MELLITIS (IDDM) in the following text.
- TYPE II DIABETES results when the body's insulin-utilizing tissues become insensitive to insulin. This can occur when insulin causes the liver to synthesize an overabundance of free fatty acids, which get stored in adipose tissue in the form of triglycerides, which can subsequently result in these triglyceride-laden tissues producing far fewer insulin receptors (i.e., thereby becoming insensitive to insulin).

The too-high sugar content in bloodstream that results from diabetes causes creation of **free radicals** (high-energy oxygen atoms bearing an "extra" electron), which can damage the eyes, kidneys, and extremity arteries (sometimes necessitating limb amputation) in one **haplotype (i.e., genetic subgroup) of people (i.e., those possessing the larger-size molecules of haptoglobin, a blood protein)**.

Some research indicates that consumption of amylose (starch only) or inulin (fructose oligosaccharide) in human diet as the primary carbohydrate source instead of glucose (or other sugars that the human body converts to glucose) can help the human body to avoid type II diabetes by avoiding gluconeogenesis.

In 1922, Canadian scientists Frederick Banting, Charles Best, J.J.R. MacLeod, and J.B. Collip succeeded in extracting insulin from the pancreas of slaughtered livestock (cows and pigs) in a form that could be injected into diabetes patients as a substitute for human insulin. The English biochemist, Fred Sanger, was first to determine the complete amino acid sequence of the insulin molecule. In 1977, the American scientist Howard Goodman, collaborating with William Rutter, announced the first cloning of insulin genes. This led to human insulin production by genetically engineered microorganisms (approved by FDA in 1982).

See also BETA CELLS, ISLETS OF LANGERHANS, HORMONE, PROTEIN, RECEPTORS, GLUCOSE (GLc), AMINO ACID, POLYPEPTIDE (PROTEIN), SEQUENCE (OF PROTEIN MOLECULE), GENETIC ENGINEERING, GLUCAGON, INSULIN-DEPENDENT DIABETES MELLITIS (IDDM), G-PROTEINS, CARBOHYDRATES, PANCREAS, AUTOIMMUNE DISEASE, INULIN, FREE RADICAL, HAPLOTYPE, OXIDATIVE STRESS, HAPTOGLOBIN, TYPE I DIABETES, TYPE II DIABETES, ADIPOSE, TRIGLYCERIDES

Insulin-Dependent Diabetes Mellitis (IDDM) An autoimmune disease in which the insulin-producing cells of the pancreas (i.e., **beta cells**, also known as ISLETS OF LANGERHANS) are attacked and destroyed by the cytotoxic T cells of the body's immune system.

See also AUTOIMMUNE DISEASE, INSULIN, ISLETS OF LANGERHANS, BETA CELLS, CYTOTOXIC T CELLS, HAPTOGLOBIN, DIABETES, TYPE I DIABETES, GLUTAMIC ACID DECARBOXYLASE (GAD)

Insulin-Like Growth Factor-1 (IGF-1) A protein hormone that is produced by the liver (when those cells have been stimulated by human growth hormone) and bone cells (when those bone cells have been stimulated by parathyroid hormone or estrogen), which is a promoter of bone formation and follicle development (in ovaries).

Another function of IGF-1 is to facilitate the transport of amino acids into cells and further inhibit protein breakdown in cells. If the body

I

is injured, IGF-1 works with platelet-derived growth factor (PDGF) to stimulate fibroblast and collagen cell division/metabolism to cause healing of wounds and bones. IGF-1 also occurs naturally in cow's milk.

See also HORMONE, HUMAN GROWTH HORMONE (HGH), CELL, ESTROGEN, FIBROBLASTS, AMINO ACID, COL-LAGEN, ESSENTIAL AMINO ACIDS, DIGESTION (WITHIN ORGANISMS), METABOLISM, PROTEIN, MESSENGER RNA (mRNA), UBIQUITIN, PLATELET-DERIVED GROWTH FACTOR (PDGF)

Insulin-Like Growth Factor-2 (IGF-2) A protein hormone that is produced by the body's brain, kidney, pancreas, and muscle tissues. IGF-2 is a primary growth factor important for early mammal development and especially for development of the liver and kidneys.

See also HORMONE, PROTEIN, EMBRYOL-OGY, GROWTH FACTOR, INSULIN-LIKE GROWTH FACTOR-1 (IGF-1)

Intact-cell MALDI-TOF-MS See ICM

Integrated Crop Management See INTE-GRATED PEST MANAGEMENT

Integrated Disease Management See INTE-GRATED PEST MANAGEMENT

Integrated Pest Management (IPM) A holistic (system) approach utilized by some farmers to try to control agricultural pests (e.g., tobacco budworm, European corn borer, soybean cyst nematode, weevils, etc.), which was initially developed as a methodology by Ray Smith and Perry Adkisson. IPM also helps to control plant diseases. For example, farmers can plant buckwheat near their corn-fields in order to help control European corn borer (ECB), a serious pest of corn (maize) *Zea mays* L. plants. Green lacewing beetles (*Chrysoperla carnea*), which prey on European corn borers, are attracted by the buckwheat and consume ECB in the corn while they live in the buckwheat areas. Because European corn borer is a vector (carrier) of **disease and mycotoxin-producing** microorganisms such as the fungi *Aspergillus flavus, Aspergillus parasiticus,* and *Fusarium* spp., this lacewing beetle (IPM) control of ECB also helps reduce those plant diseases and mycotoxins. Often utilized in conjunction with no-tillage crop production.

See also WEEVILS, *HELIOTHIS VIRESCENS (H. VIRESCENS),* EUROPEAN CORN BORER (ECB), FUNGUS, MYCOTOXINS, AFLATOXIN, LOW-TILLAGE CROP PRO-DUCTION, NO-TILLAGE CROP PRODUC-TION, SOYBEAN CYST NEMATODES (SCN), CORN, SOYBEAN PLANT, *BACIL-LUS THURINGIENSIS (B.t.)*

Integrins A class of proteins that is found on the surface (membranes) of cells and that function as cellular adhesion receptors. For example, integrin $\alpha_v\beta_3$ is a receptor on the surface of endothelial cells in growing blood vessels (e.g., the new blood vessels forming in a body with cancer to supply blood to growing tumors). It binds angiogenic endothelial cells, enabling them to form new blood vessels.

See also ADHESION MOLECULES, PRO-TEIN, GLYCOPROTEINS, CELL, RECEP-TORS, LECTINS, SELECTINS, SIGNAL TRANSDUCTION, ANGIOGENESIS, TUMOR, ENDOTHELIAL CELLS, PLASMA MEMBRANE

Intein The internal-within-protein molecule sequence that is excised (i.e., "popped out") during the protein splicing process. An intein is a protein domain in the "center" of a protein molecule.

See also SPLICING (OF PROTEIN MOLE-CULE), EXTEIN, CHEMICAL GENETICS, PROTEIN, EXCISION (OF PROTEIN MOL-ECULE), DOMAIN (OF A PROTEIN), SEQUENCE (OF A PROTEIN MOLECULE)

Intercellular Adhesion Molecule (ICAM) See ADHESION MOLECULE

Interfering RNAs See SHORT INTERFER-ING RNA (siRNA)

Interferons Discovered in 1957 by Alick Isaacs and J. Lindenman, they are a family of small (cytokines) proteins (produced by vertebrate cells following a virus infection) that **interfere** with (i.e., block) translation of viral DNA.

Via that blocking, interferons prevent synthesis of proteins needed for viral reproduction, so interferons possess potent antiviral effects. Secreted interferons bind to the plasma mem-brane of other cells in the organism and induce an antiviral state in them (conferring resis-tance to a broad spectrum of viruses).

Three classes of interferons have been isolated and purified so far: α-interferon (originally called leukocyte interferon), β-interferon (beta interferon or fibroblast interferon), and γ-interferon (gamma interferon or immune interferon, a lymphokine). These proteins have been cloned and expressed in *Escherichia coli (E. coli)*, which has enabled large quantities to be produced for evaluation of the interferons as possible antiviral and anticancer agents. To date, interferons have been used to treat Kaposi's sarcoma, hairy cell leukemia, venereal warts, multiple sclerosis, and hepatitis.

See also ALPHA INTERFERON, BETA INTERFERON, GAMMA INTERFERON, CYTOKINES, PROTEIN, LYMPHOKINES, *ESCHERICHIA COLIFORM (E. COLI)*

Interim Office of the Gene Technology Regulator (IOGTR) The regulatory body of Australia's government that was responsible for approvals of new rDNA products (e.g., new genetically engineered crops) before they could be introduced into Australia during 1999–2001. IOGTR replaced/superseded Australia's Gene Technology Office (in this role) in 1999 and was itself replaced by the Gene Technology Regulator (GTR) in 2001.

See also GENE TECHNOLOGY REGULATOR (GTR), GENE TECHNOLOGY OFFICE, GENETIC MANIPULATION ADVISORY COMMITTEE (GMAC), rDNA, DEOXYRIBONUCLEIC ACID (DNA), GENETIC ENGINEERING, RECOMBINANT DNA ADVISORY COMMITTEE (RAC), COMMISSION OF BIOMOLECULAR ENGINEERING, INDIAN DEPARTMENT OF BIOTECHNOLOGY

Interleukin-1 (IL-1) A cytokine (glycoprotein) released by activated macrophages during the inflammatory stage of immune system response to an infection, which promotes the growth of epithelial (skin) cells and white blood cells. Research has indicated that too much IL-1 is linked to the development of rheumatoid arthritis, diabetes, inflammatory bowel disease, and other autoimmune diseases.

See also MACROPHAGE, AUTOIMMUNE DISEASE, ADHESION MOLECULE, TUMOR NECROSIS FACTOR (TNF), CYTOKINES, GLYCOPROTEIN, WHITE BLOOD CELLS, ISLETS OF LANGERHANS, EPITHELIUM, INTERLEUKIN-1

RECEPTOR ANTAGONIST (IL-Ira), INTERLEUKINS

Interleukin-1 Receptor Antagonist (IL-1ra) A glycoprotein (produced by macrophages in response to presence of interleukin-1, and endotoxin in tissues) that preferentially binds to those cell receptors in the body that typically bind the lymphokine, interleukin-1 (IL-1). When manufactured by man (e.g., via genetic engineering) and injected into the body in large quantities, IL-Ira can block the deleterious effects of (too much) interleukin-1.

See also INTERLEUKIN-1 (IL-1), RECEPTORS, RECEPTOR FITTING, GLYCOPROTEIN, MACROPHAGE, ENDOTOXIN, ADHESION MOLECULE, CELLULAR IMMUNE RESPONSE, PROTEIN, LYMPHOKINES, ANTAGONISTS

Interleukin-2 (IL-2) Also known as **T cell growth factor**. A cytokine (glycoprotein) secreted by (immune system response) stimulated helper T cells, which promotes the proliferation/differentiation of more helper T cells and promotes the growth of lymphocytes to combat an infection. Interleukin-2 also stimulates the lymphocytes to produce gamma interferon. It is gamma interferon that prompts the cytotoxic T cells to attack virus-infected cells and kill the virus within them. The structure of the gene that codes for synthesis of IL-2 (by immune system cells) was determined by Tadatsugu Taniguchi in 1983.

See also IMMUNE RESPONSE, HUMORAL IMMUNITY, CYTOKINES, GLYCOPROTEIN, CYTOTOXIC T CELLS, T CELLS, HELPER T CELLS, T CELL RECEPTORS, INTERFERONS, INTERLEUKINS, GENE

Interleukin-3 (IL-3) A hematologic growth factor (glycoprotein) cytokine that stimulates the proliferation of a wide range of white blood cells (to combat an infection).

See also HEMATOLOGIC GROWTH FACTORS (HGF), GLYCOPROTEIN, CYTOKINES, WHITE BLOOD CELLS, INTERLEUKINS

Interleukin-4 (IL-4) A cytokine (glycoprotein) that stimulates production of antibody-producing B cells, Immunoglobulin-E (I_gE), and promotes cytotoxic T cell (i.e., killer T cells) growth.

See also ANTIBODY, CYTOTOXIC T CELLS, B CELLS, GLYCOPROTEIN, CYTOKINES, IMMUNOGLOBULIN, INTERLEUKINS

Interleukin-5 (IL-5) A cytokine (glycoprotein) that stimulates eosinophil growth.

See also EOSINOPHILS, PROTEIN, GLYCOPROTEIN, CYTOKINES, CELLULAR IMMUNE RESPONSE, INTERLEUKINS

Interleukin-6 (IL-6) A cytokine (glycoprotein) that is pleiotropic (i.e., stimulates several different types of immune system cells) and is a hematopoietic growth factor. For example, infections and certain physical trauma can cause the body to produce IL-6, which subsequently causes the liver to synthesize (manufacture) **C-Reactive Protein**.

See also HEMATOPOIETIC GROWTH FACTORS (HGF), GROWTH FACTOR, GLYCOPROTEIN, PLEIOTROPIC, MACROPHAGE, CYTOKINES, C-REACTIVE PROTEIN (CRP), INTERLEUKINS

Interleukin-7 (IL-7) A cytokine (glycoprotein) synthesized in the bone marrow that stimulates early (fetal) proliferation and differentiation of B cells and T cells. May be useful in regenerating lymphoid cells in patients whose immune systems have been devastated by cancer chemotherapy.

See also CYTOKINES, GLYCOPROTEIN, STEM CELL ONE, T CELLS, CANCER, INTERLEUKINS

Interleukin-8 (IL-8) A basic polypeptide (glycoprotein) with heparin-binding activity. Endogenous endothelial IL-8 appears to regulate transvenular traffic during acute inflammatory responses.

See also POLYPEPTIDE (PROTEIN), GLYCOPROTEIN, HEPARIN, ENDOTHELIAL CELLS, ENDOTHELIUM, POLYMORPHONUCLEAR LEUKOCYTES (PMN), CELLULAR IMMUNE RESPONSE, INTERLEUKINS

Interleukin-9 (IL-9) A cytokine (glycoprotein) that is released at sites in the body where inflammation has occurred.

See also CYTOKINES, GLYCOPROTEIN, CELLULAR IMMUNE RESPONSE, INTERLEUKINS

Interleukin-12 (IL-12) A cytokine (glycoprotein) produced by the body that serves to activate the immune system against certain tumors and pathogens.

See also CYTOKINES, GLYCOPROTEIN, TUMOR, TUMOR-ASSOCIATED ANTIGENS, MAJOR HISTOCOMPATIBILITY COMPLEX (MHC), T CELL RECEPTORS, CYTOTOXIC T CELLS, PATHOGEN, INTERLEUKINS, ELECTROPORATION

Interleukins A class of 24 different cytokines that "carry a signal" **between different leukocyte populations** within the immune system of an organism.

See also CYTOKINES, LEUKOCYTES, INTERLEUKIN-1 (IL-1), INTERLEUKIN-2 (IL-2), INTERLEUKIN-3 (IL-3), INTERLEUKIN-4 (IL-4), INTERLEUKIN-5 (IL-5), INTERLEUKIN-6 (IL-6), INTERLEUKIN-7 (IL-7), INTERLEUKIN-8 (IL-8), INTERLEUKIN-9 (IL-9), INTERLEUKIN-12 (IL-12)

Intermediary Metabolism The chemical reactions that take place in the cell that transform the complex molecules derived from food into the small molecules needed for the growth and maintenance of the cell.

See also METABOLISM, CELL, DIGESTION (WITHIN ORGANISMS), METABOLIC PATHWAY

International Food Biotechnology Council (IFBC) An organization that was established in 1988 by the Industrial Biotechnology Association (IBA) and the International Life Sciences Institute (ILSI) in order to "produce a (recommended) set of guidelines that could be used to assess the safety of genetically altered foods."

See also GNE, INDUSTRIAL BIOTECHNOLOGY ASSOCIATION (IBA), INTERNATIONAL LIFE SCIENCES INSTITUTE (ILSI), SENIOR ADVISORY GROUP ON BIOTECHNOLOGY, BIOTECHNOLOGY INDUSTRY ORGANIZATION (BIO), GENETIC ENGINEERING, POLYGALACTURONASE, ANTISENSE (DNA SEQUENCE), BIOTECHNOLOGY, BACTERIOCINS

International Life Sciences Institute (ILSI) A nonprofit foundation that was established in 1978 to advance the understanding of scientific issues relating to nutrition, food safety, toxicology, risk assessment, and the environment. ILSI is headquartered in Washington, D.C., and has branches in Argentina, Brazil, Europe, India, Japan, Korea, Mexico, Africa, Thailand, Singapore, China, and other countries.

International Office of Epizootics (OIE) One of the three international SPS standard-setting organizations that is recognized by the World Trade Organization (WTO), the OIE is an international veterinary organization headquartered in Paris. The OIE was established in 1924, originally as part of the League of Nations, and is the worldwide authority for development of animal health and zoonoses standards, guidelines, and recommendations.

See also SPS, INTERNATIONAL PLANT PROTECTION CONVENTION (IPPC), ZOONOSES, WORLD TRADE ORGANIZATION (WTO)

International Plant Protection Convention (IPPC) One of the three international SPS standard-setting organizations that is recognized by the World Trade Organization (WTO), the IPPC is the worldwide authority for development of plant health standards, guidelines, and recommendations (e.g., to prevent transfer of a plant disease or plant pest from one country to another). The treaty establishing the IPPC was signed in 1952 (amended in 1979 and 1997) and currently has 107 member countries (i.e., signatories to the 1979 text).

The IPPC Secretariat is within the United Nations' Food and Agriculture Organization (FAO). IPPC standards are set (and enforced) via regional SPS institutions such as the North American Plant Protection Organization (NAPPO), European Plant Protection Organization (EPPO), etc. There are currently nine RPPOs (i.e., regional plant protection organizations) under Article VIII of the 1979 IPPC text.

See also SPS, EUROPEAN PLANT PROTECTION ORGANIZATION (EPPO), INTERNATIONAL OFFICE OF EPIZOOTICS (OIE), WORLD TRADE ORGANIZATION (WTO), NORTH AMERICAN PLANT PROTECTION ORGANIZATION (NAPPO), NATIONAL PLANT PROTECTION ORGANIZATION (NPPO), QUARANTINE PEST, INTRODUCTION, ESTABLISHMENT POTENTIAL

International Society for the Advancement of Biotechnology (ISAB) A nonprofit organization of individuals that was started in 1994 "to advance and promote the general welfare of the science and commercialization of genetic engineering and industrial biotechnology."

See also GENETIC ENGINEERING, BIOTECHNOLOGY, BIOTECHNOLOGY INDUSTRY ORGANIZATION (BIO)

International Union for Protection of New Varieties of Plants (UPOV) See UNION FOR PROTECTION OF NEW VARIETIES OF PLANTS (UPOV)

Internaulin See CADHERINS

Intracellular Transport See CELL, GATED TRANSPORT, LIPIDS, MEMBRANE TRANSPORT, TRANSPORT PROTEINS

Intrinsic Protein Refers to a protein molecule that is embedded within a cell membrane (and protrudes from each side of the membrane).

See also PROTEIN, CELL, PLASMA MEMBRANE, MEMBRANES (OF A CELL), TRANSMEMBRANE PROTEINS, ION CHANNELS, IONOTROPIC

Introduction Term utilized (e.g., by the IPPC) to refer to the **entry** and **successful establishment** of a given pest (e.g., weed, insect, disease, etc.) into a (formerly) "pest-free area" (i.e., country or region where **that pest** is not yet present or is present but not widely distributed and thus officially controlled).

See also INTERNATIONAL PLANT PROTECTION CONVENTION (IPPC), ESTABLISHMENT POTENTIAL, QUARANTINE PEST, NATIONAL PLANT PROTECTION ORGANIZATION (NPPO)

Introgression The incorporation of exotic (i.e., wild-type) genes into elite germplasm (i.e., domesticated breeding lines) or of transgenes (i.e., genes from transgenic organisms) into a wild type's genome.

See also TRANSGENIC, OUTCROSSING, WILD TYPE, GENOME, GENE, TRANSLOCATION

Intron A (intervening sequence) segment of deoxyribonucleic acid (DNA) that is transcribed, but is removed from within the mRNA transcript by splicing together the sequences (exons) on either side of it (in the molecule) by snRNP during the final step of the transcription process. In the past, it was generally considered to be a "nonfunctioning" portion of the DNA molecule.

However, during the 1990s, Malcolm Simon showed that some introns contain the "markers" that scientists utilize to identify where a given gene (within DNA strand) begins and ends. For example, the genetic test (conducted on women) for presence of the "BRCA 1" gene actually detects a **DNA "marker"** in intron sequence **near** the "BRCA 1" gene and not the "BRCA 1" gene itself *per se.*

Also, sometimes a given intron remains in the transcript (e.g., via alternative splicing), resulting in a **different** protein expressed by the same gene. For example, the COX-3 enzyme and the COX-1 enzyme are both produced from the COX-1 gene. The COX-3 enzyme results when **intron 1** is retained in the mRNA transcript.

See also TRANSCRIPTION, DEOXYRIBONU-CLEIC ACID (DNA), MESSENGER RNA (mRNA), EXON, GENE, EDITING, SPLIC-ING, ALTERNATIVE SPLICING, SPLICING JUNCTIONS, MARKER (DNA SEQUENCE), BRCA GENES, ENZYME, COX-1, COX-2, COX-3, CYCLOOXYGENASE

Inulin A fructose oligosaccharide (FOS) that is naturally produced in more than 30,000 plants. Like many other FOS, consumption of inulin by humans results in several health benefits (e.g., helps prevent coronary heart disease, promotes growth of bifidobacteria in the intestines, reduces likelihood of developing diabetes, promotes absorption of calcium from foods, etc.). During 2000, the European Union's government regulatory agencies agreed to classify inulin as a water-soluble fiber (because humans cannot digest inulin).

See also FRUCTOSE OLIGOSACCHA-RIDES, WATER-SOLUBLE FIBER, BIFI-DOBACTERIA, CORONARY HEART DIS-EASE (CHD), DIABETES

Invasin A transmembrane (i.e., through the membrane of the cell) protein that enables bacterial cells to invade normal (body) cells.

See also CD4 PROTEIN, RECEPTORS, CELL, T CELL RECEPTORS, ENDOCY-TOSIS, PLASMA MEMBRANE

Inverted Micelle See also REVERSE MICELLE (RM), MICELLE

Investigational New Drug See IND

In vitro In an unnatural position (e.g., outside the body, in the test tube). *In vitro* is Latin for "in glass." For example, the testing of a substance or the experimentation in (using) a "dead" cell-free system.

See also *IN VITRO* SELECTION

In Vitro Evolution See *IN VITRO* SELEC-TION

In Vitro **Selection** A search process (e.g., for a new pharmaceutical) that first involves the construction of a large "pool" of polynucle-otide sequences (at least some of which are likely to possess the desired pharmaceutical properties) synthesized by a totally random process. This is followed by repeated cycles of screening (for those sequences possessing desired properties) and enriching and ampli-fication (of the screened/enriched sequences). Common amplification techniques include polymerase chain reaction (PCR), ligase chain reaction (LCR), self-sustained sequence rep-lication (SSR), Q-beta replicase technique, and strand displacement amplification (SDA).

See also *IN VITRO*, AMPLIFICATION, GENE AMPLIFICATION, POLYMERASE CHAIN REACTION (PCR), Q-BETA REPLICASE TECHNIQUE, NUCLEOTIDE, DEOXYRI-BONUCLEIC ACID (DNA), SYNTHESIZ-ING (OF DNA MOLECULES), OLIGONU-CLEOTIDE, DNA PROBE, GENE MACHINE, COMBINATORIAL CHEMIS-TRY

In Vivo Latin for "in living," e.g., the testing of a new pharmaceutical substance or experi-mentation in (using) a living, whole organism. An *in vivo* test is one in which an experimental substance is injected into an animal such as a rat in order to ascertain its effect on the organ-ism.

See also MODEL ORGANISM

IOGTR See INTERIM OFFICE OF THE GENE TECHNOLOGY REGULATOR (IOGTR)

Ion From the Greek *ion,* meaning "something that goes."

An ion is an atom or molecule possessing a pos-itive or a negative electrical charge. Ions are produced by the dissociation (coming apart) of (electrolyte) molecule resulting from electro-lyte dissolving in solution. One example is the dissociation of common table salt (i.e., sodium chloride) in water, which results in positively charged sodium ions (called cations) and negatively charged chloride ions (called anions). Ions play critically important roles in many biological processes such as nerve activity.

See also CHELATION, CHELATING AGENT, ION CHANNELS, CITRIC ACID, CITRATE SYNTHASE (CSb) GENE

Ion Channels Refers to specialized proteins that act as "pores" (e.g., through the plasma membrane of a cell) through which certain ions (i.e., atoms or molecules bearing an electrical charge) are allowed to pass. Examples include calcium channels, sodium channels, and potassium channels. The selectivity of ion channels can be altered when specific molecules (e.g., in the blood or digestive fluids) come in contact with the plasma membrane (i.e., G-protein receptors coupled to the ion channel).

For example, the group of pharmaceuticals known as CALCIUM CHANNEL BLOCKERS (e.g., verapamil, amlopidine, diltiazem, nifedipine, etc.) act to block or hinder the movement of calcium ions through **calcium ion channels** (i.e., "pores" that had previously allowed calcium ions to enter relevant cells [i.e., in blood vessel walls] easily).

Another example is the mode of action of the "**Cry**" (crystal-like) **proteins** that are naturally present within *Bacillus thuringiensis (B.t.)* bacteria. When eaten by certain insects (possessing alkaline digestive fluids in their stomach or gut), Cry proteins are hydrolyzed (i.e., chemically "cut") into fragments. One of those fragments — 60 kDa in size — attaches to specific receptors located on the surface (membrane) of certain cells that line the inside (i.e., epithelium) of the insect's midgut. This **attachment to the receptors** triggers ion channels in the (epithelium) cell's membrane to suddenly allow cations (i.e., atoms or molecules with positive electrical charge) to quickly flow out of the cell (which leads to the death of all gut cells that the **Cry protein piece** attached to).

See also CELL, PLASMA MEMBRANE, ION, CALCIUM CHANNEL BLOCKERS, MEMBRANE TRANSPORT, PROTEIN, CRY PROTEINS, G-PROTEINS, *BACILLUS*

THURINGIENSIS (B.t.), BACTERIA, PROTOXIN, HYDROLYZE, KILODALTON (kDa), RECEPTORS, EPITHELIUM, IONOTROPIC, GATED CHANNEL, INTRINSIC PROTEIN

Ion Trap Invented by Wolfgang Paul in 1954, it is a device that is utilized to confine ions (e.g., from a sample entering a mass spectrometer) within a small volume of space, without the use of physical walls. Instead, it utilizes three carefully placed hyperbolic electrodes to which applicable radio frequency (RF) voltage potential is applied. The ions are thereby confined within the desired volume of space by high-frequency electrical fields.

In **ion-trap-based mass spectrometers**, the voltages of the electrodes are electively changed to cause specific ions (i.e., pieces of the original sample molecules) to be ejected from the ion trap into the spectrometer's detector. As with all mass spectrometers:

- Those "pieces of sample" are separated by the differences in their mass-to-charge ratios
- Their exact mass is determined based on measurement of their mass-to-charge ratios while those "pieces" are passing through electromagnetic fields whose strength is precisely known
- The identity of the "pieces" is determined by comparison of their mass-to-charge-ratio (m/e) spectra to those within a database of known "pieces" (ions)

See also ION, MASS SPECTROMETER, MOLECULAR WEIGHT

Ion-Exchange Chromatography Separation of ionic compounds (which include nucleic acids and proteins) in a chromatographic column containing a polymeric resin (i.e., the stationary phase) having fixed charge groups. The process works in that the charges of the column (stationary phase) interact with the opposite charges of the material dissolved in the solution that is flowing through the column (mobile phase). The charge interaction between the column material and, say, the protein has the effect of slowing down the rate of

I

movement of the protein through the column. The other molecules, which do not interact with the column, meanwhile flow right on through. This then constitutes the separation process.

See also CHROMATOGRAPHY

Ionotropic Refers to a cellular receptor that impacts (mediates) that cell's processes or states, etc., via regulation of the cell's ion channels.

See also ION CHANNELS, CELL, RECEPTORS

IP-6 Inositol hexaphosphate.

See also PHYTATE

IPM See INTEGRATED PEST MANAGEMENT (IPM)

IPPC See INTERNATIONAL PLANT PROTECTION CONVENTION

iRNA Acronym for **information RNA**.

See INFORMATION RNA (iRNA)

Iron Bacteria See FERROBACTERIA

Iron Deficiency Anemia (IDA) A disease caused by lack of iron in an organism's body owing to either shortfall in diet or dietary iron not being bioavailable (digestible). For example, the phytate that is naturally present in traditional varieties of corn (maize) inhibits absorption of the iron in that corn (maize) by humans, swine, and poultry.

IDA is a major cause of childhood diseases and maternal death (i.e., death of the mother following childbirth) in many developing countries. IDA also makes people more susceptible to diphtheria.

See also GOLDEN RICE, PHYTATE, LOW-PHYTATE CORN, LOW-PHYTATE SOYBEANS, ORGANISM

Islets of Langerhans Also called **beta cells**. Cells in the pancreas that produce insulin in response to the presence of glucose (sugar) in the bloodstream. The failure of insulin production results in the disease called diabetes.

See also GLUCOSE (GLc), GLYCOLYSIS, AUTOIMMUNE DISEASE, INSULIN, INSULIN-DEPENDENT DIABETES MELLITIS (IDDM)

Isoelectric Focusing (IEF) An electrophoresis methodology in which protein molecules are moved (via application of an electrical charge/potential) through a pH gradient (e.g., in a two-dimensional gel until they reach their individual isoelectric points).

IEF is the first step in many **gene expression studies**, followed by extraction of the individual (separated) proteins for identification and quantitation (i.e., **how much** of each protein was produced by the cell, tissue, or organism being evaluated).

See also TWO-DIMENSIONAL (2-D) GEL ELECTROPHORESIS, GENE EXPRESSION ANALYSIS, PROTEIN, GENE EXPRESSION PROFILING, CELL, GENE FUNCTION ANALYSIS, ORGANISM, ISOELECTRIC POINT, CAPILLARY ELECTROPHORESIS

Isoelectric Point Refers to that point (e.g., in a two-dimensional gel) at which the charge/mass of a given protein is exactly matched by the electrical charge/potential applied to that gel. Because the isoelectric point is different for virtually every protein (e.g., in a sample applied to the gel), this enables separation of individual proteins from a (mixed) sample.

See also TWO-DIMENSIONAL (2-D) GEL ELECTROPHORESIS, PROTEIN, ISOELECTRIC FOCUSING (IEF)

Isoenzymes See ISOZYMES

Isoflavins See ISOFLAVONES

Isoflavones A group of phytochemicals (including genistein, glycitein, and daidzein) that are produced within the seeds of the soybean plant (*Glycine max* (L.) Merrill) at a typical concentration of approximately 0.04 to 0.24%. Isoflavones are also produced within other types of tissues of the soybean **plant** (e.g., to ward off infection by plant diseases such as *Phytophthera* ones) and the soybean plant's **roots** (e.g., to signal and attract the *Rhizobium japonicum* bacteria that live symbiotically among the soybean plant's roots and "fix" nitrogen from the air, thereby providing natural fertilizer for the plant). Much smaller amounts of isoflavones are produced in some wheat, lentils, chickpeas, and edible bean plants.

Evidence shows that consumption of soybean isoflavones by humans can help to lower blood content of low-density lipoproteins (LDLP) and help prevent osteoporosis, prostate enlargement, and certain types of cancer (e.g., breast cancer, colon cancer, lung cancer, prostate cancer, uterine cancer, etc.).

A human diet containing a large amount of isoflavones has been shown to increase bone density and to decrease total serum cholesterol, thereby lowering risk of osteoporosis and coronary heart disease. Isoflavones also exhibit antioxidant properties.

See also GENISTEIN (GEN), SOYBEAN PLANT, *BRADYRHIZOBIUM JAPONICUM*, PHYTOALEXINS, PHYTOCHEMICALS, LOW-DENSITY LIPOPROTEINS (LDLP), OSTEOPOROSIS, PROSTATE-SPECIFIC ANTIGEN (PSA), CANCER, SELECTIVE ESTROGEN EFFECT, STRESS PROTEINS, CHOLESTEROL, NITROGEN FIXATION, NODULATION, CORONARY HEART DISEASE (CHD), OSTEOPOROSIS, *RHIZOBIUM* (BACTERIA), *PHYTOPHTHERA MEGASPERMA* F. SP. *GLYCINEA*, *PHYTOPHTHERA* ROOT ROT, SIGNALING, SIGNALING MOLECULES, HIGH-ISOFLAVONE SOYBEANS, ANTIOXIDANTS, OXIDATIVE STRESS

Isoflavonoids See ISOFLAVONES

Isoleucine (Ile) A monocarboxylic amino acid occurring within most dietary proteins.

See also AMINO ACID, PROTEIN, ALS GENE

Isomer One of the two or more chemical substances having the same elementary percentage composition (i.e., same atoms) and molecular weight, but differing in structure and, therefore, in properties. There are many ways in which such structural differences (between the two or more isomeric molecules) occur. One example is n-butane [$CH_3 (CH_2)_2CH_3$] and isobutane [$CH_3CH(CH_3)_2$].

See also STEREOISOMERS

Isomerase An enzyme-catalyzing transformation of a compound into its positional isomer.

See also ISOMER

Isoprene The five-carbon hydrocarbon molecule: 2-methyl-1,3 butadiene. It is a recurring structural unit of the terpenoid molecules, which are either linear or cyclic. There exists a very large number of terpenes and many are major components of essential plant oils.

See also GTPases

Isotachophoresis Refers to one of the capillary electrophoresis technologies, in which the sample's components are (additionally) separated between the **leading electrolyte** (i.e., injected into the capillary tube first) and the **terminating electrolyte** (i.e., injected into the capillary tube last).

See also CAPILLARY ELECTROPHORESIS, ELECTROLYTE

Isothiocyanates See SULFORAPHANE

Isotope Refers to one of the several "varieties" of atoms that exist, of the same element, that differ from each other in the number of neutrons in the atom's nucleus. For example, the element chlorine exists primarily in two forms (isotopes) in nature — with 18 neutrons (76% of the time) and with 20 neutrons (24% of the time). The chemical properties of isotopes of a given element are virtually identical.

See also ATOMIC WEIGHT

Isozymes (Isoenzymes) Multiple forms of an enzyme that differ from each other in their substrate (substance acted upon) affinity, in their maximum activity, or in their regulatory properties.

See also ENZYME, SUBSTRATE (CHEMICAL), RIBOZYMES, PGHS

ISPM Acronym for **International Standards for Pest Management**.

See also INTERNATIONAL PLANT PROTECTION CONVENTION (IPPC)

ITP Acronym for **Isotachophoresis**.

See ISOTACHOPHORESIS

I

J

Japan Bioindustry Association An association of the largest Japanese companies that are engaged in some form of genetic engineering research or production. Similar to America's Biotechnology Industry Organization (BIO), it is headquartered in Tokyo.

See also BIOTECHNOLOGY INDUSTRY ORGANIZATION (BIO), BIOTECHNO-LOGY, GENETIC ENGINEERING, RECOMBINANT DNA (rDNA), SENIOR ADVISORY GROUP ON BIOTECHNOL-OGY (SAGB), INTERNATIONAL FOOD BIOTECHNOLOGY COUNCIL

Jasmonate Cascade Refers to the cascade of different (signaling, etc.) natural chemicals that are produced in response to certain pest insects chewing on some plant species. For example, in response to such insects chewing on the *Nicotiana attenuata* plant, the plant expresses **lipoxygenase-3** and certain other enzymes that cause production (via oxylipin pathways) of jasmonic acid, which triggers specific plant defenses (e.g., systemic acquired resistance, etc.).

See also CASCADE, SIGNALING MOLE-CULE, ENZYME, PATHWAY, JASMONIC ACID, SYSTEMIC ACQUIRED RESIS-TANCE (SAR), LIPOXYGENASE (LOX)

Jasmonic Acid Jasmonic acid is a signaling molecule in systemic acquired resistance (SAR) when SAR is triggered in plants (e.g., via spray application of harpin protein to various plants, chewing of insects on the leaves of certain plants, or the entry of certain pathogenic bacteria or fungi into plants, etc.).

See also SYSTEMIC ACQUIRED RESIS-TANCE (SAR), SIGNALING MOLECULE, SOYBEAN PLANT, FUNGUS, PATHOGEN, PROTEIN, PATHOGENESIS-RELATED PROTEINS, HARPIN, PHYTOALEXINS, JASMONATE CASCADE

Jumping Genes Genes that move (change positions) within the genome. Genes associated with transposable elements. A segment fragment of deoxyribonucleic acid (DNA) that can move from one position in the genome to another.

See also GENE, GENOME, DEOXYRIBONU-CLEIC ACID (DNA), GENETIC CODE, TRANSPOSITION, TRANSPOSON, TRANSLOCATION, INTROGRESSION, HOT SPOTS

Juncea Refers to a group of related plants; often commonly called "wild mustard."

See also BRASSICA

Junk DNA A term historically utilized by some to refer to portions of an organism's DNA that were not **obviously** genes (i.e., not transcribed into mRNA, thus not part of the DNA "tagged" or labeled with ESTs, etc.). However, it has recently been discovered that at least some of what was formerly called "junk DNA" (e.g., introns) helps enable more than one specific protein molecule to be expressed from certain genes.

See also DEOXYRIBONUCLEIC ACID (DNA), GENE, INTRON, PROTEIN, EXPRESS, EXPRESSED SEQUENCE TAG (EST), CENTRAL DOGMA (NEW)

K

KARI Acronym for either the **Kenya Agricultural Research Institute** or the **Kawanda Agricultural Research Institute in Uganda**.

Karnal Bunt A plant disease that can be caused by the smut fungus *Tilletia indica* in wheat.

See also FUNGUS, WHEAT

Karyotype A size-order alignment of an organism's chromosome pairs in the format of a (photomicrograph) chart. It enables the connecting of chromosomes to symptoms (e.g., of genetic diseases in the organism) and traits.

See also CHROMOSOMES, GENE, GENOTYPE, TRAIT, LINKAGE, LINKAGE GROUP, MUSCULAR DYSTROPHY (MD), CHROMATIDS, CHROMATIN

Karyotyper A scientist (or more frequently an automated analytical machine) that does the following:

- Takes a video picture of a given cell under a microscope
- Digitizes that picture within a computer
- "Cuts out" the individual chromosomes contained within that cell's genome
- Arranges the cell's chromosomes in pairs by size order into a chart (called a karyotype)

See also CHROMOSOMES, GENOME, KARYOTYPE

Kb An abbreviation for **1000 (kilo) base pairs of deoxyribonucleic acid (DNA).**

See also DEOXYRIBONUCLEIC ACID (DNA), KILOBASE PAIRS (Kbp)

kDa An abbreviation for **kilodalton.**

See also KILODALTON (kDa)

Kefauver Rule A 1962 U.S. law that mandates that the Food and Drug Administration (FDA) requires proof of pharmaceutical **efficacy for drugs to be sold in the U.S.**

See also FOOD AND DRUG ADMINISTRATION (FDA)

Kenya Biosafety Council Kenya's national regulatory body for granting approval to a new genetically engineered plant (e.g., a new genetically engineered crop to be planted). The Kenya Biosafety Council is analogous to Germany's ZKBS (Central Commission on Biological Safety), Australia's GMAC (Genetic Manipulation Advisory Committee), or Brazil's CTNBio (National Biosafety Commission).

See also GMAC, RECOMBINANT DNA ADVISORY COMMITTEE (RAC), ZKBS (CENTRAL COMMISSION ON BIOLOGICAL SAFETY), GENETIC ENGINEERING, CTNBio

Keratins Insoluble protective or structural proteins consisting of parallel polypeptide chains arranged in an α-helical or β-conformation.

Ketose A simple monosaccharide having its carbonyl groups at a position other than a terminal position.

See also MONOSACCHARIDES

Killer T Cell See CYTOTOXIC T CELLS

Kilobase Pairs (Kbp) A unit of DNA equal to 1000 base pairs.

See also BASE PAIR (bp), DEOXYRIBONUCLEIC ACID (DNA)

Kilodalton (kDa) A unit of mass equal to 1000 Da.

See also DALTON

Kinase Assays Refers to a variety of assays (e.g., radiolabeling, antibody-binding assays, etc.) that are utilized to assess the biological activity of compounds (e.g., certain pharmaceuticals) against kinases.

For example, the pharmaceutical Gleevec™ (imatinib mesylate) inhibits the kinase known as **Bcr-Ab1 tyrosine kinase,** which can cause excessive production of white blood cells (leukemia) if unchecked.

See also ASSAY, BIOASSAY, RADIOLABELED, LABEL (RADIOACTIVE), ANTIBODY, RADIOIMMUNOASSAY, GENE,

K

GENE EXPRESSION ANALYSIS, ENZYME, KINASES, GLEEVEC™, WHITE BLOOD CELLS, KINOME

Kinases A category of enzymes that (assist or facilitate) transfer of "phosphoryl groups" (from a molecule to another that is "targeted" by that kinase).

The subcategory known as **MAP kinases (MAPK)** help transfer certain "signals" from the cell's exterior (receptors) to its nucleus (thereby causing phosphorylation of certain protein molecules in the nucleus), resulting in changes to the cell's protein-synthesizing processes. That "transfer" occurs via a **cascade** in which each of a **series** of kinases transfers a phosphoryl group to another molecule that is itself a kinase (and that kinase then passes it to another kinase, etc.).

Such kinases signaling cascades are involved in cell apoptosis, differentiation, transcription, and other cellular processes.

See also ENZYME, PHOSPHORYLATION, PROTEIN, PROTEIN KINASES, CELL, RECEPTORS, SIGNAL TRANSDUCTION, CASCADE, MITOGEN-ACTIVATED PROTEIN KINASE CASCADE, MAPK, TYROSINE KINASE, GLEEVEC™, NUCLEUS, TYROSINE KINASE INHIBITORS (TKI), APOPTOSIS, TRANSCRIPTION, KNOCKIN, CELL DIFFERENTIATION, KINOME, AMYLOID B PROTEIN (ABP)

Kinesin A contractile (i.e., periodically contracting) protein (also called "motor protein") within cells, which transports cellular "cargo" such as vesicles or proteins complexed with chaperones along microtubules (string-like structures) within the cell. Some viruses (e.g., *Vaccinia*) also utilize kinesin to transport their viral core particle (i.e., following replication of the viral DNA in cell's nucleus) to the surface of the cell, where it is released, to infect new cells.

See also PROTEIN, CELL, VESICLE, CHAPERONES, MICROTUBULES, VIRUS, NUCLEUS, DEOXYRIBONUCLEIC ACID (DNA)

Kinome Refers to the set of all kinases present within the cells of a given organism (some time in its lifetime). For example, the human kinome is currently known to contain approximately 520 kinases. Plus, knowledge of each

kinase's function, its gene expression or activation pattern in different types of tissue (diseased and normal), and each kinase's substrate (i.e., what it chemically acts upon).

See also KINASES, KINASE ASSAYS, ENZYME, PROTEIN, CELL, GENE, GENETIC MAP, GENOMICS, ORGANISM, FUNCTIONAL GENOMICS, GENE EXPRESSION ANALYSIS, PROTEIN INTERACTION ANALYSIS, SUBSTRATE (CHEMICAL)

Knockdown Refers to a scientist's alteration of a particular gene within an organism so that the specific gene may subsequently **not be expressed** or be expressed only under (controlled) conditions selected by that scientist.

See also GENE, ORGANISM, EXPRESS, EXPRESSIVITY, RNA INTERFERENCE (RNAi), SHORT INTERFERING RNA (siRNA), SHORT HAIRPIN RNA, KNOCKOUT, HOMOLOGOUS RECOMBINATION, TRANSFECTION

Knockin Refers to a scientist's alteration of a particular gene within an organism so that specific organism gains a desired function (e.g., to be able to produce a therapeutic protein in its mammary gland, etc.).

For example, an **ASKA gene** can be "knocked in" to laboratory mice, in which the ASKA (i.e., analog sensitive kinase allele) gene codes for a kinase (in the mouse's cells) which is susceptible to modulation by certain compounds such as chemical analogs of kinases.

See also GENE, ORGANISM, PROTEIN, KINASES, GENETIC CODE, EXPRESS

Knockout Refers to one of the following:

- A scientist's alteration of a **particular gene** within an organism so that the organism loses a (specific) function (e.g., the ability to produce a given needed clotting factor in its blood, the ability to produce a given allergen in its seeds, etc.).
- The **altered organism** itself (i.e., in which the particular gene has been inactivated as detailed in the preceding text).
- A scientist's alteration of a particular protein (e.g., within an organism's cell) so that protein loses its biological

activity (e.g., the ability to cause blood clotting). That can enable detailed study of which proteins within a cell are responsible for particular diseases, etc.

Such "gene knockout" can be accomplished via any one of several different methods or technologies; such as gene silencing, cosuppression, site-directed mutagenesis (SDM), short interfering RNA (siRNA), etc.

Such "protein knockout" can be accomplished via any one of several different methods or technologies such as laser inactivation, etc.

See also GENE, ORGANISM, PROTEIN, BIOLOGICAL ACTIVITY, CELL, GENE SILENCING, COSUPPRESSION, GPA1, SITE-DIRECTED MUTAGENESIS (SDM), LASER INACTIVATION, RNA INTERFERENCE (RNAi), REDUCED-ALLERGEN SOYBEANS, SHORT INTERFERING RNA (siRNA), PROTEOMICS, DELETIONS, CRE-LOX SYSTEM

Knockout (gene) See KNOCKOUT, GENE SILENCING, GPA1, NUCLEAR TRANSFER, CRE-LOX SYSTEM, DELETIONS, RNA INTERFERENCE (RNAi)

Knottins Refers to a structural category of molecules, whose (molecule) shape resembles a knot in a rope. It was first discovered in 1982.

Examples of knottins include EETI (Ecballium elaterium trypsin inhibitors).

See also EETI

KO Acronym for **Kusabira Orange.**

See also KUSABIRA ORANGE

Konzo A term used in some countries to refer to **lathyrism.**

See also LATHYRISM, GLUCOSINOLATES

Koseisho The Japanese government agency that must approve new pharmaceutical products for sale within Japan. It is the equivalent of the U.S. Food and Drug Administration.

See also NDA (TO KOSEISHO), FOOD AND DRUG ADMINISTRATION (FDA), COMMITTEE FOR PROPRIETARY MEDICINAL PRODUCTS (CPMP), COMMITTEE ON SAFETY IN MEDICINES, MEDICINES CONTROL AGENCY (MCA), EUROPEAN MEDICINES EVALUATION AGENCY (EMEA), BUNDESGESUNDHEITSAMT (BGA)

Kozak Sequence Refers to the DNA sequence that "surrounds" (both ends of) the ATG start signal (for translation of mRNA).

See also SEQUENCE (OF A DNA MOLECULE), STARTPOINT, MESSENGER RNA (mRNA), DEOXYRIBONUCLEIC ACID (DNA)

Krebs Cycle See CITRIC ACID CYCLE

Kunitz Trypsin Inhibitor (TI) See TRYPSIN INHIBITORS

Kusabira Orange A protein that is naturally present within the stony coral *Fungia concinna*. Kusabira Orange (KO) is utilized by scientists for the following:

- Help visualize thin layers of biological tissue in fluorescence microscopy
- "Mark" certain end points in experiments (at which the orange light signals that end point was reached)

See also FLUORESCENCE, PROTEIN, TRANSFECTION, GENE EXPRESSION MARKERS, REPORTER GENE, TIRF MICROSCOPY

K

L

L-Carnitine See CARNITINE

L-Selectin Also known as the homing receptor. See also SELECTINS, LECTINS, ADHESION MOLECULES

Lab-on-a-Chip Term utilized to refer to microfluidic devices that perform applications such as nucleic acid separations, protein analysis, small-molecule organic synthesis, detection and hybridization of DNA, etc.

See also BIOCHIP, NANOTECHNOLOGY, MICROFLUIDICS, GENOSENSORS, GENE EXPRESSION, BIOSENSORS (ELECTRONIC), BIOSENSORS (CHEMICAL), GENE EXPRESSION ANALYSIS, NUCLEIC ACIDS, PROTEIN, DEOXYRIBONUCLEIC ACID (DNA), HYBRIDIZATION (MOLECULAR GENETICS)

Label (fluorescent) Refers to the practice of "attaching" a fluorophore (i.e., atom or molecule that emits fluorescent light when light of a specific wavelength is shined onto it), thereby enabling that molecule to be tracked later (e.g., when inside living cells).

See also FLUORESCENCE, CELL, FLUOROPHORE, GREEN FLUORESCENT PROTEIN, FLUORESCENCE RESONANCE ENERGY TRANSFER (FRET), LUCIFERASE, FLUORESCENCE-ACTIVATED CELL SORTER (FACS), RAPID PROTEIN FOLDING ASSAY, STREPTAVIDIN

Label (radioactive) A radioactive atom introduced into molecules in order to perform the following:

- Enable observation of that molecule's metabolic transformation (within an organism). For example, if radioactive hydrogen in the form of water (known as deuterium) is supplied to a living cell, a series of "photographs" (e.g., taken via an electron microscope, which has photographic film in it that is sensitive to radiation) will reveal how rapidly the deuterium enters the cell and into what structures within the cell the water is incorporated.

- Enable observation as to which specific substrate within a living organism or cell gets acted upon by a given compound. For example, the radiolabel (isotope) known as **phosphorous-33** can be utilized to determine which substrate gets phosphorylated via a specific kinase (e.g., as a target in an assay).

- Quantify the rate at which certain attached (non)radioactive atoms are introduced into a polymer (e.g., DNA) that is being polymerized (i.e., "manufactured") as part of a biological test or testing process (e.g., QPCR — quantitative PCR, RT-PCR — reverse transcriptase PCR, etc.).

See also AUTORADIOGRAPHY, CELL, DEOXYRIBONUCLEIC ACID (DNA), ORGANISM, SUBSTRATE (CHEMICAL), KINASES, TARGET (OF A THERAPEUTIC AGENT), HIGH-THROUGHPUT SCREENING (HTS), GENE EXPRESSION ANALYSIS, QPCR, RT-PCR, RADIOIMMUNOASSAY, RADIOIMMUNOTECHNIQUE

Labeled (molecules or cells) Also sometimes referred to as **tagged (molecules or cells)**.

See also LABEL (FLUORESCENT), LABEL (RADIOACTIVE), MOLECULAR BEACON, QUANTUM DOT, NANOPARTICLES, MICROARRAY (TESTING), DNA MICROARRAY, CELL, CELL SURFACE ENGINEERING, BIO–BAR CODES, AFFINITY TAG, AFFINITY CHROMATOGRAPHY, EXPRESSED SEQUENCE TAGS (EST), BACTERIAL EXPRESSED SEQUENCE TAGS (BEST), STREPTAVIDIN

Lac Operon An operon in *Escherichia coli (E. coli)* that codes for three enzymes involved in the metabolism of lactose.
See also OPERON, CODING SEQUENCE, *ESCHERICHIA COLIFORM (E. COLI)*

Laccase An oxidase enzyme that can perform the following:

- Break down indigo dye (used in some manufacturing processes for blue jeans).
- Catalyze certain resins (e.g., containing lignin molecules that bear phenolic hydroxyl groups) to "cure" and cause those resins to harden in place, acting as an adhesive. For example, the numerous small pieces of the so-called waste wood from lumber companies can be heated to approximately 200°C (392°F), whereupon the lignin within the wood fibers breaks into smaller molecules that bear some phenolic hydroxyl groups. Addition of laccase under appropriate conditions then results in phenoxy radical molecules, which cause the lignin-and-wood-fiber combination to harden (e.g., into a useful wood product such as a sheet of siding, within a pressurized mold).

See also ENZYME, CATALYST, LIGNINS, OXIDATION (CHEMICAL REACTION)

Lachrymal Fluid (Tears) A salty solution produced by the tear glands to bathe and lubricate the eye. Possesses antimicrobial properties.

Lactoferricin A protein compound that acts to inhibit pathogenic (i.e., disease-causing) bacteria and yeasts (e.g., in the human body).
See also PROTEIN, PATHOGEN, BACTERIA, YEAST, LACTOFERRIN

Lactoferrin A protein compound that is naturally produced in human breast milk. Also found within specific granules inside neutrophils and leukocytes, and produced in cow's milk. Consumption of lactoferrin by infants (e.g., via nursing) helps to strengthen their immune system. Consumption of lactoferrin by older humans helps their immune system to resist infectious diseases. Lactoferrin binds

free iron (e.g., in body fluids), thereby denying that iron to pathogenic bacteria (which need that iron to grow or infect).

Pepsin and some other proteases (enzymes) can convert lactoferrin to lactoferricin.
See also PROTEIN, PATHOGEN, BACTERIA, GROWTH (MICROBIAL), LACTOFERRICIN, PEPSIN, PROTEASE, HIGH-LACTOFERRIN RICE, LACTOPEROXIDASE

Lactonase An enzyme that breaks open the lactone ring in (molecular structure of) the mycotoxin **zearalenone**.
See also ENZYME, MYCOTOXIN, ZEARALENONE, TOXIN

Lactoperoxidase A protein compound (enzyme) that acts to inhibit pathogenic bacteria (e.g., in human body).
See also PROTEIN, ENZYME, PATHOGEN, BACTERIA

Lambda Bacteriophage See LAMBDA PHAGE

Lambda Phage A bacteriophage that infects *Escherichia coli (E. coli)*. It is commonly used as a vector in recombinant DNA (deoxyribonucleic acid) research.
See also PHAGE, *ESCHERICHIA COLIFORM (E. COLI)*

Langerhans Cells See DENDRITIC LANGERHANS CELLS, ISLETS OF LANGERHANS

Laser Capture Microdissection Abbreviated LCM, it refers to a methodology in which a scientist is able to extract (e.g., from living tissue) a very specific type of cell.

In the LCM procedure, the scientist covers the relevant area of tissue with a special thin thermoplastic film. Using a microscope, the scientist then shines a pulse of applicable-wavelength laser beam onto the desired cell, which causes the plastic film to fuse onto that cell. When the plastic film is subsequently lifted, the desired or fused cells are lifted out of the tissue.

LCM enables scientists to biopsy or analyze rare cells (e.g., certain malignant cells), for comparison with others (e.g., nonmalignant cells). LCM enables scientists to preserve the cell's original structure and intact molecular composition for analysis (e.g., of transcription and translation products).
See also CELL, TRANSCRIPTION, TRANSLATION

L

Laser Inactivation Refers to a "protein knockout" technique in which a chromophore (i.e., chemical that is "triggered" to react by light shined onto it) is first chemically bound to a certain protein molecule; then, a specific-wavelength laser beam is shined onto that protein-chromophore complex in order to inactivate that protein. Such inactivation results in loss of biological activity of that protein.

See also PROTEIN, KNOCKOUT, DENATURATION, CONFORMATION, PROTEIN FOLDING, PROTEIN STRUCTURE, BIOLOGICAL ACTIVITY

Lathyrism See GLUCOSINOLATES

Laurate A medium-chain-length (i.e., C12) fatty acid that is naturally produced by coconut trees, oil palm trees, and certain species of wild plants. In 1992, some canola varieties were genetically engineered so that they could also produce (desirable) laurate in their seeds.

See also FATTY ACID, FATS, CANOLA, GENETIC ENGINEERING, GENETIC CODE, LPAAT PROTEIN, ACP, LAUROYL-ACP THIOESTERASE, HIGH-LAURATE CANOLA

Lauric Acid See LAURATE

Lauroyl-ACP Thioesterase The enzyme that is required for the synthesis ("manufacturing") of laurate in plants. For example, the presence of this enzyme in the California bay tree (*Umbellularia californica*) causes its seed oil to contain as much as 45% laurate.

See also LAURATE, ENZYME, LPAAT PROTEIN, HIGH-LAURATE CANOLA

Lazaroids A class of drugs being developed to "bring back from the dead" tissues that have been (almost) killed due to a lack of oxygen (e.g., caused by a clot blocking a vital artery).

See also HUMAN SUPEROXIDE DISMUTASE (hSOD), FIBRIN, REPERFUSION

LCM Acronym for **laser capture microdissection**.

See LASER CAPTURE MICRODISSECTION

LCPUFA Acronym for **long-chain polyunsaturated fatty acids** such as the essential fatty acids eicosapentanoic acid (EPA) and docosahexanoic acid (DHA).

See also ESSENTIAL FATTY ACIDS, EICOSAPENTANOIC ACID (EPA), DOCOSAHEXANOIC ACID (DHA)

LD Acronym for **linkage disequilibrium**.

See LINKAGE DISEQUILIBRIUM

LDL See LOW-DENSITY LIPOPROTEINS (LDLP)

LDLP See LOW-DENSITY LIPOPROTEINS (LDLP)

LDLP Receptors See LOW-DENSITY LIPOPROTEINS (LDLP)

Leader See LEADER SEQUENCE

Leader Sequence (mRNA) The nontranslated sequence at the 5 end of mRNA that precedes the initiation codon.

See also MESSENGER RNA (mRNA), CODON

Leader Sequence (protein molecule) A short sequence of amino acids within a given protein molecule that determines **where** within a living cell that particular protein molecule will "reside."

See also PROTEIN, AMINO ACID, HAPERONES, SEQUENCE (OF A PROTEIN MOLECULE)

Leaky Mutants A mutant in which the mutated gene product, such as an enzyme, still possesses a fraction of its normal biological activity.

See also MUTATION, GENE, PROTEIN, BIOLOGICAL ACTIVITY, ENZYME

Lear See CANOLA

Lecithin From the Greek *lekithos*, which means "egg yolk."

See LECITHIN (Crude, Mixture), LECITHIN (Refined, Specific)

Lecithin (crude, mixture) A mixture of phospholipids (i.e., lecithin-phosphatidylcholine, cephalin, inositol phosphatides, glycerides, tocopherols, glucosides, and certain pigments). Historically, crude (mixture) lecithin has often been utilized commercially in food processing as an emulsifier, instantizing agent, and lubricating agent. Because lecithin-phosphatidylcholine naturally has a high content of linoleic acid, its consumption by humans results in a similar impact (e.g., lowered cholesterol levels in blood) as consumption of linoleic acid.

Because dietary fats are generally not absorbed directly through the intestinal wall (when eaten), they must first be emulsified to form micelles that can pass through the intestinal wall and thus be absorbed by the body. That

L

emulsification and micelle formation is aided by lecithin because it is an emulsifier. Lecithin itself (also known as phosphatidylcholine) is a source of choline when digested, and is a critical component of the lipoproteins that transport fat and cholesterol molecules in the bloodstream (e.g., from the digestive system, to body cells, to and from the liver, etc.).

Lecithin (phosphatidylcholine) promotes synthesis of high-density lipoproteins (HDLP, also known as "**good**" **cholesterol**) by the liver, when lecithin is consumed by humans, thereby helping to lower blood levels of low-density lipoproteins (LDLP, also known as "**bad**" **cholesterol**).

See also LECITHIN (refined, specific), LIPOPROTEIN, LIPIDS, CONJUGATED PROTEIN, HIGH-DENSITY LIPOPROTEINS (HDLP), LOW-DENSITY LIPOPROTEINS (LDLP), SOYBEAN PLANT, SOYBEAN OIL, CHOLINE, SIGNAL TRANSDUCTION, LINOLEIC ACID, ACETYLCHOLINE, FATS, MICELLE, DIGESTION (WITHIN ORGANISMS), CHOLESTEROL, BILE ACIDS

Lecithin (refined, specific) A by-product of the refining process for soybean oil (deoiled lecithin from processed soybeans is composed of approximately 20 to 25% phosphatidyl choline by weight). The lecithin molecule (i.e., phosphatidyl choline) naturally has a high content of linoleic acid, so consumption of lecithin by humans results in a similar impact (e.g., lowered cholesterol levels in blood) as consumption of linoleic acid.

Because dietary fats are generally not absorbed directly through the intestinal wall (when eaten), they must first be emulsified to form micelles that can pass through the intestinal wall and be absorbed by the body. That emulsification and micelle formation is aided by lecithin because it is an emulsifier. Lecithin (also known as phosphatidylcholine) is a source of choline when digested, and is a critical component of the lipoproteins that transport fat and cholesterol molecules in the bloodstream (e.g., from the digestive system, to body cells, to and from the liver, etc.).

Lecithin (phosphatidylcholine) promotes synthesis of high-density lipoproteins (i.e., HDLP, also known as "**good**" **cholesterol**) by the liver, when it is consumed by humans, thereby helping to lower blood levels of low-density lipoproteins (LDLP, also known as "**bad**" cholesterol).

Phosphatidyl choline (PC) is involved in cell signal transduction (e.g., via which a cell reacts to an external chemical "signal").

Some other common dietary sources of lecithin include eggs, red meats, spinach, and nuts.

See also LIPOPROTEIN, LIPIDS, CONJUGATED PROTEIN, HIGH-DENSITY LIPOPROTEINS (HDLP), LOW-DENSITY LIPOPROTEINS (LDLP), SOYBEAN PLANT, SOYBEAN OIL, CHOLINE, SIGNAL TRANSDUCTION, LINOLEIC ACID, ACETYLCHOLINE, LECITHIN (crude, mixture), FATS, MICELLE, DIGESTION (WITHIN ORGANISMS), CHOLESTEROL

Lectins A class of glycoproteins that have the capability to rapidly (and reversibly) combine with *specific* sugar molecules (e.g., those sugar molecules or glycoproteins on the surface of adjacent cells, within an organism). Lectins are a common component of the surface (membranes) of plant and animal cells and are so specific regarding sugar molecules that they will or will not combine with or attach to that they discriminate between different monosaccharides *and* different oligosaccharides (i.e., on the surfaces of adjacent cells within an organism).

This capability to reversibly combine with sugar (i.e., carbohydrate) molecules (on the surface of adjacent cells) is utilized by the following:

- Bacteria and other microorganisms, to adhere to (sugar molecules on surface of) host cells, as the first step in the process of infecting those host cells.
- White blood cells (e.g., lymphocytes), to adhere to the walls of blood vessels (endothelium), as the first step to leaving the bloodstream to go fight infection (pathogens, trauma) in tissue adjacent to that blood vessel. The lectin (glycoprotein) that adheres to the (endothelial sugar molecule on) blood vessel wall is called L-selectin, or the homing receptor. The two sugar molecules (glycoproteins) on the blood

vessel wall (ensothelium) are called P-selectin and E-selectin (also known as ELAM-1)

- Cancerous tumor cells, to adhere to the walls of blood vessels (endothelium) as part of the tumor-proliferation process known as metastasis (i.e., new tumors are "seeded" throughout the body via this process).

Separate and apart from these impacts, some plant lectins (e.g., in the seeds of certain plants) are toxic to some of the animals that consume these seeds.

See also PROTEIN, SUGAR MOLECULES, GLYCOPROTEIN, LEUKOCYTES, CELL, SELECTINS, LYMPHOCYTES, MONOCYTES, NEUTROPHILS, ENDOTHELIAL CELLS, ENDOTHELIUM, CANCER, METASTASIS, SIGNAL TRANSDUCTION, RICIN

Leptin A protein hormone that is produced by fat cells (adipose tissue) in the body (e.g., following consumption of food). When leptin is produced and travels to cells whose surface bears leptin receptors (e.g., in the brain), those brain cells receive signal (transduction) indicating fullness or satiety.

For example, Canadian scientists devised a test to detect which variant (SNP) of the "leptin gene" is possessed by dairy cattle breeding stock. By selecting only cattle possessing the **Leptin-tt** SNP within their DNA (i.e., SNP with lowest level of leptin production), it is expected that such cattle herds will have inherently larger appetites and, thus, larger milk production potential.

Leptin has been found to be present in the bloodstream of obese humans at a concentration of approximately four times that found in bloodstreams of lean humans. High levels of leptin present in the bloodstream disrupt some of the activities of insulin (hormone that regulates blood sugar levels), and may possibly lead to diabetes.

See also HORMONE, ADIPOKINES, PROTEIN, BIOLOGICAL ACTIVITY, GENE, SINGLE-NUCLEOTIDE POLYMORPHISMS (SNPs), INSULIN, ADIPOSE

Leptin Receptors Cellular receptors that are specific to leptin. In 1996, H. Ralph Snodgrass discovered that leptin receptors are involved in the "sorting" of immature blood cells (from bone marrow) to create subpopulations.

See also LEPTIN, RECEPTORS

Lethal Mutation Mutation of a gene to yield no, or a totally defective gene product (protein); thereby making it unable to function, and hence unable to sustain the life of the organism.

See also GENE, PROTEIN, MUTATION

Leucine (Leu) A monocarboxylic essential amino acid.

See also AMINO ACID, ESSENTIAL AMINO ACIDS, ALS GENE

Leukocytes A diverse "family" of nucleated white blood cells (including mast cells) that has many immunological functions.

See also NEUTROPHILS, INTERLEUKINS, EOSINOPHILS, BASOPHILIS, LYMPHOCYTE, B LYMPHOCYTES, MONOCYTES, GRANULOCYTES, MAST CELLS

Leukotrienes Lipid mediator molecules (synthesized from arachidonic acid via 5-lipoxygenase enzyme) that are synthesized and released by certain inflammatory cells (i.e., macrophages, polymorphonuclear leukocytes [PMN], mast cells, and T cells), which "signal" leukocytes (white blood cells) during the initial stages of an infection or an allergic reaction. Their primary mode of action is through certain G-protein-coupled receptors. When thus activated, the leukocytes migrate to the site of infection to combat the pathogens (or allergens), and mediate the inflammation.

See also EICOSANOIDS, LIPIDS, MACROPHAGES, LEUKOCYTES, RECEPTORS, POLYMORPHONUCLEAR LEUKOCYTES (PMN), MAST CELLS, SIGNALING, SIGNAL TRANSDUCTION, T CELLS, PATHOGEN, ARACHIDONIC ACID, ALLERGIES, (FOODBORNE), ALLERGIES (AIRBORNE), SIGNALING MOLECULE, G-PROTEIN-COUPLED RECEPTORS

Levorotary (L) Isomer An isomer of an optically active compound; rotates (when illuminated) the plane of plane-polarized light to the left.

See also STEREOISOMERS, DEXTROROTARY (D) ISOMER

LH See LUTEINIZING HORMONE

Library A set of cloned DNA fragments together representing the entire genome.

L

See also DEOXYRIBONUCLEIC ACID (DNA), GENOME

LIF Acronym for **laser-induced fluorescence.**
See also FLUORESCENCE, FLUORES-CENCE-ACTIVATED CELL SORTER (FACS), FLUORESCENCE *IN SITU* HYBRIDIZATION (FISH), CAPILLARY ELECTROPHORESIS

Ligand (in biochemistry) In general, a molecule or ion that can bind to (interact with) a protein molecule. For example, a pharmaceutical that binds to a receptor protein molecule on the surface of a cell may be called a ligand.

For example, the effector (inside cell) that binds to a G-protein (inside cell) after that G-protein has received (outside the cell) a chemical signal (e.g., via a hormone molecule binding onto the exterior end of a G-protein molecule) may be called a ligand.

See also PROTEIN, RECEPTORS, T CELL RECEPTORS, ENDOCYTOSIS, CD4 PROTEIN, INVASIN, LIGAND (IN CHROMATOGRAPHY), CHELATION, STRUCTURE–ACTIVITY MODELS, G-PROTEINS

Ligand (in chromatography) A term used to describe a substance (the ligand) that has the capacity for specific and noncovalent (reversible) binding to some protein. A ligand may be a coenzyme for a specific enzyme. The ligand can be covalently attached (immobilized) by means of the appropriate chemical reaction to the surface of certain porous column materials. When a mixture of proteins containing the enzyme to be isolated is passed through the column, the enzyme, which is capable of tightly binding to the ligand, does so, and is in this manner held to the column. The other proteins present, which have no specific affinity for the ligand, pass on through the column. The protein or ligand complex is then dissociated and the enzyme eluted from the column, which may be accomplished by passing more free (unbound) coenzyme through the column. The ligand may be hormones (i.e., used to isolate receptor molecules) or any other type of molecule that is capable of binding specifically and reversibly to the desired protein or protein complex.

See also AFFINITY CHROMATOGRAPHY, SUBSTRATE (IN CHROMATOGRAPHY),

CHROMATOGRAPHY, PROTEIN, PEPTIDE, ANTIBODY, MONOCLONAL ANTIBODIES (MAb)

Ligand-Activated Transcription Factors See NUCLEAR RECEPTORS

Ligase An enzyme used to catalyze the joining together (i.e., "ligating") of two separate molecules, in an energy-requiring process. For example, the joining together of two single-stranded DNA segments.

See also DEOXYRIBONUCLEIC ACID (DNA), ENZYME

Ligation The formation of a phosphodiester bond to link two adjacent bases separated by a nick in one strand of a double helix of DNA (deoxyribonucleic acid). The term can also be applied to blunt-end ligation and to the joining of RNA (ribonucleic acid) strands.

See also DEOXYRIBONUCLEIC ACID (DNA), LIGASE, EDITING, SPLICEOSOMES

Light-Chain Variable (VL) Domains The regions (domains) of the antibody (molecule's) "light chain" that vary in their amino acid sequence. The "chains" (of atoms) comprising the antibody (immunoglobulin) molecule consist of a region of variable (V) amino acid sequence and a region in which the amino acid sequence remains constant (C). An antibody molecule possesses two antigen-binding sites, and it is the variable domains of the light (VL) and heavy (VH) chains that contribute to this (antigen-binding ability).

See also ANTIBODY, IMMUNOGLOBULIN, PROTEIN, SEQUENCE (OF A PROTEIN MOLECULE), ANTIGEN, AMINO ACID, COMBINING SITE, DOMAIN (OF A PROTEIN), HEAVY-CHAIN VARIABLE (VH) DOMAINS

Lignans A category of phytochemicals that play defensive roles (e.g., against infections by bacteria, fungi, etc.) within land plants (e.g., those grown for crops). Lignans are also sometimes referred to by some people as "**phytoestrogens,**" and are typically beneficial to the health of humans who consume them. Lignans are found in virtually all fruits, vegetables, and cereals (grains), generally in the seed coats, stems, leaves, or flowers. Some of the beneficial lignans commonly consumed by humans include the following:

L

- **Sesamin**, found in seeds of the sesame plant (*Sesamum indicum*), which acts as an antioxidant
- The lignans that are found in seeds of the flax plant (*Linum usitatissimum*), and the rye plant

See also PHYTOCHEMICALS, PHYTOESTROGENS, ISOFLAVONES, ANTIOXIDANTS, OXIDATIVE STRESS

Lignins A category of **phenolic** (ring-shaped molecules) **polymeric** (i.e., composed of more than one molecular unit) **compounds** produced by land plants within the cell walls (i.e., exterior of the cell's plasma membrane) of those plants, to reinforce or strengthen those cell walls.
See also CELL, POLYMER, PLASMA MEMBRANE

Lignocellulose A complex biopolymer comprising the bulk of woody plants. It consists of polysaccharides and polymer phenols.
See also POLYSACCHARIDES, LIGNINS

Limonene See PHYTOCHEMICALS

Linkage A phenomenon discovered by Thomas Hunt Morgan in the early 1900s via his experiments with fruit flies. This term describes the tendency of genes to be inherited together as a result of their locations being physically close to each other on the same chromosome; measured by percentage recombination between loci. Because the locus (i.e., location of gene on the chromosome) determines the likelihood that two genes will go together into the offspring genome, "marker genes" that are linked to a gene (e.g., for a given trait or disease) of interest can be utilized to predict the presence of that (trait- or disease-causing) gene.
See also GENE, LOCUS, CHROMOSOMES, LINKAGE GROUP, MARKER (GENETIC MARKER), MAP DISTANCE, LINKAGE MAP, HAPLOTYPE, GENOME

Linkage Disequilibrium See LINKAGE MAP

Linkage Group Includes all loci (in a DNA molecule) that can be connected (directly or indirectly) by linkage relationships; equivalent to a chromosome.
See also LOCUS, CHROMOSOMES, LINKAGE, CHROMATIDS, CHROMATIN, LINKAGE MAP, DEOXYRIBONUCLEIC ACID (DNA)

Linkage Map A depiction of gene loci (on chromosomes) based on the frequency of recombination (of linked genes) in the offspring's genome. Close (linked) genes tend to be inherited **together**.
When that does not happen (i.e., fewer linked-together genes inherited across generations than would be expected from mathematical prediction), the phenomenon is known as **linkage disequilibrium**.
See also LINKAGE, LINKAGE GROUP, GENE, LOCUS, MARKER (GENETIC MARKER), GENOME

Linker A short synthetic duplex oligonucleotide containing the target site for some restriction enzyme. It may be added to the ends of a DNA (deoxyribonucleic acid) fragment prepared by cleavage with some other enzyme reconstructions of recombinant DNA.

Linking The process of "attaching" a drug or a toxin to a monoclonal antibody, or another homing molecule of the immune system. Because this attachment must be reversible, so that the homing molecule can release the drug or toxin after delivering that drug or toxin to the desired site in the body (e.g., delivery of a toxin to a tumor to kill the tumor), linking is a difficult process to achieve reliably.
See also IMMUNOTOXIN, CONJUGATE, MONOCLONAL ANTIBODIES (MAb), TOXIN

Linoleic Acid One of the so-called "**omega-6**" (n-6) polyunsaturated fatty acids (PUFA), it has historically constituted approximately 53% of the total fatty acid content of soybean oil. It is an essential fatty acid for humans. When consumed by humans, linoleic acid causes **LDLP cholesterol** levels in the blood to decrease, which reduces risk of coronary heart disease (CHD). The human body converts linoleic acid to the n-6 highly unsaturated fatty acid (HUFA), **arachidonic acid**.
See also POLYUNSATURATED FATTY ACIDS (PUFA), N-6 FATTY ACIDS, FATS, UNSATURATED FATTY ACIDS, ESSENTIAL FATTY ACIDS, LOW-DENSITY LIPOPROTEINS (LDLP), CHOLESTEROL, LECITHIN, CONJUGATED LINOLEIC ACID (CLA), CORONARY HEART DISEASE

L

(CHD), VOLICITIN, SOYBEAN OIL, ARACHIDONIC ACID, COSUPPRESSION

Linolenic Acid The nutritionally relevant form (i.e., an essential fatty acid) is known as α-linolenic acid. One of the so-called "**omega-3**" (n-3) polyunsaturated fatty acids (PUFA), it has historically constituted approximately 8% of the total fatty acid content of soybean oil. It is an essential fatty acid for humans (i.e., required by the human body).

The human body converts linolenic acid to the n-3 highly unsaturated fatty acids (HUFA) **docosahexanoic acid (DHA)** and **eicosapentanoic acid (EPA)**. When consumed by humans, both DHA and EPA each confer various health benefits.

See also n-3 FATTY ACIDS, POLYUNSATURATED FATTY ACIDS (PUFA), UNSATURATED FATTY ACIDS, ESSENTIAL FATTY ACIDS, CORONARY HEART DISEASE (CHD), CANCER, HIGHLY UNSATURATED FATTY ACIDS (HUFA), DOCOSAHEXANOIC ACID (DHA), EICOSAPENTANOIC ACID (EPA), FATS, GENE, FAD3 GENE, HIGH–LINOLENIC OIL SOYBEANS

Lipase An enzyme (one of a class of enzymes) that catalyzes the hydrolytic cleavage of lipid molecules (triglycerides) to yield free fatty acids. A lipase was the first enzyme to be produced via genetic engineering and marketed. Lipase also occurs naturally in cow's milk and in the intestines of many animals (where it aids or assists digestion of fats that the animal consumes).

For example, the two lipase enzymes known as **HSL (hormone-sensitive lipase)** and **ATGL (adipose triglyceride lipase)** are utilized by the human body to metabolize fats.

See also ENZYME, HYDROLYTIC CLEAVAGE, TRIGLYCERIDES, FATS, ADIPOSE, FATTY ACID, FREE FATTY ACIDS, DIGESTION (WITHIN ORGANISMS), METABOLISM

Lipid Bilayer A membrane (i.e., thin-sheet-type) structure composed of relatively small lipid molecules that possess both a **hydrophilic** (i.e., "water-loving") and a **hydrophobic** (i.e., "water-hating") moiety. Thus, these (membrane) lipids spontaneously form closed bimolecular sheets in aqueous (water-containing) media, in which the hydrophobic ends of each lipid molecule are in the center of the bimolecular membrane, and the hydrophilic ends of the lipid molecules are on the outside (i.e., touching the water molecules).

See also LIPIDS, PLASMA MEMBRANE, MOIETY

Lipid Rafts Specific domains ("islands") within a mammal cell's plasma membrane in which are embedded certain receptors or whole functional systems (e.g., signaling systems, amino acid transport systems, etc.).

See also CELL, LIPIDS, PLASMA MEMBRANE, MEMBRANE TRANSPORT, AMINO ACID, TRANSMEMBRANE PROTEINS, G-PROTEINS, RECEPTORS, NUCLEAR RECEPTORS, LIVER X RECEPTORS (LXR), FARNESOID X RECEPTORS (FXR), RETINOID X RECEPTORS (RXR), SIGNALING, SIGNAL TRANSDUCTION

Lipid Sensors See ORPHAN RECEPTORS

Lipid Vesicles See LIPOSOMES

Lipidomics The scientific study of an organism's lipids and their role in the organism's structure, metabolism, growth, health, and disease (or its resistance to disease, etc.). Some methods utilized to determine which impact results from which lipid are as follows:

- LIPID PROFILING — determination of the identities of each lipid present within a cell or tissue or organism (e.g., via mass spectrometry techniques such as MALDI-TOF-MS, etc.) and the function of each lipid.
- METABOLITE PROFILING — determination of the specific metabolic pathways (or related genes) that are "switched on," inhibited, etc., within a cell or tissue or organism (e.g., by the presence of a particular lipid).

See also LIPIDS, CELL, LIPID BILAYER, LIPASE, PLASMA MEMBRANE, FATS, LIPID SENSORS, LIPOPROTEIN, METABOLISM, MASS SPECTROMETER, MALDI-TOF-MS, PATHWAY, METABOLIC PATHWAY, METABOLITE PROFILING, GENE, ORGANISM

Lipids From the Greek word *Lipos* (fat), lipids are water-insoluble (fat) biomolecules that are highly soluble in organic solvents such as chloroform. Lipids serve as "fuel" molecules in organisms, as highly concentrated energy stores, as "signaling" molecules, and are fundamental components of cell membranes. Lipids also play important roles in signal transduction, gene transcription, and intracellular transport (e.g., movement of certain protein molecules from one part of a cell to another).

Membrane lipids are relatively small molecules that have both a hydrophilic (i.e., "water-loving") and a hydrophobic (i.e., "water-hating") moiety. These (membrane) lipids spontaneously form closed bimolecular sheets in aqueous media (water) that are barriers to the free movement (flow) of polar molecules.

See also FATS, MOIETY, LIPOPROTEIN, CHOLESTEROL, CELL, SIGNALING, SIGNALING MOLECULE, SIGNAL TRANSDUCTION, PLASMA MEMBRANE, MEMBRANE TRANSPORT, PHOSPHATIDYL SERINE, ANTIOXIDANTS, OXIDATIVE STRESS, LIPID BILAYER, LEUKOTRIENES, OLEOSOMES, GENE, TRANSCRIPTION, LIPID RAFTS, MEDIUM-CHAIN TRIACYLGLYCERIDES, LIPIDOMICS

Lipolytic Enzymes See LIPASE

Lipophilic A "fat-loving" molecule, or portion of a molecule. Relating to, or having a strong affinity for fats or other lipids.

See also LIPIDS, FATS

Lipopolysaccharide (LPS) See ENDOTOXIN

Lipoprotein A conjugated protein containing a lipid or a group of lipids. For example, **low-density lipoproteins (also known as "bad" cholesterol) are a "package" of cholesterol (lipid) surrounded by a hydrophilic protein.**

Low-density lipoproteins (LDLPs) and very-low-density lipoproteins (VLDLs) are the specific lipoproteins that are most likely to deposit cholesterol (plaque) on artery walls, which increases risk of coronary heart disease (CHD).

See also PROTEIN, LOW-DENSITY LIPOPROTEINS (LDLP), VERY-LOW-DENSITY LIPOPROTEINS (VLDL), CONJUGATED PROTEIN, HYDROPHILIC, LIPIDS, CHOLESTEROL, APOLIPOPROTEINS

Lipoprotein-Associated Coagulation (Clot) Inhibitor (LACI) A protein that prevents formation of blood clots. This occurs because LACI inhibits the controlled series of zymogen activations (enzymatic cascade) that cause the formation of fibrinogen (precursor to fibrin), subsequently leading to clot formation.

See also FIBRIN, FIBRONECTIN, ZYMOGENS

Liposomes Also called lipid vesicles or vesicle. Aqueous (i.e., watery) compartments enclosed by a lipid bilayer. They can be formed by suspending a suitable lipid, such as phosphatidyl choline, in an aqueous medium. This mixture is then sonicated (i.e., agitated by high-frequency sound waves) to give a dispersion of closed vesicles (i.e., compartments) that are quite uniform in size. Alternatively, liposomes can be prepared by rapidly mixing a solution of lipid in ethanol with water, which yields vesicles that are nearly spherical in shape and have a diameter of 500 Å. Larger vesicles (10,000 Å or 1 μm, or 0.00003937 in. in diameter) can be prepared by slowly evaporating the organic solvent from a suspension of phospholipid in a mixed solvent system. Liposomes can be made to contain certain drugs for protective, controlled-release delivery to targeted tissues. For example, pharmaceuticals that tend to be rapidly degraded in the bloodstream could be enclosed within liposomes so that more of the nondegraded pharmaceutical would remain by the time it reached the targeted tissue. The controlled-release property enables larger doses (of drugs possessing toxic side effects) to be prescribed, knowing that the drug will be released in the body over an extended period of time.

See also LIPIDS, MICRON, ANGSTROM (Å)

Lipoxidase See LIPOXYGENASE (LOX)

Lipoxygenase (LOX) A family of enzymes that include the following:

- At least one (i.e., 5-lipoxygenase) that is naturally produced within humans and some other animals; it is the primary enzyme utilized for their synthesis of leukotrienes. **See LEUKOTRIENES**.
- At least three (LOX-1, LOX-2, LOX-3) that are naturally produced within some plants. For example, lipoxygenase enzymes are produced in the seeds

L

(soybeans) of the soybean plant (*Glycine max* (L.) Merrill). Among other purposes, some lipoxygenase enzymes are utilized by some plants in their defense against certain pest insects.

For example, in response to such insects chewing on the *Nicotiana attenuata* plant, that plant expresses **lipoxygenase-3** and certain other enzymes that cause production (via oxylipin pathways) of jasmonic acid, which triggers specific plant defenses (e.g., systemic acquired resistance, etc.).

In the presence of moisture and certain other conditions, lipoxygenase enzymes catalyze a chemical reaction in which objectionable "beany" flavor can be produced from certain components of the soybean. That "beany" flavor decreases the suitability of resultant soybean raw material for the manufacture of human foods in some countries.

Prevention of the reactions that create the "beany" flavor can be accomplished via heat denaturation (of lipoxygenases present in the soybeans) or via creation of soybeans that do not contain any lipoxygenase enzymes (known as "LOX null" soybeans). Lipoxygenase enzymes also catalyze a reaction in which certain volatile chemicals are produced that inhibit growth of the *Aspergillus flavus* fungus.

See also ENZYME, LEUKOTRIENES, SOYBEAN PLANT, EXPRESS, JASMONIC ACID, CASCADE, JASMONATE CASCADE, PATHWAY, SYSTEMIC ACQUIRED RESISTANCE (SAR), LOX NULL SOYBEANS, LOX-1, LOX-2, LOX-3

Lipoxygenase Null See LOX NULL SOYBEANS, LIPOXYGENASE (LOX)

Listeria monocytogenes Refers to the family (numerous strains) of *Listeria monocytogenes* bacteria, that can grow in many different foodstuffs (e.g., meats, cheese) under specific conditions, and can cause food poisoning (listeriosis) in humans who subsequently consume these foodstuffs.

When consumed by humans, certain strains or serotypes of *Listeria monocytogenes* can cause fever, severe headaches, stiffness, nausea, diarrhea, and, possibly, miscarriages in pregnant women. Following infection of human cells by

Listeria monocytogenes, that bacteria is able to "commandeer" action in those cells, to be transported quickly within those cells (to multiply and further infect). As of January 19, 2001, all meat processed in the U.S. is required to be tested for the presence of *Listeria monocytogenes*. Recent research indicates that growth of *Listeria monocytogenes* in dairy products can be inhibited by the presence of the compound **pediocin**, which is produced by some bacteria (e.g., *L. plantarum*).

See also BACTERIA, STRAIN, SEROTYPES, CELL, ACTIN, ENTEROTOXIN, BACTERIOCINS, CADHERINS

Live Cell Array Refers to a microarray (e.g., a piece of glass, plastic, or silicon) onto which has been attached a number of living cells that are subsequently utilized to bioassay (e.g., a pharmaceutical, a toxin, etc.).

See also CELL, BIOASSAY, CELL ARRAY, MICROARRAY (TESTING), BIOSENSORS (CHEMICAL), TOXICOGENOMICS, HIGH-THROUGHPUT SCREENING (HTS)

Liver X Receptors (LXR) Refers to nuclear receptors that are primarily present within the body's tissues engaged in lipid metabolism (i.e., liver, kidney, lung, intestine, adrenals, macrophage, and adipose tissues).

Elevated levels (in the body) of certain sterols (e.g., 24(*S*), 25-epoxycholesterol or 27-hydroxycholesterol, etc.) activate the LXRs. This causes the LXRs to act as **cholesterol sensors**, transactivating a "family" of genes that collectively control the catabolism (i.e., breakdown to yield energy), transport, and elimination of cholesterol.

See also NUCLEAR RECEPTORS, LIPIDS, CHOLESTEROL, METABOLISM, MACROPHAGES, ADIPOSE, STEROLS, PROTEIN, TRANSACTIVATION, TRANSACTIVATING PROTEIN, GENE, CATABOLISM

Living Modified Organism (LMO) See GMO

LMO (Living Modified Organism) See GMO

Loci The plural of **locus**.

See LOCUS

Locus The position of a gene on a chromosome.

See also GENE, CHROMOSOMES

LOI Acronym for **loss of imprinting**.

See IMPRINTING

Long Terminal Repeat Refers to a particular sequence of (repeated) nucleotides that appear within the end portion or segment of a retrovirus element that was incorporated into the DNA of a (host) organism.

See also SEQUENCE (OF A DNA MOLECULE), DEOXYRIBONUCLEIC ACID (DNA), NUCLEOTIDE, RETROVIRUSES, ORGANISM

Loop A single-stranded region at the end of a hairpin in RNA (or single-stranded DNA). It corresponds to the sequence between inverted repeats in duplex DNA.

See also RIBONUCLEIC ACID (RNA), DEOXYRIBONUCLEIC ACID (DNA), SEQUENCE (OF A DNA MOLECULE)

LOSBM Low-oligosaccharide soybean meal.

See also LOW-STACHYOSE SOYBEANS, SOYBEAN PLANT

Loss of Imprinting See IMPRINTING

Loss-of-Function Mutations See MUTATION, KNOCKOUT, GENE SILENCING, FUNCTIONAL GENOMICS, RNA INTERFERENCE (RNAi)

Low-Density Lipoproteins (LDLP) The so-called "bad" cholesterol (i.e., LDL cholesterol), which carries cholesterol molecules from the digestive system (e.g., intestine) to body cells and can sometimes clog arteries over time (a disease called atherosclerosis or coronary heart disease). As cholesterol does not dissolve in water (which constitutes most of the volume of blood), the body turns LDL cholesterol (derived from the digestion of fatty foods) into little "packages" surrounded by a hydrophilic (i.e., "water-loving") protein. That protein "wrapper" is known as apolipoprotein B-100, or apo B-100, and it enables LDL cholesterol to be transported in the bloodstream because the apolipoprotein B-100 is attracted to water molecules in the blood. Part of the apolipoprotein B-100 molecule also will bind to special LDLP receptor molecules in the liver, which then clears those (bound) cholesterol packages out of the body as part of regular liver functions.

See also HIGH-DENSITY LIPOPROTEINS (HDLPs), HYDROPHILIC, RECEPTORS, PROTEIN, SITOSTANOL, ISOFLAVONES, WATER-SOLUBLE FIBER, CHOLESTEROL,

CORONARY HEART DISEASE (CHD), APOLIPOPROTEINS, VERY-LOW-DENSITY LIPOPROTEINS (VLDL)

Low–Linolenic-Oil Soybeans Soybeans from soybean (*Glycine max*) plant varieties that have been bred specifically to produce soybeans bearing oil that contains less than 4% linolenic acid, instead of the typical 8% linolenic acid content of soybean oil produced from traditional varieties of soybeans.

Low-linolenic soybean oil would tend to have greater flavor stability (especially at elevated temperatures utilized in frying foods) than soybean oil from traditional varieties of soybeans.

See also SOYBEAN PLANT, SOYBEAN OIL, FATTY ACID, LINOLENIC ACID, POLYUNSATURATED FATTY ACIDS (PUFA)

Low-Lipoxygenase Soybeans See LOX NULL SOYBEANS

Low-Phytate Corn Developed in the U.S. during the 1990s, these are corn (maize) hybrids possessing the Lpa1 gene, the Lpa2 gene, or the HAP (highly available phosphorous) gene (which was discovered by Victor Raboy). That gene causes corn (maize) hybrids possessing it to produce much less phytate than the 0.15% typically present in traditional varieties of corn (maize). Because phytate is not digestible in humans and other monogastric animals (e.g., swine, poultry, etc.), substituting low-phytate corn in place of traditional corn varieties in those animals' diets helps to lessen adverse environmental impact of animal feeding (e.g., phosphorous emissions in excess of annual cropland requirements).

Swine fed a diet in which traditional corn (maize) varieties have been replaced by low-phytate corn (maize) produce up to 30% less phosphorous in their manure, thereby lessening the phosphorous impact of those swine on the environment. Humans consuming a diet based heavily on corn or maize (e.g., tortillas) absorb 50% more iron when traditional corn varieties are replaced by low-phytate corn varieties. That is because the phytate (inositol hexaphosphate) molecule "binds" or chelates iron (and some other metals) within the digestive system and prevents their absorption into the body.

See also CORN, PHYTATE, HIGH-PHYTASE CORN, PHYTASE, VALUE-ENHANCED

L

GRAINS, HIGHLY AVAILABLE PHOS-PHOROUS (HAP) GENE, CHELATION, CHELATING AGENT, IRON DEFICIENCY ANEMIA (IDA)

Low-Phytate Soybeans Developed in the U.S. during the 1990s, these are soybean varieties possessing less than 0.3% (of total soybean weight) phytate, vs. the typical 0.6% phytate content of soybeans from traditional soybean varieties.

One type of low-phytate soybean is derived via a single recessive mutation (i.e., an SNP) in the gene that codes for seed-expressed **myo-inositol l-phosphate synthase**.

Because phytate (myo-inositol hexaphosphate) is not digestible in humans and other monogastric animals (e.g., swine, poultry, etc.), substituting low-phytate soybeans in place of traditional soybean varieties in those animals' diets helps to lessen adverse environmental impact of animal feeding (e.g., manure phosphorous emissions in excess of cropland requirements).

Swine fed a diet in which traditional soybean varieties have been replaced by low-phytate soybeans produce up to 20% less phosphorous in their manure, thereby lessening the phosphorous impact on the environment. Because the amino acids lysine, methionine, cysteine, arginine, and threonine all become more "bioavailable" (i.e., available for the animal to build its body tissue, or otherwise utilize) in a low-phytate diet, such diets also help reduce excess nitrogen emissions.

See also SOYBEAN PLANT, PHYTATE, MUTATION, GENE, SINGLE-NUCLEOTIDE POLYMORPHISMS (SNPs), RECESSIVE ALLELE, LOW-PHYTATE CORN, HIGH-PHYTASE CORN/SOYBEANS, LYSINE, CYSTEINE, METHIONINE, ARGININE (Arg), THREONINE, DEAMINATION

Low-Stachyose Soybeans Those soybean varieties that contain lower-than-1% levels of the relatively indigestible stachyose carbohydrate (and, thus, higher levels of easily digestible other nutrients) than traditional varieties of soybeans (which typically contain 1.4 to 4.1% stachyose in traditional soybean varieties). Compared to traditional varieties of soybeans, low-stachyose soybeans have approximately 10% more metabolizable (i.e., useable by animals) energy content and a 3% increase in amino acid digestibility.

Low-stachyose soybeans are particularly useful for feeding monogastric animals (e.g., swine, poultry, etc.) because their single stomach cannot digest stachyose. Thus, stachyose tends to "ferment" (promote excess bacterial growth) in their intestines, causing them to feel prematurely full.

See also STACHYOSE, CARBOHYDRATES (SACCHARIDES), VALUE-ENHANCED GRAINS, SOYBEAN PLANT, HIGH-SUCROSE SOYBEANS, DIGESTION (WITHIN ORGANISMS), METABOLISM

Low-Tillage Crop Production A methodology of crop production in which the farmer utilizes a minimum of mechanical cultivation (i.e., only two to four passes over the field with tillage equipment instead of the conventional five passes per year utilized for traditional crop production). This reduced mechanical tillage leaves more carbon in the (less-disturbed) soil, leaves more earthworms (*Eisenia foetida*) alive in the topsoil, and reduces soil compaction (i.e., the reduction in interstitial spaces between individual soil particles), thereby increasing the fertility of "low-till" farm fields.

The plant residue remaining on the field's surface helps to control weeds and reduce soil erosion; it also provides sites for insects to shelter and reproduce, leading to a need for increased pest control via methods such as inserting a *Bacillus thuringiensis* (*B.t.*) gene into certain crop plants. But, if a farmer needs to apply synthetic chemical pesticides, the plant residue remaining on the field's surface helps to cause breakdown of these pesticides (into substances such as carbon dioxide and water). This is because the residue helps to retain moisture in the field-surface environment, thereby enhancing growth of the types of microorganisms that help to break down pesticides.

See also NO-TILLAGE CROP PRODUCTION, GLOMALIN, EARTHWORMS, MICROORGANISMS, INTEGRATED PEST MANAGEMENT (IPM), CORN, SOYBEAN PLANT, *BACILLUS THURINGIENSIS* (*B.t.*), GENE, GENETIC ENGINEERING, EUROPEAN CORN BORER (ECB),

L

HELICOVERPA ZEA (H. ZEA), CORN ROOTWORM, COLD HARDENING

LOX Null Soybeans Refers to soybeans that do not contain any of the three lipoxygenase enzymes (thus, they result in a "null" test reading).
See also LIPOXYGENASE (LOX), LOX-1, LOX-2, LOX-3, SOYBEAN PLANT, ENZYME

LOX-1 One of the isozymes (enzyme molecule variations) of the lipoxygenase (LOX) enzyme family.
See also LIPOXYGENASE (LOX), ISOZYMES (ISOENZYMES)

LOX-2 One of the isozymes (enzyme molecule variations) of the lipoxygenase (LOX) enzyme family.
See also LIPOXYGENASE (LOX), ISOZYMES (ISOENZYMES)

LOX-3 One of the isozymes (enzyme molecule variations) of the lipoxygenase (LOX) enzyme family.
See also LIPOXYGENASE (LOX), ISOZYMES (ISOENZYMES)

LPAAT Protein A protein consisting of lysophosphatidic acid acyl transferase (enzyme), which (when present in plant) causes production of triglycerides (in the seeds) possessing saturated fatty acids in the "middle position" of the triglycerides' molecular (glycerol) "backbone." For example, canola (rapeseed) plants genetically engineered to contain LPAAT protein are able to produce high levels of saturated fatty acids (including laurate) in their oil.
See also PROTEIN, LAURATE, ENZYME, TRIGLYCERIDES, SATURATED FATTY ACIDS (SAFA), MONOUNSATURATED FATS, CANOLA, GENETIC ENGINEERING

LPE See LYSOPHOSPHATIDYLETHANOLAMINE

LPS See ENDOTOXIN

LSD1 See LYSINE-SPECIFIC DEMETHYLASE 1 (LSD1)

LTR Abbreviation for **long terminal repeat**.
See LONG TERMINAL REPEAT

Luciferase Refers to a group of enzymes that can catalyze a chemical reaction that results in the **production of light (i.e., bioluminescence)** within certain living organisms. For example, the common firefly (*Photinus pyralis*) is able to emit light from its tail (photophores) via luciferase-catalyzed bioluminescence. The ocean jellyfish known as the **sea pansy** (*Renilla reniformis*) is able to emit light via similar use of a slightly different luciferase-type molecule.
See also BIOLUMINESCENCE, LUCIFERIN, ENZYME, CATALYST, ORGANISM, NITRIC OXIDE, LUMINOPHORE

Luciferin Broadly speaking, it is any chemical substrate that becomes luminescent when catalyzed by the enzyme known as luciferase.
See also BIOLUMINESCENCE, LUMINOPHORE, LUMINESCENCE, ENZYME, CATALYST, LUCIFERASE, SUBSTRATE (CHEMICAL)

Lumen The interior opening through which blood flows, e.g., within a blood vessel.
See also ENDOTHELIUM

Luminase An enzyme that could potentially be utilized to help bleach wood pulp during the paper-making process, resulting in less adverse impact on the environment.
See also ENZYME

Luminesce See BIOLUMINESCENCE

Luminescence See BIOLUMINESCENCE

Luminescent Assays Refers to assays (i.e., tests or test techniques) that detect or measure the following via the **enzyme (e.g., luciferase)-catalyzed production of light**:

- Presence of a specific substance (e.g., bacteria ATP on surfaces in a slaughterhouse). Utilization of firefly luciferase in combination with luciferin can result in assays that can (visually) detect the presence of ATP.
- Efficacy (i.e., effectiveness) of a specific substance.

For example, one (rapid) luminescent assay utilizes two chemical reagents that first break down bacteria cell membranes, then cause ATP from those broken-open cells to luminesce. Subsequent measurement of that light is the assay's proof (e.g., that bacteria had been present on the tested surface in a slaughterhouse).
See also ASSAY, BIOLUMINESCENCE, ENZYME, BACTERIA, PLASMA MEMBRANE, ADENOSINE TRIPHOSPHATE (ATP), LUCIFERASE, LUCIFERIN

L

Luminophore Refers to any substance that becomes luminescent.

See also LUMINESCENCE, BIOLUMINES-CENCE, LUCIFERIN, LUCIFERASE, LUX PROTEINS

Lupus An autoimmune disease of the body, in which anti-DNA antibodies bind to DNA. The resulting complexes (of DNA and antibodies) travel to the kidneys via the bloodstream, and become lodged in the kidneys, where they cause inflammatory reactions (that can lead to kidney failure).

Sometimes joints, blood vessels, bone marrow, and the liver are also damaged by this disease.

See also ANTIBODY, DEOXYRIBONU-CLEIC ACID (DNA), AUTOIMMUNE DIS-EASE, SUPERANTIGENS

Lutein A carotenoid (i.e., "light-harvesting" compound utilized in photosynthesis) that is naturally produced in carrots, summer squash, broccoli, spinach, dark lettuce, and green peas. Lutein is also naturally present in the retina of the human eye. Lutein is a phytochemical or nutraceutical conducive to good eye health, and regular consumption of large amounts of lutein has been shown to reduce the risk of **age-related macular degeneration**, a leading cause of blindness in elderly people.

Research indicates that consumption of lutein by humans also reduces risk of prostate cancer and breast cancer.

See also PHYTOCHEMICALS, NUTRACEU-TICALS, CAROTENOIDS, PHOTO-SYNTHESIS

Luteinizing Hormone (LH) A reproductive hormone that acts upon the ovaries to stimulate ovulation. It is secreted by the pituitary gland.

See also HORMONE, PITUITARY GLAND, ENDOCRINE HORMONES, ESTROGEN

Luteolin See NODULATION

Lux Gene A gene within the DNA of *Vibrio fischeri*, a bacterium that lives in light-producing organs ("spotlights") of certain deep-sea fish. The lux gene codes for **lux proteins** (luminophores), which cause those bacteria (and, thus, the fish's light-producing organs) to emit light.

The lux gene can be utilized as a "reporter gene" by inserting it into the DNA of certain bacterial species that can be genetically engineered to biodegrade diesel fuel spilled in soil. When those engineered bacteria encounter diesel fuel and begin "eating" it (i.e., breaking it down), those engineered bacteria will glow (biolumi-nesce) to "report" that they are biodegrading the spilled diesel fuel.

See also GENE, REPORTER GENE, DEOX-YRIBONUCLEIC ACID (DNA), BACTERIA, BIOLUMINESCENCE, LUMINOPHORE, PROTEIN, LUX PROTEINS, GENETIC ENGINEERING, BIOREMEDIATION

Lux Proteins Refers to bioluminescent proteins found in some species of (usually deep-ocean) marine organisms. Also utilized by man to make some luminescent assays.

See also PROTEIN, BIOLUMINESCENCE, LUMINOPHORE, LUMINESCENT ASSAY, LUX GENE

LXR Acronym for **Liver X Receptors**.

See LIVER X RECEPTORS (LXR)

Lycopene An antioxidant carotenoid ("light-harvesting" pigment utilized by plants in the photosynthesis process) that is a naturally occurring phytochemical in tomatoes, watermelon, guava, pink grapefruit, and some other fruits.

Consumption of significant amounts of lyco-pene by humans causes an increase in the concentration of lycopene in the blood plasma. Lycopene is a natural constituent of blood plasma and certain tissues in the human body, but it must be consumed in the diet because the human body does not synthesize (manufacture) lycopene. Consumption of lycopene by humans has been linked to a reduction in atherosclerosis, coronary heart disease, some cancers (e.g., prostate cancer, colorectal cancer), and inhibition of **oxidation of low-density lipoproteins (LDLP).** Lycopene is also converted (in some instances) into alpha-carotene or beta-carotene. Because beta-carotene is processed into vitamin A by the human body, consumption of this phytochemical can help prevent human diseases (e.g., in developing countries) that result from deficiency of vitamin A; For example:

- Coronary heart disease
- Certain cancers (e.g., cancer of prostate, lung, etc.)
- Childhood blindness

L

- Age-related macular degeneration; a leading cause of blindness in older people
- Various childhood diseases that can cause death due to weakened immune system

Research published during 2004 indicates that the presence of lycopene in the human digestive tract induces the excretion of some cancer-inhibiting enzymes known as **Phase II detoxification enzymes**.

See also PHYTOCHEMICALS, NUTRACEUTICALS, CANCER, ANTIOXIDANTS, CAROTENOIDS, CORONARY HEART DISEASE (CHD), PLASMA, ATHEROSCLEROSIS, PROSTATE-SPECIFIC ANTIGEN (PSA), TOMATO, BETA-CAROTENE, VITAMIN, LUTEIN, PHOTOSYNTHESIS, LOW-DENSITY LIPOPROTEINS (LDLP), INDUCIBLE ENZYMES

Lymphocyte A type of cell found in the blood, spleen, lymph nodes, etc., of higher animals. They are formed very early in fetal life, arising in the liver by the sixth week of human gestation. There exist two subclasses of lymphocytes: B lymphocytes and T lymphocytes. B lymphocytes make antibodies (immunoglobulins), of which there are five classes: IgM, IgA, IgG, IgD, and IgE. The antibodies circulate in the bloodstream. T lymphocytes recognize and reject foreign tissue, modulate B cell activity, kill tumor cells, and kill host cells infected with virus. T lymphocytes are also called T cells.

The bone marrow of humans makes lymphocytes throughout its lifetime.

See also B LYMPHOCYTES, T CELLS, ANTIBODY, HELPER T CELLS (T4 CELLS), BLAST CELL, CYTOTOXIC T CELLS, ANTIGEN, DENDRITIC CELLS

Lymphokines Peptides and proteins secreted by (immune system response) stimulated T cells. These hormone-like (peptide and protein) molecules direct the movements and activities of other cells in the immune system. Some examples of lymphokines are interleukin-1, interleukin-2, tumor necrosis factor (TNF), gamma interferon, colony-stimulating factors, macrophage chemotactic factor, and lymphocyte growth factor. The suffix "-kine" comes from the Greek word *kinesis*, meaning "movement."

Lyochrome See FLAVIN

Lyophilization The process of removing water from a frozen biomaterial (e.g., a microbial culture or an aqueous protein solution) via application of a vacuum. It is a drying method for long-term preservation of proteins in the solid state, and for long-term storage of live microbial cultures.

See also CULTURE, PROTEIN

Lyse To rupture a membrane (cell). The act of lysis (rupturing a membrane).

See LYSIS

Lysine (Lys) An essential amino acid that can be obtained from many proteins by hydrolysis (i.e., cutting apart the protein molecule).

See also ESSENTIAL AMINO ACIDS, PROTEIN, OPAGUE-2, *PHOTORHABDUS LUMINESCENS*, HYDROLYSIS

Lysine-Specific Demethylase 1 (LSD1) See METHYLATED

Lysis The process of cell disintegration, membrane rupturing, or breaking-up of the cell wall.

See also CYTOLYSIS, CELL, LYSOZYME, MEMBRANE TRANSPORT, BIOCIDE, GRAM-POSITIVE (G+)

Lysogeny Refers to the ability of a bacteriophage to be able to itself become a part of a bacterium's DNA.

See also BACTERIOPHAGE, DEOXYRIBONUCLEIC ACID (DNA)

Lysophosphatidylethanolamine Also known by the abbreviation LPE and as phosphatidyl ethanolamine. It is one of the lipids (phospholipids) naturally found in soybean oil. In plants, it functions as a **signaling molecule** (e.g., speeding the ripening process).

See also LIPIDS, SOYBEAN OIL, SIGNALING MOLECULE

Lysosome A membrane-surrounded organelle within the cytoplasm of eucaryotic cells, which contains many hydrolytic enzymes. Discovered by Christian de Duve.

The lysosome internalizes and digests foreign proteins as well as cellular debris. The protein fragments (epitopes) are presented to T cells by the major histocompatibility complex (MHC) proteins on the surface of the eucaryotic cell. When a cell's exterior is mechanically wounded (e.g., by scraping), the release of calcium ions triggers fusing of lysosomes

L

with the cell's plasma membrane to quickly reseal any holes in the membrane to prevent leakage of the cell's contents.

See also CELL, ANTIGEN, MAJOR HISTO-COMPATIBILITY COMPLEX (MHC), T CELLS, PLASMA MEMBRANE, ION

Lysozyme An enzyme, naturally produced by some animals, that possesses antibacterial (i.e., bacteria-killing) properties. Discovered in 1922 by Alexander Fleming in his nasal mucus, he named it "lysozyme" from the Greek words *lyso* — because of its ability to lyse (cut) bacteria — and *zyme* — because it is an enzyme. Lysozyme lyses certain kinds of bacteria, by dissolving the polysaccharide components of the bacteria's cell wall. When the cell wall is weakened, the bacterial cell bursts because osmotic pressure (inside that bacterial cell) is greater than the weakened cell wall can contain. Tears and egg whites contain significant amounts of lysozyme, as agents to prevent bacterial infections (e.g., against bacteria entering the body via eye openings and against bacteria entering chicken embryo through the eggshell).

See also ENZYME, LYSIS, CELL, CYTOLY-SIS, POLYSACCHARIDES, BACTERIA

Lytic Infection A viral infection in which the final act of the infection is to lyse (i.e., burst or destroy) the cell. This releases the new (progeny) viruses so they can go on to infect other cells.

See also LYSE, LYSIS, VIRUS, CELL, HOLINS

L

M

M Cells The immune system cells that constitute the surface of Peyer's patches. M cells preferentially sample/evaluate certain particles (e.g., viruses) passing over the Peyer's patch, embedded in the wall of intestine, during the digestive process. Those particles that meet certain criteria (and also specific toxin molecules that adhere to the M cells) are absorbed by the M cells and their antigens "presented" to adjacent lymphoid tissue underlying the Peyer's patch.

This activates the lymphocytes present in the patches, which then migrate into the blood where they float in the tissue spaces just inside the intestinal lining. There, they secrete antibodies (primarily IgA), which are then transported into the lumen (contents) of the gut and subsequently attack (bind) the antigens.

See also PEYER'S PATCHES, VIRUS, TOXIN, ANTIGEN, LYMPHOCYTE, ANTIBODY, IMMUNOGLOBULIN

MAA Marketing Authorization Application It is the European Union (EU) equivalent of a U.S. NDA (New Drug Application). An MAA is an application to the EU's Committee for Proprietary Medicinal Products (CPMP) seeking approval of a new drug that has undergone Phase II and Phase III clinical trials.

See also NDA (TO FDA), CANDA, FOOD AND DRUG ADMINISTRATION (FDA), MAA, NDA (TO KOSEISHO), CPMP, PHASE I CLINICAL TESTING, PHASE II CLINICAL TESTS, PHASE III CLINICAL TESTS

MAB See MARKER-ASSISTED BREEDING

MAb See MONOCLONAL ANTIBODIES (MAb)

Macromolecules Large molecules with molecular weights ranging from approximately ten thousand to hundreds of millions.

See also MOLECULAR WEIGHT

Macrophage A phagocytic cell that is the counterpart of the monocyte. A monocyte that has left the bloodstream and has moved into the tissues. Macrophages have basically the same functions as monocytes, but they carry these out in the tissues. In summary, they engulf and kill microorganisms, present antigen to the lymphocytes, kill certain tumor cells, and their secretions (e.g., leukotrienes) regulate inflammation. Macrophages utilize nitric oxide and hydrogen peroxide (which they synthesize) to kill the microorganisms they engulf (via oxidation), and the nitric oxide also helps to regulate the immune system. In the spleen, macrophages engulf and destroy old red blood cells. When they reside in the bone marrow, they store iron and then transfer it to red blood cells. In the lungs and GI tract, they are scavengers and keep tissues clean. They also serve as a reservoir for the AIDS virus. They (and other phagocytic cells) are largely responsible for the localization and degradation of foreign materials at inflammatory sites.

Macrophages display chemotaxis (i.e., the sensing of, and movement toward or away from, a specific chemical). For example, consumption (in food or feed) of mannanoligosaccharides by mammals causes macrophages (within that mammal's bloodstream) to depart from the bloodstream and move toward the gastrointestinal tract (tissues) where those macrophages eliminate some pathogens (i.e., those growing or reproducing in the gastrointestinal tract).

See also CELL, CELLULAR IMMUNE RESPONSE, CHEMOTAXIS, ONOCYTES, PHAGOCYTE, ADHESION MOLECULE, LYSOSOME, NITRIC OXIDE, NITRIC OXIDE SYNTHASE, MANNANOLIGOSACCHARIDES (MOS), PATHOGEN, LEUKOTRIENES, INTERLEUKIN-1 (IL-1), PHOSPHATIDYL SERINE

Macrophage Colony-Stimulating Factor (M-CSF) A colony-stimulating factor (CSF) that stimulates production of macrophages in the body.

M

See also COLONY-STIMULATING FACTORS (CSFs), MACROPHAGE

MACS Acronym for **magnetic cell sorting**. See MAGNETIC PARTICLES

Magainins Discovered within frog skin tissues by Michael Zasloff in 1987, magainins are antimicrobial, amphopathic peptides that lyse (i.e., burst) certain cells on contact by "worming" their hydrophobic portion into the cell's membrane, which creates a transmembrane (i.e., through the surface) pore (allowing ions to flow into the cell, causing osmotic bursting). Magainins are selective against bacteria, fungi, and protozoa cells (the word magainin comes from the Hebrew word for "shield").

See also AMPHIPHILIC MOLECULES, CELL, PEPTIDE, BACTERIA, FUNGUS, ANTIBIOTICS, PLASMA MEMBRANE

"Magic Bullet" When this term was first coined by Paul Ehrlich in 1905, it initially referred only to antibodies (e.g., because antibodies seek their own target without damaging other nearby tissues).

However, over time, this term has come to be applied to immunotoxins and other immunoconjugates (i.e., toxic or pharmacological molecules that are "attached" to an antibody that "steers/guides" the toxic or pharmacological molecule to the intended "target" in the body such as a tumor). During 2005, Stephen Russell was able to modify a measles virus so that:

- It expressed an antibody that targeted an antigen on the surface of a cancer tumor's cells in a mouse, thereby causing the (injected) virus to accumulate on the cancerous cells.
- It "infected" those cancerous cells, and killed them without harming adjacent healthy tissue.

See also ANTIBODY, IMMUNOCONJUGATE, IMMUNOTOXIN, GENISTEIN, RICIN, MONOCLONAL ANTIBODIES (MAb), HER-2 GENE, VIROTHERAPY, CELL, ANTIGEN, CANCER, TUMOR

Magnetic Antibodies See MAGNETIC PARTICLES

Magnetic Beads See MAGNETIC PARTICLES

Magnetic Cell Sorting See MAGNETIC PARTICLES

Magnetic Labeling See MAGNETIC PARTICLES

Magnetic Particles Refers to various tiny pieces of naturally magnetic materials that are bonded (attached) to **capture molecules** such as specific molecular ligands, receptors, aptamers, antigens, antibodies (e.g., monoclonal antibodies that are specific to a particular type of cell), etc.

These can then be mixed with a large population of many cell types (e.g., crude tissue samples, cells grown in a vat or reactor, etc.), in which the **now-magnetic capture molecules** will attach themselves to **only the desired cells**, then the desired cells are separated out using a magnetic field (and the magnetic particles/antibodies are subsequently removed from those cells). For example, magnetic nanoparticles (100-nm diameter) attached to **antibodies against epithelial cells** can be utilized to detect metastasis of cancer in a human. The magnetized antibodies attach themselves to epithelial cells (a biomarker of metastasis) in a blood sample, enabling the epithelial cells to be detected/counted by doctors.

In a similar fashion, specific nucleic acids/DNA can be attached to magnetic particles. These can then be mixed with a mixture of nucleic acids/DNA whereby the magnetic particles will attach themselves (via hybridization) to only the desired nucleic acids/DNA; then they are separated out using a magnetic field.

See also CAPTURE MOLECULE, ANTIBODY, MONOCLONAL ANTIBODIES (MAb), CELL, IMMUNOCONJUGATE, CELL SORTING, NUCLEIC ACIDS, DEOXYRIBONUCLEIC ACID (DNA), HYBRIDIZATION (MOLECULAR GENETICS), HYBRIDIZATION SURFACES, BIO–BAR CODES, NANOPARTICLES, LIGAND (IN BIOCHEMISTRY), RECEPTORS, APTAMERS, ANTIGEN, CANCER, METASTASIS, BIOMARKERS

Maillard Reaction Refers to a set of chemical reactions that occur when certain foodstuffs are cooked at temperatures exceeding 121°C

M

(250°F). Certain amino acids within the food-stuffs react with sugars to produce flavorful chemical compounds (e.g., melanoidins). Carefully controlled Maillard reactions of soybean meal can also be utilized to produce a **ruminal-bypass feed** ingredient. Such feed (protein) would be protected from breakdown in the rumen (e.g., of a dairy cow) so that optimal digestion would occur in the cow's intestine (abomasum).

See also AMINO ACID, MELANOIDINS, PROTEIN, SOYBEAN PLANT, SOY PROTEIN, RUMEN (OF CATTLE)

Maize See CORN

Major Histocompatibility Antigen — Class I A "family" of glycoproteins that appear on the surfaces of most cells of an organism that help enable that organism's immune system to distinguish "self" (cells) from "nonself" (e.g., invading pathogens).

See also GLYCOPROTEIN, CELL, ORGANISM, PATHOGEN, MAJOR HISTOCOMPATIBILITY COMPLEX (MHC), MAJOR HISTOCOMPATIBILITY ANTIGEN — CLASS II

Major Histocompatibility Antigen — Class II A "family" of glycoproteins that appear only on the surface of specific lymphocyte cells (dendritic cells) and on the surface of certain macrophages within an organism.

See also GLYCOPROTEIN, CELL, LYMPHOCYTE, DENDRITIC CELLS, MACROPHAGE, ORGANISM, MAJOR HISTOCOMPATIBILITY COMPLEX (MHC), MAJOR HISTOCOMPATIBILITY ANTIGEN — CLASS II

Major Histocompatibility Complex (MHC) A genetic loci or chromosomal region (approximately 3000 Kb) that encodes for three classes of transmembrane (cell) proteins. MHC I proteins (located on the surface of nearly all cells) present foreign epitopes (i.e., fragments of antigens that have been ingested; peptides) to cytotoxic T cells (killer T cells). MHC II proteins (located on the surface of immune system lymphocyte/dendritic cells and phagocytes) present foreign epitopes to helper T cells. The **presenting** of epitopes induces the organism's immune response.

MHC III proteins are components of the complement cascade. Genes in the MHC must be matched (between an organ donor and organ recipient) to prevent rejection of organ transplants.

See also COMPLEMENT CASCADE, LOCI, LOCUS, CHROMOSOMES, GRAFT-VERSUS-HOST DISEASE (GVHD), Kb, LYMPHOCYTE, DENDRITIC CELLS, MACROPHAGE, PROTEIN, CELL, T CELL RECEPTORS, ANTIGEN, T CELLS, CYTOTOXIC T CELLS, EPITOPE, HUMORAL IMMUNITY, GENE, TUMOR-ASSOCIATED ANTIGENS, HUMAN LEUKOCYTE ANTIGENS (HLA), CELLULAR IMMUNE RESPONSE

MAL (Multiple Aleurone Layer) Gene A gene in corn (maize) that (when present in the DNA of a given plant) causes the plant to produce seed that contains higher-than-normal levels of calcium, magnesium, iron, zinc, and manganese. These higher mineral levels are particularly useful for feeding swine, because traditional Number 2 yellow (dent) corn does not contain enough for optimal pig growth.

See also GENE, DEOXYRIBONUCLEIC ACID (DNA), HIGH-METHIONINE CORN, HIGH-LYSINE CORN, FLOURY-2, OPAGUE-2

MALDI-TOF-MS Acronym for **matrix-associated laser desorption ionization time of flight mass spectrometry,** a mass spectrometry methodology/technology that was initially developed by Franz Hillenkamp for analysis of biological molecules.

MALDI-TOF-MS can establish, in seconds, the identity, purity, etc., of a sample of proteins, oligonucleotide, or (poly)peptides. It also aids the identification of Gram-positive microorganisms, or characterization of genetic materials (e.g., DNA, RNA, etc.) on hybridization surfaces.

MALDI-TOF utilizes measurement of the **time for particles (e.g., proteins) to transit a specific distance** after being "dislodged" from within a specific point on the anode where each was placed (e.g., by a robot arm, which picks proteins, for instance, out of the gel after running them through two-dimensional gel electrophoresis to separate from others in a sample).

After being placed by the robot arm onto the anode and dried into crystalline matrix

M

adhered to its surface, MALDI-TOF-MS dislodges (molecules) from ("adhered") surface by vaporization with a specific amount of laser energy to precisely determine the molecular weight (e.g., of proteins, etc.).

See also MASS SPECTROMETER, MICRO-ORGANISM, OLIGONUCLEOTIDE, GRAM-POSITIVE, RIBONUCLEIC ACID (RNA), HYBRIDIZATION SURFACES, DEOXYRIBONUCLEIC ACID (DNA), *IN SILICO* BIOLOGY, PROTEIN, PEPTIDE, TWO-DIMENSIONAL (2-D) GEL ELECTROPHORESIS, ICM

Male-sterile See BARNASE

Malonyl-CoA See FATS

Mammalian Cell Culture Technology to artificially cultivate cells of mammal origin in a laboratory or production-scale device (i.e., *in vitro*). Can be either a batch or continuous process device. The first mammalian cell culture was performed by a neurobiologist named R.G. Harrison in 1907 when he added chopped-up spinal cord tissue to clotted (blood) plasma in a humidified growth chamber. The nerve cells from this spinal cord tissue successfully grew, divided, and extended long fibers into the clot. Many improvements to the cell culture process have been made over the years, including special growth media (fluids that bathe the cultured cells with the right amounts of amino acids, salts, and other minerals).

See also CONTINUOUS PERFUSION, DISSOCIATING ENZYMES, CHO CELLS, HARVESTING ENZYMES, *IN VITRO*, PLASMA, CELL, MEDIUM, AMINO ACID

Mannan Oligosaccharides See MANNANO-LIGOSACCHARIDES (MOS)

Mannanoligosaccharides (MOS) A "family" of oligosaccharides that can be produced in commercial quantities via certain yeast cells. When consumed (e.g., by humans or monogastric livestock such as swine or poultry), mannose sugars in the MOS stimulate the liver to secrete the mannose-binding protein. Mannose-binding protein enters the digestive system and binds to the (mannose-containing) capsule (surface membrane) of pathogenic bacteria. That binding to pathogens triggers the immune system's complement cascade to combat these pathogenic bacteria.

Consumption of mannanoligosaccharides by mammals also causes macrophages to move toward the gastrointestinal tract (in the body's tissues), where they eliminate some pathogens (i.e., those that grow/reproduce in the gastrointestinal tract).

See also OLIGOSACCHARIDES, FRUCTOSE OLIGOSACCHARIDES, SUGAR MOLECULES, YEAST, COMPLEMENT CASCADE, PATHOGENIC, BACTERIA, IMMUNE RESPONSE, COMPLEMENT, CAPSULE, MACROPHAGE, FOSHU, NUTRACEUTICALS

Mannogalactan See HIGH-MANNOGALACTAN SOYBEANS

Map Distance A number proportional to the frequency of recombination between two genes. One map unit corresponds to a recombination frequency of 1%.

See also GENETICS, GENETIC CODE, GENETIC MAP, GENE, LINKAGE, QUANTITATIVE TRAIT LOCI (QTL)

MAPK Acronym for **mitogen-activated protein kinase**.

See also MITOGEN-ACTIVATED PROTEIN KINASE CASCADE

MAPK System See MITOGEN-ACTIVATED PROTEIN KINASE CASCADE

Mapping (of genome) See GENETICS, GENETIC CODE, GENETIC MAP, QUANTITATIVE TRAIT LOCI, POSITION EFFECT

Marker (DNA marker) A DNA fragment of known size used to calibrate an electrophoretic gel.

See also ELECTROPHORESIS, TWO-DIMENSIONAL (2-D) GEL ELECTROPHORESIS, DEOXYRIBONUCLEIC ACID (DNA)

Marker (DNA sequence) A specific sequence of DNA that is virtually always associated with a specified trait, because of "linkage" between that DNA sequence (the "marker") and the genes that cause that particular trait. Such markers have been utilized to aid or speed up the process of plant (e.g., crop) breeding since the mid-1970s via **marker-assisted selection**.

See also DEOXYRIBONUCLEIC ACID (DNA), TRAIT, LINKAGE, LINKAGE GROUP, LINKAGE MAP, GENE, SEQUENCE (OF A DNA MOLECULE),

M

MARKER-ASSISTED SELECTION, YSTR DNA

Marker (genetic marker) A trait that can be observed to occur or not to occur in an organism, for example, bacteria or plants. Genetic markers include the following traits:

- Expression of luciferase-catalyzed bioluminescence in leaf cells (causing leaves to glow when illuminated by certain light sources)
- Resistance to specific antibiotics
- The nature of the cell wall and capsule characteristics
- Requirements for a particular growth factor and carbohydrate utilization

For example, if a culture of dividing (growing) bacteria that is not resistant to a particular antibiotic (i.e., lacks the trait of antibiotic resistance) is exposed to only the DNA isolated from bacteria that are resistant to the antibiotic, then a fraction of the cells exposed will directly incorporate this trait (some DNA) into their genome, hence acquiring the trait. The first genetically engineered plants bearing a marker gene were field tested in 1986.
See also ALLELE, GENETIC ENGINEERING, POSITIVE AND NEGATIVE SELECTION (PNS), TRANSFORMATION, TRANSFECTION, NPTII GENE, BIOLUMINESCENCE, MARKER-ASSISTED SELECTION, GUS GENE, bla GENE, RECOMBINASE

Marker-Assisted Breeding See MARKER-ASSISTED SELECTION

Marker-Assisted Selection The utilization of DNA sequence "markers" by commercial breeders to select the organisms (e.g., crops, livestock, etc.) that possess genes for a particular performance trait (e.g., rapid growth, high yield, etc.) desired — for subsequent breeding/propagation. Marker-assisted selection has been utilized in many plant-breeding programs (e.g., crop) since the mid-1970s.
See also DEOXYRIBONUCLEIC ACID (DNA), SEQUENCE (OF A DNA MOLECULE), MARKER (DNA SEQUENCE), GENE, TRAIT, GENETIC MAP, LINKAGE, LINKAGE GROUP, MOLECULAR BREEDING™, LINKAGE MAP, QUANTITATIVE TRAIT LOCI (QTL)

MARS Acronym for **marker-assisted recurrent selection**. Refers to the cycle utilized within MAS (marker-assisted selection) formal breeding programs (e.g., conducted by modern crop seed companies) to help the plant breeder to more rapidly increase the frequency of favorable-trait (desired) genes in the DNA of the breeding population.
See also MARKER-ASSISTED SELECTION, GENE, TRAIT, DEOXYRIBONUCLEIC ACID (DNA)

MAS See MARKER-ASSISTED SELECTION

Mass Applied Genomics See GENOMICS, BIOCHIPS, MICROARRAYS (TESTING), BIOINFORMATICS

Mass Spectrometer An analytical device that can be used to determine the molecular weights (mass) of proteins and nucleic acids, the sequence of (composition and order of amino acids comprising) protein molecules, the chemical composition of virtually any biomaterial (e.g., lipids), and the rapid identification of intact gram-negative and gram-positive microorganisms (the latter, using matrix-assisted laser desorption ionization time of flight mass spectrometry).
The exact mass of such charged particles (e.g., ions) is based on measurement of their mass-to-charge ratios (while the particles are passing through magnetic and electrical fields whose strengths are precisely known).
To utilize a mass spectrometer to identify each protein present within a given sample, the protein molecules are first separated (e.g., via two-dimensional gel electrophoresis or via liquid chromatography). Next, these protein molecules are **very specifically** reduced, alkylated, and broken (in specifically known ways, via enzymes) into peptides. When passed through the mass spectrometer, the peptides (and, by derivation, the initial proteins), are identified by comparing their mass/charge spectra to those within a database of known proteins (i.e., which were earlier passed through the mass spectrometer).
See also GRAM NEGATIVE, GRAM POSITIVE, MOLECULAR WEIGHT, ION, SEQUENCING (OF DNA MOLECULES), PROTEIN, AMINO ACID, NUCLEIC ACIDS, GENE MACHINE, MALDI-TOF-MS,

M

TWO-DIMENSIONAL (2-D) GEL ELEC-TROPHORESIS, CHROMATOGRAPHY, REDUCTION (IN A CHEMICAL REAC-TION), PEPTIDE, ENZYME, LIPIDS, ION TRAP

Massively Parallel Signature Sequencing Refers to a form of gene expression analysis in which a given cell's small RNA molecules (21 to 24 ribonucleotides in length) can be thoroughly profiled. This profiling is accomplished by the following steps:

- Cloning each (known) small RNA molecule of that organism/cell and attaching it to a single bead of approximately 5-μm size
- Placing such RNA-attached beads into a suitable container and flowing the relevant cellular (fluid) sample around those beads
- Determining the amounts of each small RNA molecule that hybridizes to each bead

Because the *known* small RNA molecule depicted in the first step acts as a **sequence tag** for the agglomeration on each bead, the respective amounts of each of the cell's small RNA molecules can be subsequently determined.

See also GENE, GENE EXPRESSION ANALYSIS, CELL, RIBONUCLEIC ACID (RNA), NUCLEOTIDE, CLONE (A MOLECULE), MICRON, HYBRIDIZATION (MOLECULAR GENETICS), HYBRIDIZATION SURFACES

Mast Cells Fixed (noncirculating) leukocyte cells that are present in many different kinds of body tissues. When two IgE molecules of the same antibody "dock" at adjacent receptor sites on a mast cell, and then they capture an allergen (e.g., a particle of pollen) between them, a chemical-energetic signal is sent to the interior (inside the mast cell) portion of receptor molecules, which causes that portion of the molecule to change (i.e., transduction). This signal transduction causes a protein named "syk" to set off a chemical chain reaction inside the mast cell, thereby causing the cell to release leukotrienes, histamine, serotonin, bradykinin, and "slow-reacting substance." Release of these chemicals into the

body causes the blood vessels to become more permeable (leaky) and the nose to run, and itchy and watery eyes. These chemicals also cause smooth muscle contraction, which causes sneezing, breath constriction, coughing, wheezing, etc.

See also BASOPHILS, ANTIGEN, ANTIBODY, RECEPTORS, SIGNAL TRANSDUCTION, HISTAMINE, ALLERGIES (FOODBORNE), SIGNALING, LEUKOTRIENES, LEUKOCYTES

Matrix Metalloproteinases (MMP) A family of enzymes that contain the zinc metal ion (Zn^{2+}) at their active sites. Among this family are the collagenases.

See also ENZYME, ION, ACTIVE SITE, CATALYTIC SITE, STROMELYSIN (MMP-3), COLLAGENASE

Matrix-Assisted Laser Desorption/Ionization Time of Flight Mass Spectrometry See MALDI-TOF-MS

Maximum Residue Level (MRL) Term used for an officially established upper allowable limit of a given compound (e.g., a synthetic hormone) in a particular product such as meat. For example, in 1994, the Codex Alimentarius Commission in Rome, Italy, decided to establish maximum residue levels for each of five growth promotants that are commonly utilized by the U.S. beef industry. Because the World Trade Organization (WTO) subsequently stated that it would respect MRLs, a WTO member nation cannot legally refuse to allow import of meat products on growth-promotant-content basis if the content of the promotant contained in the meat is less than its maximum residue level.

See also GROWTH HORMONE, GROWTH FACTOR, CODEX ALIMENTARIUS COMMISSION, WORLD TRADE ORGANIZATION (WTO)

Maysin A chemical that is naturally produced in low amounts within most varieties of corn/maize (*Zea Mays L.*) plants. During the 1980s and 1990s, certain corn/maize varieties with very high maysin content were developed in the U.S. Because maysin "binds up" certain (essential) amino acids in the gut of the corn earworm (*Helicoverpa zea*) caterpillar (larvae), these insects stop growing when they are consuming a large amount of maysin.

M

See also CORN, *HELICOVERPA ZEA (H. ZEA)*, AMINO ACIDS, ESSENTIAL AMINO ACIDS, HIGH-MAYSIN CORN

MCA See MEDICINES CONTROL AGENCY (MCA)

MCT Acronym for **medium-chain triacylglycerides**.
See MEDIUM-CHAIN TRIACYLGLY-CERIDES

MEA Acronym for **multilateral environmental agreement**; an agreement (e.g., treaty) between a number of nations that is intended to protect/benefit the environment.
See also CONVENTION ON BIOLOGICAL DIVERSITY (CBD)

Medicines Control Agency (MCA) The British government agency that, in concert with the Committee on Safety in Medicines, regulates the approval and sale of pharmaceutical products in the U.K.
See also COMMITTEE ON SAFETY IN MEDICINES, FOOD AND DRUG ADMINISTRATION (FDA), COMMITTEE FOR PROPRIETARY MEDICINAL PRODUCTS (CPMP), KOSEISHO, NDA (TO KOSEISHO), IND, BUNDESGESUNDHEITSAMT (BGA)

Medifoods See NUTRACEUTICALS, PHYTOCHEMICALS

Medium A substance used to provide nutrients for cell growth. It may be liquid (e.g., broth) or solid (e.g., agar).
See also CULTURE MEDIUM, AGAR, MAMMALIAN CELL CULTURE

Medium-Chain Saturated Fats See MEDIUM-CHAIN TRIACYLGLYCERIDES

Medium-Chain Triacylglycerides Refers to a category of saturated fatty acid molecule (fragments or derivatives). When consumed by humans, **medium-chain triacylglycerols (MCTs)** are more rapidly digested, metabolized, and absorbed than the corresponding full-length fatty acid molecules (triacylglycerols). For this reason, MCTs are utilized to deliver lipid nourishment to people (e.g., certain hospital patients) whose bodies suffer from lipid nutrient maladsorption.
Research indicates that consumption of MCTs increases the body's caloric consumption more than long-chain triacylglycerols.
See also FATS, FATTY ACID, LIPIDS, SATURATED FATTY ACIDS (SAFA), TRIA-

CYLGLYCERIDES, TRIGLYCERIDES, DIGESTION (WITHIN ORGANISMS)

Medium-Chain Triglycerides See MEDIUM-CHAIN TRIACYLGLYCERIDES

Mega-Yeast Artificial Chromosomes (Mega YAC) A large (i.e., greater than 500 bp in length) piece of DNA that has been cloned (made) inside a living yeast cell. While most bacterial vectors cannot carry DNA pieces that are larger than 50 bp and "standard" YACs typically cannot carry DNA pieces that are larger than 500 bp, mega YACs can carry DNA pieces (chromosomes) as large as 1,000,000 bp in length.
See also YEAST, CHROMOSOMES, HUMAN ARTIFICIAL CHROMOSOMES (HAC), *ARABIDOPSIS THALIANA*, DEOXYRIBONUCLEIC ACID (DNA), CLONE (A MOLECULE), VECTOR, BASE PAIR (bp), YEAST ARTIFICIAL CHROMOSOMES (YAC)

Megabase A unit of length for DNA equal to 1,000,000 bp.
See also DEOXYRIBONUCLEIC ACID (DNA), BASE PAIR (BP)

Megakaryocyte-Stimulating Factor (MSF) A colony-stimulating factor (protein) involved in the regulation of platelet production, white-blood-cell production, and red-blood-cell production from stem cells in bone marrow.
See also COLONY-STIMULATING FACTORS (CSFs), PLATELETS, STEM CELLS

Meiosis Discovered by Edouard Van Beneden in the 1870s, meiosis is the sequence of complex cell nucleus changes resulting in the production of cells (as gametes) with half the number of chromosomes present in the original cell and typically involving an actual **reduction division** in which the chromosomes join in pairs with homologous chromosomes (of maternal and paternal origin) without undergoing prior splitting and then separate (i.e., pulled apart by actin and microtubules within the cell) so that one member of each pair enters each product cell nucleus and undergoes a second division not involving reduction. Occurs by two successive divisions (meiosis I and meiosis II) that reduce the starting number of $4n$ chromosomes to $1n$ in each of the four product cells. Product cells may mature to germ cells (sperm or eggs).

M

See also OOCYTES, CELL, CHROMOSOME, NUCLEUS, MICROTUBULES, ACTIN, MOTOR PROTEINS

Melanoidins A class of flavorful chemicals that are formed as reaction products during the **Maillard reaction**. Melanoidins act as strong antioxidants in the human body.

See also ANTIOXIDANTS, MAILLARD REACTION

Melanoma A potentially fatal skin cancer in which melanocytes (i.e., pigment-manufacturing cells in the skin) grow and proliferate rapidly to form cancerous tumors.

See also CANCER, TUMOR, ELECTROPORATION

Melting (of DNA) Melting DNA means to heat-denature it. When this happens, the hydrogen bonds holding the DNA molecule together in the normal way are disrupted, allowing a more random polymer structure to exist.

See also DENATURED DNA

Melting (of a substance other than DNA) To change from a solid to a nonsolid (e.g., liquid) state by the addition of heat (to the solid substance).

Melting Temperature (of DNA) (Tm) The midpoint of the temperature range over which DNA is denatured.

See also MELTING (OF DNA)

Membrane Channels See PLASMA MEMBRANE, ION, AQUAPORINS, MEMBRANE TRANSPORTER PROTEIN, CALCIUM ION CHANNELS, POTASSIUM ION CHANNELS

Membrane Transport The facilitated transport of a solute across a membrane, usually by a specific membrane protein (e.g., adhesion molecule, receptor, etc.).

See also ENDOCYTOSIS, EXOCYTOSIS, SIGNAL TRANSDUCTION, G-PROTEINS, VAGINOSIS, RECEPTORS, ADHESION MOLECULE, VESICULAR TRANSPORT, GATED TRANSPORT, CALCIUM CHANNEL BLOCKERS, LIPIDS, CAGE CARRIER, GATED CHANNEL, TRANSLOCATION (OF PROTEIN MOLECULES), AQUAPORINS

Membrane Transporter Protein A class of transmembrane proteins (i.e., protein molecules embedded in a cell's membrane,

extending through both sides of the membrane), which function to **transport certain molecules through the cell's membrane**. Such molecules thus transported include the following:

- Sugar molecules (utilized by the cell as fuel)
- Inorganic ions (that catalyze certain cellular processes)
- Polypeptides (e.g., "manufactured" in the cell's ribosomes and then secreted from cell to perform some function elsewhere in the body of the organism)
- Anticancer drugs
- Antibiotics

See also PROTEIN, CELL, PLASMA MEMBRANE, MEMBRANE TRANSPORT, RIBOSOMES, POLYPEPTIDE (PROTEIN), ABC TRANSPORTERS, TRANSLOCATION (OF PROTEIN MOLECULES)

Membranes (of a cell) Refers to the thin "skinlike" structures that surround the exterior of a cell (i.e., plasma membrane) and also surround various specialized bodies (e.g., nucleus, mitochondria, etc.) **within** the cell itself (e.g., the membrane that surrounds the cell's nucleus is called the "nuclear envelope").

Membranes are lipoidal, **i.e., made of lipoidal (fatlike) material in which proteins and protein complexes are embedded.** For example, protein molecules known as receptors are embedded in the **plasma membrane (i.e., the outermost membrane of the cell)** and in the nuclear envelope.

See also CELL, CECROPHINS (LYTIC PROTEINS), MAGAININS, PLASMA MEMBRANE, TRANSMEMBRANE PROTEINS, ION CHANNELS, RECEPTORS, NUCLEAR RECEPTORS

MEMS (nanotechnology) Acronym utilized by Americans to refer to **"microelectromechanical systems"** (Europeans tend to refer to this as "microsystems technology" [MST]).

See also NANOTECHNOLOGY, BIOCHIP, GENOSENSORS, BIOSENSORS (ELECTRONIC), BIOSENSORS (CHEMICAL), NANOCRYSTAL MOLECULES MICROFLUIDICS, QUANTUM WIRE, QUANTUM

M

DOT, MOLECULAR MACHINES, BIOMO-
TORS, BIOMEMS

mEPSPS The "**m**" **variant** of (the many forms
of) the enzyme **5-enolpyruvyl-shikimate-3-
phosphate synthase**. mEPSPS is unaffected
by glyphosate-containing or sulfosate-containing herbicides, so introduction of the gene
(coding for mEPSPS) into crop plants (e.g.,
corn/maize) makes these crop plants essentially impervious to glyphosate-containing or
sulfosate-containing herbicides.

See also ENZYME, GENE, GENETIC ENGI-
NEERING, EPSP SYNTHASE, GLYPHO-
SATE, SULFOSATE, CORN, HERBICIDE-
TOLERANT CROP, ARO A

Mesenchymal Adult Stem Cells See MESO-
DERMAL ADULT STEM CELLS

Mesenchymal Stem Cell (MSC) Refers to a
pluripotent stem cell that differentiates (and
migrates where needed) to become connective
tissue within the body of an organism.

See also CELL, STEM CELLS, PLURIPO-
TENT STEM CELLS, CELL DIFFERENTI-
ATION, CELL MOTILITY

Mesodermal Adult Stem Cells Certain stem
cells present within (adult) bodies of organisms that can be differentiated (via chemical
signals) to give rise to bone, muscle, and fat
cells.

See also STEM CELLS, MULTIPOTENT
ADULT STEM CELLS, CELL, ORGAN-
ISM, SIGNALING

Mesophile An organism that grows best in the
temperature range of 25°C (77°F) to 40°C
(104°F).

See also THERMOPHILE, PSYCHROPHILE

Mesoscale See NANOSCIENCE

Messenger RNA (mRNA) Messenger ribonucleic acid, first identified by Francis Crick,
Sydney Brenner, and Matthew Meselson.
Messenger RNA (mRNA) is the intermediary
molecule between DNA and ribosomes (in a
cell) that synthesize (i.e., manufacture) the
proteins coded for by the cell's DNA. On
receiving the "message" encoded in the DNA,
the messenger RNA passes through the ribosomes (similar to the manner in which a reel
of punched paper passes through an old player
piano), giving the ribosomes the specifications
for making the coded-for proteins. This process
is aided by transfer RNA (tRNA) molecules,

which forage for amino acids that float around
in the cell (outside of the cell's nucleus and
ribosomes). The tRNA molecules attach to
and escort individual amino acids to the ribosome, as and when the mRNA directs. Each
of the 20 different amino acids has at least one
of its own purpose-built tRNA molecules,
which possess a three-letter code of nucleotides at the stem of the cloverleaf-shaped
rRNA molecule.

The ribosome has room for only two tRNA
molecules at a time. The mRNA molecule
(that itself is passing through the ribosome)
calls over the first tRNA molecule, which
brings with it the specified amino acid. Short
sections of the mRNA and tRNA molecules
lock together inside the ribosome (because
where these two molecules meet, their three
nucleotides are complementary), the whole
(locked together) apparatus shifts along by
three notches (i.e., nucleotides), and a second
tRNA molecule (bearing another amino acid)
slips in next to the first tRNA molecule. Next,
the first amino acid (brought in by the first
tRNA molecule) jumps over to the second
tRNA molecule; joining to the amino acid that
was brought in by the second tRNA molecule,
thus making the start of a protein (i.e., a poly
amino acid molecule, also known as polypeptide or protein molecule). The empty (first)
tRNA molecule falls out of the ribosome, and
the whole (locked together) apparatus (i.e.,
mRNA plus second tRNA molecule) moves
three more notches (i.e., nucleotides) along
the mRNA molecule to make room for a third
tRNA molecule bearing another amino acid,
and so on.

This process of creating ever-longer chains of
amino acids continues to repeat itself inside
the ribosome until the protein (coded for by
the DNA, which code was transferred to
mRNA, which transferred it to the ribosome)
is completed.

See also TRANSCRIPTION, COMPLEMEN-
TARY DNA (c-DNA), CENTRAL DOGMA,
DEOXYRIBONUCLEIC ACID (DNA), RIBO-
NUCLEIC ACID (RNA), NUCLEIC ACIDS,
CODING SEQUENCE, GENETIC CODE,
CELL, INFORMATIONAL MOLECULES,
CODON, RIBOSOMES, POLYRIBOSOME
(POLYSOME), rRNA (RIBOSOMAL RNA),

M

NUCLEOTIDE, POLYMER, TRANSFER RNA (tRNA), PROTEIN, AMINO ACID, POLYPEPTIDE (PROTEIN), ANTISENSE (DNA SEQUENCE)

Messenger™ See HARPIN

Metabolic Engineering The selective, deliberate alteration of an organism's metabolic pathways via genetic engineering of the genes that define or control the organism's metabolism. Some reasons for the metabolic engineering of an organism include the following:

- Altering cell "behavior" and organism metabolic patterns to induce production of proteins/polypeptides and metabolites that are desired by mankind (e.g., "golden rice").
- Altering cell "behavior" and organism metabolic patterns to induce a given organism to consume or accumulate toxic wastes or valuable materials (e.g., gold) that are present at a site in low concentration or highly dispersed.
- Altering cell "behavior" and organism metabolic patterns to cure disease. For example, in 2004 Koji Yanai et al. utilized metabolic engineering of *Rosellinia sp.* filamentous fungi to make a more potent version of the naturally occurring compound known as **PF1022A**, which can be used to kill parasitic nematodes.

See also METABOLISM, INTERMEDIARY METABOLISM, CELL, PATHWAY, METABOLIC PATHWAY, FLUX, GENETIC ENGINEERING, ORGANISM, GENE, GENE SPLICING, PROTEIN, FUNGUS, PHYTOMANUFACTURING, POLYPEPTIDES, BIOLEACHING, BIODESULFURIZATION, BIORECOVERY, BIOREMEDIATION, GOLDEN RICE, PHYTOREMEDIATION, CELL SURFACE ENGINEERING, METABONOMICS, METABOLITE PROFILING, NEMATODES

Metabolic Flux Analysis See FLUX

Metabolic Pathway Refers to a particular pathway (i.e., series of chemical reactions, each of which is dependent on previous ones) within the overall process of metabolism in an organism. For example, when humans consume the herb known as Saint John's Wort (*Hypericum perforatum*), certain components in that herb induce a (new) metabolic pathway — catalyzed by cytochrome P450 enzymes — that (more) rapidly metabolizes (i.e., breaks down) a number of commercial pharmaceuticals (thereby lowering the effectiveness of a given dose of that particular pharmaceutical).

See also METABOLISM, PATHWAY, ORGANISM, INTERMEDIARY METABOLISM, CYTOCHROME P450, CYTOCHROME P450 3A4, CATALYST, GOLDEN RICE, FLUX, METABONOMICS, METABOLITE PROFILING

Metabolism The entire set of enzyme-catalyzed transformations of organic nutrient molecules (to sustain life) in living cells. Conversion of food and water into nutrients that can be used by the body's cells *and* the use of these nutrients by these cells (to sustain life, grow, etc.).

See also ENZYME, CELL, INTERMEDIARY METABOLISM, METABOLITE, COMBINATORIAL BIOLOGY, CITRIC ACID, AFLATOXIN, *FUSARIUM*, CYTOCHROME P4503A4, PATHWAY, METABOLIC PATHWAY, FLUX, METABONOMICS, METABOLITE PROFILING

Metabolite A chemical intermediate in the enzyme-catalyzed chemical reactions of metabolism.

See also METABOLISM, ENZYME, CELL, INTERMEDIARY METABOLISM, AFLATOXIN, *FUSARIUM*, METABONOMICS, METABOLITE PROFILING

Metabolite Profiling Determination of specifically which metabolic pathways (and/or related genes) are "switched on" (e.g., within a cell, tissue, or organism), thereby enabling precise definition of the **metabonomic condition** of that cell/tissue/organism at that moment in time (e.g., cellular response to an environmental stimulus or a genetic modification).

See also METABOLISM, METABOLITE, GENE, METABOLOME, METABOLIC PATHWAY, METABOLIC ENGINEERING, CELL, ORGANISM, METABONOMICS

Metabolome The complete set/complement of all metabolite and other molecules

M

(e.g., metabolon) involved in, or produced during, a cell's metabolism.

See also METABOLISM, METABOLITES, METABOLON, CELL

Metabolomics Refers to metabonomics of a given **single cell** or within a given **single cell type**.

See also METABONOMICS, CELL, METABOLITE PROFILING, METABOLOME

Metabolon A large agglomeration (within cell) of the enzymes involved (i.e., sequentially) in a metabolic pathway in an organism.

See also ENZYME, METABOLISM, PATHWAY, METABOLIC PATHWAY, ORGANISM, FLUX

Metabonomic Signature Refers to the complete set of metabolites (both **quantitative** compounds — metabolites' amounts — and also **qualitative** metabolic pathways) of a cell/tissue/organism at a specific moment in time.

See also METABOLISM, METABOLITE, METABOLIC PATHWAY, METABOLIC ENGINEERING, METABONOMICS, CELL, ORGANISM

Metabonomics The scientific study (e.g., delineation, measurement, etc.) of an organism's **metabolic response** (e.g., delineation of its metabolic pathways and measurement of all metabolites, etc.) to an environmental stimulus or a genetic modification.

See Also METABOLISM, METABOLITE, METABOLIC PATHWAY, ORGANISM, GENETIC ENGINEERING, METABOLIC ENGINEERING, ACTIVATOR (OF GENE), METABONOMIC SIGNATURE, BIOMARKERS

Metalloenzyme An enzyme having a metal ion as its prosthetic group.

See also ENZYME, PROSTHETIC GROUP, METALLOPROTEINS

Metalloproteins A term that is utilized to refer to any protein molecule that contains within it (i.e., in "peptide chain") a metal atom (e.g., zinc, iron, copper, etc.). Approximately one third of all proteins are metalloproteins. Those that contain a zinc atom (Zn^{2+}) are generally enzymes (thus called **metalloenzymes**) because zinc acts as a catalyst.

See also PROTEIN, PEPTIDE, ENZYME, CATALYST, METALLOENZYME

Metamodel Methods (of bioinformatics) These refer to methods utilized to integrate data that has been independently generated/created (and generally stored in separate database models) via independent **genomics** research projects, **combinatorial chemistry** projects, **high-throughput screening** projects (e.g., via biochip use), etc.

Metamodel methods sometimes reveal important interrelationships that were not apparent in the **individual** models (i.e., created solely for the GENOMICS project data, or created solely for the COMBINATORIAL CHEMISTRY project data, or created solely for the HIGH-THROUGHPUT SCREENING project data, etc.).

See also BIOINFORMATICS, GENOMICS, FUNCTIONAL GENOMICS, STRUCTURAL GENOMICS, COMBINATORIAL CHEMISTRY, HIGH-THROUGHPUT SCREENING, BIOCHIP

Metanomics See METABONOMICS, METABOLOMICS

Metastasis The process by which a given cancer (e.g., initial tumor) spreads from the site of its initial formation (in body) to other parts of the body.

One symptom of metastasis beginning or occurring in humans is the presence of epithelial cells in the bloodstream. That is because a transition of **epithelial cells becoming mesenchymal** (thereby enabling cell motility) is the typical first step of cancer metastasis. Transforming growth factor-beta (TGF-beta), exuded by cancerous tumor, leads epithelial tissue to dissolve the tight junctions between cells (e.g., in epithelium), and these cells then undergo morphogenesis to mesenchymal phenotype, as a prelude to cancer "invasion" of adjacent tissues.

See also CANCER, CELL, EPITHELIUM, OLIGOSACCHARIDES, LECTINS, ANGIOGENESIS, ANTIANGIOGENESIS, GENISTEIN (Gen), ISOFLAVONES, PHENOTYPE, HAPLOTYPE, TRANSFORMING GROWTH FACTOR-BETA (TGF-BETA)

Meter A unit of measurement that was first created by French scientists during the 1670s. It was initially defined to be one ten-millionth of the distance from Earth's equator to its poles.

See also NANOMETERS (nm)

M

Methionine (Met) An essential amino acid that furnishes (the organism with) both labile methyl groups and sulfur necessary for normal metabolism.
See also ESSENTIAL AMINO ACIDS, METABOLISM, CYSTINE, HIGH-METHIONINE CORN

Methyl Jasmonate The volatile chemical compound that results when methyl groups (CH_3) are chemically added to a molecule of jasmonic acid.
See also JASMONIC ACID

Methyl Salicylate The volatile chemical compound that results when methyl groups (CH_3) are added to a molecule of salicylic acid. In 1997, Ilya Raskin showed that methyl salicylate emitted by one tobacco plant (e.g., under "attack" by insects, fungi, bacteria, or viruses) could cause other nearby tobacco plants to "turn on" their self-defense mechanism (systemic acquired resistance).
See also SALICYLIC ACID (SA), BACTERIA, SYSTEMIC ACQUIRED RESISTANCE (SAR), FUNGUS

Methylated Refers to either of the following:

- A DNA molecule that is saturated with methyl groups (i.e., methyl submolecule groups, $-CH_3$, have attached themselves to the DNA molecule at all possible locations). Generally, when a DNA molecule is methylated, the genes comprising that DNA molecule are "turned off" (i.e., inactivated).
or
- A histone (i.e., the protein portion of a chromosome that the DNA condenses around) in which a protruding amino acid (e.g., lysine) has a methyl group attached to it. Generally, when a histone is methylated, the genes regulated by that histone are upregulated/"turned on."

In 2004, Yang Shi discovered an enzyme named LSD1 that demethylates (i.e., "cuts" methyl group off) histone's protruding lysine amino acid. That demethylation results in repression of the genes regulated by that histone.

See also DNA METHYLATION, DEOXYRIBONUCLEIC ACID (DNA), TRANSCRIPTION, MESSENGER RNA (mRNA), GENE, GENETIC CODE, GENE EXPRESSION, EXPRESSIVITY, P53 GENE, TUMOR SUPPRESSOR GENES, IMPRINTING, PROTEIN, HISTONES, CHROMOSOMES, AMINO ACID, LYSINE (Lys), UPREGULATION, POSITIVE CONTROL, TRANSCRIPTIONAL ACTIVATOR, ENZYME, REPRESSION (OF GENE TRANSCRIPTION/TRANSLATION), DEMETHYLATION, LYSINE-SPECIFIC DEMETHYLASE 1 (LSD1)

MFA Acronym for **metabolic flux analysis**.
See FLUX

MGED Acronym for **Microarray Gene Expression Data Society.** It consists of scientists who are attempting to jointly create a set guidelines (known as MIAME standards) governing the types of information to record/publish concerning experiments in which DNA microarrays are utilized. The goal is to make it easier to analyze and compare the results achieved by differing researchers utilizing different microarrays.
See also MICROARRAY (TESTING), DEOXYRIBONUCLEIC ACID (DNA), DNA MICROARRAY, GENE, EXPRESS, GENE EXPRESSION ANALYSIS, BIOINFORMATICS

MHC See MAJOR HISTOCOMPATIBILITY COMPLEX (MHC)

MHC I See MAJOR HISTOCOMPATIBILITY COMPLEX (MHC), MAJOR HISTOCOMPATIBILITY ANTIGEN — CLASS I

MHC II See MAJOR HISTOCOMPATIBILITY COMPLEX (MHC), MAJOR HISTOCOMPATIBILITY ANTIGEN — CLASS II

MIAME Acronym for **minimum information about a microarray experiment**.
See MGED

Micelle The spherical structure formed by the association of a number of amphiphilic molecules dissolved in water. Structurally, the outer surface of the micelle (sphere) is covered with the polar domains (head groups) that are directed towards (stick into) the water whereas the interior of the micelle contains the nonpolar domains (tails) that self-associate to create an "oil droplet" microenvironment. Micelles may be used to solubilize nonwater (oil) soluble or

M

sparingly-water-soluble molecules in water. They may be formed by ionic or nonionic surfactants.

See also AMPHIPHILIC MOLECULES, SUPERCRITICAL CARBON DIOXIDE, CRITICAL MICELLE CONCENTRATION, REVERSE MICELLE (RM), SURFACTANT, FATS, SELF-ASSEMBLY

Micro Sensors See BIOCHIP, MICROARRAY (TESTING), BIOSENSOR

Micro Total Analysis Systems Abbreviated μTAS or mTAS.

See GENE EXPRESSION ANALYSIS, BIOCHIP, GENOSENSORS, NANOTECHNOLOGY, BIOSENSORS (ELECTRONIC), BIOSENSORS (CHEMICAL), LAB-ON-A-CHIP

Micro Total Analytical Systems See MICRO TOTAL ANALYSIS SYSTEMS

Microaerophile An organism that grows best in the presence of a small amount of oxygen.

See also ORGANISM, MICROORGANISM, FACULTATIVE ANAEROBE

Microarray (testing) Refers to a piece of glass, plastic, or silicon, onto which has been placed a large number of biosensors at known, specific locations. These microarrays (sometimes called "biochips" or "DNA chips") can then be utilized to test a single biological sample for a variety of attributes or effects.

For example, by placing protein-detection molecules (e.g., ligands, dyes which change color, fluoresce, or cause electronic signal on contact with specific protein molecules) onto a microarray, a scientist can perform GENE EXPRESSION ANALYSIS (i.e., evaluation of the protein expression and **expression levels** of genes in a biological sample).

Another application would be to place (cellular) receptors, nucleic acids/probes, oligonucleotides, adhesion molecules, messenger RNA (specific to which gene is "turned on" in a given disease state), cDNA (complementary to mRNA coded for by each gene that is "turned on"), oligosaccharides and other relevant carbohydrate molecules, or cells (indicating which cellular pathway is "turned on," etc.) onto a microarray to utilize that microarray to screen for proteins or other chemical compounds that act against a disease (i.e., therapeutic target), as indicated by (the relevant component from biological sample)

adhesion or hybridization to a specific spot (location) on the microarray where a specific (target molecule) was earlier placed/attached. The "detection event" (e.g., hybridization of sample molecules to cDNA, etc.) is indicated to the scientist via "tagging"/"labeling" of the sample molecules prior to testing. For example:

- Fluorescent Tags reveal the location (and thus the cDNA molecule) on the biochip that the sample molecule hybridized to, when the biochip is scanned with a laser of appropriate wavelength.
- Radioactive Labels reveal the location (and thus the cDNA molecule) on the biochip that the sample molecule hybridized to, when the biochip is utilized to expose or develop relevant photographic film.
- Enzymatic reveals the location (and thus the target molecule) on the biochip that the sample molecule hybridized to, adhered to, etc., when the biochip is scanned (e.g., to detect location of the product of the enzyme "tag" that is released when the sample molecule hybridizes to or adheres to the specific target molecule on the biochip).

"Quantum dots" could potentially be used on microarrays in place of cellular receptors in the future.

See also DNA CHIP, MULTIPLEXED (ASSAY), BIOCHIPS, GENE, CODING SEQUENCE, GENE EXPRESSION, GENE EXPRESSION ANALYSIS, GENOSENSORS, NANOTECHNOLOGY, GENOMICS, FUNCTIONAL GENOMICS, BIOSENSORS (ELECTRONIC), BIOSENSORS (CHEMICAL), HIGH-THROUGHPUT SCREENING (HTS), TARGET–LIGAND INTERACTION SCREENING, OLIGOSACCHARIDES, OLIGOSACCHARIDE MICROARRAYS, FLUORESCENCE, ADME/Tox, RECEPTORS, BIORECEPTORS, COMBINATORIAL CHEMISTRY, TARGET (OF A THERAPEUTIC AGENT), IMMUNOSENSOR, TARGET (OF A HERBICIDE OR INSECTICIDE), ADHESION MOLECULE, MICROFLUIDICS, BIOELECTRONICS,

M

ASSAY, BIOASSAY, MESSENGER RNA (mRNA), CHARACTERIZATION ASSAY, PROBE, HYBRIDIZATION (MOLECULAR BIOLOGY), BIOINFORMATICS, CELL ARRAY, HYBRIDIZATION SURFACES, PATHWAY, DEOXYRIBONUCLEIC ACID (DNA), QUANTUM DOT, NANOPARTICLES, PROTEIN MICROARRAYS, PROTEOME CHIP, DIP-PEN NANOLITHOGRAPHY, SNP CHIP, IMMOBILIZATION

Microbe A microscopic organism; a term applied particularly to bacteria. The word "microbe" was coined by Sedillot, a colleague of Louis Pasteur.

See also BACTERIA, GENETICALLY ENGINEERED MICROBIAL PESTICIDES (GEMP), PHYTOALEXINS

Microbial Physiology The cell structure, growth factors, metabolism, and genetics of microorganisms.

See also MICROORGANISM, CELL, METABOLISM, GENETICS, MICROBIOLOGY

Microbial Source Tracking (MST) The process of systematically determining the **original source** (in a specific environment) **of a microbe** (e.g., the one that has caused a given disease outbreak). Some of the technologies utilized in MST include genetic fingerprinting, polymerase chain reaction (PCR), serotyping, etc.

See also MICROBE, PATHOGEN, POLYMERASE CHAIN REACTION (PCR) TECHNIQUE, SEROTYPES

Microbicide Any chemical that will kill microorganisms. Used synonymously with the terms "biocide" and "bactericide."

See also MICROORGANISM, BIOCIDE

Microbiology The science dealing with the structure, classification, physiology, and distribution of microorganisms, and with their technical and medical significance. The term microorganism is applied to the simple unicellular and structurally similar representatives of the plant and animal kingdoms. With few exceptions, the unicellular organisms are invisible to the naked eye and generally have dimensions of between a fraction of a micrometer and 200 μm.

See also MICRON

Microchannel Fluidic Devices See MICROFLUIDICS

Microelectromechanical Systems See MEMS (NANOTECHNOLOGY)

Microfilaments Very thin filaments found in the cytoplasm of cells.

See also CELL, CYTOPLASM, MICROTUBULES

Microfluidic Chips See BIOCHIP, MICROFLUIDICS, NANOTECHNOLOGY

Microfluidics Refers to the science and properties of fluids when flowing through **very small passages** (e.g., micron or nanometer dimensions) and in **very small amounts** (e.g., femtogram quantities).

For example, to move fluid (samples), **microfluidic chips** utilize either capillary action or else they "pump" fluid (through microchannels in those chips) electrokinetically (i.e., cause the flow to occur by applying a controlled electrical field so liquid is attracted to electrical charge, and thereby flows). Such pumping could also be utilized to deliver certain medicines in very small, precisely timed, and metered doses (e.g., if the microfluidic chip is embedded into diseased tissue within the body).

Another potential application of this pumping could be to perform multiple chemical analyses (e.g., of body fluids within diseased tissues), in which case such microfluidic chips are known as "**lab-on-a-chip**" (laboratory-on-a-chip) analytical devices.

See also BIOCHIP, NANOTECHNOLOGY, MICROARRAY (TESTING), NANOSCIENCE, MICRON

Microgram 10^{-6} g or 2.527×10^{-8} oz (avoirdupois).

Micromachining Refers to the technology and tools/methods utilized to create the very small parts, grooves (in chips/arrays), etc., in NEMS (nanoelectromechanical systems), biochips, microarrays, and other devices in the field of nanotechnology.

See also NANOTECHNOLOGY, NANOELECTROMECHANICAL SYSTEMS (NEMS), BIOCHIP, MICROARRAY (TESTING), DIP-PEN NANOLITHOGRAPHY

Micromodification Term utilized by some people to refer to posttranslational modification of protein molecules.

See also POSTTRANSLATIONAL MODIFICATION OF PROTEIN, TRANSLATION

M

Micron Also called micrometer. A unit of length convenient for describing cellular dimensions; the Greek letter μ is used as its symbol. A micron is equal to 10^{-3} mm (millimeter) or 104 (Angstroms) or 0.00003937 in.
See also MICROBIOLOGY, CELL, MICRO-FLUIDICS

Microorganism Any organism of microscopic size (i.e., requires a microscope to be seen by man). First viewed by Antoni van Leeuenhoek in 1676. Some microorganisms are pathogenic (i.e., disease causing) and some are not.
See also MICROBIOLOGY, BACTERIA, PATHOGENIC, NEMATODES, CAPSULE

Microparticles Refers to the metal particles (<1 μm in diameter) that are coated with genes and "shot" into cells with the Biolistic^R gene gun.
See also BIOLISTIC^R GENE GUN, VECTORS, MICRON, GENE

Microphage See POLYMORPHONUCLEAR LEUKOCYTES

Micropropagation A technique used by man to replicate (mass produce) a given (e.g., valuable) plant by making genetic clones ("copies") of that original plant.
See also CLONE (AN ORGANISM), GENETICS

MicroRNA See MICRORNAs

MicroRNAs Refers to either of the following:

- Naturally occurring small segments of RNA (approximately 22 nucleotides in length) that play an important role in gene regulation (i.e., "turning on" or "turning off" genes) via binding to and impacting the translation of specific mRNAs. MicroRNAs thereby help regulate an organism's early development, cell differentiation, and apoptosis. MicroRNAs are directly coded for by an organism's genes. It is estimated that approximately 30% of human genes are regulated by microRNAs. or
- Small, chemically synthesized RNA segments that are designed to mimic the products (i.e., siRNA segments) of Dicer enzymes, in terms of causing RNA interference.

Research indicates that microRNAs can also cause the following:

- Some genes within certain invading (e.g., pathogenic) viruses to shut down (via RNA silencing), thereby preventing infection of the host
- Some genes within a plant's DNA to revert to (grandparent's) wild-type version of the gene when both parents' DNA contained a mutated version of the gene

See also RIBONUCLEIC ACID (RNA), MESSENGER RNA (mRNA), TRANSLATION, DEOXYRIBONUCLEIC ACID (DNA), GENE, GENE EXPRESSION, REGULATORY GENES, RNA INTERFERENCE (RNAi), ORGANISM, EMBRYOLOGY, DIFFERENTIATION, CELL DIFFERENTIATION, WILD TYPE, MUTATION, CODING SEQUENCE, APOPTOSIS, DICER ENZYMES, SHORT INTERFERING RNA (siRNA), PATHOGEN, VIRUS

Microsatellite DNA Pieces of the same small segment (i.e., a DNA sequence) that are "repeated" (appear repeatedly in sequence within the DNA molecule) adjacent to a specific gene within the DNA molecule. Thus, these "microsatellites" are linked to that specific gene.
See also DEOXYRIBONUCLEIC ACID (DNA), LINKAGE, SEQUENCE (OF A DNA MOLECULE), SATELLITE DNA, GENE, LINKAGE GROUP

Microsystems Technology See MST (NANOTECHNOLOGY)

Microtubules Tiny hollow filaments (i.e., string-like structures) within eucaryotic cells, which are made of tubulin (α and β proteins). Some microtubules give the cell its shape (e.g., act as structural components of cell). Other microtubules are the "towropes" utilized to move proteins within cells via vesicular transport (vesicles are small hollow structures that contain these protein molecules). Microtubules also "tow" apart the paired chromosomes within nuclear DNA of cells undergoing meiosis.
Microtubule proteins present in bacterial cells include **FtsZ**. Microtubules also "power" flagella (i.e., the whiplike structures used by

M

sperm and some bacteria to "swim") and cilia (i.e., the tiny hairlike projections that line many mucosal surfaces in humans and that "sweep" dust particles, etc., to clean the mucosal surfaces).

Within neurons (cells of the mammalian nervous system), microtubules transport messenger RNAs (mRNA) from the nucleus (where they are "manufactured") to the ribosomes in the dendrites (i.e., long extensions of the neuron cell), where the mRNAs are "translated" into protein molecules (i.e., proteins are "manufactured" by ribosome).

See also CELL, MEIOSIS, NUCLEAR DNA, DEOXYRIBONUCLEIC ACID (DNA), BACTERIA, FLAGELLA, CILIA, NEURON, MESSENGER RNA (mRNA), NUCLEUS, RIBOSOMES, DENDRITES, PROTEIN, VESICULAR TRANSPORT (OF A PROTEIN), MreB, ParM, PLASMID, EUCARYOTE, ANALOGUE, CYTOSKELETON

Mid-Oleic Sunflowers Refers to sunflower (*Helianthus annus* L.) plant varieties that have been bred so their seeds contain 50-75% oleic acid within the oil in those seeds vs. the historical average of 20% oleic acid in the oil of traditional sunflower (crop) plant varieties.

See also FATTY ACID, OLEIC ACID, HIGH-OLEIC SUNFLOWERS, HIGH-OLEIC OIL SOYBEANS

Mid-Oleic Vegetable Oils Refers to any of the vegetable oils (other than sunflower oil) that contain 50 to 70% oleic acid. The range of **oleic acid content** is slightly different for mid-oleic sunflower oil definition.

See also MID-OLEIC SUNFLOWERS, FATTY ACID, OLEIC AID

Mimetics See BIOMIMETIC MATERIALS

Minimized Domains See MINIMIZED PROTEINS

Minimized Proteins The domain/active site of a (former) native protein after all or most of its extraneous (unneeded) portions (peptides) have been removed. In 1995, Brian Cunningham and James A. Wells reduced the 28-residue (peptide) protein (hormone) **atrial natriuretic factor** to 15-residues (peptides) size **without reducing its potency (biological activity).**

Minimized proteins that retain their potency hold the potential for medicines possessing a greater serum lifetime (when injected into a patient's body), and as "models" for the creation of organic-chemical-synthesized mimetic drugs possessing the same therapeutic effect as the native protein did.

See also PROTEIN, PEPTIDE, ACTIVE SITE, ENZYME, CATALYTIC SITE, DOMAIN (OF A PROTEIN), HORMONE, ATRIAL NATRIURETIC FACTOR, BIOMIMETIC MATERIALS, SERUM LIFETIME, BIOLOGICAL ACTIVITY, NANOBODIES

Minimum Tillage See LOW-TILLAGE CROP PRODUCTION, NO-TILLAGE CROP PRODUCTION

Miniprotein Domains See MINIMIZED DOMAINS

Miniproteins See MINIMIZED PROTEINS

miRNAs Acronym for **microRNAs.**

See MICRORNAs

Mismatch Repair Refers to cellular enzyme systems that repair any nucleotide-insertion errors (i.e., resulting from the DNA replication process) via excising (i.e., cutting out) the incorrect DNA sequence and replacing it with correct DNA sequence.

See also CELL, ENZYME, NUCLEOTIDE, DEOXYRIBONUCLEIC ACID (DNA), DNA REPAIR, REPLICATION (OF DNA), SEQUENCE (OF A DNA MOLECULE), UNWINDING PROTEIN

Mitochondria Granular or rod-shaped bodies (organelles) in a cell's cytoplasm that contain the zyme systems required in the citric acid cycle, electron transport, beta-oxidation of fatty acids, and synthesis of ATP via oxidative phosphorylation.

See also ZYME SYSTEMS, CELL, MITOCHONDRIAL DNA, CARNITINE, UBIQUINONE, ADENOSINE TRIPHOSPHATE, FATTY ACIDS, FATS, PHOSPHOLIPIDS, CYTOCHROME, CYTOPLASM, CITRIC ACID CYCLE, ATP, AcCoA

Mitochondrial DNA The DNA within an organism's (e.g., human) cells that is located inside the mitochondria (organelles), and not inside the cell nucleus. Mitochondrial DNA is only passed down from **mother** to offspring, not from father to offspring, as with **nuclear DNA**.

See also DEOXYRIBONUCLEIC ACID (DNA), CELL, MITOCHONDRIA, NUCLEUS, CYTOPLASMIC DNA

M

Mitogen A substance (e.g., growth factor, hormone, etc.) that initiates cell division within the body. For example, most angiogenic growth factors (e.g., fibroblast growth factor) stimulate cell division of the endothelial cells that line blood vessel walls.
See also MITOSIS, GROWTH FACTOR, HORMONE, ANGIOGENIC GROWTH FACTORS, ENDOTHELIAL CELLS, MAPK, MITOGEN-ACTIVATED PROTEIN KINASE CASCADE

Mitogen-Activated Protein Kinase Cascade A cellular signaling pathway via which many fundamental cell processes such as differentiation, transcription, proliferation, apoptosis, etc., are controlled. For example, cell proliferation is promoted by growth factors' activation of receptor tyrosine kinases, which then "recruit" *ras*-**family small G proteins** to the cell's internal plasma membrane surface, followed by activation of other cellular kinases (thereby causing phosphorylation of certain proteins in the cell's nucleus), resulting in changes to the cell's protein-synthesizing processes.
In certain plants, exposure to cold temperatures can cause oxidative stress. This oxidative stress can then initiate activation of the mitogen-activated protein kinase (MAPK) cascade, resulting in production of several **stress responsive proteins** (e.g., heat-shock proteins). These "stress proteins" help protect such plants from cold temperatures.
See also CASCADE, KINASES, RECEPTORS, MITOGEN, PROTEIN, CELL, DIFFERENTIATION, APOPTOSIS, TRANSCRIPTION, GROWTH FACTORS, *ras* PROTEIN, G-PROTEINS, PHOSPHORYLATION, NUCLEUS, CELL DIFFERENTIATION, TRANSLATION, COLD HARDENING, OXIDATIVE STRESS, STRESS PROTEINS

Mitosis A process of cell duplication or reproduction during which one cell gives rise to two identical daughter cells.
See also MITOGEN, TUBULIN

Mixed-Function Oxygenases Enzymes catalyzing simultaneous oxidation of two substances by oxygen, one of which is usually NADPH or NADH.
See also NADPH, NADH, OXIDATION, ENZYME

Model Organism Refers to an organism that is utilized (e.g., in scientific experiments) to conduct tests, etc., in an attempt to infer results applicable to larger, more complex organisms. For example:

- The use of the microscopic roundworm *C. elegans* in high-throughput screening to attempt to find pharmaceuticals that will be useful for humans
- The use of the zebra fish (*Danio rerio*) for research on embryonic development applicable to all vertebrates

See also ORGANISM, DROSOPHILA, *CAENORHABDITIS ELEGANS (C. elegans)*, HIGH-THROUGHPUT SCREENING (HTS), *ARABIDOPSIS THALIANA*, HOMOLOGOUS (CHROMOSOMES OR GENES), ORTHOLOG, PHYLOGENETIC PROFILING

Moiety Referring to a part or portion of a molecule, generally complex, having a characteristic chemical or pharmacological property.
See also ANALOGUE, PHARMACOPHORE

Mold See FUNGUS

Mole An Avogadro's number ($6.022141527 \times 10^{23}$) of whatever units are being considered. One gram molecular weight of an element or a compound (i.e., same number of grams of an element or a compound as that substance's molecular weight, equal to 6.023×10^{23} molecules).
See also MOLECULAR WEIGHT

Molecular Beacon Term that is used to refer to specific **oligonucleotides possessing a "hairpin loop" and bearing a fluorescent dye**. A "quencher dye" located on a **nearby portion of the hairpin loop** prevents fluorescence until the hairpin loop is opened up. Molecular beacons (sometimes called **fluorogenic probes**) are utilized (e.g., in **high-throughput screening** or **high-throughput identification**) to detect the presence of a desired "target" molecule. When the "target" (i.e., a molecule possessing the desired functional group or desired property) is present within a given sample being evaluated, the "hairpin loop" opens up because a portion of it forms a stronger bond to the "target" (than to the rest of the loop), thereby allowing the fluorescent dye to emit light.

M

See also OLIGONUCLEOTIDE, HAIRPIN LOOP, FLUORESCENCE, TARGET (OF A THERAPEUTIC AGENT), TARGET (OF A HERBICIDE OR INSECTICIDE), HIGH-THROUGHPUT IDENTIFICATION, HIGH-THROUGHPUT SCREENING (HTS)

Molecular Biology A term coined by Vannevar Bush during the 1940s that eventually came to mean the study and manipulation of molecules that constitute or interact with cells. Molecular biology as a distinct scientific discipline originated largely as a result of a decision to provide "support for the application of new physical and chemical techniques to biology" during the 1930s by Warren Weaver, director of the biology (funding) program at Rockefeller Foundation (a philanthropic organization).

See also MOLECULAR GENETICS, GENETICS, GENETIC ENGINEERING, BIOLOGICAL ACTIVITY, BIOPOLYMER, BIOGENESIS, BIOCHEMISTRY, DEOXYRIBONUCLEIC ACID (DNA), MITOSIS, MEIOSIS

Molecular Breeding™ A trademarked term that refers to certain "**molecular evolution**" technologies developed by Maxygen Company.

This term is also sometimes used to refer to the utilization of molecular genetics and **marker-assisted selection** in a breeding program (e.g., within a seed company or within a university) to select the organisms (e.g., crop varieties) that possess genes for a particular trait (e.g., higher yield, disease resistance, etc.).

See also MARKER-ASSISTED SELECTION, MOLECULAR EVOLUTION, GENE, TRAIT, MARKER (DNA SEQUENCE), QUANTITATIVE TRAIT LOCI (QTL)

Molecular Bridge Refers to the use of high-affinity molecules such as biotin and streptavidin or other surface treatments in order to "attach" something (e.g., quantum dot, nanoshell, enzyme, probe, etc.) to specific molecules (e.g., antibody targeted to tumor, etc.) or to a specific surface (e.g., the surface of a biosensor, biochip/microarray, etc.).

See also ANTIBODY, STREPTAVIDIN, QUANTUM DOT, NANOSHELLS, LIGAND (IN BIOCHEMISTRY), ENZYME, PROBE, TUMOR, BIOSENSORS (CHEMICAL), BIOSENSORS (ELECTRONIC), BIOCHIPS, MICROARRAY (TESTING), HYBRIDIZATION SURFACES, PROTEOME CHIP, BIOTIN

Molecular Chaperones See CHAPERONES, PROTEIN FOLDING

Molecular Diversity Sometimes referred to as "irrational drug design," this refers to the drug design technique of generating large numbers of diverse candidate molecules (e.g., pieces of DNA, RNA, proteins, or other organic moieties) at random (via a variety of methods). These diverse candidate molecules are then tested to see which is best at working against a disease/condition (e.g., fitting a cell receptor or category of receptors relevant to the disease in question). Molecular candidates that show promise (e.g., via a "pretty good fit" to receptor) are then produced in larger quantities (e.g., via polymerase chain reaction techniques) along with additional molecules that are similar though slightly different in structure (e.g., via site-directed mutagenesis) in an attempt to create a molecule that is a "perfect fit" (e.g., to receptor).

See also RATIONAL DRUG DESIGN, DEOXYRIBONUCLEIC ACID (DNA), RIBONUCLEIC ACID (RNA), RECEPTORS, RECEPTOR FITTING (RF), RECEPTOR MAPPING (RM), MOIETY, POLYMERASE CHAIN REACTION (PCR), SITE-DIRECTED MUTAGENESIS, DIVERSITY BIOTECHNOLOGY CONSORTIUM, COMBINATORIAL CHEMISTRY, COMBINATORIAL BIOLOGY

Molecular Evolution See COMBINATORIAL CHEMISTRY

Molecular Fingerprinting See COMBINATORIAL CHEMISTRY

Molecular Genetics The science dealing with the study of the nature and biochemistry of the genetic material. Includes the technologies of genetic engineering.

See also GENETICS, GENETIC ENGINEERING, MOLECULAR BIOLOGY, BIOLOGICAL ACTIVITY, BIOPOLYMER, BIOGENESIS, BIOCHEMISTRY, DEOXYRIBONUCLEIC ACID (DNA), MITOSIS, MEIOSIS, MOLECULAR DIVERSITY, CENTRAL DOGMA

Molecular Lithography See BIOELECTRONICS, NANOLITHOGRAPHY

M

Molecular Machines Refer to nanometer-dimension "machines" capable of doing various tasks.
See also NANOTECHNOLOGY, NANOMETERS (nm), BIOMOTORS, NANOBOTS, NANOELECTROMECHANICAL SYSTEM (NEMS), NANOSCIENCE

Molecular Pharming™ A trademark of the Groupe Limagrain Company, it refers to the production of pharmaceuticals and certain other chemicals (e.g., intermediate chemicals utilized to manufacture pharmaceuticals) in agronomic plants (that have been genetically engineered).
See also ANTIBIOTIC, GENETIC ENGINEERING, PHYTOCHEMICALS, EDIBLE VACCINES, CORN, PLANTIBODIES™

Molecular Profiling See GENE EXPRESSION PROFILING, METABOLITE PROFILING, GENE EXPRESSION ANALYSIS

Molecular Sieves Refer to structures bearing pores/channels whose internal diameters are smaller than 0.5 nm and thus can be utilized to separate small molecules (in a solution) from "large" molecules in the solution.
See also NANOMETERS (nm), NANOTUBE, CARBON NANOTUBES, NANOTUBE MEMBRANES

Molecular Weight The sum of the atomic weights of the constituent atoms in a molecule.
See also ATOMIC WEIGHT

Monarch Butterfly Refers to the insect (*Lepidoptera: Danaidae* or *Danaus plexippus*) whose pupae (caterpillars) feed exclusively on the tissue of the plant known as **common milkweed** (*Asclepias syriaca*) and whose territory extends from northern Mexico to approximately Canada's southern border.
See also *BACILLUS THURINGIENSIS (B.t.)*, *B.T. KURSTAKI, B.T. TOLWORTHI*, CRY1A (b) PROTEIN

Monoclonal Antibodies (MAb) Discovered and developed in the 1970s by Cesar Milstein and Georges Kohler, monoclonal antibodies are derived from a single source or clone of cells that recognize only one kind of antigen. Made by fusing myeloma cancer cells (that multiply very fast) with antibody-producing cells and then spreading the resulting conjugate colony so thin that each cell can be grown into a whole, separate colony (i.e., cloning). In this way, one gets whole batches of the same (monoclonal) antibody, which are all specific to the same antigen. Monoclonal antibodies have found markets in diagnostic kits, pharmaceuticals (e.g., trastuzumab, rituximab, bevacizumab, adalimumab, infliximab, etc.), imaging agents, and in purification processes. One example of a diagnostic use is the invention in 1997 by Bruno Oesch of a monoclonal-antibody-based rapid test to detect the prion (PrP 5c) that causes bovine spongiform encephalopathy (BSE) in cattle.
During the 1990s, scientists were able to insert gene cassettes into plants to cause them to produce such antibodies in plant tissue (e.g., seeds).
See also ASCITES, MYELOMA, TUMOR, CORN, IMMUNOTOXIN, BLAST CELL, ANTIGEN, ANTIBODY, SINGLE-DOMAIN ANTIBODIES (dAbs), MURINE, CATALYTIC ANTIBODY, SEMISYNTHETIC CATALYTIC ANTIBODY, ANGIOGENESIS INHIBITORS, BSE, PRION, GENE, HER-2 GENE, RHEUMATOID ARTHRITIS, ADALIMUMAB, INFLIXIMAB, RITUXIMAB, HUMANIZED ANTIBODY, TRASTUZUMAB, PLANTIBODIES, CYTOSKELETON, CASSETTE

Monocytes Also called monocyte macrophages. The round-nucleated cells that circulate in the blood.
In summary, they engulf and kill microorganisms, present antigen to the lymphocytes, kill certain tumor cells, and are involved in the regulation of inflammation. These cells are often the first to encounter a foreign substance or pathogen or normal cell debris in the body. When they do, the material is taken up (engulfed) and degraded by means of oxidative and hydrolytic enzymatic attack. Peptides that result from the degradation of foreign protein are then bound to a monocyte protein called class II MHC (major histocompatibility complex), and this self-foreign complex then migrates to the surface of the cell, where it is embedded into the cell membrane in such a way as to present the peptide to the outside of the cell. This positioning allows T lymphocytes to recognize (inspect) the peptide. Whereas self-peptides derived from normal cellular debris are ignored, foreign peptides activate precursors of helper T cells to further mature into active, lymphokine-secreting

M

helper T lymphocytes, also known as TH cells. When monocytes move out of the bloodstream and into the tissues, they are then called macrophages.

See also MACROPHAGE, CELLULAR IMMUNE RESPONSE, PATHOGEN, MHC

Monoecious A category of plants (e.g., the soybean plant is one) that possess both male and female reproductive structures on the same plant. Thus, such plants are capable of self-pollination. For example, 95% of the pollen from a soybean plant (*Glycine max*) does not leave the flower that it was produced in. Virtually none of a given soybean plant's pollen leaves the plant that it was produced in.

See also SOYBEAN PLANT, BARNASE

Monomer The basic molecular subunit from which, by repetition of a single reaction, polymers are made. For example, amino acids (monomers) link together via condensation reactions to yield polypeptides or proteins (polymers). A monomer is analogous to a link (monomer) in a metal chain (polymer).

See also POLYMER

Monosaccharides The chemical building blocks of carbohydrates, hence known as "simple sugars." They are classified by the number of carbon atoms in the (monosaccharide) molecule. For example, pentoses have five and hexoses have six carbon atoms. They normally form ring structures. The empirical formula for monosaccharides is $(CH_2O)_n$.

See also OLIGOSACCHARIDES, CARBOHYDRATES, SUGAR MOLECULES

Monounsaturated Fats Fat molecules possessing one less than the maximum possible number of hydrogen atoms (on that given fat molecule). Diets that are high in monounsaturated fat content have been shown to reduce low-density lipoprotein ("bad cholesterol") levels in blood content, while leaving blood levels of high-density lipoproteins ("good cholesterol") essentially unchanged.

See also FATTY ACID, SATURATED FATTY ACIDS, DEHYDROGENATION, UNSATURATED FATTY ACID, LOW-DENSITY LIPOPROTEINS (LDLP), HIGH-DENSITY LIPOPROTEINS (HDLPs), OLEIC ACID, FATS

Monounsaturated Fatty Acids (MUFA) Refer to the category of those fatty acids (e.g., oleic acid) that possess one less than the maximum possible number of hydrogen atoms (e.g., possible to be attached to the molecular structure of oleic acid, in this example).

Enzymes (e.g., Δ12 desaturase) present in some oilseed plants (e.g., soybean, corn/maize, canola, etc.) convert some MUFAs to polyunsaturated fatty acids (PUFAs) within their developing seeds.

Diets that are high in monounsaturated fatty acid content have been shown to reduce low-density lipoprotein (i.e., so-called "bad cholesterol") levels in blood content while simultaneously leaving blood levels of high-density lipoproteins (i.e., "good cholesterol") essentially unchanged. Soybean oil has historically averaged approximately 24.5% of monounsaturated fatty acids content by weight.

See also MONOUNSATURATED FATS, FATTY ACID, UNSATURATED FATTY ACID, SOYBEAN OIL, OLEIC ACID, LOW-DENSITY LIPOPROTEINS (LDLP), DELTA 12 DESATURASE, POLYUNSATURATED FATTY ACIDS (PUFA)

Morphogenetic An adjective referring to the formation and differentiation of tissues and organs in an organism.

See also MORPHOLOGY, STEM CELLS, TOTIPOTENT STEM CELLS

Morpholino Refers to a methodology utilized for gene silencing.

See GENE SILENCING

Morphology First used in print by the poet Johann Wolfgang von Goethe, this word is utilized to refer to the form or structure of an organism or any of its parts.

See also TRAIT, PHENOTYPE

MOS See MANNANOLIGOSACCHARIDES

Motor Proteins Refers to specialist protein molecules (e.g., kinesin, myosin, actin, etc.) within cells, which transport various items (e.g., newly made protein molecules, organelles, etc.) from one part of the cell to another. Some of them sometimes also move the entire cell to another location inside the organism (e.g., via "towropes" called **filopodia**).

See also PROTEIN, KINESIN, MYOSIN, ACTIN, CELL, ORGANELLES, ORGANISM

Mouse-Ear Cress A common name for *Arabidopsis thaliana* utilized in some countries.

See *ARABIDOPSIS THALIANA*

M

MPSS Acronym for **massively parallel signature sequencing**.
See MASSIVELY PARALLEL SIGNATURE SEQUENCING

MRA See MUTUAL RECOGNITION AGREEMENTS, MUTUAL RECOGNITION ARRANGEMENTS

MreB A contractile (i.e., periodically contracting) string-like protein that is present in at least the rod-shaped bacteria (probably some other bacterial types too); they are present just beneath the surface (membrane) of these bacteria. MreB filaments thus give rod-shaped bacteria their shape.
See also PROTEIN, MOTOR PROTEINS, BACTERIA

MRL See MAXIMUM RESIDUE LEVEL

mRNA See MESSENGER RNA

MS Acronym for **mass spectrometer**.
See MASS SPECTROMETER

MSA Acronym for **molecular self-assembly**.
See SELF-ASSEMBLY (OF A LARGE MOLECULAR STRUCTURE), SELF-ASSEMBLING MOLECULAR MACHINES

MSF See MEGAKARYOCYTE-STIMULATING FACTOR

MST (microbes) See MICROBIAL SOURCE TRACKING

MST (nanotechnology) Acronym utilized by Europeans to refer to **"microsystems technology"** (i.e., their common term for "microelectromechanical systems" — MEMS).
See also NANOTECHNOLOGY, BIOCHIP, GENOSENSORS, BIOSENSORS (ELECTRONIC), BIOSENSORS (CHEMICAL), QUANTUM WIRE, QUANTUM DOT, NANOCRYSTAL MOLECULES, MICROFLUIDICS, BIOMOTORS, MOLECULAR MACHINES

MTAS See MICRO TOTAL ANALYSIS SYSTEMS

mTAS Acronym for **micro total analysis systems**.
See MICRO TOTAL ANALYSIS SYSTEMS

mtDNA Acronym for **mitochondrial DNA**.
See MITOCHONDRIAL DNA

MUFA See MONOUNSATURATED FATTY ACIDS (MUFA)

Multicopy Plasmids Plasmids that are present inside bacteria in quantities greater than one plasmid per (host) cell.

See also PLASMID, VECTOR, COPY NUMBER

Multi-Drug Resistance See P-GLYCOPROTEIN, FLUX, ANTIBIOTIC RESISTANCE

Multienzyme System A sequence of related enzymes participating in a given metabolic (chemical reaction) pathway.

Multigenic See POLYGENIC

Multiple Sclerosis A disease in which the human body's immune cells attack myelin (i.e., the "insulation" that surrounds nerve fibers in the spinal cord and brain) and acetyl choline receptors. That leads to recurrent muscle weakness, loss of muscle control, and (potentially) eventual paralysis.
Research published in 2001 indicated that women whose blood contained significant levels of antibodies to Epstein-Barr virus were four times more likely to develop multiple sclerosis, than women without significant blood levels of those antibodies.
Some research has implicated degradation of myelin (during midlife) with Alzheimer's disease.
See also AUTOIMMUNE DISEASE, THYMUS, ACETYLCHOLINE, RECEPTORS, IMMUNE RESPONSE, NEUROTRANSMITTER, EXCITATORY AMINO ACIDS (EAAs), ANTIBODY, VIRUS, ALZHEIMER'S DISEASE

Multiplex Assay Refers to an assay that generates **more than one data point** in each (assay) evaluation that is performed. For example, fluorescence mapping (i.e., scanning an x-y plane within the tissue at varying depths with a microscope/light of selected wavelength) is designed to cause/detect any fluorescence resulting from a biological event of interest (e.g., the binding of a particular protein to a given cell receptor, the expression of particular genes, etc.).
See also ASSAY, BIOASSAY, CELL, FLUORESCENCE, FLUORESCENCE MAPPING, RECEPTORS, HIGH-CONTENT SCREENING, HIGH-THROUGHPUT SCREENING (HTS), TARGET–LIGAND INTERACTION SCREENING, GENE, GENE EXPRESSION PROFILING, CELLULAR PATHWAY MAPPING, METABOLOMICS, MULTIPLEXED (ASSAY)

Multiplexed (assay) Refers to an assay that simultaneously measures several different aspects (e.g., several different proteins

M

produced within a cell, several different products produced in the same chemical reaction, etc.).

See also ASSAY, PROTEIN, CELL, MICROARRAY (TESTING), HIGH-CONTENT SCREENING, MULTIPLEX ASSAY

Multipotent Refers to the property of certain cells (e.g., stromal cells, some adult stem cells, etc.) to be differentiated (i.e., via chemical signals) so that they then give rise to one of several different cell/tissue types. For example, **stromal cells** within mammary tissue can be influenced by the presence of conjugated linoleic acid (CLA) to become fat cells (adipose tissue). Otherwise, stromal cells tend to become **blood-vessel-lining** cells (endothelial cells) or **connective-tissue-producing** cells (fibroblasts).

See also CELL, ADULT STEM CELL, MULTIPOTENT ADULT STEM CELL, SIGNALING, DIFFERENTIATION, CONJUGATED LINOLEIC ACID (CLA), ADIPOSE, ENDOTHELIAL CELLS, FIBROBLASTS

Multipotent Adult Stem Cell Certain stem cells present within (adult) bodies of organisms can be differentiated (via chemical signals) to give rise to a variety of different cell/tissue types (e.g., bone, cartilage, fat, muscle, red blood cells, B cells, T cells, etc.).

For example, adipose (body fat) cells have been removed from the bodies of some mammals by researchers and subsequently coaxed into expressing genes and otherwise exhibiting characteristics of (differentiated) bone cells, cartilage cells, muscle cells, etc.

See also STEM CELLS, CELL, MULTIPOTENT, DIFFERENTIATION, ORGANISM, SIGNALING, RED BLOOD CELLS, B CELLS, T CELLS, MESODERMAL ADULT STEM CELLS, ADIPOSE, GENE, EXPRESS, GENE EXPRESSION ANALYSIS

Murine Of, or pertaining to, mice. For example, the first monoclonal antibodies were produced using cells from mice. This frequently caused adverse immune responses to monoclonal antibodies when they were injected into the human body (e.g., thus limiting their use in therapeutic purposes). However, researchers have recently discovered how to make monoclonal antibodies in human cells.

See also MONOCLONAL ANTIBODIES (MAb)

Muscular Dystrophy (MD) A genetic disease caused by a defect in the X chromosome (resulting in nonexpression of the Duchenne muscular dystrophy gene), first recognized by G.A.B. Duchenne in 1858. The disease afflicts males almost exclusively because males have only one X chromosome, whereas females inherit two copies of the X chromosome and have a backup in case one X chromosome is damaged (as is the case for MD victims). In 1981, Kay E. Davies used DNA probes (genetic probes) to discover that the Duchenne muscular dystrophy (DMD) gene must lie somewhere between two unique (to MD victims) segments on the upper, shorter arm of the X chromosome.

See also DNA PROBE, CHROMOSOMES, KARYOTYPE, CHROMATIDS, CHROMATIN, SINGLE-NUCLEOTIDE POLYMORPHISMS (SNPs)

Mutagen A chemical substance capable of producing a genetic mutation (change) by causing changes in the DNA of living organisms. For example, Gary Shaw discovered in 1996 that women who smoke cigarettes during their pregnancies are twice as likely to have babies with the genetic deformity known as cleft lip and palate. If those women have a particularly susceptible (to smoke) gene variant (allele) within their DNA, they are as much as eight times as likely to have babies with cleft lip and palate.

According to the World Health Organization (WHO), 60 to 80% of all known mutagens are also carcinogens (i.e., cancer causing).

See also MUTATION, GENE, GENETICS, HEREDITY, GENETIC CODE, CANCER, CARCINOGEN, ALLELE, DEOXYRIBONUCLEIC ACID (DNA), ONCOGENES, MUTANT, TOXICOGENOMICS, ANTIOXIDANTS

Mutant An altered cell or organism resulting from mutation (an alteration) of the original wild (normal) type. A change from the normal to the unique or abnormal.

For example, in 1970, an **orange**-colored wild cauliflower was discovered growing in Bradford Marsh in Canada. Its orange color resulted from a mutation that caused it to

M

produce approximately 100 times more beta-carotene than original (wild-type) cauliflower. If that particular mutation was of a **single nucleotide** in the cauliflower's DNA (e.g., caused by ultraviolet radiation striking it), then it is a **point mutation**.

See also CELL, ORGANISM, MUTAGEN, MUTATION, HEREDITY, WILD TYPE, BETA-CAROTENE, POINT MUTATION, DEOXYRIBONUCLEIC ACID (DNA), NUCLEOTIDE

Mutase An enzyme-catalyzing transposition of a functional group in the substrate (substance acted upon by the enzyme). Intramolecular transfer of a chemical group from one position (i.e., carbon atom) to another within the same molecule. An example of a mutase is phosphoglucomutase. It has a molecular weight of about 60,000 Da with about 600 amino acid residues (monomers). The mutase can interchange (move) a phosphate unit between the 1 and 6 positions. The 1 refers to a carbon atom designated as "#1" and the 6 refers to a different carbon atom designated as "#6."

Mutation From the Latin term *mutare,* meaning "to change." Any change that alters the sequence of the nucleotide bases in the genetic material (DNA) of an organism or cell, with alteration occurring either by displacement, addition, deletion, cross linking, or other destruction. The mutation alteration to the DNA sequence would alter its meaning, that is, its ability to produce the normal amount or normal kind of protein, so the (organism or cell) is itself altered. Such an altered organism is called a mutant.

See also MUTANT, INFORMATIONAL MOLECULES, HEREDITY, GENETIC CODE, GENETIC MAP, PROTEIN, DEOXYRIBONUCLEIC ACID (DNA)

Mutation Breeding Refers to several techniques involving induced mutations that were utilized by some crop plant breeders (e.g., primarily in the 1960s and 1970s) to introduce desirable genes into the plants they were working with; for example, genes to confer the following qualities:

- Resistance to plant diseases
- Increased yield per acre/hectare
- Improvements in composition

These were not present within the historic/natural germplasm of that plant species.

These **new-to-that-species** genes were "created" via any of the following:

- Soaking its seeds or pollen in mutation-causing chemicals (i.e., mutagens) such as colchicine or sodium azide.
- Via bombardment of seeds with x-rays.
- Via bombardment of seed with *fast neutron* radiation (i.e., causes deletion of approximately 1000 bp of DNA each time).
- Via bombardment of seed with gamma radiation (i.e., causes deletion of several hundred bp of DNA each time). For example, cauliflower was the result of such a naturally occurring mutation (to wild cabbage).

These were followed by grow-out of the resultant plants and selection of the particular mutation (i.e., beneficial trait) desired by the plant breeder. That plant was then propagated via straightforward breeding to yield seeds that are still sown today.

See also TRADITIONAL BREEDING METHODS, MUTATION, MUTAGEN, GENE, TRAIT, WHEAT, BARLEY, POINT MUTATION, COLCHICINE, BASE PAIR (BP), DELETIONS

Mutual Recognition Agreements (MRAs) Legal agreements (e.g., treaties) between two or more nations, to recognize and respect each other's approval process (e.g., for new crops derived via biotechnology).

See also GMO, COMMITTEE FOR VETERINARY MEDICINAL PRODUCTS (CVMP), ORGANIZATION FOR ECONOMIC COOPERATION AND DEVELOPMENT (OECD), EVENT, EUROPEAN MEDICINES EVALUATION AGENCY (EMEA), COMMITTEE FOR PROPRIETARY MEDICINAL PRODUCTS (CPMP), UNION FOR PROTECTION OF NEW VARIETIES OF PLANTS (UPOV)

Mutual Recognition Arrangements See MUTUAL RECOGNITION AGREEMENTS (MRAs)

M

Mycelia The fine, thread-like filaments that are sent out into the surrounding soil by mycorrhizal species of fungi.
See also MYCORRHIZAE

Mycobacterium tuberculosis The pathogen that causes tuberculosis, a human disease in which the lungs are destroyed as this bacteria grows (within lung tissue). In 1998, scientists completed sequencing of the genome of *Mycobacterium tuberculosis.* Recently, a new strain of *Mycobacterium tuberculosis* has begun to infect some people. This pathogen is resistant to virtually all commercial antibiotics.
See also BACTERIA, PATHOGEN, SEQUENCING (OF DNA MOLECULES), ANTIBIOTIC, ANTIBIOTIC RESISTANCE, GENOME, STRAIN

Mycorrhizae Refers to the symbiotic (i.e., mutually beneficial) relationship that exists between certain plants and the specific soil-dwelling species of fungi dwelling among the roots of those particular plants. The fungi provide certain minerals (e.g., phosphorous) to the plant roots (that the fungi's mycelia are able to extract from the soil). In return, the plant roots provide certain nutrients (e.g., sugar molecules) needed by those fungi. In some cases, the fungal mycelia (i.e., filaments sent out some distance into the surrounding soil) will transfer certain nutrients (e.g., some sugar molecules) from one plant to another.
In some cases, the mycorrhizae will:

- Help to protect certain plants from some pathogens
- Transform/render certain toxins present in the soil (e.g., some heavy

metals) to be unavailable for uptake by the host plant's roots

See also SYMBIOTIC, FUNGUS, SPECIES, MYCELIA, SUGAR MOLECULES, PATHOGEN, GLOMALIN

Mycotoxins Toxins produced by fungi. More than 350 different mycotoxins are known to man, but the first ones to be isolated and scientifically characterized (i.e., described) were the **aflatoxins**, in 1961. The second group of mycotoxins to be isolated and characterized were the **ochratoxins**, in 1965. Almost all mycotoxins possess the capacity to harmfully alter the immune systems of animals. Consumption by animals (including humans) of certain mycotoxins (e.g., via eating infected corn/maize, wheat, certain tree nuts, peanuts, cottonseed products, etc.) can result in liver toxicity, gastrointestinal lesions, cancer, muscle necrosis, etc.
See also TOXIN, FUNGUS, *FUSARIUM*, AFLATOXIN, VOMITOXIN, *FUSARIUM MONILIFORME*, FUMONISINS, ZEARALENONE, OCHRATOXINS, PATULIN, ERGOTAMINE, P53 GENE

Myeloma A tumor cell line derived from a lymphocyte. It usually produces a single type of immunoglobulin.
See also HYBRIDOMA, LYMPHOCYTE, AGING

Myoelectric Signals The nerve signals that are sent by the body to control muscle movement.

Myo-Inositol Hexaphosphate See PHYTATE

Myristoylation Transformation of proteins in cells in such a manner that these cells then cause cancer.
See also CANCER

M

N

N Glycosylation See GLYCOSYLATION

n-3 Fatty Acids Also known as "omega-3" fatty acids. Research indicates there are human health benefits (e.g., antithrombotic, reduce/avoid coronary heart disease) if the ratio of **n-6** to **n-3** fatty acids contained in the diet is higher than 3, but less than 10. Soybean oil has an **n-6/n-3 ratio** of approximately **7:1**.

Examples of **n-3 fatty acids** include linolenic acid (C18:3n-3), eicosapentanoic acid, and docosahexanoic acid. Research indicates that human consumption of n-3 fatty acids imparts antithrombotic and anti-inflammatory health benefits; it also lowers levels of triglycerides content in the bloodstream. At least some n-3 fatty acids are essential for membrane synthesis within the human brain and retina, and some have been shown to be essential for neural development.

During 2000, research results that indicated a 66% reduction in probability for children developing "**juvenile**" **(type 1) diabetes** if their mothers consumed significant quantities of n-3 fatty acids during the pregnancy were published.

See also POLYUNSATURATED FATTY ACIDS (PUFA), DOCOSAHEXANOIC ACID (DHA), EICOSAPENTANOIC ACID (EPA), LINOLENIC ACID, SOYBEAN OIL, STEARIDONIC ACID, THROMBOSIS, TRIGLYCERIDES, CORONARY HEART DISEASE (CHD), DIABETES, INSULIN

n-6 Fatty Acids Also known as "omega-6" fatty acids. Research indicates there are human health benefits (e.g., antithrombotic, reduced or no coronary heart disease) if the ratio of **n-6** to **n-3** fatty acids contained in the diet is higher than 3, but less than 10. Soybean oil has an **n-6/n-3 ratio** of approximately **7:1**.

Examples of **n-6 fatty acids** include linoleic acid (C18:2n-6). Research indicates that consumption of n-6 fatty acids has been related to decreased cholesterol levels in the bloodstream and decreased incidence of coronary heart disease (CHD).

See also POLYUNSATURATED FATTY ACIDS (PUFA), ARACHIDONIC ACID, LINOLEIC ACID, SOYBEAN OIL, THROMBOSIS, CORONARY HEART DISEASE (CHD), CHOLESTEROL

N-cofilin See CELL MOTILITY

NAD (NADH, NADP, NADPH) Nicotinamide adenine dinucleotide, also known as diphosphopyridine nucleotide, codehydrogenase 1, coenzyme 1, and coenzymase by its discoverers, Arthur Harden and William Young. $C_{21}H_{27}O_{14}N_7P_2$ is an organic coenzyme (molecule) that functions as a distinct yet integral part of certain enzymes. NAD plays a role in certain enzymes concerned with oxidation–reduction reactions. (NADH: nicotinamide adenine dinucleotide, reduced; NADP: nicotinamide adenine dinucleotide phosphate; NADPH: nicotinamide adenine dinucleotide phosphate [reduced]).

See also ENZYME, COENZYME, OXIDATION-REDUCTION REACTION, NITRIC OXIDE SYNTHASE, SIRTUINS

NADA (New Animal Drug Application) An application to the U.S. Food and Drug Administration (FDA) to begin testing or studies of a new drug for animals (e.g., livestock) that might (eventually) lead to its FDA approval.

See also IND

NADH Nicotine adenine dinucleotide, reduced.

See NAD

NADP Nicotine adenine dinucleotide phosphate.

See NAD, NITRIC OXIDE SYNTHASE

NADPH Nicotinamide adenine dinucleotide phosphate, reduced.

See NAD

Naive T Cells See DENDRITIC CELLS

Naked DNA See NAKED GENE

Naked Gene A bare gene (strand of DNA that codes for a protein) that has been extracted from an organism or has been otherwise derived (e.g., synthesized from sequence data). During the 1990s, the following were discovered:

- Injecting the Duchenne muscular dystrophy "naked gene" into muscle tissue in the bodies of people suffering from muscular dystrophy (MD) resulted in temporary production of the relevant protein in that muscle tissue (i.e., temporary MD symptom reduction).
- Injecting the VEGF "naked gene" into relevant tissue in the bodies of people suffering from inadequate local blood supply (e.g., the shortage of blood flow to heart, known as myocardial ischemia, lack of blood flow in legs or other extremities, etc.) resulted in (new) growth of blood vessels or endothelium, and reduction in symptoms of those inadequate-blood-supply conditions.
- Injecting the "naked gene" for the relevant antigen of certain pathogens into some tissues in the organism (usual disease host) sometimes resulted in those (host organism) tissues taking up the "naked gene" and expressing some of the (pathogen's) antigens such that the (putative host organism's) immune system initiates an immune response (thereby resulting in vaccination against the disease conferred by pathogen). When that happens, such "naked genes" are referred to as "DNA vaccines."

See GENE, DEOXYRIBONUCLEIC ACID (DNA), PROTEIN, ORGANISM, SYNTHESIZING (OF DNA MOLECULES), SEQUENCING (OF DNA MOLECULES), DUCHENNE MUSCULAR DYSTROPHY GENE, MUSCULAR DYSTROPHY (MD), VASCULAR ENDOTHELIAL GROWTH FACTOR (VEGF), PATHOGEN, EXPRESS, DNA VACCINES, IMMUNE RESPONSE, CELLULAR IMMUNE RESPONSE, HUMORAL IMMUNITY, ANTIBODY, DNA VECTOR

Nanobiology See NANOTECHNOLOGY, NANOCOMPOSITES, NANOCAPSULES, BIOINORGANIC, NANOCRYSTALS, NANOELECTROMECHANICAL SYSTEM (NEMS)

Nanobodies Refers to the smallest possible portion of an antibody that will bind to an antigen or hapten. Although nanobodies are not made naturally (i.e., the body always makes complete or full-sized antibodies), nanobodies (approximately 120 amino acids in length) can be made via genetically engineered cells grown via cell culture. Because nanobodies are able to survive highly acidic conditions (e.g., passage through the stomach) without losing their biological activity, they could potentially be utilized in orally administered pharmaceuticals.

See also ANTIBODY, ANTIGEN, HAPTEN, COMBINING SITE, PROTEIN, AMINO ACID, GENETIC ENGINEERING, CELL, CELL CULTURE, BIOLOGICAL ACTIVITY, ORALLY ADMINISTERED, PRODRUG THERAPY

Nanobots Refers to very small "robots" whose dimensions are on the order of nanometers (nm). These could perform specific tasks.

See also NANOELECTROMECHANICAL SYSTEM (NEMS), NANOSCIENCE, MEMS (NANOTECHNOLOGY), BIOMEMS, NANOMETERS (nm), NANOTECHNOLOGY, SELF-ASSEMBLING MOLECULAR MACHINES

Nanocapsules Refers to nanometer-sized, hollow, spherically-shaped objects that can be utilized to encapsulate small amounts of pharmaceuticals, enzymes or other catalysts, etc.

See also NANOSHELLS, DENDRIMERS, NANOCOCHLEATES, SELF-ASSEMBLY (OF A LARGE MOLECULAR STRUCTURE), NANOMETERS (nm), NANOSCIENCE, NANOTECHNOLOGY, ENZYME, CATALYST

Nanocochleates See PHOSPHATIDYL SERINE

Nanocomposites Nanometer-scale composite structures composed of organic molecules intimately incorporated with inorganic molecules. For example, Abalone shellfish make mother-of-pearl shells via an intimate combination of protein and calcium carbonate (in the form of multiple-sided microscopic "tablets").

Researchers are working on making semiconductor devices (chips) containing peptides and other organic molecules attached to silicon or gallium arsenide. Also, they are working on nanoelectromechanical systems (NEMS), which would have tiny "moving parts" to be able to do "work" on nanometer length scale. See also NANOMETERS (nm), NANOTECHNOLOGY, PROTEIN, BIOCHIP, PEPTIDE, BIOSENSORS (ELECTRONIC), BIOINORGANIC, NANOELECTROMECHANICAL SYSTEM (NEMS)

Nanocrystal Molecules Coined by researchers A. Paul Alivisatos and Peter G. Schultz, it is a term used to describe double-stranded DNA molecules that **have attached to them** several multiatom clusters of gold. As of 1996, these researchers were trying to create nanometer-scale electrical circuits, semiconductors, etc. A separate methodology, researched by Chad A. Mirkin et al., utilizes strands of DNA to reversibly assemble gold nanoparticles (nanometer-scale multiatom particles) into supramolecular (many molecule) agglomerations, in which the gold particles are separated from each other by a distance of approximately 60. The aggregation of these DNA–metal nanoparticles causes a visible color change to occur. As of 1996, these researchers were working to create simple and rapid tests that would indicate the presence of a virus (e.g., HIV-1 or HIV- 2) via a visible color change. Such a test would use two noncomplementary DNA sequences, each of which has attached to it a gold nanoparticle (via a thiol group). The two sequences would be selected for their ability to latch onto a target sequence in the desired virus, but they would be unable to combine with each other, because they are noncomplementary. When double-stranded DNA molecules possessing two "sticky ends" (that are complementary to the sequences attached to virus) are added, the resultant color change indicates presence of a virus.
See also DOUBLE HELIX, DEOXYRIBONUCLEIC ACID (DNA), ANGSTROM (Å), NANOMETERS (nm), HYBRIDIZATION SURFACES, BASE PAIR (bp), SELF-ASSEMBLY, NANOTECHNOLOGY, STICKY ENDS, HYBRIDIZATION (MOLECULAR GENETICS), SEQUENCE (OF A DNA MOLECULE),

VIRUS, BIOSENSORS (CHEMICAL), BIOCHIP, MICROFLUIDICS, NANOCRYSTALS

Nanocrystals A term that refers to any crystalline structure possessing dimensions (e.g., overall width) measured in terms of nanometers.
See also NANOMETERS (nm), QUANTUM DOT, NANOSCIENCE, NANOTECHNOLOGY, NANOCRYSTAL MOLECULES, NANOCOMPOSITES

Nanoelectromechanical System (NEMS) Refers to working (i.e., those with moving "mechanical parts") systems on a scale of nanometers (nm).
For example, in 2000, Carlo Montemagno and colleagues assembled a NEMS, in which a tiny metal "propeller" was caused to spin within the domain of the enzyme ATP synthase. The metal propeller was attached (via a biotin–streptavidin "molecular linkage") to the one subunit (designated alpha) of ATP synthase that rotates within the other (hollow) part of ATP synthase molecule — when ATP is "fed" to a free-standing (i.e., not in cell) molecule of ATP synthase.
See also NANOMETERS (nm), ATP SYNTHASE, ENZYME, ADENOSINE TRIPHOSPHATE (ATP), BIOTIN, AVIDIN, NANOCOMPOSITES, NANOSCIENCE, MICROMACHINING, SELF-ASSEMBLING MOLECULAR MACHINES, DIRECTED SELF-ASSEMBLY

Nanofibers See SELF-ASSEMBLY (OF A LARGE MOLECULAR STRUCTURE)

Nanofluidics See MICROFLUIDICS

Nanogram (ng) 10^{-9} or 3.527×10^{-11} oz. (avoirdupois).

Nanolithography Refers to the practice of using an atomic force microscope tip to apply specific (e.g., DNA) molecules to surfaces such as metals, oxides, etc. Nanolithography can be used to direct (via DNA interactions) the assembly of tiny structures such as gene chips, catalysts, nanoscale circuits, etc.
See also DEOXYRIBONUCLEIC ACID (DNA), ATOMIC FORCE MICROSCOPY, HYBRIDIZATION (MOLECULAR GENETICS), HYBRIDIZATION SURFACES, GENE CHIPS, CATALYST, DIRECTED SELF-ASSEMBLY, BIOELECTRONICS, SELF-ASSEMBLING MOLECULAR MACHINES, TEMPLATE

N

Nanometers (nm) 10^{-9} m. Often used to express wavelengths of light (e.g., in a spectrophotometer) or to express dimensions of nanocomposites, devices (e.g., of miniature "machines" called nanoelectromechanical systems), etc., in the field of nanotechnology.
See also SPECTROPHOTOMETER, NANOTECHNOLOGY, NANOCOMPOSITES, NANOELECTROMECHANICAL SYSTEM (NEMS), MICROFLUIDICS, METER

Nanoparticles Term that refers to a variety of nanometer-sized particles (e.g., nanocrystals, quantum dots, etc.). Depending on the materials used to construct nanoparticles, their uses include:

- Imaging tissues within the body — When injected and subsequently "illuminated" by light of specific wavelength, relevant quantum dots emit light in colors, which vary depending on the particular tissue they happen to reside in.

- Detection of cancer metastasis — Magnetic nanoparticles (100-nm diameter) attached to **antibodies against epithelial cells** can be utilized to detect metastasis of cancer in a human. The magnetized antibodies attach themselves to epithelial cells (a biomarker of metastasis) in a blood sample, enabling the epithelial cells to be detected or counted by doctors.

- Detection of DNA hybridization — When relevant DNA molecules or segments are "labeled" in advance with **superparamagnetic particles**, those "labeled DNA segments" can be utilized in **magnetic DNA microarrays** to detect when or which DNA segments are hybridized (by DNA within samples being analyzed).

- Treating some diseases via creation of nanoshells—When covered with applicable "molecular bridges" so they accumulate inside tumors after being injected, certain nanoshells can subsequently be heated by shining near-infrared light through the tissues, thereby destroying the tumors without harming adjacent tissues.

See also NANOMETERS (nm), NANOCRYSTALS, QUANTUM DOT, NANOCRYSTAL MOLECULES, CANCER, METASTASIS, BIOMARKERS, MAGNETIC PARTICLES, DEOXYRIBONUCLEIC ACID (DNA), SEQUENCE (OF A DNA MOLECULE), HYBRIDIZATION (MOLECULAR GENETICS), DNA PROFILING, MICROARRAY (TESTING), BIO-BAR CODES, NANOTECHNOLOGY, NANOCOCHLEATES, NANOSHELLS

Nanopore A device that can distinguish between different DNA strands (molecules) that differ (from each other) by a single nucleotide (in the makeup of those molecular strands). Developed by Hagan Bayley, David Deamer, and Mark Akeson in 2001, it consists of an artificial membrane (lipid bilayer) with a "hole" (nanopore) punctured in it by the protein alpha-hemolysin.

Because a DNA molecule moving through such a "nanopore" temporarily blocks the nanopore (until it dissociates into a single DNA strand and "slides" through), an electrical current or voltage applied to that nanopore varies (in amplitude, modulation, duration, etc.) as the DNA strand "slides through" in a way that provides information (e.g., to scientist) about the nucleotides that make up that DNA strand. It is expected that nanopores will also be used for DNA sequencing.
See also NANOSCIENCE, NANOMETERS (nm), NANOTECHNOLOGY, PLASMA MEMBRANE, MICELLE, DEOXYRIBONUCLEIC ACID (DNA), NUCLEOTIDE, SINGLE-NUCLEOTIDE POLYMORPHISM (SNP), ION CHANNELS, SEQUENCING (OF DNA MOLECULES)

Nanopore Detection See NANOPORE

Nanoscience A term utilized to refer to the science underlying nanotechnology, nanocrystals, nanocrystal molecules, nanocomposites, quantum dots, nanoelectromechanical systems (NEMS), etc.

"Nanoscale" materials (i.e., whose dimensions are approximately 1 to 100 nm) generally possess different chemical and physical properties than "bulk" materials. For example, when bulk gold metal is formed into nanoscale rods, the intensity of its fluorescence increases by a factor of approximately 10 million. Another example is that silicon nanocrystals (i.e.,

N

quantum dots) dispersed in a silicon dioxide matrix, emit larger-than-typical-for-silicon amounts of light, when stimulated (i.e., bombarded) with pulses of ultraviolet light.

See also NANOTECHNOLOGY, CARBON NANOTUBES, NANOPARTICLES, NANOCRYSTALS, QUANTUM DOT, NANOCRYSTAL MOLECULES, NANOCOMPOSITES, NANOELECTROMECHANICAL SYSTEM (NEMS), SELF-ASSEMBLY (OF A LARGE MOLECULAR STRUCTURE), NANOPORE, OPTICAL TWEEZER, MICROFLUIDICS, TEMPLATE, SELF-ASSEMBLING MOLECULAR MACHINES, SCANNING TUNNELING MICROSCOPE, ATOMIC FORCE MICROSCOPE, NANOCOCHLEATES, SURFACE PLASMONS, NANOCAPSULES, BIONANOTECHNOLOGY

Nanoshells Refers to nanometer-scale crystalline structures that are formed in the shape of hollow balls. For example, nanoshells can be manufactured by surrounding cobalt nanoparticles with sulfur (in a 9:8 ratio). When the proper reaction conditions are subsequently applied to this 9:8 cobalt–sulfur mixture, the Kirkendall effect causes the cobalt atoms within the nanoparticle to diffuse out to (and react with) the sulfur atoms faster than the sulfur atoms diffuse in to the nanoparticle. The end result is a spherical nanoshell comprised of the compound Co_9S_8.

One potential application of certain nanoshells is to inject them into a cancer patient's bloodstream. For that application, nanoshells are made of materials or thicknesses selected to absorb specific wavelengths of infrared light (to which human tissue is transparent) and are "surface modified" (via attachment of **molecular bridges** to surface) so that they will accumulate inside tumors. Once the nanoshells have accumulated within the tumor, subsequent shining of intense near-infrared light of the appropriate wavelength at that tumor causes the nanoshells to heat up and kill the tumor tissue without harm to adjacent noncancerous tissue.

Another version of that (tumor-destroying) application is to manufacture such nanoshells from magnetic elements and then cause them to heat up in the tumor via application of oscillating magnetic fields.

The self-assembling capsid (hard outer spherical protein shell) of certain viruses can also be considered to be a "nanoshell" (when empty of contents). During 2004, Gijs Wuite determined using an atomic force microscope that the capsid of one particular spherical virus possesses a **Young's modulus (measure of "hardness")** that is similar to the Young's modulus of some hard synthetic plastics. Such nanoshells might be used to deliver certain pharmaceuticals to only specific body tissues.

See also NANOSCIENCE, NANOMETERS (nm), NANOTECHNOLOGY, NANOPARTICLES, CANCER, LIGAND (IN BIOCHEMISTRY), VIRUS, CAPSID, TOBACCO MOSAIC VIRUS (TMV), SELF-ASSEMBLY (OF A LARGE MOLECULAR STRUCTURE), MOLECULAR BRIDGE

Nanotechnology From the Latin *nanus,* meaning "dwarf"; so it literally means "dwarf technology." The word was originally coined by Norio Taniguchi, in 1974, to refer to high-precision machining. However, Richard Feynman and K. Eric Drexler later popularized the concept of nanotechnology as a new and developing technology in which man manipulates objects whose dimensions are approximately 1 to 100 nm. Theoretically, it is possible that in the future a variety of synthetic "nanoassemblers," i.e., tiny (molecular) machines smaller than a grain of sand) would manufacture those things that are produced today in factories. For example, enzyme molecules function essentially as jigs and machine tools to shape large molecules as they are formed in biochemical reactions. The technology also encompasses BIOCHIPS, BIOSENSORS, and manipulating atoms and molecules in order to form (build) bigger but still vanishingly small functional structures and machines.

See also ENZYME, GENOSENSORS, NANOMETERS (nm), CARBON NANOTUBES, BIOSENSORS (ELECTRONIC), BIOCHIP, MICROFLUIDICS, NANOPARTICLES, NANOCRYSTALS, NANOCRYSTAL MOLECULES, BIOSENSORS (CHEMICAL), QUANTUM DOT, NANOCOMPOSITES, NANOELECTROMECHANICAL SYSTEM (NEMS), NANOWIRE, SELF-ASSEMBLY (OF A LARGE MOLECULAR STRUCTURE), TEMPLATE, MOLECULAR SIEVES,

NANOPORE, BIOMEMS, OPTICAL TWEE-
ZER, DIRECTED SELF-ASSEMBLY, SELF-
ASSEMBLING MOLECULAR MACHINES,
DIP-PEN NANOLITHOGRAPHY, NANOCO-
CHLEATES, NANOSHELLS, SURFACE
PLASMONS, NANOCAPSULES, BIONAN-
OTECHNOLOGY

Nanotube Refers to a tiny tube whose diameter is measured in nanometers. For example,
during 2001–2002, Charles R. Martin et al.
were able to manufacture antibody-laced nanotube membranes via the following:

- First creating alumina films, which
  naturally possess cylindrical pores
  extending through the film
- Then "growing" silica nanotubes
  within those pores, using special
  sol–gel chemistry methods
- Then coating the interior surfaces of
  the silica nanotubes with aldehyde
  silanes
- And finally, reacting the free amino
  sites (on antibody fragments — raised
  against one of the enantiomers in a
  racemic mixture) with the aldehydes
  (on the aldehyde silane molecules),
  thereby attaching antibodies to the
  interior surfaces of the nanotubes.

Thus constructed, the antibody-laced nanotube
membranes were utilized by those scientists
to separate out the desired enantiomer from a
racemic mixture (racemate).

Another example of the use of nanotubes is the
2004 discovery by Thomas Webster and colleagues that coating a titanium object (e.g.,
the stem of an artificial hip joint) with nanotubes constructed from "rings" comprised of
guanine and cytosine result in significantly
improved attachment (to the artificial hip) by
bone osteoblast cells as the bone grows around
the stem following hip replacement surgery.

See also NANOSCIENCE, NANOMETERS
(nm), NANOTECHNOLOGY, ANTIBODY,
AMINO ACID, ENANTIOMERS, RACE-
MATE, ENANTIOPURE, ULTRAFILTRA-
TION, SELF-ASSEMBLY (OF A LARGE
MOLECULAR STRUCTURE), GUANINE,
CYTOSINE

Nanotube Membranes See NANOTUBE,
CARBON NANOTUBES

Nanowire Term utilized to describe (relatively)
long and narrow electrical conductors whose
dimensions are measured in nanometers (nm).
For example, during 2003, Susan L. Lindquist
utilized yeast amyloid proteins (which self-
assemble into 60- to 300-nm-long fibers) to
create **nanowires**, by subsequently coating
those fibers with gold and silver. Other potential materials with which nanowires can be
manufactured include carbon nanotubes.

One of the ways to precisely handle nanowires
(possibly to thereby "build" electrical circuits)
is to attach tiny pieces of nickel metal to each
end of the nanowire. Because nickel is ferromag-
netic, magnetic field lines of force can then be
utilized to precisely move and position the
nanowires.

See also BIOELECTRONICS, NANOME-
TERS (nm), CARBON NANOTUBES,
SELF-ASSEMBLY (OF A LARGE MOLEC-
ULAR STRUCTURE), NANOTECHNOL-
OGY, TEMPLATE

Napole Gene See REDEMENT NAPOLE
(RN) GENE

Naringen A glycosylated flavone that is naturally present in oranges and other citrus fruits.
See also GLYCOSYLATION, FLAVONOLS

NARK Gene A gene within the DNA of the
soybean plant (*Glycine max* (L.) Merrill) that
controls the growth of root nodules in which
nitrogen fixation takes place. This gene was
identified by Peter Gresshoff in 2002, and its
acronym stands for **Nodule Autoregulation
Receptor Kinase**.

When *Bradyrhizobium japonicum* bacteria
(attracted to the vicinity of soybean plant's
roots by the isoflavones those roots exude)
are exposed to isoflavones, those bacteria's
nod genes code for production of specific
chemical compounds, which then trigger
NARK gene to cause the soybean plant roots
to create or grow nodules that the bacteria
subsequently move into and begin to fix
nitrogen.

See also GENE, DEOXYRIBONUCLEIC ACID
(DNA), SOYBEAN PLANT, NODULATION,
NITROGEN FIXATION, *BRADYRHIZO-
BIUM JAPONICUM*, ISOFLAVONES, NOD
GENES, RECEPTORS

NAS See NATIONAL ACADEMY OF SCI-
ENCES

National Academy of Sciences (NAS) A private, self-perpetuating society of distinguished scholars in scientific and engineering research, dedicated to the advancement of science and technology and their use for the general welfare. Under the authority of its congressional charter of 1863, NAS has a working mandate that calls upon it to advise the U.S. federal government on scientific and technical matters.
See also VITAMIN E

National Cancer Institute (NCI) One of the National Institutes of Health.
See NATIONAL INSTITUTES OF HEALTH (NIH)

National Heart, Lung, and Blood Institute (NHLBI) One of the National Institutes of Health.
See NATIONAL INSTITUTES OF HEALTH (NIH)

National Institute of Allergy and Infectious Diseases (NIAID) The main agency of the National Institutes of Health.
See NATIONAL INSTITUTES OF HEALTH (NIH)

National Institute of General Medical Sciences (NIGMS) One of the National Institutes of Health.
See NATIONAL INSTITUTES OF HEALTH (NIH)

National Institutes of Health (NIH) The major U.S. government sponsor of biotechnology research. It is composed of a group of government institutes that each focus on specific medical areas.
See also RECOMBINANT DNA ADVISORY COMMITTEE (RAC)

National Plant Protection Organization (NPPO) Refers to the official service (agency) established by a nation's government to discharge the functions specified by the International Plant Protection Convention (IPPC). Examples of those functions include the enforcement of phytosanitary regulations (e.g., to prevent plant diseases being accidentally brought into a country).
See also INTERNATIONAL PLANT PROTECTION CONVENTION (IPPC), SPS

Native Conformation The normal, biologically active conformation (i.e., the three-dimensional arrangement of its atoms) of a protein molecule.

See also CONFORMATION

Native Structure See NATIVE CONFORMATION

Naturaceuticals See NUTRACEUTICALS

Natural Killer Cells These cells are involved in tumor surveillance. They also kill virus-laden cells.

NCI See NATIONAL CANCER INSTITUTE (NCI)

NDA (to FDA) New Drug Application (to the U.S. Food and Drug Administration). A (paper) application to the U.S. Food and Drug Administration (FDA) seeking approval of a new drug that has undergone Phase 2 and Phase 3 clinical trials. An NDA is submitted in the form of (thousands of) pages of (clinical and other) data, along with various analyses (e.g., statistical) of that data for efficacy, safety, etc.
See also CANDA, FOOD AND DRUG ADMINISTRATION (FDA), MAA, NDA (TO KOSEISHO), PHASE I CLINICAL TESTING

NDA (to Koseisho) New Drug Application. It is the Japanese equivalent of a U.S. IND (investigational new drug) application. to the Koseisho, the Japanese equivalent of the U.S. Food and Drug Administration (FDA).
See also IND, KOSEISHO, FOOD AND DRUG ADMINISTRATION (FDA)

Near-Infrared Spectroscopy (NIR) Refers to analytical instruments that shine light (possessing wavelengths between that of visible light and infrared light spectrum) onto samples (e.g., kernels of grain) and measure the reflected or transmitted (near-infrared) light in order to quickly determine the amounts of protein, fat, moisture, lignans, etc., present in the sample.
In certain samples, the near-infrared light causes cells or (specific molecules) to fluoresce (as light of very defined wavelength), which can be subsequently utilized for measurement or identification of compounds within the sample. NIR is also being developed for use in the following:

- Quantifying (e.g., amounts that are present within the sample) of immunoassays
- Predicting (e.g., the total amount of digestible energy [DE] or actual metabolizable energy [AME] in a

sample of animal feed) from those quantified amounts.

- Detection of specific molecules (e.g., in DNA sequencing process).

See also PROTEIN, FATS, LIGNANS, IMMUNOASSAY, FLUORESCENCE, SEQUENCING (OF DNA MOLECULES)

Near-Infrared Transmission (NIT) Refers to certain analytical instruments that shine light (possessing wavelengths between that of visible light and infrared spectrum) through samples (e.g., kernels of grain) in order to quickly determine the amounts of protein, fat, moisture, lignans, etc. present in the sample.

See also PROTEIN, FATS, LIGNANS, NEAR-INFRARED SPECTROSCOPY (NIR)

Necrosis Refers to cell death caused by physical injury to the cell (e.g., exposure to toxin, exposure to ultraviolet light, lack of oxygen, etc.).

See also CELL, TOXIN, RESPIRATION, TUMOR NECROSIS FACTOR

Neem Tree A tropical tree (*Azadirachta indica*) found in tropical countries, including India, Somalia, Mauritania, and Australia, that resists insect (e.g., whiteflies, mealybugs, aphids, mites) depradations and certain fungal diseases (e.g., rusts, powdery mildew, etc.) via secretions of liquids that contain **Azadirachtin** (an insect-repelling chemical).

See also AZADIRACHTIN, FUNGUS

Negative Control Refers to the "turning off" or decrease (i.e., downregulation) of a given gene's transcription (i.e., coding for production of relevant protein) in an organism because of the binding (to DNA) of negative regulatory elements.

See also GENE, TRANSCRIPTION, KNOCKDOWN, KNOCKOUT, DOWNREGULATING, RIBOSWITCHES, METHYLATED

Negative Supercoiling Comprises the twisting of a duplex of DNA (deoxyribonucleic acid) in space in a sense opposite to the turns of the strands in the double helix.

See also DOUBLE HELIX

Nematodes Microscopic roundworms, which are the most abundant multicelled creatures on Earth. They are primarily found living in soil. One nematode named *Caenorhabditis elegans (C. elegans)* is commonly used by

scientists in genetics experiments; so a large database of its genetics has been accumulated by the world's scientific community. For example, of the nearly 300 "disease-causing" genes in the human genome, more than half of them have an analogous gene within the genome of *C. elegans*. One Antarctic nematode (*Panagrolaimus davidi*) is able to survive Antarctic winters by **drying out and achieving a state of "suspended animation" (anhydrobiosis)** for as long as 39 years.

See also CELL, *CAENORHABDITIS ELEGANS (C. elegans)*, GENETICS, GENE, GENOME, GENETIC MAP, MODEL ORGANISM, SOYBEAN CYST NEMATODES (SCN), CYSTX

NEMS See NANOELECTROMECHANICAL SYSTEM (NEMS)

Neoantigen An antigen that is expressed by an organism's cells after transformation (e.g., of a cell) by an oncogenic virus.

See also ANTIGEN, ORGANISM, CELL, VIRUS, ONCOGENES

Neoplasia New growth.

See also NEOPLASTIC GROWTH

Neoplasm Refers to new uncontrolled growth of tissue (e.g., a tumor).

See NEOPLASTIC GROWTH

Neoplastic Growth A new growth of animal or plant tissue resembling (more or less) the tissue from which it arises but having biochemicals distinct from that of the parent cell. The neoplastic tissue is a mutant version of the original and appears to serve no physiological function in the same sense as did the original tissue. It may be benign or malignant (i.e., a cancerous tumor).

See also TUMOR, CANCER, SELECTIVE APOPTOTIC ANTINEOPLASTIC DRUG (SAAND), METASTASIS

Nerve Growth Factor (NGF) A protein produced by the salivary glands (and also in tumors) that greatly increases growth or reproduction of nerve cells and guides the formation of neural networks. In the brain, NGF is thought to increase the production of the messenger chemical, acetylcholine, by protecting and stimulating neurons that produce acetylcholine. Because those (acetylcholine-producing) neurons are typically the first to be destroyed in Alzheimer's disease, NGF holds potential to be used to counteract (some of) the effects of the disease. NGF is also necessary for normal development of the hypothalamus, a brain structure that regulates a number of hormones. Human T cells appear to have receptors for NGF, which could explain the "mind–body connection" between a person's emotional well-being and physical health (i.e., NGF may be a go-between for the brain and the immune system). NGF was discovered by Rita Levi-Montalcini in 1954.

See also GROWTH FACTOR, EPIDERMAL GROWTH FACTOR (EGF), HYPOTHALAMUS, HORMONE, PROTEIN, ALZHEIMER'S DISEASE

Nested PCR Refers to a specific PCR (polymerase chain reaction) technique of two **consecutive-run PCRs**, in which the second PCR amplifies (i.e., makes multiple copies of) a DNA sequence within the product (amplicon) of the first PCR.

See also POLYMERASE CHAIN REACTION (PCR), POLYMERASE CHAIN REACTION (PCR) TECHNIQUE, SEQUENCE (OF A DNA MOLECULE), DEOXYRIBONUCLEIC ACID (DNA), AMPLICON

Neu5Gc A gene that is present within the DNA of most animals but not in human DNA. The Neu5Gc gene controls production or expression of sialic acid (e.g., on surfaces of some cells in the organism).

See also GENE, DEOXYRIBONUCLEIC ACID (DNA), SIALIC ACID

Neuraminidase (NA) A transmembrane (i.e., through the membrane) glycoprotein enzyme that appears in the (external) membrane of the influenza virus.

See also ENZYME, GLYCOPROTEIN, VIRUS

Neuron Cells of the nervous system, which transmit nerve impulses (nerve impulses are electrical signals conducted by the flow of ions across the plasma membrane of neuron cells). Neurons are involved in controlling movement (known as motor control), emotions, and memory.

There are approximately 100 billion neurons in the typical human brain. The nerve impulses within them move at a speed of approximately 400 km/h (300 mi/h).

See also NEUROTRANSMITTER, ACETYLCHOLINE, SEROTONIN, CELL,

PARKINSON'S DISEASE, PLASMA MEMBRANE, ION, DENDRITES

Neurotransmitter An organic, low-molecular-weight compound that is secreted from the (axon) terminal end of a neuron (in response to the arrival of an electrical impulse) into the liquid-filled gap that exists between neurons. The transmitter molecule then diffuses across the small gap and attaches to the next neuron. This attachment causes structural changes in the membrane of the neuron and initiates the conductance of an electrical impulse. In this way, an electrical impulse is transmitted (via this "cascade") along a neuron network, in which the neurons themselves are not in physical contact. A neurotransmitter serves to transmit a nerve impulse between different neurons. Examples of neurotransmitters include dopamine, norepinephrine, etc. A shortage of dopamine in the brain causes Parkinson's disease.

See also MOLECULAR WEIGHT, NEURON, SEROTONIN, ACETYLCHOLINE, PARKINSON'S DISEASE, CASCADE, DENDRITES, GATED CHANNEL

Neutraceuticals See NUTRACEUTICALS

Neutriceuticals See NUTRACEUTICALS

Neutrophils Phagocytic (ingesting and scavenging) white blood cells that are produced in the bone marrow. They ingest and destroy invading microorganisms and facilitate postinfection tissue repair.

Upon ingestion of pathogens, the neutrophil generates reactive oxygen species such as O_2^- (also known as free radicals). O_2^- causes an influx of potassium ions into the portion of the neutrophil that contains the pathogen, which thereby releases proteases from existing granules ("storage" sites) in the neutrophil. The proteases then kill the pathogen.

In addition to generating proteases, neutrophils can secrete collagenase and plasminogen activator. They are the immune system's "first line" of defense against invading pathogens, and large reserves are called forth within hours of the start of a "pathogen invasion."

See also PATHOGEN, COLLAGENASE, MICROORGANISM, FREE RADICAL, ION, PROTEASE, PHAGOCYTOSIS, INNATE IMMUNE SYSTEM

N

New Drug Application See NDA (TO KOSEISHO), NDA (TO FDA), MAA, IND, CANDA

NFκB Abbreviation for **nuclear factor-κB**, a "family" of nuclear transcription factors that help cells regulate the expression of genes that do the following:

- Induce inflammation (sometimes leading to onset of autoimmune disease, NFκB proteins are overexpressed)
- Sometimes induce tumorigenesis
- Sometimes induce apoptosis
- Sometimes induce viral replication within cells

See also TRANSCRIPTION FACTORS, NUCLEAR DNA, DEOXYRIBONUCLEIC ACID (DNA), GENE, CELL, GENE EXPRESSION, TRANSCRIPTION, EXPRESS, GENE EXPRESSION CASCADE, AUTOIMMUNE DISEASE, TUMOR, APOPTOSIS, VIRUS, ADIPONECTIN

NIAID See NATIONAL INSTITUTE OF ALLERGY AND INFECTIOUS DISEASES

Nick A break in one strand of a double-stranded DNA molecule. One of the phosphodiester bonds between two adjacent nucleotides is ruptured. No bases are removed from the strand; it is just opened at that point.

See also DEOXYRIBONUCLEIC ACID (DNA)

Nicotine Adenine Dinucleotide (NAD) See NAD

Nicotine Adenine Dinucleotide Phosphate (NADP) See NAD

Nicotine Adenine Dinucleotide Phosphate, reduced (NADPH) See NAD

Nicotine Adenine Dinucleotide, reduced (NADH) See NAD

NIH See NATIONAL INSTITUTES OF HEALTH (NIH)

NIHRAC See RECOMBINANT DNA ADVISORY COMMITTEE (RAC)

Ninhydrin Reaction A color reaction given by amino acids and peptides on heating with the chemical ninhydrin. The technique is widely used for the detection and quantitation (measurement) of amino acids and peptides. The concentration of amino acid in a solution (of hydrochloric acid) is proportional to the optical absorbance of the solution after heating it with ninhydrin. α-Amino acids give an intense blue color, and amino acids (such as proline) give a yellow color. One is able to determine the concentration of a protein or peptide and also obtain an idea of the type of protein or peptide that is present.

See also ABSORBANCE (A), AMINO ACID, PEPTIDE

Nisin A powerful antibacterial peptide, first isolated in 1944 from *Lactococcus lactis* bacteria. Because nisin kills the human pathogenic *Salmonella* and *Clostridium* bacteria, it has been utilized by man as a food preservative for cheese and other dairy products for four decades.

The nisin molecule acts via binding tightly to **Lipid II**, which is a precursor molecule utilized by at least some bacteria to build or repair their cytoplasmic membrane (outer cell wall). Because nisin prevents such cell wall building or repair in those pathogenic bacteria, their cytoplasmic membrane weakens and becomes more permeable (i.e., "leaky"), and they die.

See also PEPTIDE, CELL, BACTERIA, ANTIBIOTIC, PATHOGEN, PATHOGENIC, SALMONELLA, *CLOSTRIDIUM*, LIPIDS, LIPID BILAYER, CYTOPLASMIC MEMBRANE

Nitrate Bacteria See NITRATES, NITRITES, BACTERIA

Nitrate Reduction The reduction of nitrate to nitrite or ammonia by an organism.

See also NITRATES, REDUCTION (IN A CHEMICAL REACTION), NITRITES

Nitrates Refers to nitrogen compounds that exist in a chemical form which plant roots are able to take in (i.e., utilized by the plant to make nitrogen-containing molecules such as proteins). Nitrates are produced from nitrogen that has been taken out of the following:

- The atmosphere by nitrogen-fixing bacteria (living in the roots of legume plants such as the soybean, etc.)
- Nitrites (in soil) by nitrate bacteria
- The atmosphere by blue-green algae

See also PROTEIN, NITROGEN FIXATION, SOYBEAN PLANT, NITRITES

Nitric Oxide Abbreviated **NO**, it is a molecule produced in the body of an organism (including plants), which can act as:

- A signaling molecule (e.g., it signals to cause a firefly's tail to begin the chemical reaction of luciferin with luciferase, which results in the light emission known as bioluminescence)
- Fostering the formation of new blood vessels (a process known as angiogenesis) in an animal's body
- Fostering the body's wound-healing process
- An oxidant utilized against pathogens by the immune system
- An instigator of (destructive) free radicals within the body
- An **inducer of genes** (e.g., in soybean plants) **that cause production of certain chemical compounds** that protect the organism (e.g., soybean plant) from bacterial diseases

As a **signaling molecule**, or "messenger molecule," nitric oxide is utilized by the human body for control of blood pressure (i.e., when the endothelial cells that line blood vessels produce NO, which causes neighboring smooth-muscle cells to relax so that the entire blood vessel dilates, thereby lowering blood pressure and protecting the lining from macrophage adhesion or initiation of plaque deposit).

Nitric oxide is also utilized by the human body for immune system regulation, and its synthesis in macrophages is required for macrophages to kill pathogens and tumor cells (by oxidizing them after the macrophage has engulfed them). During the 1980s, John Garthwaite and Solomon H. Snyder showed that nitric oxide is an important messenger molecule utilized in neural signaling (i.e., NO is an important signaling molecule in the human brain).

Nitric oxide increases the effectiveness of reactive free radicals (e.g., superoxide O^-_2) in killing any infected cells within a soybean plant.

Nitric oxide also induces certain genes to code for the production of certain chemical compounds that protect the soybean plant and some other plants from bacterial plant diseases.

See also SIGNALING MOLECULE, SIGNALING, OXIDIZING AGENT, PATHOGEN, IMMUNE RESPONSE, HUMAN SUPEROXIDE DISMUTASE (hSOD), SIGNAL TRANSDUCTION, NITRIC OXIDE SYNTHASE, SOYBEAN PLANT, PROTEIN, INDUCERS, GENE, CODING SEQUENCE, FREE RADICAL, ENDOTHELIAL CELLS, ENDOTHELIUM, MACROPHAGE, ADIPOSE, PATHOGEN, BACTERIA, TUMOR, NEUROTRANSMITTER, BIOLUMINESCENCE, ANGIOGENESIS, CHEMOTAXIS

Nitric Oxide Synthase An enzyme that catalyzes the reaction that the body (of animals or plants) utilizes to make nitric oxide from L-arginine (via cleavage of that molecule). The cofactor for that reaction is nicotine adenine dinucleotide phosphate (NADP).

See also ENDOTHELIAL NITRIC OXIDE SYNTHASE (eNOS), ENZYME, NITRIC OXIDE, COFACTOR, NAD (NADH, NADP, NADPH), ARGININE (Arg), LEVOROTARY (L) ISOMER, HYDROLYTIC CLEAVAGE, ENDOTHELIAL CELLS, ENDOTHELIUM, MACROPHAGE

Nitrification The oxidation of ammonia (e.g., from ammonia-containing substances such as liquid wastes excreted by animals, decomposed animals and plants, etc.) to nitrates by a microorganism.

See also NITRATES, NITRITES, OXIDATION (CHEMICAL REACTION)

Nitrifying Bacteria See NITRITES

Nitrilase An enzyme that catalyzes the degradation (i.e., breaking down) of bromoxynil (an active ingredient in some herbicides). Nitrilase is naturally produced in the soil bacteria *Klebsiella pneumoniae* ssp. *Ozaenae*. If the gene (called **BXN**) that codes for the production of nitrilase is inserted via genetic engineering into crop plants, the resultant **plant production of nitrilase** would enable such plants to survive post emergence applications of bromoxynil-containing herbicides.

See also ENZYME, BACTERIA, BROMOXYNYL, GENE, CODING SEQUENCE, GENETIC ENGINEERING

Nitrites Refers to nitrogen compounds that exist in a chemical form which plant roots are unable to take in. After conversion to **nitrates** via internal respiration by nitrate bacteria (in soil), the nitrates can be taken in by plant roots (i.e., utilized by the plant to make nitrogen-containing molecules such as proteins).

Nitrites are made (via internal respiration) by nitrifying bacteria (e.g., in soil) from ammonia-containing substances (e.g., liquid wastes excreted by animals, decomposed animals and plants, etc.).

See also NITRATES, PROTEIN, RESPIRATION

Nitrogen Cycle The cycling of various forms of biologically available nitrogen through the plant, animal, and microbial worlds (kingdoms), as well as the atmosphere and geosphere.

See also NITRATES, NITRITES, NITRIFICATION, DENITRIFICATION, NITROGEN FIXATION

Nitrogen Fixation Conversion of atmospheric nitrogen (N_2) into ammonium ion (NH_4^+); a soluble, biologically available form (nitrate) that plants can utilize to synthesize ("manufacture") amino acids and other nitrogen-containing compounds.

First explained during the 1880s by Mikhail Voronin and Hermann Hellriegel, the conversion is carried out by nitrogen-fixing organisms (e.g., *Rhizobium* bacteria) that live symbiotically in the roots of legume plants, e.g., alfalfa or soybeans. This is one of nature's ways of fertilizing (e.g., traditional varieties of soybeans typically leave approximately 40 lb of residual nitrogen per acre (44 kg per hectare) in fields at the end of the growing season).

When insufficient nitrogen fixation occurs (when only nonlegume plants are grown), the soil is not able to produce maximum crop yields, and farmers may need to spread onto the field fixed nitrogen in the form of the fertilizer **anhydrous ammonia**, **ammonium nitrate**, or **sodium nitrate**.

See also NITRATES, SYMBIOTIC, GENISTEIN (Gen), BACTERIA, SOYBEAN PLANT, NITROGENASE SYSTEM, NITROGEN CYCLE, ISOFLAVONES, HEMAGGLUTININ (HA), NODULATION, *RHIZOBIUM* (BACTERIA), *BRADYRHIZOBIUM JAPONICUM*, AMINO ACID, ION

Nitrogen Metabolism See GLUTAMATE DEHYDROGENASE

Nitrogenase System A system of enzymes capable of reducing atmospheric nitrogen to ammonium ion (NH_4^+) in the presence of ATP. Ammonium ion is a soluble form, which plants can utilize.

See also REDUCTION (IN A CHEMICAL REACTION), ENZYME, NITROGEN FIXATION, ION

NMR Acronym for **Nuclear Magnetic Resonance**.

See NUCLEAR MAGNETIC RESONANCE

NO See NITRIC OXIDE

No-Tillage Crop Production A methodology of crop production in which the farmer utilizes virtually no mechanical cultivation (i.e., only one pass over the field with a planter, instead of the conventional four passes per year with mechanical cultivator equipment plus one pass with a planter, used for traditional crop production). This reduction in field soil disturbance leaves more carbon in the soil (thereby reducing "greenhouse gases" in the atmosphere), leaves more earthworms (e.g., *Eisenia foetida*) per cubic foot (or per cubic meter) living in the topsoil, and reduces soil compaction (i.e., the reduction of interstitial spaces between individual soil particles), thereby increasing the fertility of such "no till" farm fields.

The plant residue remaining on the field's surface helps to control weeds and reduce soil erosion (by 90 to 95% versus traditional mechanical tillage); it also provides sites for insects to shelter and reproduce, leading to a need for increased insect control via methods such as inserting a *Bacillus thuringiensis (B.t.)* gene into certain crop plants or utilizing integrated pest management (IPM). But if a farmer needs to apply synthetic chemical pesticides, the plant residue remaining of field's surface helps to cause breakdown (into substances such as carbon dioxide and water) of pesticides. That is because that plant residue helps to retain moisture in the field surface, thereby enhancing growth of the microorganisms that help break down pesticides.

Use of no-tillage crop production (a methodology) helps farmers to reduce the incidence of certain plant diseases such as *white mold disease*.

See also INTEGRATED PEST MANAGE-
MENT (IPM), CORN, GLOMALIN, SOY-
BEAN PLANT, *BACILLUS THURINGIENSIS
(B.t.)*, GENE, GENETIC ENGINEERING,
EUROPEAN CORN BORER (ECB), *HELI-
COVERPA ZEA (H. ZEA)*, CORN ROOT-
WORM, COLD HARDENING, MICROOR-
GANISM, LOW-TILLAGE CROP
PRODUCTION, EARTHWORMS, WHITE
MOLD DISEASE, DROUGHT TOLER-
ANCE

Nod Gene See NODULATION

Nod Genes Refers to a category of genes
present within the DNA of certain soil-dwelling *Rhizobium* bacteria. When those bacteria
are in the presence of specific "signaling molecules" (e.g., isoflavones produced by roots of
soybean plant, or luteolin produced by roots
of alfalfa plant), nod genes code for the production (by those bacteria) of specific chemical compounds when then trigger relevant
plant genes (e.g., NARK gene in soybean
plant) to cause the plant roots to create or grow
nodules (which the bacteria subsequently
move into and begin to "fix" nitrogen).

See also GENE, DEOXYRIBONUCLEIC
ACID (DNA), *RHIZOBIUM* (BACTERIA),
SOYBEAN PLANT, NODULATION,
ISOFLAVONES, NARK GENE, NITROGEN
FIXATION

Nodulation The process in which certain
strains of soil-dwelling *Rhizobium* bacteria
colonize the roots of specific plants (i.e., the
legumes) such as soybean (*Glycine max* (L.))
or alfalfa. As part of that process the following
take place:

- *Rhizobium* bacteria are attracted to
  the vicinity of the plant's roots. For
  the **soybean plant** (*Glycine max*
  (L.)), this is accomplished by the
  soybean plant synthesizing the signaling molecules known as **isoflavones,** which attract *Bradyrhizobium
  japonicum* bacteria. For the **alfalfa
  plant**, this is accomplished by the
  alfalfa plant synthesizing luteolin
  molecules, which attract *Sinorhizo-
  bium meliloti* bacteria.
- Certain genes (called nod) within the
  relevant *Rhizobium* bacteria are

expressed (resulting in the synthesis
of specific chemical compounds).
- When the plant roots detect those
  chemical compounds, certain genes
  (called NARK) within those roots are
  expressed (resulting in the formation
  of **nodules** on those roots).
- The relevant *Rhizobium* bacteria
  move in and inhabit those plant root
  nodules, where the bacteria then
  "fix" nitrogen from the atmosphere,
  which converts that nitrogen into a
  chemical form (i.e., nitrates) that is
  available for use by plants (as fertilizer or plant food).

See also *RHIZOBIUM* (BACTERIA),
CHEMOTAXIS, SOYBEAN PLANT,
BRADYRHIZOBIUM JAPONICUM, ISO-
FLAVONES, GENISTEIN (Gen), TRAN-
SCRIPTION FACTORS, GENE, GENE
EXPRESSION, SIGNALING MOLECULE,
NOD GENES, NARK GENE, NITROGEN
FIXATION, SYMBIOTIC, HEMAG-
GLUTININ (HA)

Nonstarch Polysaccharides Term (abbreviated **NSP**) that refers to **polysaccharide molecules (in plant seeds) other than starch**.
These include arabinoxylans, pectins, beta
glucans, and alpha galactosides (e.g., raffinose, stachyose, verbascose).

See also POLYSACCHARIDES, STACHYOSE

Nonessential Amino Acids Amino acids of
proteins that can be made (biochemically synthesized within the body) by humans and certain other vertebrate animals from simple
chemical precursors (in contrast to the essential amino acids). These amino acids are thus
not required in the diet (of humans and those
other vertebrates).

See also ESSENTIAL AMINO ACIDS,
AMINO ACID, PROTEIN

Nonheme-Iron Proteins Proteins containing
iron but no porphyrin groups (within which
iron atoms are held) in their structure.

See also HEME

Nonpolar Group A hydrophobic ("water-hating") group on a molecule, usually hydrocarbon (composed of hydrogen and carbon
atoms) in nature. These groups are more at
home in a nonpolar (oil-like) environment.

See also POLAR GROUP, AMPHIPATHIC MOLECULES, AMPHOTERIC COMPOUND

Nonsense Codon A triplet of nucleotides that does not code for an amino acid. Any one of three triplets (U-A-G, U-A-A, or U-G-A) that cause termination of protein synthesis (in ribosome) and thus the release from ribosome of a (completely translated) protein molecule. U-A-G is known as **amber** and U-A-A is known as **ochre**.

See also GENETIC CODE, CODON, TERMINATION CODON (SEQUENCE), TRANSLATION, RIBOSOMES, PROTEIN

Nonsense Mutation A mutation that converts a codon that specifies an amino acid into one that does not specify any amino acid. A change in the nucleotide sequence of a codon that may result in the termination of a polypeptide chain.

See also NONSENSE CODON, GENETIC CODE, CODON

Nontranscribed Spacer A region between transcription units in a tandem gene cluster.

See also TRANSCRIPTION, MESSENGER RNA (mRNA), GENETIC CODE, GENE SPLICING, GENE

North American Plant Protection Organization (NAPPO) One of the international SPS standard-setting organizations that develops plant health standards, guidelines, and recommendations (e.g., to prevent transfer of a disease from one country to another). Subsidiary to the International Plant Protection Convention (IPPC), it covers the countries of North America. Its secretariat is located in Nepean, Canada.

See also INTERNATIONAL PLANT PROTECTION CONVENTION (IPPC), EUROPEAN PLANT PROTECTION ORGANIZATION (EPPO), SPS

Northern Blotting A research test or methodology used to transfer RNA fragments from an agarose gel (perhaps following gel electrophoresis) to a filter paper without changing the relative positions of the RNA fragments (e.g., re electrophoresis separation grid).

See also RIBONUCLEIC ACID (RNA), GEL ELECTROPHORESIS, AGAROSE, CHROMATOGRAPHY, FIELD INVERSION GEL ELECTROPHORESIS

Northern Corn Rootworm Latin name *Diabrotica barberi*.

See CORN ROOTWORM

NOS Terminator A **termination codon** (sequence of DNA) that is frequently utilized in genetic engineering of plants to "terminate" expression of the inserted gene (i.e., to **halt synthesis** of desired protein in the plant after the desired protein synthesis has occurred).

The NOS terminator was originally extracted from the bacterial species *Agrobacterium tumefaciens*.

See also TERMINATION CODON (TERMINATOR SEQUENCE), SEQUENCE (OF A DNA MOLECULE), DEOXYRIBONUCLEIC ACID (DNA), GENETIC ENGINEERING, EXPRESS, GENE, PROTEIN, SYNTHESIZING (OF PROTEIN MOLECULE), *AGROBACTERIUM TUMEFACIENS*, BACTERIA, CONTROL SEQUENCES

NPTII See NPTII GENE

NPTII Gene A marker gene that codes for (i.e., "causes manufacture of") the enzyme **neomycin phosphotransferase II**, which can inactivate the antibiotic **kanamycin**. The NPTII gene is commonly utilized as a "marker gene" for genetically engineered plants. Neomycin phosphotransferase confers kanamycin resistance on cells expressing it (i.e., cells that contain the NPTII gene in addition to the other genes inserted along with it) so that those (engineered) cells will live in a laboratory vessel containing kanamycin.

See also GENE, MARKER (GENETIC MARKER), CODING SEQUENCE, ENZYME, CELL, GENETIC ENGINEERING

NSP See NONSTARCH POLYSACCHARIDES

NT An acronym for **Nuclear Transfer**.

See NUCLEAR TRANSFER

nt An abbreviation for **nucleotide**.

See NUCLEOTIDE

Nuclear DNA The DNA that is contained within the nucleus of a cell.

See also DEOXYRIBONUCLEIC ACID (DNA), CELL, GENOME, NUCLEUS, NUCLEAR TRANSFER

Nuclear Envelope See MEMBRANE (OF A CELL)

Nuclear Hormone Receptors Refers to receptors in a cell's outer membrane that serve to convey the "signal" received (when certain hormones and vitamins latch onto those receptors) all the way into the cell's nucleus. Within the cell's nucleus, they serve as transcription activators or factors that regulate the expression of certain specific genes.

See also RECEPTORS, NUCLEAR RECEPTORS, CELL, PLASMA MEMBRANE, NUCLEUS, HORMONE, VITAMIN, SIGNALING, SIGNAL TRANSDUCTION, G-PROTEINS, TRANSCRIPTION, TRANSCRIPTION FACTORS, TRANSCRIPTION ACTIVATORS, GENE, EXPRESS, EXPRESSIVITY

Nuclear Magnetic Resonance The acronym is **NMR**. It is a spectrometry tool or methodology that can be utilized by scientists to determine several fundamental properties of complex or large biomolecules. NMR machines send a very specifically shaped pulse of radio frequency (RF) energy at the **precise resonance frequency (known as Larmor frequency)** needed to "pump" (i.e., add) energy to the **precessional motion** ("**rotation**") of the atomic nuclei within the sample (biomolecule) being examined within a magnetic field.

Those pulses cause the relevant atoms' **nuclear magnetic moments** to either turn in space by 90° or to turn by 180°. The former causes the sample's atomic nuclei to send out a signal known as a **free induction decay**; the latter causes the sample's atomic nuclei to send out detectable **spin echos**, which are detected by the NMR machine and turned into useful data.

See also QUANTITATIVE STRUCTURE–ACTIVITY RELATIONSHIP (QSAR)

Nuclear Matrix Proteins Protein molecules that are present in cancerous cells but not in normal (nonmutated) cells.

See also PROTEIN, CELL, MUTATION, MUTANT, MYRISTOYLATION, NEOPLASTIC GROWTH, PARP

Nuclear Receptors Receptors in a cell's outer membrane that serve to convey a "signal" from outside the cell all the way into the cell's nucleus. They function as ligand-activated transcription factors, which thus serve within cells as transcription activators or factors that regulate the expression of certain specific genes (i.e., those affecting cell or life processes such as fatty acid metabolism, reproduction, and general development of the organism). Each nuclear receptor contains two zinc finger proteins, which target **hormone response elements** (i.e., specific DNA sequences that initiate the activation of applicable genes for that particular receptor).

See also RECEPTORS, SIGNALING, SIGNAL TRANSDUCTION, NUCLEUS, G-PROTEINS, ORPHAN RECEPTORS, RETINOID X RECEPTORS (RXR), ENDOCYTOSIS, VAGINOSIS, CD4 PROTEIN, PROTEIN, ORGANISM, CELL, GENE, EXPRESS, GENE EXPRESSION, ZINC FINGER PROTEINS, TRANSCRIPTION, TRANSCRIPTION FACTORS, TRANSCRIPTION ACTIVATORS, FATTY ACID, METABOLISM, LIGAND (IN BIOCHEMISTRY), POLYUNSATURATED FATTY ACIDS (PUFA), MEMBRANES (OF A CELL), PLASMA MEMBRANE, LIPID RAFTS, FARNESOID X RECEPTORS (FXR), LIVER X RECEPTORS (LXR)

Nuclear Transfer A method of cloning a living organism, in which that organism's entire genetic information is conveyed via transfer of an (adult) cell nucleus into an unfertilized egg (from another animal of the same species) whose nucleus had previously been removed. This was the method utilized to produce "Dolly," the first cloned sheep, in 1996. It is possible to also delete or substitute genes (e.g., brought in from another species) as part of the nuclear transfer process, so nuclear transfer can be utilized to produce transgenic organisms or "**knockout**" **organisms**.

See also CLONE (AN ORGANISM), CELL, NUCLEUS, GENOME, NUCLEAR DNA, DEOXYRIBONUCLEIC ACID (DNA), GENE, SPECIES, TRANSGENIC (ORGANISM), KNOCK OUT (GENE), GENETIC ENGINEERING

Nuclease An enzyme capable of hydrolyzing the internucleotide linkages of a nucleic acid (e.g., DNA or RNA). Nucleases present in cells tend to degrade (i.e., hydrolyze and cleave) artificially inserted DNA strands, making genetic targeting more difficult.

See also GENETIC TARGETING, HYDROL-YSIS, DEOXYRIBONUCLEIC ACID (DNA), RIBONUCLEIC ACID (RNA), ANTISENSE (DNA SEQUENCE)

Nucleic Acid Probes See DNA PROBE, NUCLEIC ACIDS, POLYMERASE CHAIN REACTION (PCR), RAPID MICROBIAL DETECTION (RMD)

Nucleic Acids A nucleotide polymer. A large, chain-like molecule containing phosphate groups, sugar groups, purine and pyrimidine bases. Two types are ribonucleic acid (RNA), and deoxyribonucleic acid (DNA). The bases involved are adenine, guanine, cytosine, and thymine (uracil in RNA).

Nucleic acids are either the specific (genetic) informational molecule (i.e., DNA), or act as agent (i.e., RNA) in causing that information to be expressed (e.g., as a protein).

See also NUCLEOTIDE, POLYMER, INFOR-MATIONAL MOLECULES, GENE, GENETIC CODE, DEOXYRIBONUCLEIC ACID (DNA), RIBONUCLEIC ACID (RNA), EXPRESS, EXTENSION (IN NUCLEIC ACIDS)

Nucleoid The compact body that contains the genome in a bacterium.

See also GENOME

Nucleolus A round, granular structure situated in the nucleus of eucaryotic cells. It is involved in rRNA (ribosomal RNA) synthesis and ribosome formation.

See also RIBOSOMES, NUCLEUS

Nucleophilic Group An electron-rich group with a strong tendency to donate electrons to an electron-deficient nucleus.

See also POLAR GROUP, NONPOLAR GROUP

Nucleoplasm The protoplasm present within a cell's nucleus.

See also CELL, NUCLEUS, PROTOPLASM

Nucleoproteins Complexes made up of nucleic acid and protein. These two substances are apparently not linked by strong chemical bonds but are held together by salt linkages and other weak bonds. Most viruses consist entirely of nucleoproteins, although some viruses also contain fatty substances. Nucleoproteins also occur in animal and plant cells and in bacteria.

See also PROTEIN, NUCLEIC ACIDS, VIRUS

Nucleoside A "hybrid" molecule consisting of a purine (adenine and guanine) or pyrimidine (thymine, uracil, or cytosine) base covalently linked to a five-membered sugar ring (ribose in the case of RNA and deoxyribose in the case of DNA).

See also NUCLEOTIDE, ADENINE, GUA-NINE, GUANOSINE, URIDINE, RIBONU-CLEIC ACID (RNA), DEOXYRIBONU-CLEIC ACID (DNA)

Nucleoside Diphosphate Sugar A coenzyme-like carrier of a sugar molecule functioning in the enzymatic synthesis of polysaccharides and sugar derivatives.

See also POLYSACCHARIDES

Nucleosome Spherical particles composed of a special class of basic proteins (histone) in combination with DNA (146 bp of DNA are wrapped 1.75 times around a "core" of histone proteins). The particles are approximately 12.5 nm in diameter and are connected to each other by DNA filaments. Under an electron microscope they appear somewhat like a string of pearls.

Nucleosomes are the basic structural unit of the chromosome and are sometimes called **chromosomal packing units**.

See also CHROMATIN, HISTONES, PRO-TEIN, DEOXYRIBONUCLEIC ACID (DNA), BASE PAIR (bp), CHROMO-SOMES, NANOMETERS (nm)

Nucleotide An ester of a nucleoside and phosphoric acid. Nucleotides are nucleosides that have a phosphate group attached to one or more of the hydroxyl groups of the sugar (ribose or deoxyribose). In short, a nucleotide is a hybrid molecule consisting of a purine or pyrimidine base covalently linked to a five-membered sugar ring that is covalently linked to a phosphate group. Whereas (polymerized) nucleotides are the structural units of a nucleic acid, free nucleotides that are not an integral part of nucleic acids are also found in tissues and play important roles in the cell, e.g., ATP and cyclic AMP. Two nucleotides form each "rung of the ladder" within DNA molecules.

See also ATP, CYCLIC AMP, BASE (NUCLE-OTIDE), NUCLEOSIDE, NUCLEIC ACIDS, MESSENGER RNA (mRNA), RIBONU-CLEIC ACID (RNA), DEOXYRIBONU-CLEIC ACID (DNA), TRANSVERSION

N

Nucleus Discovered by Robert Brown in the early 1800s, it is the usually spherical body within each living cell that contains its hereditary biological material (e.g., DNA, genes, chromosomes, etc.) and controls the cell's life functions (e.g., metabolism, growth, and reproduction). The nucleus is a highly differentiated, relatively large organelle lying in the cytoplasm of the cell. The nucleus is surrounded by a (nuclear) membrane, which is quite similar to the plasma (cell) membrane except that the nuclear membrane contains holes or pores. It is characterized by its high content of chromatin, which contains most of the cell's DNA. That chromatin is normally (when cell is not in process of dividing) distributed throughout the nucleus in a diffuse manner.

See also GENOME, CELL, GENE, GENETIC CODE, RNA, HEREDITY, DEOXYRIBONUCLEIC ACID (DNA), CHROMOSOMES, MEIOSIS, NUCLEAR TRANSFER, METABOLISM, CHROMATIDS, CHROMATIN, PLASMA MEMBRANE, ORGANELLES, NUCLEAR RECEPTORS

Nutraceuticals Coined in 1989 by Stephen DeFelice, this term is used to refer to either a food or portion of food (e.g., a vitamin, essential amino acid, etc.) that possesses medical or health benefits (when consumed). For example, saponins (present in beans, spinach, tomatoes, potatoes, alfalfa, clover, etc.) possess some cancer prevention properties. Also sometimes called pharmafoods, functional foods, or designer foods, these are food products that have been designed to contain specific concentrations and/or proportions of certain nutrients (e.g., vitamins, amino acids, etc.) that are critical to good health.

See also ESSENTIAL AMINO ACIDS, AMINO ACID, VITAMIN, FOOD GOOD MANUFACTURING PRACTICE (FGMP), SAPONINS, ESSENTIAL NUTRIENTS, PHYTOCHEMICALS, ANTIOXIDANTS, ISOFLAVONES, GENISTEIN (Gen), RESVERATROL, PHYTOSTEROLS, BETA-CAROTENE, LYCOPENE, CAROTENOIDS, LUTEIN, ANTHOCYANINS, VITAMIN E, XANTHOPHYLLS, STEROLS, SITOSTEROLS, SITOSTANOLS, ELLAGIC ACID, ALICIN, PROANTHOCYANIDINS, POLYPHENOLS, ZEAXANTHIN, PHYTO-MANUFACTURING

Nutriceuticals See NUTRACEUTICALS

Nutricines See NUTRACEUTICALS

Nutrient Enhanced™ A phrase that is now a trademark of Garst Seed Company, it refers to plants that have been modified to possess novel traits that make those plants more economically valuable for nutritional uses (e.g., higher-than-normal protein content in certain feed grains).

See also VALUE-ENHANCED GRAINS, HIGH-OIL CORN, PROTEIN, GENETIC ENGINEERING, HIGH-LYSINE CORN, HIGH-METHIONINE CORN, PLANT'S NOVEL TRAIT (PNT), HIGH-PHYTASE CORN AND SOYBEANS

Nutrigenomics See NUTRITIONAL GENOMICS

Nutritional Epigenetics See EPIGENETIC

Nutritional Genomics Refers to the study of the biological impacts of certain foods or food ingredients on the body **owing specifically to the different genomes (DNA) of those individual organisms that consume those foods or ingredients**. The subgroup consisting of all those individuals whose genome (DNA) causes their body to respond in a specific way to a given food or ingredient is known as a HAPLOTYPE. A haplotype could (theoretically) be as small as one individual (e.g., one man possessing a certain genome), because that man's particular response to a food or ingredient could result from one single-nucleotide polymorphism (SNP) that only his genome possesses.

Thus, nutritional genomics applies to the genetically determined **biological impact of a given food or ingredient within a specific haplotype**. For example, research indicates that consumption of oleic acid by women whose genome possesses the *Her-2/neu* (breast-cancer-promoting gene) SNP, results in downregulation of expression of that *Her-2/neu* gene.

See also GENOME, PHARMACOGENOMICS, GENOMICS, DEOXYRIBONUCLEIC ACID (DNA), GENE, HAPLOTYPE, SINGLE-NUCLEOTIDE POLYMORPHISMS (SNPs), CODING SEQUENCE, EXPRESS, DOWN-REGULATING, BIOLOGICAL ACTIVITY, ORGANISM, HER-2 GENE, OLEIC ACID

O

O Glycosylation See GLYCOSYLATION (TO GLYCOSYLATE)

O'Farrell Gels Refers to **two-dimensional gel electrophoresis**, discovered by Patrick O'Farrell in 1975. See TWO-DIMENSIONAL (2-D) GEL ELECTROPHORESIS

OAB (Office of Agricultural Biotechnology) A unit of the U.S. Department of Agriculture that is in charge of a part of the federal regulatory process for biotechnology (e.g., field tests of transgenic plants).

See also TOXIC SUBSTANCES CONTROL ACT (TSCA), RECOMBINANT DNA ADVISORY COMMITTEE (RAC), FOOD AND DRUG ADMINISTRATION (FDA), TRANSGENIC

Ochratoxins A term that refers to a group of related mycotoxins (i.e., toxic metabolites produced by fungi) that are produced by some *Aspergillus* species and some *Penicillium* species of fungi (e.g., *Aspergillus ochraceus* [alutaceus], *Penicillium verrucosum*, *Penicillium viridicatum*).

These particular fungi tend to produce ochratoxins when the they grow in damaged grain (e.g., during grain storage), especially when the grain temperature is above 4°C (40°F) and grain moisture content is above 18%.

Ochratoxin A (OTA) is a very carcinogenic (cancer-causing) toxin, which also can cause kidney damage when consumed by humans. When dairy cattle consume ochratoxin-A-containing grain, the ochratoxin A soon appears in the milk produced by those cows.

See also MYCOTOXINS, TOXIN, FUNGUS, *PENICILLIUM, CARCINOGEN*

Octadecanoid–Jasmonate Signal Complex A **chemical signal** that is created and emitted by certain plants in response to being wounded (e.g., via chewing) by insects. The octadecanoid–jasmonate signal complex then causes the production and emission of volatile chemicals such as volicitin, which attract certain types of wasps that are natural enemies of the

insects that initially wounded the plants. Thus, the octadecanoid–jasmonate signal complex is crucial part of an (indirect) defense mechanism of such plants.

See also SIGNALING MOLECULE, SIGNALING, EUROPEAN CORN BORER, INTEGRATED PEST MANAGEMENT (IPM), VOLICITIN

OD See OPTICAL DENSITY

Odorant-Binding Protein A protein that enhances people's ability to smell odorants in trace quantities that are much lower than those needed to activate olfactory (i.e., smelling) nerves. The protein accomplishes this by latching on to (odorant) molecules and enhancing their aroma. Hence, it acts as a kind of "helper" entity in bringing about the ability to smell certain odorants present in low concentration.

See also PROTEIN

OECD See ORGANIZATION FOR ECONOMIC COOPERATION AND DEVELOPMENT

Office International des Epizootics See INTERNATIONAL OFFICE OF EPIZOOTICS (OIE)

OGM See GMO

OH43 A gene in plants (e.g., corn or maize) that causes production of a seed coat that is more resistant to tearing. Greater tear resistance results in a lower incidence of fungi infestation in seed, which results in less mycotoxin production in seed.

See also GENE, FUNGUS, AFLATOXIN, MYCOTOXINS

OIE Acronym for **Office International des Epizootics**.

See INTERNATIONAL OFFICE OF EPIZOOTICS (OIE)

OIF See OSTEOINDUCTIVE FACTOR

Oils See FATTY ACID

Oleate A term utilized by some to refer to **oleic acid**.

See OLEIC ACID

Oleic Acid A fatty acid that is naturally present in the fat of animals and also in oils extracted from oilseed plants (e.g., soybean, canola, etc.). For example, the soybean oil produced from traditional varieties of soybeans tends to contain 24% oleic acid. Research indicates that consumption of adequate amounts of oleic acid helps to reduce (over)expression of the Her-2/neu gene and thereby confer some protection against breast cancer.

See also MONOUNSATURATED FATS, FATTY ACID, FATS, CANOLA, SOYBEAN PLANT, SOYBEAN OIL, HIGH-OLEIC OIL SOYBEANS, GENE, EXPRESS, EXPRESSIVITY, COSUPPRESSION, CANCER, HER-2/NEU GENE, DOWNREGULATING

Oleosomes The **storage bodies** for lipids (fats) in the seeds of certain plants.

See also LIPIDS, FATS, FATTY ACID

Oligionucleotide See OLIGONUCLEOTIDE

Oligofructans See FRUCTAN, FRUCTOSE OLIGOSACCHARIDES

Oligofructose See FRUCTOSE OLIGOSACCHARIDES

Oligomer A relatively short (the prefix "oligo-" means few, or slight) chain molecule (polymer) that is made up of repeating units (e.g., XAX-AXAXA or XXAAXXAAXXAA, etc.). Short polymers consisting of only two repeating units are called *dimers*, and those of three repeating units are called *trimers*. Longer units are called polymers (i.e., many units). As a rule of thumb, oligomers consisting of eleven or more repeating units are called *polymers*.

See also POLYMER

Oligonucleotide Synonymous with oligodeoxyribonucleotide, they are short chains of nucleotides (i.e., single-stranded DNA or RNA) that have been synthesized (i.e., made by man or inside living cells) by chemically linking together a number of specific nucleotides. When made by man, oligonucleotides (also called, simply, "oligos") are used as synthetic (i.e., synthetic) genes, DNA probes, and in site-directed mutagenesis.

See also NUCLEOTIDE, GENE, DNA PROBE, OLIGOMER, SITE-DIRECTED MUTAGENESIS, GENE MACHINE, DEOXYRIBONUCLEIC ACID (DNA), RIBONUCLEIC ACID, SYNTHESIZING (OF DNA MOLECULES)

Oligonucleotide Probes Short-chain fragments of DNA that are used in various gene analysis tests (e.g., the single base change in DNA that causes sickle cell anemia).

See also OLIGONUCLEOTIDE, DEOXYRIBONUCLEIC ACID (DNA), DNA PROBE, GENE MACHINE

Oligopeptide A relatively-short-chain molecule that is made up of amino acids linked by peptide bonds.

See also PEPTIDE, POLYPEPTIDE (PROTEIN), OLIGOMER, AMINO ACID

Oligos Term utilized to refer to manmade "chains" (nucleic acids) consisting of 18 to 30 nucleotides. They are utilized as synthetic genes, DNA probes, "bio-bar codes" on nanoparticle probes, primers, siRNA, and in site-directed mutagenesis. Oligos can modulate (i.e., increase or decrease) gene expression in cells by directly interacting with the cell's DNA or mRNA.

See also OLIGONUCLEOTIDE, NUCLEIC ACIDS, NUCLEOTIDE, GENE, DNA PROBE, PRIMER (DNA), DEOXYRIBONUCLEIC ACID (DNA), RIBONUCLEIC ACID (RNA), SHORT INTERFERING RNA (siRNA), SITE-DIRECTED MUTAGENESIS (SDM), CELL, BIO–BAR CODES, EXPRESS, EXPRESSIVITY

Oligosaccharide Microarrays See MICROARRAY (TESTING)

Oligosaccharides Relatively short molecular chains made up of 10 to 100 simple sugar (saccharide) units. These sugar (i.e., carbohydrate) chains are frequently attached to protein molecules. When this happens, the resulting molecule is known as a glycoprotein, that is, a hybrid molecule that is part protein and part sugar. The oligosaccharide portion affects a protein's conformations and biological activity. The oligosaccharide (carbohydrate) portion of a glycoprotein functions as a mediator of cellular uptake of that glycoprotein. Glycosylation thus affects the length of time the molecule resides in the bloodstream before it is taken out of circulation (serum lifetime). It is thought that blood group (e.g., A, B, O, etc.) is based on an oligosaccharide concept. For example, different oligosaccharide "branches" on a given glycoprotein (e.g., tissue plasminogen activator) could cause that glycoprotein to be perceived by the body's immune system to be another (incorrect) blood type, thus provoking an immune response against it. Oligosaccharides play a critical role in numerous disease processes (e.g., bacterial and viral infection processes, cancer metastasis processes, inflammation processes, etc.). For example, oligosaccharide "chains" extending from the exterior membrane **plasma membrane** of cells are utilized by bacteria (and inflammation-triggering immune system cells) to **latch on to** cells and facilitate entry into cells.

See also POLYSACCHARIDES, CELL, CONFORMATION, MONOSACCHARIDES, FURANOSE, PENTOSE, PYRANOSE, GLYCOGEN, GLYCOFORM, FRUCTOSE OLIGOSACCHARIDES, GLYCOPROTEIN, SIALIC ACID, MANNANOLIGOSACCHARIDES, TISSUE PLASMINOGEN ACTIVATOR (tPA), OLIGOMER, SEROLOGY, HUMORAL IMMUNITY, CELLULAR IMMUNE RESPONSE, METASTASIS, ADHESION MOLECULES, HEMAGGLUTININ (HA), TRANSGALACTO-OLIGOSACCHARIDES

Omega-3 Fatty Acids More properly called "*n*-3 fatty acids."

See n-3 FATTY ACIDS

Omega-6 Fatty Acids More properly called "*n*-6 fatty acids."

See n-6 FATTY ACIDS

Oncogenes Genes within a cell's DNA that code for receptors (proteins on outer surface of cell membrane) for a cellular growth factor (e.g., epidermal growth factor). Via that coding of applicable receptors (or other protein molecules that are part of the signal transduction process of a cell), oncogenes "turn on" the process of cell division (replication) at appropriate times during the life of each cell in an organism. When oncogenes are mutated (e.g., via exposure to cigarette smoke or ultraviolet light, etc.), those oncogenes can become cancer-causing genes, some of which (e.g., erythroblastosis virus gene) are almost identical to the gene for epidermal growth factor (EGF) receptor (i.e., oncogene is a "deformed copy" of that gene). Such mutated oncogenes code for (i.e., cause to be made) proteins (e.g., protein kinases, protein phosphorylating enzymes, etc.) that trigger uncontrolled cell growth. They sometimes may consist of a human chromosome that has viral nucleic acid material incorporated into it and is a permanent part of that chromosome.

See also GENE, CELL, DEOXYRIBONUCLEIC ACID (DNA), BRCA GENES, HER-2 GENE, *ras* GENE, MEIOSIS, CARCINOGEN, RIBOSOMES, PROTEIN, TYROSINE KINASE, ENZYME, CHROMOSOME, PLASMA MEMBRANE, EPIDERMAL GROWTH FACTOR (EGF), SIGNAL TRANSDUCTION, CODING SEQUENCE, TUMOR, CANCER, PROTO-ONCOGENES, GENETIC CODE, RECEPTORS, MUTAGEN

Oocytes The cells, produced by an organism's ovaries, that eventually become an ovum ("egg cell") via meiosis.

See also MEIOSIS, CELL, ORGANISM

Opague-2 A gene in corn (maize) that (when present in the DNA of a given plant) causes that plant to produce seed that contains higher-than-normal levels of lysine, calcium, magnesium, iron, zinc, and manganese.

See also LYSINE (Lys), HIGH-METHIONINE CORN, ESSENTIAL AMINO ACIDS, CORN, VALUE-ENHANCED GRAINS, HIGH-LYSINE CORN, DEOXYRIBONUCLEIC ACID (DNA), GENE, MAL (MULTIPLE ALEURONE LAYER) GENE

Open Reading Frame (ORF) Region of a gene (DNA) that contains a series of triplet (bases) coding for amino acids without any termination codons. The ORF sequence is potentially translatable into a protein, but the presence of an open reading frame (sequence) does not guarantee that a protein molecule will be produced (by cell ribosome).

See also GENE, DEOXYRIBONUCLEIC ACID (DNA), AMINO ACID, PROTEIN, CODING SEQUENCE, GENETIC CODE, TRANSLATION, CELL, RIBOSOMES

Operator Also known as the "**o locus.**" The site on the DNA to which a repressor molecule binds to prevent the initiation of transcription. The operator locus is a distinct entity and exists independently of the structural genes and the regulatory gene. It is the structural or biochemical "switch" with which the operon is turned on or off, and it controls the transcription of an entire group of coordinately induced genes. One type of mutation of the operator locus is called operator constitutive mutants. Constitutive mutants continually churn out the protein characteristic for that operon because the operon unit cannot be **turned off** by the repressor molecule.

See also OPERON, PROMOTER, REGULATORY GENES, REPRESSION (OF GENE TRANSCRIPTION/TRANSLATION), REPRESSOR (PROTEIN), STRUCTURAL GENE, STRUCTURAL GENOMICS

Operon A gene unit consisting of one or more genes that specify a polypeptide and an operator unit that regulates the structural gene, that is, the production of messenger RNA (mRNA) and hence, ultimately, of a number of proteins. Generally an operon is defined as a group of functionally related structural genes mapping (that is, being) close to each other in the chromosome and **being controlled by the same (one) operator**. If the operator is "turned on," then the DNA of the genes comprising the operon will be transcribed into mRNA, and eventually specific proteins are produced. If, on the other hand, the operator is "turned off," then transcription of the genes does not occur and the production of the operon-specific proteins does not occur.

See also DEOXYRIBONUCLEIC ACID (DNA), GENE, OPERATOR, TRANSCRIPTION, POLYPEPTIDE, PROTEIN, MESSENGER RNA (mRNA), CHROMOSOME

Opsonin A protein present within blood that makes pathogens and other microorganisms more easily engulfed (e.g., by macrophages, etc.).

See also PROTEIN, PATHOGEN, PHAGOCYTE, MACROPHAGE, MICROORGANISM

Opsonization Refers to (immune response) **covering of a pathogen or other microorganism** in the bloodstream **with opsonin** in order to render that pathogen or microorganism more susceptible to being engulfed or destroyed (e.g., by macrophages, etc.).

See also OPSONIN, IMMUNE RESPONSE, PATHOGEN, PHAGOCYTE, MACROPHAGE

Optical Activity The capacity of a substance to rotate the plane of polarization of plane-polarized light when examined in an instrument known as a polarimeter. All compounds that are capable of existing in two forms that are nonsuperimposable mirror images of each other exhibit optical activity. Such compounds are called stereoisomers (or enantiomers or chiral molecules), and the two forms arise because compounds having asymmetric carbon atoms to which other atoms are connected may arrange themselves in two different ways.

See also STEREOISOMERS, ENANTIOMERS, CHIRAL COMPOUND

Optical Density (OD) The absorbance of light of a specific wavelength by molecules normally dissolved in a solution. Light absorption depends on the concentration of the absorbing compound (chemical entity) in the solution, the thickness of the sample being illuminated, and the chemical nature of the absorbing compound. An analytical instrument known as a spectrophotometer is used to (quantitatively) express the amount of a substance (dissolved) in a solution. Mathematically, this is accomplished using the Beer–Lambert law.

See also SPECTROPHOTOMETER, ABSORBANCE (Å)

Optical Tweezer Invented in 1986 by A. Ashkin, this refers to the use of laser or highly focused infrared light beams to "trap" a tiny object (e.g., biomolecules, dendrimers, supramolecular assemblies, etc.) in three-dimensional space, holding them against gravity, Brownian (molecular) motion, etc., for measurements or to be otherwise manipulated. That is accomplished by shining the light beam through a narrow aperture, thereby directing its "radiation pressure" against the tiny object.

See also NANOTECHNOLOGY, DENDRIMERS, SUPRAMOLECULAR ASSEMBLY, SELF-ASSEMBLING MOLECULAR MACHINES

Optimum Foods See NUTRACEUTICALS, PHYTOCHEMICALS

Optimum pH The pH (level of acidity) at which maximum growth occurs, maximal enzymatic activity occurs, or any reaction occurs maximally.

See also ENZYME

Optimum Temperature The temperature at which the maximum growth occurs, maximal enzymatic activity occurs, or any reaction occurs maximally.

See also ENZYME, ENSILING

Optrode A fiber-optic sensor made by coating the tip of a (glass) optic fiber with an antibody that fluoresces when the antibody comes in contact with its corresponding antigen. Alternatively, the fiber tip is sometimes coated with a dye that fluoresces when the dye comes in contact with specific chemicals (e.g., oxygen, glucose, etc.). Functionally, a beam of light is sent down the fiber and strikes ("pumps") the fluorescent complex, which then fluoresces (releases light of a specific wavelength). The light produced by fluorescence travels back up the same optic fiber and is detected by a spectrophotometer upon its return. By application of the Beer–Lambert law, quantitative detection or measurement of the antigen or chemical *in vivo* in, for example, a patient's bloodstream is possible.

See also ANTIGEN, *IN VIVO*, ANTIBODY, GLUCOSE (GLc), SPECTROPHOTOMETER

Oral Cancer Also sometimes known as "cancer of the mouth," this is a cancer involving the tissues lining the human mouth. Causes include consumption by humans of carcinogens (e.g., tobacco products, certain mycotoxins, etc.). Oral cancerous cells arise from precancerous mouth lesions known as oral leukoplakia. During 2000, research by Frank Meyskins and William Armstrong indicated that consumption of Bowman–Birk trypsin inhibitor (BB T.I.) derived from soybeans, in a manner that "bathes" mouth tissues in BB T.I. (for an extended period of time), inhibits the development of oral leukoplakia.

See also CANCER, TUMOR, MUTAGEN, MYCOTOXINS, TRYPSIN INHIBITORS

Oral Leukoplakia See ORAL CANCER

Oral Tolerance See GLUTAMIC ACID DECARBOXYLASE (GAD)

Orally Administered Refers to the ability of compounds (e.g., pharmaceuticals) to be delivered to the body via the digestive system, and still retain their efficacy (biological activity). One method to accomplish that (i.e., protect the compound from being broken down by the digestive system prior to the compound arriving at the site within body where needed) is to encapsulate molecules of the compound within a phosphatidyl serine "nanocoating" (known as a **nanocochleate**).

See also BIOLOGICAL ACTIVITY, PHOSPHATIDYL SERINE, PEYER'S PATCHES, NANOBODIES

ORF See OPEN READING FRAME (ORF)

Organelles Membrane-surrounded structures found in eucaryotic cells; they contain enzymes and other components required for specialized cell function (e.g., ribosomes for protein synthesis or lysosomes for enzymatic hydrolysis). Some organelles such as mitochondria and chloroplasts contain DNA and can replicate autonomously (from the rest of the cell).

See also NUCLEUS, EUCARYOTE, ENZYME, RIBOSOMES, LYSOSOME

Organism Refers to any living plant, animal, bacteria, fungus, virus, etc. Also (e.g., in certain international treaties such as the Convention on Biological Diversity), this term includes things (e.g., seeds, spores, and eggs) **possessing the potential to become** plants, animals, fungi, etc.

See also BIOLOGY, BACTERIA, FUNGUS, VIRUS, CONVENTION ON BIOLOGICAL DIVERSITY (CBD)

Organismos Geneticamente Modificados See GMO

Organization for Economic Cooperation and Development (OECD) An international organization comprised of the world's wealthiest (most developed) nations, originally established in 1960 to study trade and related matters. In 1991, the OECD's Group of National Experts on Safety in Biotechnology (GNE) completed a document entitled "Report on the Concepts and Principles Underpinning Safety Evaluations of Food Derived from Modern Biotechnology." The "aim of that document was to elaborate the scientific principles to be considered (i.e., by OECD member nations' regulatory agencies) in evaluating the safety of new foods and food components" (e.g., genetically modified soybeans, corn or maize, potatoes, etc.).

See also BIOTECHNOLOGY, SOYBEAN PLANT, GNE, CANOLA, MUTUAL RECOGNITION AGREEMENTS (MRA)

Organogenesis The production of entire organs, usually from basic cells, such as fibroblasts, and structural material such as collagen.
See also COLLAGEN, FIBROBLASTS

Origin Point or region where DNA (deoxyribonucleic acid) replication is begun. Often abbreviated "Ori."
See also DEOXYRIBONUCLEIC ACID (DNA), REPLICATION (OF VIRUS), REPLICATION FORK

Orphan Drug The name of the legal status granted (to certain pharmaceuticals) by the U.S. Food and Drug Administration's (FDA) Office of Orphan Products Development. This classification provides the sponsors of those pharmaceuticals with special tax benefits and other financial incentives (e.g., market monopoly for a limited time). If companies feel that they possess a cure (i.e., a drug) for a certain disease but the number of potential patients is below a certain number and there is potential competition from rival companies, then the high cost of developing and shepherding the drug through the FDA would be such that the company would not be able to regain its development costs and make a profit. Hence, orphan drug status was designed to encourage drug development efforts for otherwise noneconomic pharmaceuticals with less than 200,000 patients a year.
See also FOOD AND DRUG ADMINISTRATION (FDA)

Orphan Genes Genes within an organism's genome or DNA that have no apparent function.
See also GENE, ORGANISM, GENOME, DEOXYRIBONUCLEIC ACID (DNA), FUNCTIONAL GENOMICS

Orphan Receptors Refers to nuclear receptors (i.e., embedded in surface of cell's plasma membrane) that are **not** coupled to G-protein (cell) system complexes. **Orphan receptors** include receptors for fatty acids (PPARs), bile acids (FXR), xenobiotics/toxins (PXR/SXR), etc. Many of the orphan receptors **function as lipid sensors that respond to lipid concentrations in cells (e.g., resulting from lipid consumption in diet)** and cause changes in gene expression to protect cells from lipid overload.
See also BIORECEPTORS, RECEPTORS, NUCLEAR RECEPTORS, RETINOID X RECEPTORS RXR), CELL, PLASMA MEMBRANE, G-PROTEINS, LIPIDS, FATTY ACIDS, ADHESION MOLECULE, MICROARRAY (TESTING), BIOCHIPS, HIGH-THROUGHPUT SCREENING (HTS), TARGET–LIGAND INTERACTION SCREENING, LIGAND (IN BIOCHEMISTRY), BIOASSAY, GENE EXPRESSION ANALYSIS, TARGET (OF A THERAPEUTIC AGENT)

Ortholog Refers to a gene (e.g., within the DNA of a small or simple **model organism**) that has the following features:

- Is also present (or at least a very similar sequence gene is) within the DNA of another species (e.g., a more complex species) at an analogous location (e.g., at a particular distance from a certain end of the other organism's DNA molecule)
- Possesses a similar function to that of the analogous gene in the more complex organism (e.g., human)

Identification and study of such a gene (within a model organism) enables the properties or function of its analogous **ortholog gene** in the more complex organism to be inferred. For example, the **Sir2** gene within the organism *Saccharomyces cerevisiae* is an ortholog of the **SirT1** gene in mammals.
See also GENE, DEOXYRIBONUCLEIC ACID (DNA), SEQUENCE (OF A DNA MOLECULE), MODEL ORGANISM, PHYLOGENETIC PROFILING, FUNCTIONAL GENOMICS, SIR2 GENE, SIRT1 GENE

Orthophosphate Cleavage Enzymatic cleavage of one of the phosphate ester bonds of ATP to yield ADP and a single phosphate molecule known as orthophosphate (designated as P_i). The cleavage of the phosphate bond is energy yielding and is (except in the case of a futile cycle) coupled enzymatically to reactions that utilize energy to run the cell. An orthophosphate cleavage reaction releases relatively less energy than does a corresponding pyrophosphate cleavage reaction.
See also ADENOSINE DIPHOSPHATE (ADP), ADENOSINE TRIPHOSPHATE (ATP), FUTILE CYCLE, PYROPHOSPHATE CLEAVAGE

Osmosis Bulk flow of water through a semipermeable (or more accurately, differentially permeable) membrane into another (aqueous) phase
containing more of a solute (dissolved compound). As an example, let us set up an osmot-
ically active system. There are two solutions, A
and B. Solution A has less salt dissolved in it
than solution B, and furthermore the two solutions are separated by a differentially permeable
membrane (this looks like a plastic film). Water
molecules (and only water molecules) will flow
from solution A through the membrane and into
solution B. The reason for this is that the membrane allows free passage only to water molecules. The bulk flow of water has the effect of
diluting solution B while concentrating solution
A. Water will flow from solution A to solution
B until the salt concentrations of both solutions
arc equal. Osmosis is therefore a process in
which water passes from regions of low salt concentration to regions of high salt concentration.
The process can be viewed as equalizing the
number of water and solute molecules on both
sides of the membrane.
See also OSMOTIC PRESSURE

Osmotic Pressure May be defined as the
hydrostatic pressure that must be applied to a
solution on one side of a semipermeable membrane (solution B in the example for osmosis)
in order to offset the flow of solvent (water) from
the other side (solution A in the example for
osmosis). It is a measure of the tendency or
"strength" of water to flow from a region of low
salt concentration (and conversely high water
concentration) to regions of high salt concentration (and conversely low water concentration).
See also OSMOSIS

Osmotins A category of proteins, which are
produced by some organisms as a natural
defense against pathogenic fungi.
See also CECROPHINS, MAGAININS,
ORGANISM, FUNGUS, PATHOGENIC

Osteoarthritis A disease that affects primarily
women older than 45 yr, in which cartilage
within the body's joints breaks down.
Osteoarthritis encompasses approximately half
of all cases of arthritis.

Osteoinductive Factor (OIF) A protein that
induces the growth of both cartilage-forming
cells and bone-forming cells (e.g., after a
bone has been broken). When applied in the

presence of **transforming growth factor-
beta, type 2** (another protein), osteoinductive
factor first causes connective tissue cells to
grow together to form a matrix of cartilage
(e.g., across the bone break), and then bone
cells slowly replace that cartilage. Osteoinductive factor also seems to thwart the type
of cell that tears down bone formation, so
OIF may someday be used to combat
osteoporosis.
See also GROWTH FACTOR, TRANSFORM-
ING GROWTH FACTOR-BETA (TGF-
BETA), FIBROBLASTS, FIBROBLAST
GROWTH FACTOR (FGF), OSTEOPOROSIS

Osteoporosis A disease of humans in which
the bones gradually weaken and become brit-
tle. A diet containing a large amount of soy
isoflavones (i.e., especially genistein) has
been shown to increase bone density, thereby
lowering the risk of osteoporosis.
Groups that are especially at risk for osteoporosis include postmenopausal women (particularly of Caucasian or Asian ethnicity), those
who have undergone early menopause (i.e.,
prior to age 45), those who smoke, those who
consume excessive amounts of alcohol, and
those who consume excessive amounts of certain pharmaceuticals (e.g., steroids such as
prednisone, thyroid hormone, etc.).
See also OSTEOINDUCTIVE FACTOR (OIF),
GENISTEIN (Gen), SOY PROTEIN,
ISOFLAVONES, STEROID, SOYBEAN
PLANT, HIGH-ISOFLAVONE SOYBEANS,
HAPLOTYPE

OTA Acronym for **Ochratoxin A**.
See OCHRATOXINS

Outcrossing The transfer of a given gene or
genes (e.g., one synthesized by man and
inserted into a plant via genetic engineering)
from a domesticated organism (e.g., crop
plant) to a wild type (relative of the plant).
See also GENE, INTROGRESSION, SYN-
THESIZING (OF DNA MOLECULES),
GENETIC ENGINEERING, WILD TYPE

Overlapping Gene Refers to a gene whose
sequence at least partially overlaps that of
another gene (adjacent to the first within the
DNA of an organism).
See also GENE, SEQUENCE (OF A DNA
MOLECULE), ORGANISM, DEOXYRIBO-
NUCLEIC ACID (DNA)

Overwinding Positive supercoiling. Winding that applies further tension in the direction of winding of the two strands about each other in the duplex.

See also DEOXYRIBONUCLEIC ACID (DNA), SUPERCOILING, DOUBLE HELIX, DUPLEX

Oxalate A salt or ester of oxalic acid.

See also CALCIUM OXALATE

Oxalate Oxidase (OxOx) An enzyme that catalyzes the breakdown of oxalic acid.

Because certain pathogenic fungi (e.g., *Sclerotina sclerotiorum*) produce oxalic acid to help those fungi "invade" specific crop plants' tissues, the production of OxOx by those crop plants would make them resistant to those pathogenic fungi. The crop plant wheat (*Triticum aestivum*) possesses a gene that codes for the production of OxOx.

See also ENZYME, FUNGUS, OXALIC ACID, PATHOGEN, GENE, CODING SEQUENCE

Oxalic Acid An acid that is naturally produced by some organisms. Oxalic acid is exuded by some pathogenic fungi species to help them invade plant tissues (i.e., as part of the fungal "infection" process).

See also ACID, FUNGUS, ORGANISM, PATHOGEN, OXALATE OXIDASE (OxOx)

Oxidant See OXIDIZING AGENT

Oxidation (chemical reaction) Loss of electrons from a compound (or element) in a chemical reaction. When one compound is oxidized, another compound is reduced. That is, the other compound must "pick up" the electrons that the first has lost.

See also OXIDATION-REDUCTION REACTION, HYDROGENATION, OXIDATION (OF FATS/OILS/LIPIDS)

Oxidation (of fats, oils, or lipids) A chemical transformation of fat or lipid molecules, in which oxygen (e.g., from air) is combined with those molecules. As a result of that (oxidation chemical reaction), various chemical entities are created (e.g., peroxides, aldehydes, etc.), which possess objectionable flavors or odors and are harmful to animals that consume such (rancid) fats or oils.

See also FATS, FATTY ACID, LIPIDS, PLASMA MEMBRANE, OXIDATION (CHEMICAL REACTION), OXIDATIVE STRESS, HYDROLYSIS

Oxidation (of fatty acids) See CARNITINE

Oxidation–Reduction Reaction A chemical reaction in which electrons are transferred from a donor to an acceptor molecule or atom.

See also OXIDATION (CHEMICAL REACTION), OXIDIZING AGENT, REDUCTION (IN A CHEMICAL REACTION)

Oxidative Phosphorylation The enzymatic phosphorylation of ADP to ATP coupled to electron transport from a substrate to molecular oxygen. The synthesis (production) of ATP from the starting materials of ADP and inorganic phosphate (orthophosphate).

See also ADENOSINE DIPHOSPHATE (ADP), ADENOSINE TRIPHOSPHATE (ATP), ORTHOPHOSPHATE CLEAVAGE

Oxidative Stress The physiological stress or damage that results from the (chemical reaction) breakdown of all or part of an organism, via oxidation reactions. For example, oxidative stress appears to be present in the brains of all persons with neurodegenerative diseases (e.g., Alzheimer's disease, Parkinson's disease, etc.).

One common result of such oxidation reactions is the generation (within an organism's body) of reactive oxygen species (e.g., "free radicals") that can adversely affect the following:

- Endothelial function (i.e., the inner lining of blood vessels)
- Platelet aggregation (e.g., inappropriate blood clotting or clumping)
- Atherosclerosis (i.e., buildup of oxidized fatty deposits known as plaque on internal walls of arteries)
- Myocardial function (e.g., heart failure)
- Eye and kidney tissue (especially in diabetics)

A key indicator of oxidative stress is the peroxidation of membrane lipids to form mono- and bifunctional aldehydes (e.g., 4-hydroxy-2-nonenal, also known as HNE).

See also ORGANISM, OXIDATION (CHEMICAL REACTION), ALZHEIMER'S DISEASE, PARKINSON'S DISEASE, CELL, ANTIOXIDANTS, PLASMA MEMBRANE, LIPIDS, GLUTATHIONE, CAROTENOIDS, ENDOTHELIAL CELLS, PLATELETS, ATHEROSCLEROSIS,

INSULIN, CORONARY HEART DISEASE (CHD), HAPTOGLOBIN, COLD HARDENING, MITOGEN-ACTIVATED PROTEIN KINASE CASCADE

Oxidizing Agent (Oxidant) The acceptor of electrons in an oxidation–reduction reaction. The oxidant is reduced by the end of the chemical reaction. That is, the oxidizing agent is the entity that seeks and accepts electrons. Electron acceptance is, by definition, reduction.
See also OXIDATION–REDUCTION REACTION, PEROXIDASE

Oxygen Free Radical See FREE RADICAL

Oxygenase An enzyme catalyzing a reaction in which oxygen is introduced into an acceptor molecule.

P

P34 Protein One of the primary storage proteins in soybean seeds, it can also cause an allergic response in some people (e.g., approximately 1% of humans) who consume it. During 2001–2002, Eliot Herman and Rick Helm utilized genetic engineering to induce "gene silencing" of P34 protein production to create a **reduced-allergen soybean** variety. The resultant biotechnology-derived soybeans contain the same total amount of protein, because production of the other proteins increased exactly enough to offset the (now absent) P34 protein in the resultant seeds.

See also PROTEIN, STORAGE PROTEINS, SOYBEAN PLANT, ALLERGIES (FOOD-BORNE), REDUCED-ALLERGEN SOYBEANS, GENE, GENETIC ENGINEERING, GENE SILENCING, RNA INTERFERENCE (RNAi), COSUPPRESSION, BIOTECHNOLOGY

p53 Gene Discovered in 1978 by David Lane, it is a tumor suppressor gene that controls passage of a given cell from the **"GI" phase** to the **"s"** (i.e., DNA synthesis) phase. The p53 protein that is coded for by the p53 gene is a transcription factor (i.e., it "reads" DNA to determine if it is damaged and then acts to control cell division, whereas the p53 gene codes for more production of additional p53 protein). The p53 gene was discovered in 1993 by Arnold J. Levine and colleagues to be responsible for approximately 50% of all human cancer tumors (when the gene is damaged or mutated).

Normally, the p53 gene codes for (i.e., causes to be manufactured in cell) the p53 protein, which acts to prevent cells from dividing uncontrollably when the cell's DNA has been damaged (e.g., via exposure to cigarette smoke, ultraviolet light, certain mycotoxins, etc.). If in spite of the presence of p53 protein a cell begins to divide uncontrollably following damage to its DNA, the p53 gene can cause apoptosis, which is also known as "programmed cell death" (to try to prevent tumors).

When even slightly methylated (e.g., a single methyl molecular group attached to a cytosine base in the p53 gene at a site adjacent to DNA damage), carcinogens such as those within cigarette smoke or aflatoxin are attracted to that site and insert themselves between adjacent base pairs in the DNA, thereby preventing normal DNA repair.

See also GENE, TUMOR SUPPRESSOR GENES, *ras* GENE, GENETIC CODE, MEIOSIS, DEOXYRIBONUCLEIC ACID (DNA), CARCINOGEN, MYCOTOXINS, RIBOSOMES, ONCOGENES, TRANSCRIPTION FACTORS, CANCER, TUMOR, p53 PROTEIN, PROTO-ONCOGENES, PROTEIN, APOPTOSIS, METHYLATED, CYTOSINE, DNA REPAIR

p53 Protein A tumor suppressor protein, sometimes called the **master transcription factor** or the "guardian of the genome," but whose amino acid sequence alterations (resulting from damage or mutation to the p53 gene) are believed to be responsible for up to 50% of all human cancer tumors. The p53 protein has four domains, one of which (i.e., the core domain) binds to specific sequences of the cell's DNA in order to prevent the cell from dividing uncontrollably when its DNA has been damaged (e.g., via exposure to cigarette smoke, ultraviolet light, or other carcinogen), until it can be repaired.

As the amount of DNA within a given (damaged) cell increases, the concentration of p53 protein also increases. Because p53 protein is a transcription factor (i.e., it "reads" DNA to determine if it is damaged and then acts to control cell division, whereas the p53 gene codes for production of more p53), p53 is very efficient at preventing and inhibiting tumors.

However, if the cell's DNA **cannot be repaired**, the p53 protein can cause **apoptosis** ("programmed cell death") **to prevent development of (cancerous) tumors**. The p53 protein does this by inducing expression of relevant apoptosis-causing genes (e.g., *noxa*, *puma* [bbc3], etc.).

See also GENE, p53 GENE, TUMOR SUP-
PRESSOR GENES, *ras* GENE, *ras* PRO-
TEIN, GENETIC CODE, MEIOSIS, CAR-
CINOGEN, DEOXYRIBONUCLEIC ACID
(DNA), AFLATOXIN, RIBOSOMES,
ONCOGENES, CANCER, TUMOR,
PROTO-ONCOGENES, PROTEIN, TRAN-
SCRIPTION FACTORS, DOMAIN (OF A
PROTEIN), APOPTOSIS

P Element A transposon whose genes (i.e.,
within this transposon) resist rearrangement during the process (i.e., transposition) of the P element being incorporated into a new location
within an organism's genome (i.e., its deoxyribonucleic acid or DNA). In addition to "carrying" genes to a new location in the genome, the
P element itself codes for transposase (an
enzyme that makes transposition possible).

See also TRANSPOSON, GENE, ENZYME,
TRANSPOSITION, TRANSPOSASE,
DEOXYRIBONUCLEIC ACID (DNA),
GENOME

P. gossypiella See *PECTINOPHORA GOS-
SYPIELLA*

P-Glycoprotein Refers to a specific glycosylated protein (e.g., in the cells of certain cancer
tumors) that sometimes acts as a "pump" to
remove specific chemicals (e.g., chemotherapy drugs) from within tumor cells.

See also PROTEIN, GLYCOSYLATION,
GLYCOPROTEIN, CELL, CANCER,
TUMOR, MULTI-DRUG RESISTANCE

P-Selectin Formerly known as GMP-140 and
PADGEM, it is a selectin molecule that is synthesized by endothelial cells before adjacent
tissues are infected. Thus "stored in advance,"
the endothelial cells can present P-selectin molecules on the internal surface of the endothelium
within minutes after an infection of adjacent
tissue begins. This presentation of P-selectin
molecules attracts leukocytes to the site of the
infection and draws them out of the bloodstream (the leukocytes "squeeze" between
adjacent endothelial cells).

See also SELECTINS, LECTINS, ELAM-1,
ADHESION MOLECULE, LEUKOCYTES,
ENDOTHELIUM

Paclitaxel An anticancer compound (pharmaceutical) that was originally isolated from the
Pacific yew tree (*Taxus brevifolia*), although
it is made synthetically today.

In 1966, Maurice Wall first identified antitumor
effects in an extract from *Taxus brevifolia*. In
1992, the U.S. Food and Drug Administration
approved paclitaxel for use in treating recurrent ovarian cancer. Other anticancer uses
were later approved.

When injected into the human body, paclitaxel
also inhibits growth of the parasitic microorganism *Toxoplasma gondii*, which can cause
loss of sight and neurological disease in
humans if not controlled.

See also CANCER, TAXOL, FOOD AND
DRUG ADMINISTRATION (FDA), CHE-
MOTHERAPY, TUBULIN, MICROOR-
GANISM, GROWTH (MICROBIAL)

PAF Acronym for **platelet activating factor**.
See CHOLINE

PAGE See POLYACRYLAMIDE GEL ELEC-
TROPHORESIS (PAGE)

Palindrome A DNA molecule sequence that is
the same when one strand of the molecule is
read left to right and the other strand is read
right to left.

See also DEOXYRIBONUCLEIC ACID
(DNA), READING FRAME

Palmitate See PALMITIC ACID

Palmitic Acid A saturated fatty acid containing 16 carbon atoms in its molecular "backbone"; it tends to increase cholesterol levels
in the bloodstream when consumed by
humans.

It has been shown that feeding of extruded
(whole) high-oleic-oil soybeans to dairy cattle
did decrease the content of palmitic acid in
their milk.

See also FATTY ACID, SATURATED FATTY
ACIDS (SAFA), CHOLESTEROL, HIGH-
OLEIC-OIL SOYBEANS

Pancreas An organ (gland) located near the
stomach that secretes insulin and glucagon
into the bloodstream and digestive fluids into
the intestines.

See also DNase, INSULIN, GLUCAGON,
BETA CELLS, TYPE I DIABETES, TYPE II
DIABETES, DIABETES

Papovavirus A class of animal viruses, e.g.,
SV40 and polyoma.

See also VIRUS

Parkinson's Disease A disease of the human
brain in which the nerve cells (neurons) associated with emotions and the neurons that are

involved in controlling movement (motor control) die.

Discovered in 1919 by doctors treating an epidemic of encephalitis lethargica (onset of Parkinson's disease commonly follows that encephalitis, but it can also be induced by certain drugs, etc.). The (natural) cause of Parkinson's disease (i.e., causing a dwindling supply of dopamine in the brain) is unknown, though it can be induced by drug misuse. When a human brain is functioning normally, cells within a region of the brain called the **substantia nigra** initiate motor (i.e., muscle) activity by releasing the chemical "messenger" known as dopamine. In the brain of a person suffering from Parkinson's disease, the dopamine-producing cells die, causing a progressive loss of motor control.

See also NEUROTRANSMITTER, CILIARY NEUROTROPHIC FACTOR (CNTF), SIGNALING, GLIAL-DERIVED NEUROTROPHIC FACTOR (GDNF), OXIDATIVE STRESS, NEURON, ALPHA-SYNUCLEIN

ParM A contractile (i.e., periodically contracting) protein that is present in at least some bacteria. Via its contractions during meiosis, ParM is involved in those cells' separation of nuclear DNA (i.e., prior to cell division).

See also PROTEIN, MOTOR PROTEINS, BACTERIA, MEIOSIS, DEOXYRIBONUCLEIC ACID (DNA)

PARP Acronym for **poly ADP-ribose polymerase** (an enzyme naturally present in human cells, which is involved in control of apoptosis, among other cellular processes). This enzyme can be commercially produced (e.g., to manufacture tests) by genetically engineered hamster cells grown in cell culture. This enzyme can be utilized to determine if a given substance (e.g., industrial chemical) is carcinogenic to humans.

See also ENZYME, ADENOSINE DIPHOSPHATE (ADP), RIBOSE, POLYMERASE, CELL, APOPTOSIS, CELL CULTURE, MAMMALIAN CELL CULTURE, CHO CELLS, CARCINOGEN, CANCER, NUCLEAR MATRIX PROTEINS, GENETIC ENGINEERING, AMES TEST, CASPASES

Particle Cannon See BIOLISTIC® GENE GUN, MICROPARTICLES

Particle Gun See BIOLISTIC® GENE GUN, MICROPARTICLES, "SHOTGUN" METHOD

Partition Coefficient A constant (number) that expresses the ratio in which a given solute will be partitioned (i.e., distributed) between two given immiscible liquids (e.g., oil and water) at equilibrium.

Partitioning Agent Any one of a number of chemical compounds (e.g., certain hormones, conjugated fatty acids, etc.) that cause a given animal's metabolism to deposit significantly more lean muscle tissue and significantly less fat tissue in the (growing) animal's body.

See also BOVINE SOMATOTROPIN (BST), PORCINE SOMATOTROPIN (PST), CONJUGATED LINOLEIC ACID (CLA), CARNITINE, METABOLISM, FATS

Passive Immunity An immune response (to a pathogen) that results from injecting *another* organism's antibodies or T lymphocytes into the organism that is being challenged by the pathogen.

See also POLYCLONAL ANTIBODIES, HUMORAL IMMUNITY, ANTIBODY, COMPLEMENT, COMPLEMENT CASCADE, IMMUNOGLOBULIN, PATHOGEN, ANTIGEN, MONOCLONAL ANTIBODIES (MAb), LYMPHOCYTE, T CELLS

PAT Gene A dominant gene **isolated from the *Streptomyces viridochromogenes* bacterium** that codes for (i.e., causes production of) the enzyme **phosphinothricin acetyl transferase (PAT)**. When the PAT gene is inserted into a plant's genome, it imparts resistance to glufosinate-ammonium-containing herbicides. Because the glufosinate-ammonium herbicides act via inhibition of glutamine synthetase (an enzyme that catalyzes the synthesis of glutamine), this inhibition of enzyme kills plants (e.g., weeds). That is because glutamine is crucial for plants to synthesize critically needed amino acids. The PAT gene is also often used by genetic engineers as a marker gene.

See also GENE, GENOME, GENETIC ENGINEERING, MARKER (GENETIC MARKER), BAR GENE, DOMINANT ALLELE, ESSENTIAL AMINO ACIDS, HERBICIDE-TOLERANT CROP, GTS, SOYBEAN

PLANT, CANOLA, CORN, GLUTAMINE, GLUTAMINE SYNTHETASE, PHOSPHINO-THRICIN, PHOSPHINOTHRICIN ACETYL-TRANSFERASE (PAT)

Patch-Clamp Recording See WHOLE-CELL PATCH-CLAMP RECORDING

Pathogen Refers to a virus, bacterium, parasitic protozoan, or other microorganism that causes infectious disease by invading the body of an organism (e.g., animal, plant, etc.) known as the host. It should be noted that infection is not synonymous with **disease,** because infection does not always lead to injury of the host.

See also VIRUS, BACTERIA, PROTOZOA, MICROORGANISM, STRESS PROTEINS, ANTIGEN, IMMUNE RESPONSE, PHY-TOALEXINS, PATHOGENESIS-RELATED PROTEINS, QUORUM SENSING

Pathogenesis-Related Proteins Protective (i.e., disease-fighting) proteins that are produced within certain plants in response to the entry into plant of plant pathogens (e.g., bacteria, fungi, etc., that infect and cause disease in plants).

One pathogenesis-related protein is chitinase, a protein enzyme that degrades (breaks down) the chitin within cell walls of pathogenic fungi. Production of pathogenesis-related proteins is often initiated by **signaling molecules** (e.g., harpin) produced **by the pathogens**.

See also PROTEIN, PATHOGEN, BACTERIA, FUNGUS, CHITINASE, CHITIN, CELL, ENZYME, SIGNALING, SIGNALING MOLECULE, HARPIN, HYPERSENSI-TIVE RESPONSE

Pathogenic Disease causing.

See also PATHOGEN

Pathway A sequential series of chemical reactions, each of which is dependent on previous ones in the pathway (e.g., the third reaction requires chemical product produced by first and second chemical reactions) that, overall, yields a beneficial impact.

For example, metabolism (i.e., the entire set of enzyme-catalyzed chemical reactions that converts food into nutrients which can be used by the body's cells, **and** the use of those nutrients by the cells to sustain life, grow, etc.) occurs via a very specific METABOLIC PATHWAY.

See also METABOLISM, ACC SYNTHASE, R GENES, PATHWAY FEEDBACK MECHANISMS, RETINOID X RECEP-TORS (RXR), MITOGEN-ACTIVATED PROTEIN KINASE CASCADE

Pathway Feedback Mechanisms Chemical mechanisms (e.g., series of chemical reactions) that hinder (or increase rate of) a given PATHWAY.

For example, when the body of bacteria need **catabolism (i.e., energy production)** to be slowed down, it uses the mechanism of **catabolite repression** (to slow down catabolism via chemical reactions).

See also PATHWAY, METABOLISM, CATAB-OLISM, CATABOLITE REPRESSION

Pattern Biomarkers Refers to the pattern (group) of genes that are **jointly** turned on/off/up/down as a result of a disease (endpoint or progression), toxicity of a compound (e.g., pharmaceutical ingested), etc.

In metabonomics, the term PATTERN BIO-MARKER refers to the resultant **several compounds** (e.g., metabolites) and not to the genes.

See also BIOMARKERS, GENE, EXPRESS, EXPRESSIVITY, GENE EXPRESSION ANALYSIS, METABONOMICS

Patulin A term that refers to a particular myc-otoxin (i.e., toxic metabolite produced by fungi) that is produced especially by the fungus *Penicillium expansum*. The fungus tends to grow (postharvest) in apples under certain conditions, causing "soft rot" or "blue mold rot."

Research indicates that patulin can cause adverse impacts on the immune system and mutations, and can have neurotoxic effects.

See also MYCOTOXINS, TOXIN, FUNGUS, *PENICILLIUM*, MUTATION, MUTAGEN

PBEF Acronym for **pre-B cell colony-enhancing factor**.

See VISFATIN, PRE-B CELL COLONY-ENHANCING FACTOR

PBR The intellectual property rights that are legally accorded to plant breeders by laws, treaties, etc. Similar to patent law for inventors.

See also PLANT BREEDER'S RIGHTS (PBR), PLANT'S NOVEL TRAIT (PNT), PLANT VARIETY PROTECTION ACT (PVP), EUROPEAN PATENT CONVEN-TION, EUROPEAN PATENT OFFICE (EPO), U.S. PATENT AND TRADEMARK OFFICE (USPTO)

pBR322 An *Escherichia coli (E. coli)* plasmid cloning vector that contains the ampicillin resistance and tetracycline resistance genes. It consists of a circle of double-stranded DNA.
See also *ESCHERICHIA COLIFORM (E. COLI)*, PLASMID, VECTOR, DEOXYRIBONUCLEIC ACID (DNA)

PC Phosphatidyl choline.
See LECITHIN (REFINED, SPECIFIC), LECITHIN (CRUDE, MIXTURE)

PCC See PROTEIN-CONDUCTING CHANNEL

PCD Acronym for **programmed cell death**.
See PROGRAMMED CELL DEATH

PCR See POLYMERASE CHAIN REACTION (PCR)

PDCAAS See PROTEIN-DIGESTIBILITY-CORRECTED AMINO ACID SCORING (PDCAAS)

PDE See PHOSPHODIESTERASES

PDGF See PLATELET-DERIVED GROWTH FACTOR (PDGF)

PDWGF See PLATELET-DERIVED WOUND GROWTH FACTOR (PDWGF)

Pectinophora gossypiella Also known as the pink bollworm, this is one of three insect species that are called "bollworms" (when they are on cotton plants). The holes that they chew in cotton plant's bolls have been shown to enable the fungus *Aspergillas flavus* to infect those plants.
See also *B.t. KURSTAKI, HELICOVERPA ZEA (H. zea), HELIOTHIS VIRESCENS*, BRIGHT GREENISH-YELLOW FLUORESCENCE (BGYF)

PEG-SOD (Polyethylene Glycol Superoxide Dismutase) A modified version of the enzyme human superoxide dismutase (hSOD) in which polyethylene glycol (a polymer made up of ethylene glycol monomers) is combined with the hSOD molecule. The PEG seems to wrap around or about the enzyme in such a way that the whole complex is able to exist in the blood for longer periods of time than the unmodified hSOD enzyme. This is because the PEG effectively camouflages the hSOD molecule and hence protects it from being inactivated by the body's own defense mechanisms in the bloodstream. This technology is important in that hSOD is used to fight certain diseases by injecting it into the body. However, the SOD must be present in the body for extended periods of time in order to effectively work, and because the injected SOD is a foreign molecule the body tries to destroy it (and hence its function) as quickly as possible.
See also HUMAN SUPEROXIDE DISMUTASE (hSOD), CATALASE, ENZYME

Pegylation See APTAMERS, PEG-SOD (POLYETHYLENE GLYCOL SUPEROXIDE DISMUTASE)

Penicillin G (Benzylpenicillin) The original penicillin (antibiotic) molecule discovered by Alexander Fleming in 1928 in a petri dish (experiment) "spoiled" by accidental introduction of a mold. Fleming named the antibiotic after the particular mold (*Penicillium notatum*) that had produced it.
During the 1940s, scientists at the U.S. Department of Agriculture in Peoria (IL) discovered how to produce commercial quantities of Penicillin G by utilizing the fungus *Penicillium chrysogenum*, which they found growing on a cantaloupe in Peoria. Penicillin kills bacteria by blocking an enzyme that is crucial to growth and repair of the bacteria's cell wall (peptidoglycan layer). But penicillin does not harm other species, so it is species specific to certain pathogenic bacteria (e.g., streptococcus, meningococcus, and the diphtheria bacillus).
See also ANTIBIOTIC, FUNGUS, BACTERIA, ENZYME, SPECIES SPECIFIC, *PENICILLIUM*, BETA-LACTAM ANTIBIOTICS, BACILLUS

Penicillinases (E.C. 3.5.2.6) Also known as β-lactamases, these are enzymes that hydrolyze (break down) the β-lactam ring (portion) of the penicillin molecule's structure. Some microorganisms (e.g., pathogenic bacteria) are able to produce these enzymes as a defense to penicillin and cephalosporin antibiotics (drugs).
See also ENZYME, HYDROLYZE, PENICILLIN G (BENZYLPENICILLIN), PATHOGENIC, BACTERIA, ANTIBIOTIC, ANTIBIOTIC RESISTANCE

Penicillium Refers to the genus of fungi (mold) that belongs to the category *Deutromycotina* and often causes food spoilage. Some of the genus have been utilized commercially to produce antibiotics.

P

See also GENUS, FUNGUS, OCHRATOXINS, ANTIBIOTIC, PENICILLIN G (BENZYL-PENICILLIN)

Pentose A simple sugar (monosaccharide molecule) whose backbone structure contains five carbon atoms. There exists many different pentoses. Some examples of pentoses are ribose, arabinose, and xylose.

See also MONOSACCHARIDES

Pepsin A crystallizable proteinase (enzyme) that in an acidic medium digests (breaks down) most proteins to polypeptides. It is secreted by glands in the mucous membrane of the stomach of higher animals. In combination with dilute hydrochloric acid, it is the chief active principal (component) of gastric juice. Also used in manufacturing peptones and in digesting gelatin for the recovery (i.e., recycling) of silver from photographic film.

See also DIGESTION (WITHIN ORGANISMS), PROTEIN, PEPTIDE, LACTOFERRIN, PEPTONE

Peptidase An enzyme that hydrolyzes (cleaves) a peptide bond.

See also PEPTIDE BOND, PEPSIN, PEPTONE, PEPTIDE MAPPING ("FINGERPRINTING")

Peptide Two or more amino acids covalently joined by peptide bonds. An oligomer component of a polypeptide. A dipeptide, for example, consists of two (di) amino acids joined together by a peptide bond or linkage. By analogy, this structure would correspond to two joined links of a chain.

See also POLYPEPTIDE (PROTEIN), OLIGOMER, AMINO ACID

Peptide Bond A covalent bond (linkage) between the α-amino group of one amino acid and the α-carboxyl group of another amino acid. This is the linkage or bond that holds the amino acids (chain links) together in a polypeptide chain. It is the all-important bond that holds the amino acid monomers together to form the polymer known as a polypeptide.

See also PEPTIDE, POLYPEPTIDE (PROTEIN), OLIGOMER, PEPTIDYL TRANSFERASE, CARBOXYL TERMINUS (OF A PROTEIN MOLECULE)

Peptide Mapping (Fingerprinting) Refers to the characteristic pattern of peptides (i.e., pieces that make up a protein molecule) resulting from partial hydrolysis (cleavage, digestion) of a protein. The pattern (fingerprint) is obtained by separating the peptides via two-dimensional chromatography, in which the peptides are first subjected to chromatography using one solution that separates many, but not all peptides. The chromatogram is then turned 90°, and is again chromatographed using a second solution, which then separates all of the peptides, thereby producing the final "fingerprint" of the protein.

See also CHROMATOGRAPHY, PEPTIDE, PROTEIN, HYDROLYSIS, MASS SPECTROMETER

Peptide Nanotube See SELF-ASSEMBLY (OF A LARGE MOLECULAR STRUCTURE)

Peptido-Mimetic See BIOMIMETIC MATERIALS, PEPTIDE

Peptidoglycan Refers to a polymer ("molecular chain") that comprises equal amounts of peptides and polysaccharide units.

See also PEPTIDE, GLYCAN, POLYMER, POLYSACCHARIDES

Peptidyl Transferase An enzyme within the ribosome that catalyzes the formation of peptide bonds (within protein molecule) as protein molecules are being synthesized (i.e., "manufactured") during the process of translation.

See also ENZYME, RIBOSOMES, PEPTIDE BOND, PROTEIN, GENE, TRANSLATION

Peptone A protein that has been partially hydrolyzed (i.e., cleaved) by the peptidase pepsin.

See also PROTEIN, HYDROLYTIC CLEAVAGE, PEPTIDASE, PEPSIN, PEPTIDE MAPPING ("FINGERPRINTING")

Perforin A 70 kDa (kilodalton) protein that is instrumental in the lysis of infected cells. A series of reactions occur on the surface of a cell, which result in the polymerization of certain monomers to form transmembrane (i.e., through the membrane) pores 100 Å (angstroms) wide, which allows ions to rush into the cell (owing to osmotic pressure) and thus burst (lyse) that cell, so the (formerly) internal pathogens can be attacked by the body's immune system. Perforin is a protein that is akin to the C9 component of the complement.

See also OSMOTIC PRESSURE, COMPLEMENT, COMPLEMENT CASCADE, kDa, CYTOTOXIC T CELLS, CECROPHINS, MAGAININS, OSMOTINS

Periodicity The number of base pairs per turn of the DNA double helix.

See also DEOXYRIBONUCLEIC ACID (DNA)

Periodontium Tissue that anchors teeth in the jaw. Regrowth of periodontal tissue can be stimulated by a combination of platelet-derived growth factor and insulin-like growth factor-1.

See also PLATELET-DERIVED GROWTH FACTOR (PDGF), INSULIN-LIKE GROWTH FACTOR-1 (IGF-1)

Peritoneal Cavity/Membrane The smooth, transparent, serous membrane that lines the cavity of the abdomen of a mammal.

Peroxidase An enzyme that catalyzes the **oxidation of a substrate with hydrogen peroxide** (as the electron acceptor, the hydrogen peroxide is **reduced**).

Peroxidase is naturally produced in soybeans by approximately half of all commercial soybean varieties. Peroxidase very effectively inhibits (stops) growth of any *Aspergillus flavus* fungi that might be present (e.g., in the soil). Peroxidase can be used to replace more toxic and environmentally problematic chemicals in certain industrial processes. Among other applications, peroxidase can replace formaldehyde use in paints, varnishes, glues, and computer chip manufacturing.

See also ENZYME, OXIDIZING AGENT (OXIDANT), OXIDATION, SUBSTRATE (CHEMICAL), OXIDATION–REDUCTION REACTION

Peroxisome See PPAR

Persistence The tendency of a compound (e.g., an insecticide) to resist degradation by biological means (e.g., metabolism by microorganisms) after it has been introduced into the environment (e.g., sprayed onto a field) or by physical means (e.g., degradation caused by exposure to sunlight, moisture, etc.).

See also METABOLISM, MICROORGANISM, BIODEGRADABLE

Personalized Medicine See PHARMACOGENOMICS

Pest-Free Area See INTRODUCTION, PEST RISK ANALYSIS (PRA)

Pest Risk Analysis (PRA) A process delineated by the IPPC (International Plant Protection Convention), consisting of:

- Analyzing risk — identification of potential pests and pathways by which a pest (e.g., weed, insect, disease, etc.) might enter a "**pest-free area**," and determination of whether a pest is a "**quarantine pest**" and evaluation of its potential "**introduction**" to that area
- Assessing pest risk — determination of whether a given pest is a "**quarantine pest**" and evaluation of the potential for that pest to be "**introduced**" into a "**pest-free area**"
- Managing pest risk — the decision-making process and measures instituted to reduce the risk of a "**quarantine pest**" being "**introduced**" into a "**pest-free area**"

See also INTERNATIONAL PLANT PROTECTION CONVENTION (IPPC), QUARANTINE PEST, INTRODUCTION, ESTABLISHMENT POTENTIAL

Peyer's Patches A specific set of lymphoid organs found in the intestinal wall of many mammals. These patches filter out antigens that enter the intestine in food or come from bacteria growing in the intestine and "present" those intact antigens to adjacent lymphoid tissues via special **M cells** of the Peyer's patches. This activates the lymphocytes in the patches, which then migrate out of the node and into the blood where they float in the tissue spaces just inside the intestinal lining. There they secrete antibodies (primarily IgA), which are then transported into the lumen (contents) of the gut and subsequently attack (bind) the antigens.

See also HUMORAL IMMUNITY, ANTIGEN, LYMPHOCYTE, ANTIBODY, IMMUNOGLOBULIN, M CELLS, EDIBLE VACCINES

Pfiesteria piscicida A single-celled microscopic algae that has a predator–prey relationship with fish in its ecosystem. During a large part of its life cycle, *Pfiesteria piscicida* exists in a nontoxic cyst form at the bottom of a river. When the cysts detect certain substances (e.g., excreta) emitted by live fish, the *Pfiesteria piscicida* transform into an amoeboid or dinoflagellate form, which secretes a water-soluble neurotoxin into the water (which incapacitates nearby fish). The *Pfiesteria piscicida* next attach themselves to those fish, excrete a lipid-soluble toxin that destroys the epidermal layer of the fish's skin, allowing the *Pfiesteria piscicida* to begin "eating" the fish's tissue. Human exposure to the neurotoxin apparently causes short-term memory loss.

See also ECOLOGY, CELL, TOXIN, LIPIDS

PGHS Abbreviation for **prostaglandin H synthase**, an enzyme that is colloquially referred to as **cyclooxygenase** or COX. PGHS exists in two different forms (isozymes) — PGHS-1 (COX-1) and PGHS-2 (COX-2).

PHA See POLYHYDROXYALKANOIC ACID (PHA)

Phage Abbreviation for **bacteriophage**, another name for a specific type of virus. A virus that attacks bacteria is known as a bacteriophage. Bacteriophages are frequently used as vectors for carrying (foreign) DNA into cells by genetic engineers.

See also BACTERIOPHAGE, VECTOR, GENETIC ENGINEERING, TRANSFECTION, DEOXYRIBONUCLEIC ACID (DNA), PHAGE DISPLAY

Phage Display A methodology in which capsid proteins (i.e., on the surface of bacteriophages) are attached to selected peptides. Because determination of each bacteriophage's DNA (gene) sequence thus determines the peptide (sequence) that is "displayed" on its surface, large "libraries" of phage-displayed peptides can be created (e.g., to be utilized by scientists in the screening of candidate compounds, etc., in the search for new pharmaceuticals). For example, the pharmaceutical ADALIMUMAB (Humira™) was developed using phage display technology.

See also PROTEIN, CAPSID, BACTERIOPHAGE, GENETIC ENGINEERING, TRANSFECTION, VECTOR, PEPTIDE, LIBRARY, ADALIMUMAB, GENE, DEOXYRIBONUCLEIC ACID (DNA)

Phagocyte A cell such as a leukocyte that engulfs and digests cells, cell debris, microorganisms, and other foreign bodies in the bloodstream and tissues (phagocytosis). The ingested material is then degraded via enzymes. A whole class of cells is known to be phagocytic.

See also MACROPHAGE, MICROPHAGE, MONOCYTES, T CELLS, POLYMORPHONUCLEAR LEUKOCYTES (PMN),

CELLULAR IMMUNE RESPONSE, POLYMORPHONUCLEAR GRANULOCYTES, LYSOSOME

Phagocytosis A process by which certain immune system cells (e.g., macrophages, polymorphonuclear leukocytes, etc.) extend toward and engulf (by surrounding and enveloping) specific cells (e.g., pathogens that are invading that organism). Subsequent to engulfing, such immune system cells later fuse with lysosomes, resulting in the digestion/destruction of the engulfed pathogen.

See also CELLULAR IMMUNE RESPONSE, PHAGOCYTE, MACROPHAGE, LYSOSOME, PATHOGEN

Pharmacoenvirogenetics A word coined in 2000 by Tim Studt to describe the fact that **environmental factors** interact with a given individual's (human/animal/plant) genetic makeup (i.e., genome) to determine the individual's (body's) response to a given pharmaceutical (and/or progression of a disease). The environmental factors the individual is exposed to include:

- Foods eaten.
- Stress.
- Air and water pollution.
- Temperature and humidity.
- Geographical elevation.
- Bacteria. For example, when *Rhizobium japonicum* bacteria grow in the soil near the roots of a soybean plant (*Glycine max* (L.)), which causes certain specific genes in the soybean plant to be expressed (i.e., "turned on") so that soybean plant's roots **become more hospitable as a "home" for the bacteria to live** in symbiotically (in nodules on the roots) with the soybean plant.

See also PHARMACOKINETICS, GENETICS, PHARMACOLOGY, PHARMACOGENETICS, ABSORPTION, METABOLISM, SNP, ALLELE, HAPLOTYPE, HAPTOGLOBIN, *RHIZOBIUM* (BACTERIA), NODULATION, SYMBIOTIC, CENTRAL DOGMA (NEW), ACCLIMATIZATION

Pharmacogenetics A branch of pharmacokinetics that deals with the reactions between drugs, or free radicals, or synthetic food ingredients, and **specific individuals** owing to the genetics of those individuals.

The subgroup of individuals whose DNA causes their bodies to respond in a specific way to a given drug or synthetic food ingredient is known as a haplotype. For example, one haplotype (subgroup) of **pediatric leukemia** patients suffers severe and life-threatening reactions to some commonly used leukemia treatment drugs because of the variation (i.e., SNP) in the **thiopurine S-methyl transferase gene** (allele) in their genome.

Another example is that consumption of the tyrosine kinase inhibitor drug **gefinitib** (Iressa) helps to control tumors of non-small-cell lung cancer in people who possess a mutation (i.e., the SNP that codes for the epidermal growth factor receptor) within their lung cancer tumors.

Also, consumption of the pharmaceuticals tolbutamide, warfarin, or phenytoin can be riskier for people who possess a mutation (i.e., an SNP that codes for less or no expression of CYP2C9) within their liver tissue. That is because the CYP269 enzyme causes rapid metabolism of tolbutamide, warfarin, phenytoin (and some other pharmaceuticals), so the "typical dose" could result in higher-than-expected bloodstream levels of these pharmaceuticals in people possessing that particular SNP.

Consumption of sodium-containing food ingredients tends to cause dangerous increase in blood pressure (hypertension) among the African-Americans, more often than among other ethnic groups living in the U.S.

See also PHARMACOKINETICS, PHARMACOGENOMICS, GENETICS, PHARMACOLOGY, ABSORPTION, METABOLISM, HAPLOTYPE, DEOXYRIBONUCLEIC ACID (DNA), GENE, MUTATION, SNP, ALLELE, CODING SEQUENCE, EXPRESS, EXPRESSIVITY, ENZYME, CYTOCHROME P450 (CYP), CANCER, HAPTOGLOBIN, TRANSVERSION, FLUORESCENCE *IN SITU* HYBRIDIZATION (FISH), TYROSINE KINASE INHIBITORS (TKI), RECEPTORS, EPIDERMAL GROWTH FACTOR RECEPTOR (EGF)

Pharmacogenomics A branch of pharmacokinetics that deals with the biological impacts of pharmaceuticals or synthetic food ingredients and the **specific differences in response/reaction** of living structures (e.g., tissues, organs, etc.) **owing to different genomes (DNA) of the individual organisms that consume those pharmaceuticals or food ingredients**. The subgroup consisting of all those individuals whose genome (DNA) causes their body to respond in a specific way to a given pharmaceutical, free radical, or synthetic food ingredient is known as a haplotype. A haplotype could (theoretically) be as small as one individual (e.g., one woman possessing a specific type of genome, because that woman's specific response to a pharmaceutical could result from one single-nucleotide polymorphism (SNP) that only her genome possesses).

Thus, pharmacogenomics is the **pharmacokinetics (of a given pharmaceutical or food ingredient) within a specific haplotype**. For example, some ethnic minorities, genders, and some individuals have very different biological reactions/responses to certain pharmaceuticals, e.g., the painkiller morphine works better in women, aspirin "thins" men's blood better than women's blood, the painkiller ibuprofen works better in men, the AstraZeneca tyrosine kinase inhibitor drug **gefinitib** (Iressa™) works to control tumors of non-small-cell lung cancer in patients whose lung cancer tumors possess the **SNP that codes for the epidermal growth factor receptor**, the blood-thinning drug warfarin can cause life-threatening internal bleeding in patients possessing certain SNPs (i.e., approximately one in every 250 people), the diuretic drug thiazide works to control hypertension in 60% of U.S. African-Americans but only 8% of U.S. Caucasion people, etc., and food ingredients (e.g., monosodium glutamate, lactase, ethanol, etc.) impact some ethnic minorities more than the majority of humans. This is due to the fact that different genes within their genomes (DNA) cause synthesis of certain different proteins (generally enzymes), thereby causing the body tissues of those individuals to react differently to specific pharmaceuticals or food ingredients in terms of the following:

P

- Absorption — transport of the drug (pharmaceutical) or food ingredient into the bloodstream (e.g., from the intestinal tract, in the case of food ingredients or orally administered drugs).
- Distribution — initial physical disposition/behavior of the substance in the body after the substance enters the body tissues. For example, does the substance preferentially concentrate in the fat cells (adipose tissue) of the body or in other specific tissues?
- Metabolism — breakdown of the substance (if breakdown does occur) into other chemical compounds and the ultimate disposition in body of those compounds (or the original substance, if breakdown does not occur).
- Elimination — the speed and thoroughness with which the substance is excreted or is otherwise removed from the body.

See also PHARMACOKINETICS, GENOMICS, PHARMACOLOGY, ADME TESTS, ABSORPTION, METABOLISM, GENOME, DEOXYRIBONUCLEIC ACID (DNA), DIGESTION (WITHIN ORGANISMS), PHASE I CLINICAL TESTING, HAPLOTYPE, CONSENSUS SEQUENCE, PHARMACOGENETICS, GENE, ALLELE, SINGLE-NUCLEOTIDE POLYMORPHISMS (SNPs), PROTEIN, ENZYME, HAPTOGLOBIN, ADIPOSE, FLUORESCENCE *IN SITU* HYBRIDIZATION (FISH), TYROSINE KINASE INHIBITORS (TKI), RECEPTORS, EPIDERMAL GROWTH FACTOR (EGF)

Pharmacokinetics (Pharmacodynamics) A branch of pharmacology dealing with the reactions between drugs or synthetic food ingredients and living structures (e.g., tissues, organs). The study of the following:

- Absorption — transport of the drug (pharmaceutical) or food ingredient into the bloodstream (e.g., from the intestinal tract in the case of food ingredients)
- Distribution — initial physical disposition/behavior of the substance in the body after the substance enters the body. For example, does the substance preferentially concentrate in the fat cells of the body?
- Metabolism — breakdown of the substance (if breakdown does occur) into other compounds and ultimate disposition of those compounds (or the original substance if breakdown does not occur). For example, some pharmaceuticals break down into smaller compounds, one of which then acts upon the relevant body cells (e.g., to relieve pain, lower blood pressure, etc.).
- Elimination — the speed and thoroughness with which the substance is excreted or otherwise removed from the body.

In short, pharmacokinetics deals with what happens to a substance that is introduced into a living system. For example, how quickly it is broken down, to what intermediates and metabolites is it broken down, and what the pathway of this breakdown is.

See also PHARMACOLOGY, ADME TESTS, ABSORPTION, METABOLISM, INTERMEDIARY METABOLISM, DIGESTION (WITHIN ORGANISMS), PHASE I CLINICAL TESTING, PHARMACOGENOMICS, PHARMACOGENETICS, PHARMACOENVIROGENETICS, PATHWAY

Pharmacology The study of chemicals (e.g., pharmaceuticals) and their effects on living organisms.

See also PHARMACOKINETICS, PHARMACOGENOMICS, PHARMACOGENETICS

Pharmacophore The portion of a molecule (e.g., a pharmaceutical) that is responsible for its biological activity (i.e., therapeutic action on recipient's tissue, etc.).

See also BIOLOGICAL ACTIVITY, ACTIVE SITE, CATALYTIC SITE, MINIPROTEINS

Pharming Refers to the production of pharmaceuticals (or intermediate chemicals utilized to manufacture pharmaceuticals) in agronomic plants (that have been genetically engineered).

See also GENETIC ENGINEERING, PLANTIBODIES™, PLANTIGENS, EDIBLE VACCINES

Phase I Clinical Testing The first in a series of human tests of new pharmaceuticals, mandated by the U.S. Food and Drug Administration (FDA). The primary purpose of the Phase I clinical test is to detect if the new pharmaceutical is toxic or otherwise harmful to normal, healthy humans. The conclusion of Phase I testing leads to Phase II and Phase III testing.

During the 1990s, the FDA began to require the inclusion of ethnic minorities and women (in addition to men) as subjects in these tests to enable pharmacogenomics (i.e., the testing to determine if a given pharmaceutical causes nontypical response in the bodies of members of these subgroups).

See also FOOD AND DRUG ADMINISTRA-TION (FDA), KEFAUVER RULE, KOSEISHO, BUNDESGESUNDHEIT-SAMT (BGA), COMMITTEE FOR PROPRI-ETARY MEDICINAL PRODUCTS (CPMP), IND, IND EXEMPTION, PHARMACOGE-NOMICS, HAPLOTYPE, PHASE II CLINI-CAL TESTS, FLUORESCENCE *IN SITU* HYBRIDIZATION (FISH)

Phase I Detoxification Enzymes See INDU-CIBLE ENZYMES

Phase II Clinical Tests The second in a series of human tests of new pharmaceuticals, mandated by the U.S. Food and Drug Administration (FDA). The primary purpose of the Phase II clinical tests is to determine the pharmaceutical's **efficacy** (i.e., does it work?). Successful conclusion of Phase II tests allows Phase III clinical tests to begin.

See also PHASE I CLINICAL TESTING, FOOD AND DRUG ADMINISTRATION (FDA), KEFAUVER RULE, KOSEISHO, BUNDESGESUNDHEITSAMT (BGA), COMMITTEE FOR PROPRIETARY MEDIC-INAL PRODUCTS (CPMP), IND, IND EXEMPTION, FLUORESCENCE *IN SITU* HYBRIDIZATION (FISH)

Phase II Detoxification Enzymes See INDUCIBLE ENZYMES

Phase III Clinical Tests The third in a series of human tests of new phamaceuticals, mandated by the U.S. Food and Drug Administration (FDA). The primary purpose of Phase III clinical tests is to verify proper dosage of a new pharmaceutical.

See also PHASE I CLINICAL TESTING, PHASE II CLINICAL TESTS, FOOD AND DRUG ADMINISTRATION (FDA), KEFAU-VER RULE, KOSEISHO, BUNDESGE-SUNDHEITSAMT (BGA), COMMITTEE FOR PROPRIETARY MEDICINAL PROD-UCTS (CPMP)

Phaseolus vulgaris Term refers to the broad "family" of edible beans that includes kidney beans, pinto beans, snap beans, etc.

See also AMYLASE INHIBITORS

PHB See POLYHYDROXYLBUTYLATE

Phenolic Hormones A category of compounds found in the human body, which are synthesized (i.e., "manufactured") by the body from certain phenolic dietary substances (phytochemicals) such as isoflavones.

Research indicates that phenolic hormones act to prevent a number of cancers such as those of the prostate, breast, large bowel, etc.

See also HORMONE, PHYTOCHEMICALS, ISOFLAVONES, CANCER, SELECTIVE ESTROGEN EFFECT

Phenomics Utilized to refer to the relationship between genomics and phenotype/traits.

See also FUNCTIONAL GENOMICS, PHE-NOTYPE, TRAIT, GENE FUNCTION ANALYSIS

Phenotype Coined in 1909 by Wilhelm Johannsen, this term refers to the outward appearance (structure) or other visible characteristics of an organism (which, of course, is determined by the DNA of its genotype). This also includes (and determines) how that organism's body responds to a given physical agent (e.g., a pharmaceutical, a toxin, sunlight, etc.). For example, genetically fair-skinned people tend to get sunburned easier and faster than other people.

See also GENOTYPE, DEOXYRIBONU-CLEIC ACID (DNA), MORPHOLOGY, GENE, HAPLOTYPE, GENE EXPRESSION PROFILING

Phenylalanine (Phe) An essential amino acid. L-Phenylalanine is one of the raw materials used to manufacture NutraSweet® (NutraSweet Co.) synthetic sweetener.

See also LEVOROTARY (L) ISOMER, ESSEN-TIAL AMINO ACIDS, STEREOISOMERS

Pheromones From the Greek words "pherein" (to carry) and "hormon" (to excite), they are

P

sex hormones emitted by insects and animals and spread through the air by the wind and diffusion for the purposes of attracting the opposite sex. Some pheromones have been produced artificially and are used in lure traps to attract and catch male insects so as to prevent their mating with females (i.e., a biological pesticide). Pheromone traps for Japanese beetles are commonplace in infested areas (e.g., when utilizing integrated pest management). It is envisioned that commercial exploitation of this area of science will increase.

See also HORMONE, INTEGRATED PEST MANAGEMENT (IPM)

Philadelphia Chromosome Refers to a particular human chromosome that is (visibly) distorted by the **mutated gene** that results in the disease known as chronic myelogenous leukemia (abbreviated **CML**, also known as chronic myeloid leukemia). This is because the gene codes for extensive production of the tyrosine kinase known as Bcr-Ab1, an enzyme that causes neoplastic (aberrant) cell growth and cell division. As a result, people with CML disease tend to have 10 to 25 times more white blood cells than normal.

The pharmaceutical known as Gleevec™ induces **apoptosis — "programmed" (self-destruct) cell death** — in the cells that have the Philadelphia chromosome, thus leading to cessation of CML.

See also CHROMOSOMES, KARYOTYPE, KARYOTYPER, GENE, CODING SEQUENCE, MUTATION, CANCER, CELL, WHITE BLOOD CELLS, GLEEVEC™, APOPTOSIS

Phosphate Transporter Genes Genes within the genomes of at least some plants that code for proteins that enable or increase the ability of those plants to extract and utilize **phosphate (form of phosphorous)** from the soil. Because all plants require phosphorous for proper growth and functioning but most plants are not inherently very adept at extracting and utilizing soil phosphate, adding (more) phosphate transporter genes to a given (crop) plant is likely to increase the plant's growth and yield (e.g., of seeds).

See also GENE, GENETIC ENGINEERING

Phosphate-Group Energy The decrease in free energy as 1 mol of a phosphorylated compound at 1.0 M concentration undergoes hydrolysis to equilibrium at pH 7.0 and 25°C (77°F); the energy that is available to do biochemical work. The energy arises from the breakage (cleavage) of a **phosphate-to-phosphate** bond.

See also FREE ENERGY, HYDROLYSIS, FATS, MOLE, PHOSPHOLIPIDS

Phosphatidyl Choline See LECITHIN

Phosphatidyl Serine A lipid that is naturally produced in soybeans, certain green leafy vegetables, and some meats. Research indicates that human consumption of large enough amounts of phosphatidyl serine can help to improve brain function.

During 2003, the U.S. Food and Drug Administration (FDA) approved a qualified (label) health claim that associates consumption of phosphatidyl serine with reduced risk of cognitive dysfunction in people and reduced risk of dementia in elderly people.

Because phosphatidyl serine in healthy living cells is only present within the "interior layer" of the cell's plasma membrane, one way that **a cell undergoing apoptosis** is marked for degradation/clean-up (i.e., done by macrophages) is the presence of phosphatidyl serine on the exterior surface of the cell's plasma membrane.

Some formerly injected pharmaceuticals (e.g., Amphotericin B) can be rendered to be orally administrable via encapsulation inside a coating of phosphatidyl serine (i.e., known as a nanocochleate).

See also LIPIDS, SOYBEAN PLANT, FOOD AND DRUG ADMINISTRATION (FDA), CELL, PLASMA MEMBRANE, APOPTOSIS, MACROPHAGE, ORALLY ADMINISTERED, NANOCOCHLEATES

Phosphatidylserine See PHOSPHATIDYL SERINE

Phosphinothricin Another name for the herbicide active ingredient **glufosinate**.

See also GLUFOSINATE, PHOSPHINOTHRICIN ACETYLTRANSFERASE (PAT), PAT GENE, BAR GENE

Phosphinothricin Acetyltransferase (PAT)
An enzyme that degrades (breaks down) phosphinothricin (also known as glufosinate), which is an active ingredient in some herbicides.

PAT is naturally produced in some strains of soil bacteria (e.g., *Streptomyces viridochromogenes*).

If a gene (called the "PAT gene") that codes for the production of phosphinothricin acetyltransferase is inserted via genetic engineering into a crop plant's genome, it would enable the plants to survive postemergence applications of phosphinothricin-containing herbicides.

See also ENZYME, PHOSPHINOTHRICIN, GLUFOSINATE, BACTERIA, GENE, PAT GENE, GENETIC ENGINEERING, GENOME, BAR GENE, MARKER (GENETIC MARKER)

Phosphinotricine See PHOSPHINOTHRICIN

Phosphodiesterases A category of enzymes that inhibit apoptosis. The abbreviation for this term (category) is **PDE**

See also ENZYME, APOPTOSIS

Phospholipids The principal class of lipids that are present in cell membranes; phospholipids are diglycerides (i.e., two fatty acids attached to a glycerol "**molecular backbone**") to which a phosphate group is also attached.

The principal sites in plants of lipid and fatty acid biosynthesis (i.e., "manufacturing") are the endoplasmic reticulum, chloroplasts, and the mitochondria.

See also LIPIDS, PLASMA MEMBRANE, CELL, FATS, FATTY ACID, PHOSPHATE-GROUP ENERGY, ENDOPLASMIC RETICULUM (ER), CHLOROPLASTS, MITOCHONDRIA, CHOLINE

Phosphorylation The introduction of a phosphate group into a molecule. Formation of a phosphate derivative of a biomolecule, usually by enzymatic transfer of a phosphate group from ATP.

See also ADENOSINE TRIPHOSPHATE (ATP), KINASES

Phosphorylation Potential Abbreviated ΔG_p, it is the actual free-energy change of ATP hydrolysis under a given set of conditions.

See also PHOSPHORYLATION, FREE ENERGY, HYDROLYSIS, ADENOSINE TRIPHOSPHATE (ATP)

Photolyases A class of enzymes that are present in plants, frogs, fish, and snakes, which harness the energy of ultraviolet and near-ultraviolet light to repair damaged DNA within cells.

See also ENZYME, DNA REPAIR

Photon A single unit of light energy.

See also PHOTOSYNTHESIS, PHOTOSYNTHETIC PHOSPHORYLATION

Photoperiod The optimum length or period of illumination required for the growth and maturation of a plant. The photoperiod is distinct from photosynthesis.

See also PHYTOCHROME, CENTRAL DOGMA (NEW)

Photophore See BIOLUMINESCENCE

Photophosphorylation See CYCLIC PHOTOPHOSPHORYLATION

Photorhabdus luminescens A soil-dwelling bacterium that produces certain toxins (effective against a variety of insect pests), antibiotics, antifungal compounds, lipases, proteases, and bioluminescent (light-producing) compounds.

Photorhabdus luminescens naturally colonizes the gut of the heterorhabditis nematode, which attacks certain insect pests (e.g., tobacco hornworm, mealworm, cockroaches, etc.). When the nematode enters the insects, the *Photorhabdus luminescens* is released inside the insect, which it subsequently kills via the toxins secreted by *Photorhabdus luminescens*.

Photorhabdus luminescens synthesizes (i.e., "manufactures") a protein that is high in methionine and lysine content and constitutes approximately 50% of the **total protein content** of *Photorhabdus luminescens*.

See also BACTERIA, ANTIBIOTIC, TOXIN, LIPASE, PROTEASE, BIOLUMINESCENCE, CORN, PROTEIN, METHIONINE, LYSINE

Photosynthesis The synthesis (production) of bioorganic compounds (molecules) using light energy as the power source. The synthesis of carbohydrates (hexose) occurs via a complicated, multistep process involving reactions that occur both in the light (light reactions) and in the dark (dark reactions). In eucaryotic cells, the photosynthetic machinery necessary to capture light energy and subsequently utilize it is contained in structures called chloroplasts, which contain the molecule that initially captures light energy, called chlorophyll. Chlorophyll appears green. Green plants synthesize carbohydrates from carbon dioxide and water, which are used as a hydrogen source. The synthesis reaction, which is light driven, liberates oxygen in the process. Other organisms use this oxygen to sustain life.

From initial carbohydrates, plants subsequently also synthesize (i.e., manufacture) other compounds (e.g., fatty acids, amino acids, etc.). Plants are not the only users of photosynthesis. Other organisms such as green sulfur bacteria and purple bacteria also carry out photosynthesis, but they use other compounds besides water as a hydrogen source.

See also CARBOHYDRATES, CHLORO-PLASTS, ORGANISM, EUCARYOTE, HEXOSE, CYCLIC PHOTOPHOSPHORY-LATION, CAROTENOIDS, GOLDEN RICE, FATTY ACIDS, AMINO ACIDS, BACTERIA

Photosynthetic Phosphorylation Also called **photophosphorylation**, it is the formation of ATP from the starting compounds ADP and inorganic phosphate (P_i). The formation is coupled to light-dependent electron flow in photosynthetic organisms.

See also PHOTON, PHOTOSYNTHESIS, ADENOSINE TRIPHOSPHATE (ATP), ADENOSINE DIPHOSPHATE (ADP), CYCLIC PHOTOPHOSPHORYLATION

Phylogenetic Profiling A research methodology that is utilized to try to predict the **function of a protein molecule** within a larger, complex organism (e.g., a human) from the function of a similar or related protein molecule in a smaller or simple organism (e.g., a "model organism") that is easier to study.

See also PROTEIN, ORGANISM, MODEL ORGANISM, ORTHOLOG

Physical Map (of genome) A diagram showing the linear order of genes or genetic markers on the genome, with units indicating the actual distance between the genes or markers.

See also GENETIC MAP, GENE, GENOME, POSITION EFFECT

Physiology The branch of biology dealing with the study of the functioning of living things. The scope of physiology includes all life: animals, plants, microorganisms, and viruses.

Phytase A digestive enzyme that is present in the digestive systems of many plant-eating animals to enable breakdown of phytate (also known as "phytic acid"). Phytase is sometimes

present within the plant material consumed by animals. For example, phytase is naturally produced in the seed coat of wheat.

See also ENZYME, DIGESTION (WITHIN ORGANISMS), PHYTATE, HIGH-PHYTASE CORN AND SOYBEANS, LOW-PHYTATE CORN, LOW-PHYTATE SOYBEANS

Phytate A chemically complex (large molecule) substance (inositol hexaphosphate) that is the dominant (i.e., 60% to 80%) chemical form of phosphorus present within cereal grains, oilseeds, and their by-products. Monogastric animals (e.g., swine, poultry) cannot digest and utilize the phosphorous within phytate, because they lack the phytase enzyme in their digestive system; so phosphorus (phytate) is excreted into the environment. When the phytase enzyme is present in the ration of a monogastric animal at a high enough level, the animal is then able to digest the phytate (thereby "releasing" most of that phosphorus for absorption by the body of the animal).

However, the cleaved-off, "free" inositol that was "liberated" from six phosphate atoms per molecule of phytate then can quickly chelate (i.e., "combine" with) other minerals in the feed ration (e.g., iron, calcium, zinc, etc.).

Thus, **low-phytate** crop varieties (i.e., containing inherently smaller amounts of inositol) are less likely to chelate important dietary minerals such as iron (which can exacerbate malnutrition in typically iron-poor diets such as those found in developing countries, where adequate iron content/iron fortification of human diets is not common).

In adult humans (e.g., those past childbearing age), the chelating ("combining-with") property of the phytate source inositol causes it to act as a beneficial antioxidant in the human body, which can help to protect against certain cancers (e.g., prostate cancer).

See also PHYTASE, LOW-PHYTATE CORN, LOW-PHYTATE SOYBEANS, ENZYME, DIGESTION (WITHIN ORGANISMS), HIGH-PHYTASE CORN AND SOYBEANS, PROSTATE, CANCER, ANTIOXIDANTS, CHELATION, IRON DEFICIENCY ANE-MIA (IDA)

Phytic Acid Also known as **phytate** or inositol hexaphosphate.

See PHYTATE

Phytoalexins From the Greek words *phyton* meaning "plant" and *alexein* meaning "to defend."

Term utilized to refer to chemical compounds (e.g., enzymes, etc.) that are produced by certain plants in response to the presence of infectious agents (e.g., fungus, bacteria) or their products.

Phytoalexins possess antimicrobial (i.e., fungus-killing, bacteria-killing) properties, so they can help plants to protect themselves against those microorganisms.

See also PHYTOTOXIN, ISOFLAVONES, ALLELOPATHY, STRESS PROTEINS, PHARMACOENVIROGENETICS, ANTIBIOTIC, PHYTOCHEMICALS, ENZYME, FUNGUS, BACTERIA, ISOFLAVONES, PATHOGENIC, MICROBE, MICROBICIDE, SALICYLIC ACID (SA), PATHOGENESIS-RELATED PROTEINS, SYSTEMIC ACQUIRED RESISTANCE (SAR)

Phytochemicals A term used to refer to certain biologically active chemical compounds that occur in fruits, vegetables, grains, herbs, flowers, bark, etc. Phytochemicals act to repel or control insects, prevent plant diseases, control fungi and adjacent weeds. Phytochemicals sometimes confer beneficial health effects on the animals (e.g., humans) that consume the plant (portions) containing those phytochemicals.

Some examples of phytochemicals are vitamin C in citrus fruits, beta-carotene in carrots and other orange vegetables, *d*-limonene in orange peels, tannins in green tea, capsaicin in chili peppers, n-3 (omega-3) fatty acids in soybean oil and fish oil, **genistein, saponins, vitamin E, and phytosterols in soybeans**, etc.

Beta-carotene has been found to aid eyesight and may help prevent lung cancer. *d*-limonene has been found to protect rats against breast cancer. Tannins appear to help prevent stomach cancer. Quercitin appears to help prevent prostate cancer. Capsaicin can reduce arthritis pain. n-3 (omega-3) fatty acids help to lower triglyceride levels in the blood. Genistein appears to block growth of breast cancer tumors, prostate cancer tumors, and to prevent the loss of bone density that leads to the disease osteoporosis. Tocotrienols act as antioxidants and also inhibit synthesis of cholesterol (in humans).

See also CANCER, DEXTROROTARY (D) ISOMER, FATTY ACID, LINOLENIC ACID, LINOLEIC ACID, GENISTEIN (Gen), BIOLOGICAL ACTIVITY, MOLECULAR PHARMING, FLAVONOIDS, RESVERATROL, NUTRACEUTICALS, CHOLESTEROL, n-3 FATTY ACIDS, PHYTOTOXIN, ALLELOPATHY, ANTIBIOTIC, PHYTOALEXINS, ANTIOXIDANTS, ABRIN, RICIN, *PFIESTERIA PISCICIDA*, PHYTOSTEROLS, LIGNANS, POLYPHENOLS, GLYCYRRHIZIC ACID, SAPONINS, FRUCTOSE OLIGOSACCHARIDES, LYCOPENE, LUTEIN, ANTHOCYANIN, SOYBEAN PLANT, SOYBEAN OIL, VITAMIN E, XANTHOPHYLLS, SITOSTEROLS, CAROTENOIDS, STEROLS, ALICIN, ELLAGIC ACID, PROANTHOCYANIDINS, CAFFEINE, QUERCITIN, ROSEMARINIC ACID, ZEAXANTHIN, CATECHINS, PHOSPHATIDYL SERINE, SULFORAPHANE

Phytochrome A protein plant pigment that serves to direct the course of plant growth and development and differentiation in a plant. The response is independent of photosynthesis, e.g., in the photoperiod (i.e., length of light period) response.

See also PHOTOPERIOD, PROTEIN, PHOTOSYNTHESIS, PLANT HORMONE

Phytoene See GOLDEN RICE, LYCOPENE, CAROTENOIDS

Phytoestrogens Compounds possessing molecular structures that are somewhat similar to that of estrogen, and that are naturally found in all plants. As a result, every vegetable, fruit, cereal, and legume contains at least one type of "phytoestrogen."

For example, flavones and flavonols are beneficial phytoestrogens (mostly red-and yellow-colored pigments) found in colored vegetables and fruits (e.g., in red grapes, yellow grapefruit, oranges, etc.).

See also PHYTOCHEMICALS, FLAVONOIDS, FLAVONOLS, LIGNANS, SELECTIVE ESTROGEN EFFECT, ISOFLAVONES, ESTROGEN

Phytohormone See PLANT HORMONE

Phytomanufacturing Refers to the production of valuable substances (e.g., polyhydroxybutylate biodegradable plastic, industrial-process enzymes, etc.) in plants (e.g., genetically engineered plants).

See also POLYHYDROXYLBUTYLATE (PHB), BIOPOLYMER, POLYHYDROXY-ALKANOIC ACID (PHA), EXTREM-OZYMES, NUTRACEUTICALS

Phytonutrients See PHYTOCHEMICALS

Phytopharmaceuticals See PHYTOCHEMICALS, NUTRACEUTICALS, PHYTO-MANUFACTURING

Phytophthora A genus of fungus-like organisms (oomycetes). The word is derived from the Greek words for **plant destroyer**.

See also FUNGUS

***Phytophthora megasperma* f. sp. Glycinea** A strain of phytophthora fungus that can infect the soybean plant (*Glycine max* (L.) *Merrill*) under certain conditions and thereby cause the plant's stem and root to degrade (so-called rot).

See also FUNGUS, PATHOGENIC, SOYBEAN PLANT, STRAIN, ISOFLAVONES

Phytophthora Root Rot A plant disease that is caused by a certain phytophthora fungus (*Phytophthora sojae*). Some soybean varieties are genetically resistant to as many as 21 races or strains of phytophthora fungi.

See also FUNGUS, RPS1c GENE, RPS1k GENE, GENOTYPE, STRAIN, PATHO-GENIC, SOYBEAN PLANT, RPS6 GENE, ISOFLAVONES

Phytophthora sojae See PHYTOPHTHORA ROOT ROT

Phytoplankton Algae that float or are freely suspended in the water.

Phytoremediation Refers to the use of specific plants to remove contaminants or pollutants from either soil (e.g., polluted fields) or water resources (e.g., polluted lakes). For example, the Brazil water hyacinth (*Eichhornia crassipes*) naturally accumulates in its tissues toxic metals such as lead, arsenic, cadmium, mercury, nickel, copper, etc., and so it has been utilized as a "biofilter" (e.g., in India).

Insertion of the *Escherichia coliform* bacteria gene known as **gsh 11** into the plant known as Indian mustard causes the plant to accumulate 40 to 90% higher amounts of cadmium (from cadmium-tainted soil) in its tissues than before, so such genetically engineered plants can be utilized to extract cadmium from polluted sites.

See also BIOREMEDIATION, BIORECOVERY, *ESCHERICHIA COLIFORM*, BACTE-RIA, GENE, GENETIC ENGINEERING, ENDOPHYTE

Phytosterols A group of phytochemicals (i.e., solid alcohols consisting of ring-structured molecules) that are present in seeds produced by certain plants (e.g., the soybean plant *Glycine max* (L.)).

Evidence shows that human consumption of certain phytosterols can help to prevent certain types of cancers (e.g., cancers of the colon, prostate, breast), and can help lower total serum cholesterol and low-density lipoproteins' (LDLP) levels, thereby reducing the risk of coronary heart disease (CHD). Evidence also indicates that the phytosterols (e.g., campesterol, stigmasterol, beta-sitosterol) interfere with absorption of dietary cholesterol by the intestines and decrease the body's recovery and reuse of cholesterol-containing bile salts, which causes more cholesterol to be excreted from the body than previously.

In 2000, the researcher Joseph Judd fed phytosterols extracted from soybeans (*Glycine max* (L.)) to human volunteers who were consuming a "low-fat" diet. Their total blood serum cholesterol and low-density lipoprotein (LDLP) levels decreased by more than 10% in a short time.

During 2003, the U.S. Food and Drug Administration (FDA) approved a (label) health claim that associates consumption of phytosterols (added into a broad range of food products) with reduced coronary heart disease (CHD) in humans.

See also PHYTOCHEMICALS, STEROLS, SITOSTANOL, SOYBEAN PLANT, LOW-DENSITY LIPOPROTEINS (LDLP), CHO-LESTEROL, CAMPESTEROL, STIGMAS-TEROL, BETA-SITOSTEROL, SITOS-TEROL, CORONARY HEART DISEASE (CHD), FOOD AND DRUG ADMINISTRA-TION (FDA)

Phytotoxin Any toxic compound produced by a plant.

See also ALLELOPATHY, ANTIBIOTIC, PHYTOCHEMICALS, PHYTOALEXINS, TOXIN, ABRIN, RICIN, *PFIESTERIA PIS-CICIDA*, SOLANINE, GLUCOSAMINES,

PSORALENE, GLUCOSINOLATES, GOS-
SYPOL, ALKALOIDS

Picogram (pg) 10^{-12} g or 3.527×10^{-14} oz
(avoirdupois).

See also MICROGRAM

Picorna A "family" of the smallest known
viruses. The viruses of this family are a cause
of the common cold and hepatitis A in
humans, one form of hoof-and-mouth disease
in animals, and at least one disease in corn
(maize).

In 1994, Dr. Asim Dasgupta discovered a cellular molecule within ordinary baker's yeast
that prevents picorna virus reproduction. This
advance could lead to the creation of a treatment, in the future, to cure one or more of the
aforementioned diseases after infection has
begun.

See also VIRUS, CLADISTICS, CLADES

Pink Bollworm See *PECTINOPHORA GOS-
SYPIELLA*

**Pink-Pigmented Facultative Methylotroph
(PPFM)** A type of bacteria that is naturally
present in virtually all plants, PPFM produces
cytokinin, which aids the cell division
(growth) process in plants. PPFM also produces a chemical substance similar to vitamin
B-12. In 1996, Joe Polacco discovered that
impregnation of aged seeds with PPFM
improved the germination (sprouting) rate of
the seeds.

See also BACTERIA, MITOSIS, CELL DIF-
FERENTIATION, VITAMIN

Pituitary Gland One of the endocrine glands,
it lies beneath the hypothalamus (at the base
of the brain). Along with the other endocrine
glands, the pituitary helps to control long-term
bodily processes. This control is accomplished via interdependent secretion of hormones along with the other glands comprising
the total endocrine system.

For example, the pituitary helps to control the
body's growth from birth until the end of
puberty, by secreting growth hormone (GH).
Secretion of GH by the pituitary is itself governed by the hormone known as growth-hormone-releasing factor (GHRF), received by
the pituitary gland from the hypothalamus.
The pituitary gland also helps to control reproduction (e.g., development and growth of ovaries, timing of ovulation, maturation of

oocytes, etc.) by secreting two gonadotropic
(reproductive) hormones named luteinizing
hormone (LH) and follicle-stimulating hormone (FSH). Secretion of LH and FSH by the
pituitary is itself governed by the hormones
gonadotropin-releasing hormone (GnRH,
received by pituitary from the hypothalamus)
and estrogen/progesterone (received by pituitary from the ovaries).

See also ENDOCRINE GLANDS, ENDO-
CRINE HORMONES, HORMONE,
ENDOCRINOLOGY, HYPOTHALAMUS,
FOLLICLE-STIMULATING HORMONE
(FSH), ESTROGEN, GROWTH-HOR-
MONE-RELEASING FACTOR (GRF or
GHRF), GROWTH HORMONE (GH)

Plant Breeder's Rights (PBR) The intellectual property rights that are legally accorded
to plant breeders by various laws, international treaties, etc. Similar to patent law for
inventors.

See also PLANT'S NOVEL TRAIT (PNT),
PLANT VARIETY PROTECTION ACT
(PVP), PLANT PROTECTION ACT, EURO-
PEAN PATENT CONVENTION, EURO-
PEAN PATENT OFFICE (EPO), U.S.
PATENT AND TRADEMARK OFFICE
(USPTO), UNION FOR PROTECTION OF
NEW VARIETIES OF PLANTS (UPOV),
COMMUNITY PLANT VARIETY OFFICE

Plant Hormone An organic compound that is
synthesized in minute quantities by certain
plants. It influences and regulates plant physiological processes. Also called a **phytochrome**. The four general types of hormones
that together influence cell division, enlargement, and differentiation are the auxins, gibberellins, kinins, and abscisic acid.

See also HORMONE, GIBBERELLINS, PHY-
TOCHROME, GPA1, ETHYLENE, LYSO-
PHOSPHATIDYLETHANOLAMINE

Plant Protection Act A law passed by Congress in 1930 that enabled intellectual property protection via patents for new plants
(developed by scientists) that are propagated
asexually (e.g., via grafting).

See also U.S. PATENT AND TRADEMARK
OFFICE (USPTO), EUROPEAN PATENT
CONVENTION, EUROPEAN PATENT
OFFICE (EPO), PLANT'S NOVEL TRAIT
(PNT), PLANT BREEDER'S RIGHTS

P

(PBR), COMMUNITY PLANT VARIETY OFFICE, PLANT VARIETY PROTECTION ACT (PVP)

Plant Sterols See PHYTOSTEROLS

Plant Variety Protection Act (PVP) A law passed by Congress in 1970 that enables intellectual property protection (analogous to copyright protection) for new seed plants and seeds in America.

See also U.S. PATENT AND TRADEMARK OFFICE (USPTO), EUROPEAN PATENT CONVENTION, EUROPEAN PATENT OFFICE (EPO), PLANT'S NOVEL TRAIT (PNT), PLANT BREEDER'S RIGHTS (PBR), PLANT PROTECTION ACT, UNION FOR PROTECTION OF NEW VARIETIES OF PLANTS (UPOV), COMMUNITY PLANT VARIETY OFFICE

Plant's Novel Trait (PNT) The new (novel) trait added to a plant (e.g., crop plant such as cotton, corn/maize, soybean, etc.). Example novel traits are **herbicide tolerance** (via inserted CP4 EPSPS gene, PAT gene, etc.), **insect resistance** (via inserted *B.t.* gene, *Photorhabdus luminescens* gene, etc.), **resistance to aluminum toxicity** (via inserted CSb gene, etc.), among others.

See also TRAIT, CORN, SOYBEAN PLANT, CP4 EPSPS, GENE, PAT GENE, *B.t.*, *BACILLUS THURINGIENSIS (B.t.)*, EVENT, CITRATE SYNTHASE (CSb) GENE, GENETIC ENGINEERING, *AGROBACTERIUM TUMEFACIENS*, *PHOTORHABDUS LUMINESCENS*

Plantibodies™ A trademark owned by EPIcyte Pharmaceutical, Inc.

It refers to antibodies (e.g., akin to mammalian ones) produced in plants that are genetically engineered to produce those (specific) antibodies. That process (i.e., genetically engineering plants to cause them to produce **plantibodies**) was invented during the 1990s by Andrew Hiatt and Mich Hein.

Although plants do not always glycosylate (i.e., attach oligosaccharide units to protein molecules such as these antibodies) in the same manner as animal cells, an **antibody against the HSV-2 pathogen expressed in genetically engineered soybean plants has proven comparable to the same antibody expressed in genetically engineered animal cells**.

See also ANTIBODY, GENETIC ENGINEERING, GLYCOSYLATION, OLIGOSACCHARIDES, EXPRESS, SOYBEAN PLANT, PATHOGEN, MOLECULAR PHARMING™, PHARMING

Plantigens Antigens (e.g., of pathogenic bacteria) produced in plants that are genetically engineered to produce those (specific) antigens. That process (i.e., genetically engineering plants to cause them to produce specific antigens) can be utilized to produce **edible vaccines** for the **pathogenic bacteria possessing these antigens**. Then, people could be "vaccinated" against disease merely by eating the genetically engineered plant (e.g., banana).

See also ANTIGEN, PATHOGENIC, BACTERIA, VACCINE, GENETIC ENGINEERING, EDIBLE VACCINES, PHARMING

Plaque Refers to deposits of (oxidized) cholesterol intermixed with smooth-muscle cells and some macrophages, lining the inside of certain blood vessels. These deposits can result in the disease **atherosclerosis**, and/or adversely increase blood platelet aggregation (e.g., clotting or thrombosis).

See also VITAMIN E, ATHEROSCLEROSIS, THROMBOSIS, ARTERIOSCLEROSIS, CHOLESTEROL, ADIPOSE, MACROPHAGE, EPITHELIUM, ENDOTHELIN, APO A-1 MILANO

Plasma A pale, amber-colored fluid constituting the fluid portion of the blood in which are suspended the cellular elements. Plasma contains 8 to 9% solids. Of these, 85% are proteins consisting of three major groups, which are fibrinogen, albumin, and globulin. The other components are the lipids, which include the neutral fats, fatty acids, lecithin, and cholesterol. Also present are sodium, chloride and bicarbonate, potassium, calcium, lycopene, and magnesium. A most essential function of plasma is the maintenance of blood pressure and the exchange (with tissues) of nutrients for waste.

See also ABSORPTION, HOMEOSTASIS, LYCOPENE

Plasma Cell An antibody-producing B lymphocyte.

See also B LYMPHOCYTES, ANTIBODY

Plasma Membrane From the Greek word *plasm*, meaning "something formed."

Also known as a **plasmalemma**, it is a thin structure that completely surrounds the cell as a sort of "skin." This membrane may be seen with the aid of an electron microscope. The entire membrane appears to be about 100 Å (0.1 mm) thick and is composed of two dark lines each about 30 Å thick which are, however, separated by a lighter area. This trilaminar "sandwich" structure is referred to as the unit membrane.

The plasma membrane is composed of lipoidal (fatlike) material in which proteins and protein complexes and whole functional systems are embedded within specific regions known as **lipid rafts** (flat "islands" within the plasma membrane) or **caveolae** (cavelike structures within the plasma membrane). For example, the folate receptor (i.e., the cellular receptor for the B vitamin folic acid) is embedded in caveolae.

In the plasma membrane are incorporated such energy-dependent transport systems as Na^+ and K^+ transporting ATPase and amino acid transport systems. Besides the cell, membranes surround systems such as the endoplasmic reticulum, vacuoles, lysosomes, Golgi bodies, mitochondria, chloroplasts, and the nucleus, to mention just a few. The plasma membrane and membranes in general function in part as a permeability barrier to the free movement of substances between the inside and exterior of the cell or organelles that they surround.

See also CELL, PROTEIN, CECROPHINS (LYTIC PROTEINS), MAGAININS, MEMBRANES (OF A CELL), GOLGI BODIES, ENDOPLASMIC RETICULUM (ER), LYSOSOMES, TRANSMEMBRANE PROTEINS, RECEPTORS, LIPIDS, LIPID BILAYER, LIPID RAFTS, CAVEOLAE, MEMBRANE TRANSPORT, ATPase, AMINO ACID, VITAMIN, INTRINSIC PROTEIN, PHOSPHATIDYL SERINE, AQUAPORINS

Plasma Protein Binding See ADME TESTS, ADME/Tox

Plasmalemma See PLASMA MEMBRANE

Plasmid An independent, stable, self-replicating piece of DNA in bacterial cells that is not a part of the normal cell genome and that never becomes integrated into the host chromosome. This is in contrast to a similar genetic element known as an episome plasmid that may exist independently of the chromosome or may become integrated into the host chromosome. Plasmids are known to confer resistance to antibiotics and may be transferred by cell-to-cell contact (by conjugation via the sex pilus) or by viral-mediated transduction. Plasmids are commonly used in recombinant DNA experiments as acceptors of foreign DNA. Known forms of plasmids include both linear and circular molecules.

See also EPISOME, VECTOR, COPY NUMBER, MULTICOPY PLASMIDS, DEOXYRIBONUCLEIC ACID (DNA), CELL, GENOME, CHROMOSOME, ANTIBIOTIC, Ti PLASMID, MreB, ParM

Plasmocyte Another name for a blast cell.
See BLAST CELL

Plastid From the Greek word *plastis,* meaning "builder."

It is an independent, stable, self-replicating organelle containing a piece of DNA, inside a plant cell's cytoplasm. Plastids, which include both chloroplasts and chromoplasts, are not a part of the reproduction cell genome (i.e., in nucleus). Because there can exist up to 10,000 plastids in a given plant cell, the insertion of a gene (e.g., via genetic engineering) into plastids can result in a higher yield (of the specific protein coded for by that gene) than is achieved via insertion of the gene into the cell's nuclear DNA.

Prior to 2000, it had proved almost impossible for scientists to genetically engineer the plastids of plants other than the tobacco plant. However, during 2000, the plastids in the tomato plant (*Lycopersicon esculentum*) were successfully genetically engineered.

See also DEOXYRIBONUCLEIC ACID (DNA), CELL, CYTOPLASM, NUCLEAR DNA, COPY NUMBER, GENOME, PROMOTER, GENE, GENETIC ENGINEERING, FATS, CHLOROPLASTS, TOMATO, PLASTIDOME

Plastidome The complete set of plastid compounds contained within a cell.
See also PLASTID, CELL

Platelet Activating Factor (PAF) See CHOLINE

Platelet-Derived Growth Factor (PDGF)
An angiogenic growth factor produced by the blood's platelet cells that attracts the growth of capillaries into the vicinity of a fresh

wound. This action releases still other growth factors and starts the process of building a fibrin network to support the subsequent (blood) clot. PDGF is a competence factor (i.e., a growth factor that is required to make a cell able or competent to react to other growth factors). PDGF is normally contained within the platelet cells, so it does not circulate in the blood in a form enabling it to be freely available to its "target cells." This "containment" of PDGF in platelets ensures site-specific delivery of the PDGF directly to a wound site, so stimulus (i.e., of capillary growth) is localized to the actual wound site. After PDGF has caused the formation of the initial clot at a wound site, PDGF attracts connective tissue cells into the vicinity of the wound (to start the tissue-repair process). PDGF also acts as a mitogen (substance causing cell to divide and thus multiply) for connective tissue cells, granulocytes, and monocytes (each of which is involved in the wound's healing process).

See also ANGIOGENIC GROWTH FACTORS, FIBRIN, FIBRONECTIN, PLATELETS, MITOGEN, GRANULOCYTES, MONOCYTES, CYCLOOXYGENASE

Platelet-Derived Wound Growth Factor (PDWGF) See PLATELET-DERIVED GROWTH FACTOR (PDGF)

Platelet-Derived Wound-Healing Factor (PDWHF) See PLATELET-DERIVED GROWTH FACTOR (PDGF)

Platelets Disk-shaped blood cells that stick to the (microscopically "jagged") edges of wounds. The aggregation of platelets at the wound site leads to blood clotting, forming a temporary wound covering. During this blood-clotting process, the platelets release platelet-derived growth factor (PDGF), which attracts fibroblasts to the wound area (for subsequent healing process).

See also FIBRIN, FIBRONECTIN, PLATELET-DERIVED GROWTH FACTOR (PDGF), FIBROBLASTS, CYCLOOXYGENASE, CHOLINE, OXIDATIVE STRESS

Plectonemic Coiling Refers to the **intertwining** (within cell) of a double helix (DNA) molecule in such a manner that correction of that intertwining requires "unwinding" of the double helix molecule (DNA).

See also DEOXYRIBONUCLEIC ACID (DNA), DOUBLE HELIX, CELL, UNWINDING PROTEIN

Pleiotropic Adjective used to describe a gene that affects more than one trait (apparently unrelated) characteristic of the phenotype (appearance of an organism). For example, biologist David Ho in 1993 discovered a single gene in the barley (*Hordeum vulgare*) plant that controls the traits of the plant's height, drought resistance, strength, and time to maturity.

See also GENE, GENETIC CODE, DEOXYRIBONUCLEIC ACID (DNA), INFORMATIONAL MOLECULES, PHENOTYPE

Pluripotent Stem Cells Refers to those stem cells from which each of the human body's 210 different types of tissues could arise.

See also STEM CELLS, STEM CELL GROWTH FACTOR (SCF), DIFFERENTIATION, HUMAN EMBRYONIC STEM CELLS, ERYTHROPOIESIS, MESENCHYMAL STEM CELL (MSC)

PMP Acronym for **plant-made pharmaceuticals**.

See PHARMING

PNT See PLANT'S NOVEL TRAIT (PNT)

Point Mutation A mutation consisting of a change of only one nucleotide in a DNA molecule. At "hot spots" (i.e., certain locations on the DNA within some organisms), numerous point mutations can occur.

In the case of single-nucleotide polymorphisms (SNPs), the **same** point mutation occurs at the same location (on the DNA within some organisms) across a population of individuals of that organism.

See also MUTATION, HEREDITY, MUTANT, MUTAGEN, DEOXYRIBONUCLEIC ACID (DNA), NUCLEOTIDE, HOT SPOTS, BASE EXCISION SEQUENCE SCANNING (BESS), ORGANISM, SITE-DIRECTED MUTAGENESIS (SDM), SINGLE-NUCLEOTIDE POLYMORPHISMS (SNPs), TRADITIONAL BREEDING METHODS

"Points to Consider" Document See POINTS TO CONSIDER IN THE MANUFACTURE AND TESTING OF MONOCLONAL ANTIBODY PRODUCTS FOR HUMAN USE

Points to Consider in the Manufacture and Testing of Monoclonal Antibody Products for Human Use The Food and Drug Administration's (FDA's) governing rules for IND (investigational new drug) submission for monoclonal antibody (MAb) based pharmaceuticals.
See also IND

Polar Group A hydrophilic ("water-loving") portion of a molecule; it may carry an electrical charge. A group that "likes" to be in the presence of water molecules or other polar compounds.
See also NONPOLAR GROUP, POLARITY (CHEMICAL), POLAR MOLECULE (DIPOLE), AMPHIPATHIC MOLECULES, AMPHOTERIC COMPOUND, LIPID BILAYER

Polar Molecule (Dipole) A molecule in which the centers of positive and negative (electrical) charge do not coincide, so that one end of the molecule carries a positive (or partial positive) charge and the other end a negative (or partial negative) charge.
See also POLARITY (CHEMICAL), POLAR GROUP, ION-EXCHANGE CHROMATOGRAPHY, NONPOLAR GROUP

Polar Mutation A mutation in one gene which, because transcription occurs only in one direction, reduces the expression of subsequent genes in the same transcription unit further down the line.
See also TRANSCRIPTION, TRANSLATION, EXPRESS, NUCLEIC ACIDS

Polarimeter An instrument used for measuring the degree of rotation of plane-polarized light by an optically active compound or solution.
See also STEREOISOMERS, OPTICAL ACTIVITY, LEVOROTARY (L) ISOMER, DEXTROROTARY (D) ISOMER

Polarity (chemical) The degree to which an atom or molecule bears an electrical charge or a partial electrical charge. In general, the more polar (i.e., separation or partial separation of charge) a molecule is, the more hydrophilic ("water loving") it is. Polarity results from an uneven distribution of electrons between the atoms comprising a molecule.
See also POLAR GROUP, HYDROPHILIC, POLAR MOLECULE (DIPOLE)

Polarity (genetic) Having to do with the one-way nature, or unidirectionality, of gene transcription in an operon unit. That is, the region near the operator is always transcribed before the more distant regions. By analogy, transcription begins at the left end of an operon unit and proceeds (reads, transcribes) toward the right end of the operon unit. The distinction between the 5' and the 3' ends of nucleic acids.
See also POLAR MUTATION, TRANSCRIPTION

Polyacrylamide Gel A "sieving" gel used in electrophoresis.
See also POLYACRYLAMIDE GEL ELECTROPHORESIS (PAGE)

Polyacrylamide Gel Electrophoresis (PAGE) A form of chromatography in which molecules are separated on the basis of size and charge. The stationary phase (the polyacrylamide gel) is a polymerized version of acrylamide monomers. The gel looks and feels like Jello™. On a molecular basis, it consists of an intertwined and cross-linked mesh of polyacrylamide strings. As can be imagined, there are tiny "holes" in the gel (as in a plastic mesh bag) and with enough cross-linking, the size of the holes begins to approach the size of the molecules that are to be separated. Because some molecules will be larger than others, some of them will be able to pass through the gel matrix more easily. This is part of the basis for separation. It should be noted at this point that if the gel is cross-linked enough and the holes in that gel are smaller than the molecules to be separated, then the molecules will not be able to penetrate into the gel and no separation can occur. The charge on the molecule also plays a role in the separation. Functionally, the gel serves to hold and separate the molecules. Although details are not presented here, after the gel has been prepared (poured and cross-linked), a small amount of the solution containing the molecules to be separated is placed into wells (grooves to hold the liquid) on the gel and the system is subjected to an electric current. Over the course of minutes to hours, molecules bearing different charge/mass separate.
See also BIOLUMINESCENCE, CHROMATOGRAPHY, TWO-DIMENSIONAL (2-D) GEL ELECTROPHORESIS, FIELD INVERSION GEL ELECTROPHORESIS (FIGE), ELECTROPHORESIS

Polyadenylation The addition of a sequence of polyadenylic acid to the 3′ end of a eucaryotic mRNA after its transcription (posttranscriptional).

See also MESSENGER RNA (mRNA), TRANSCRIPTION

Polycation Conjugate Refers to a synthetic macromolecule that possesses several positive charges (cations), which is attached (conjugated) to a specific protein that binds to a cell receptor (it thereby gets "admitted" into the cell's interior). Some polycation conjugates can be utilized (e.g., in gene therapy) to deliver genes into cells.

See also CATION, POLYMER, VECTOR, CONJUGATE, PROTEIN, MACROMOLECULES, CELL, RECEPTORS, GENE, GENE THERAPY

Polycistronic Coding regions representing more than one gene in mRNA (i.e., they code for two or more polypeptide chains). Many mRNA molecules in procaryotes are polycistronic.

See also RIBOSOMES, PROCARYOTES

Polyclonal Antibodies (used in humans) A mixture of antibody molecules that are specific for given antigens, which have been purified from an immunized (to that given antigen) animal's blood. Such antibodies are polyclonal in that they are the products of many different populations of antibody-producing cells (within the animal's body). Hence, they differ somewhat in their precise specificity and affinity for the antigen.

Decades ago, antibodies (then called antitoxin) that were purified from an immunized animal's blood (e.g., a horse) were injected into humans suffering from certain diseases (e.g., diphtheria). In these cases, the pathogen had caused disease by secreting large amounts of toxin into the victim's bloodstream. The antitoxin combined quantitatively (e.g., 1:1, 2:1, 1:2, 1:3, 3:1, etc.) with the toxin and neutralized it (for those few diseases for which it was applicable). Vaccines are now generally used instead, because of the adverse immune response caused by the horse's blood (antigens).

During 2003, polyclonal antibodies from (immunized) goat blood serum were utilized by Angus Dalgleish to treat some multiple sclerosis patients, with good results reported.

See also ANTIBODY, PASSIVE IMMUNITY, MONOCLONAL ANTIBODIES (MAb), ANTIGEN, PATHOGEN, TOXIN, MULTIPLE SCLEROSIS

Polyclonal Response (of immune system to a given pathogen) Because a given pathogen generally has several antigenic sites on its surface, the B lymphocytes (activated by helper T cells in response to a pathogen invading the body) synthesize several (subtly different) antibodies against that pathogen. And because the antibodies are made by different cells, the response is known as polyclonal.

See also PATHOGEN, ANTIGEN, ANTIBODY, HAPTEN, EPITOPE, HELPER T CELLS (T4 CELLS), LYMPHOCYTE, B LYMPHOCYTES, LYMPHOKINES

Polyethylene Glycol Superoxide Dismutase (PEG-SOD) See PEG-SOD (POLYETHYLENE GLYCOL SUPEROXIDE DISMUTASE), HUMAN SUPEROXIDE DISMUTASE (hSOD)

Polygalacturonase (PG) An enzyme (e.g., present in tomatoes) that starts the breakdown (softening) of the fruit tissue. Recent advances make it possible to significantly delay the softening (i.e., spoilage) process by reducing the production of polygalacturonase through genetic engineering of the plant. In 1986, William Hiatt of the American company Calgene discovered the gene for polygalacturonase, which led to that company commercializing a tomato variety that had been genetically engineered to reduce production of polygalacturonase in that particular variety of tomato (in 1994).

See also EPSP SYNTHASE, GENETIC ENGINEERING, ANTISENSE (DNA SEQUENCE), ENZYME, GENE, ACC SYNTHASE

Polygenic A trait or end product (e.g., in a grain-produced crop) that requires simultaneous expression of more than one gene. For example, the level of protein produced in soybeans is controlled by five genes.

See also POLYHYDROXYLBUTYLATE (PHB), PROTEIN, SOYBEAN PLANT, GENE, TRAIT, SOYBEAN OIL, BCE4, *ARABIDOPSIS THALIANA*, PLASTID

Polyhydroxyalkanoates See POLYHYDROXYALKANOIC ACID (PHA)

Polyhydroxyalkanoic Acid (PHA) A "family" of chemically related "energy storage"

substances (i.e., polyesters) that are naturally produced by certain bacteria (90 strains are known). When PHA is removed from the bacteria and purified, this substance has physical properties quite similar to thermoplastics such as polystyrene. PHA can quickly be broken down by soil microorganisms, so PHA is a biodegradable plastic.

During the 1990s, Daniel Solaiman and coworkers at the U.S. Department of Agriculture developed some bacteria strains (e.g., *Bacillus thermoleovorans*) that can produce PHA utilizing vegetable oils (e.g., soybean oil) as a major part of their "diet" (energy source). The precise chemical composition (and physical characteristics) of the PHA thereby produced varies according to the particular vegetable oil that is used as the **energy source** for those bacteria. For example, PHA thus produced utilizing soybean oil is very amorphous (formable).

In 1994, researchers transferred genes for the production of one PHA into the weed plant *Arabidopsis thaliana* and the crop plant rapeseed (canola). In 1997, researchers transferred **phaB** and **phaC** genes into the crop plant cotton (*Gossypium hirsutum*), which caused the transformed plants to express (i.e., produce) PHA inside the fibers (seed hair cells) in amount of 0.34% of the fiber weight. The PHA resulted in a fabric (i.e., cotton-PHA "blend") possessing better insulation properties than traditional cotton fabric.

See also POLYHYDROXYLBUTYLATE (PHB), STARCH, BACTERIA, BIOPOLYMER, *ARABIDOPSIS THALIANA*, CANOLA, GENE, TRANSFORMATION, EXPRESS, BIODEGRADABLE, MICROORGANISM, SOYBEAN OIL

Polyhydroxylbutylate (PHB) One of the PHAs, polyhydroxybutylate is an "energy storage" substance that is naturally produced by certain bacteria, yeasts, and plants. When removed from the bacteria and purified, this substance has physical properties quite similar to thermoplastics such as polystyrene. PHB can quickly be broken down by soil microorganisms, so PHB is a biodegradable plastic. Three separate enzymes are utilized by the organism in order to make the PHB molecule. In 1994, researchers succeeded in transferring

genes for PHB production into the weed plant *Arabidopsis thaliana* and the crop plant rapeseed (canola).

Later (in 1997), researchers transferred **phaB** and **phaC** genes into the crop plant cotton (*Gossypium hirsutum*), which caused those transformed plants to express (produce) PHA inside the fibers (seed hair cells) in amount of 0.34% of the fiber weight. The PHA resulted in a fabric (i.e., cotton-PHA "blend") possessing better insulation properties than traditional cotton fabric.

See also STARCH, BACTERIA, BIOPOLYMER, ENZYME, POLYGENIC, MICROORGANISM, POLYHYDROXYALKANOIC ACID (PHA), CANOLA, *ARABIDOPSIS THALIANA*, GENE, EXPRESS, BIODEGRADABLE

Polymer A molecule possessing a regular, repeating, covalently bonded arrangement of smaller units called monomers. By analogy, a chain (polymer) that is composed of links (monomer) hooked together.

See also OLIGOMER, PROTEIN, NUCLEIC ACIDS

Polymerase Refers to an enzyme that catalyzes the assembly of nucleotides into RNA (RNA polymerase) and of deoxynucleotides into DNA (DNA polymerase).

See also DNA POLYMERASE, RNA POLYMERASE, REVERSE TRANSCRIPTASES, DNA, RNA, *TAQ*

Polymerase Chain Reaction (PCR) A reaction that uses the enzyme DNA polymerase to catalyze the formation of more DNA strands from an original one by the execution of repeated cycles of DNA synthesis. Functionally, this is accomplished by heating and melting double-stranded (hydrogen-bonded) DNA into single-stranded (non-hydrogen-bonded) DNA and producing an oligonucleotide primer complementary to each DNA strand. The primers bind to the DNA and mark it in such a way that the addition of DNA polymerase and deoxynucleoside triphosphates cause a new strand of DNA to form that is complementary to the target section of DNA. The process described previously is repeated (trait, product, etc.) again and again to produce millions of **copies (amplicons)** of the desired strand of DNA. PCR and its registered

P

trademarks are the property of F. Hoffmann-La Roche, Basel, Switzerland.

See also POLYMERASE CHAIN REACTION (PCR) TECHNIQUE, NESTED PCR, DEOXYRIBONUCLEIC ACID (DNA), DNA PROBE, PROBE, Q-BETA REPLICASE TECHNIQUE, COCLONING (OF MOLECULES), POSITIVE AND NEGATIVE SELECTION (PNS), AMPLICON, NESTED PCR, PRIMER (DNA), CAPILLARY ELECTROPHORESIS

Polymerase Chain Reaction (PCR) Technique Developed in 1984 and 1985 by Kary B. Mullis, Randall K. Saiki, Stephen J. Scharf, Fred A. Faloona, Glenn Horn, Henry A. Erlich, and Norman Arnheim, the PCR technique is an *in vitro* method that greatly amplifies (makes millions of copies of) DNA sequences that otherwise could not be detected or studied. It can be utilized to amplify a given DNA sequence that constitutes less than one part per million of initial sample (e.g., a 100-bp target DNA sequence within the genome of one of the higher organisms, which can contain up to 500 million bp). The procedure alleviates the necessity of *in vivo* replication of a target DNA sequence, or of replication of one-of-a-kind tiny DNA samples (e.g., from a crime scene).

See also *IN VITRO*, *IN VIVO*, POLYMERASE CHAIN REACTION (PCR), AMPLICON, NESTED PCR, DEOXYRIBONUCLEIC ACID (DNA), BASE PAIR (bp), GENOME, SEQUENCE (OF A DNA MOLECULE), *TAQ*, DNA POLYMERASE, PRIMER (DNA)

Polymorphism (chemical) The property of a chemical substance crystallizing (or simply existing) in two or more forms having different structures. For example, diamond and graphite are two different structures (manifestations) of the element carbon. Deoxyribonucleic acid (DNA) is a polymorphic compound because the polymer can take on different forms.

See also A-DNA, B-DNA, Z-DNA, DEOXYRIBONUCLEIC ACID (DNA), DNA PROFILING, POLYMORPHISM (GENETIC)

Polymorphism (genetic) A name applied to a condition in which a species of plant or animal is represented by several distinct, nonintegrating forms or types unrelated to age or sex. The

differences are often in coloration, though any characteristic of the organism may be involved (e.g., nuclei shape for polymorphonuclear leukocytes).

See also POLYMORPHONUCLEAR LEUKOCYTES (PMN), POLYMORPHONUCLEAR GRANULOCYTES, SINGLE-NUCLEOTIDE POLYMORPHISMS (SNPs), POLYMORPHISM (CHEMICAL)

Polymorphonuclear Granulocytes Neutrophils, eosinophils, and basophils are collectively known as polymorphonuclear granulocytes. This is due to the fact that collectively their nuclei are segmented into lobes and they have granule-like inclusions within their cytoplasm.

See also GRANULOCYTES, BASOPHILS, EOSINOPHILS, NEUTROPHILS, CYTOPLASM

Polymorphonuclear Leukocytes (PMN) Formerly named **microphages**, they are phagocytic (i.e., foreign-particle-ingesting) white blood cells that have a lobed nucleus. For example, during an attack of the common cold (when virus first invades mucous membranes of the human nose), the body responds by making interleukin-8 (IL-8) — a glycoprotein that attracts large quantities of polymorphonuclear leukocytes to the mucous membranes of the nose (to try to combat the infection).

Another example is when polymorphonuclear leukocytes (PMN) migrate into a female pig's uterus within 6 h after semen is introduced via breeding. PMN remove excess sperm and bacteria, resulting in a "**friendly**" **environment** for embryos to develop in the uterus.

See also CELLULAR IMMUNE RESPONSE, LEUKOTRIENES, LEUKOCYTES, PHAGOCYTOSIS, POLYMORPHISM (GENETIC), VIRUS, BACTERIA, GLYCOPROTEIN, INTERLEUKIN-8 (IL-8), CELL, NUCLEUS, PLASMA MEMBRANE

Polypeptide (protein) A molecular chain of amino acids linked by peptide bonds. Synonymous with protein. Via the synthesis (of this "chain") performed by ribosomes, each polypeptide (protein) in nature is the ultimate expression product of a gene. All of the amino acids commonly found in proteins have an asymmetric carbon atom, except the amino acid glycine. Thus, the polypeptide is potentially chiral in nature.

See also PROTEIN, AMINO ACID, GENE, PEPTIDE, STEREOISOMERS, CHIRAL COMPOUND, EXPRESS, RIBOSOMES, POLYRIBOSOME (POLYSOME), MESSENGER RNA (mRNA)

Polyribosome (polysome) A complex of a messenger RNA (mRNA) molecule on which ribosomes (ribosomal RNA; rRNA) are anchored. A number of ribosomes bound to only a single mRNA molecule. One mRNA molecule hence functions as a template for a number of polypeptide chains at a time.

See also RIBOSOMES, rRNA (RIBOSOMAL RNA), MESSENGER RNA (mRNA)

Polysaccharides Linear and/or branched (structure) macromolecules (i.e., large molecules) composed of many monosaccharide units (monomers such as glucose) linked by glycosidic bonds.

See also GLYCOSIDE, MONOSACCHARIDES, AMYLOSE, AMYLOPECTIN

Polysome See POLYRIBOSOME

Polyunsaturated Fatty Acids (PUFA) Unsaturated fatty acids, possessing more than one molecular double bond in their molecular "backbone" (i.e., they contain **at least two less than the maximum possible number of hydrogen atoms**).

Enzymes (e.g., Δ 12 desaturase) present in some oilseed plants (e.g., soybean, canola, corn/maize, etc.) convert some monounsaturated fatty acids (e.g., oleic acid) to some polyunsaturated fatty acids (e.g., linoleic acid) within their developing seeds. For example, soybean oil contains (historical average) 60% polyunsaturated fatty acids.

Extensive research shows that polyunsaturated fatty acids (PUFA) impart a variety of health benefits to humans who consume them. In general, these health benefits include anti-inflammatory and anti-hypertensive (i.e., prevention of high blood pressure) effects, reduction in cancer risk, reduction in the blood cholesterol levels, reduction in the risk of coronary heart disease (CHD), and aiding in the development of retina and brain tissues.

For example, the **n-3** ("omega-3") PUFAs possess antithrombotic effects and also reduce blood concentrations of triglycerides. High dietary levels (in human diet) of the **n-6** ("omega-6") PUFAs have been related to a decreased risk of coronary heart disease (CHD).

Research indicates that some of the beneficial effects of PUFAs occur via PUFA interactions with several types of nuclear receptors (present in cells of some human tissues), which results in **(PUFA-) modulation** of certain genes' expression in those cells.

See also UNSATURATED FATTY ACID, ESSENTIAL FATTY ACIDS, THROMBOSIS, TRIGLYCERIDES, CORONARY HEART DISEASE (CHD), CANCER, n-3 FATTY ACIDS, SOYBEAN OIL, n-6 FATTY ACIDS, ENZYME, DOCOSAHEXANOIC ACID (DHA), HIGHLY UNSATURATED FATTY ACIDS (HUFA), EICOSAPENTANOIC ACID (EPA), CONJUGATED LINOLEIC ACID (CLA), CELL, GENE, RECEPTORS, NUCLEAR RECEPTORS, DEOXYRIBONUCLEIC ACID (DNA), EXPRESS, GENE EXPRESSION, TRANSCRIPTION FACTORS, SOYBEAN PLANT, OLEIC ACID, LINOLEIC ACID, LINOLENIC ACID

Porcine Somatotropin (PST) A hormone produced in the pituitary gland of pigs that increases a swine's muscle tissue production efficiency. Injecting this hormone causes a faster-growing, leaner pig.

Porin A transmembrane (i.e., through the cell's membrane) protein that forms pores through the membrane. Porins are present in the outer membranes of bacteria and mitochondria.

See also PROTEIN, CELL, MEMBRANES (OF A CELL), PLASMA MEMBRANE, TRANSMEMBRANE PROTEINS, BACTERIA, MITOCHONDRIA

Porphyrins Complex nitrogenous compounds containing four substituted pyrroles covalently joined into a ring structure. When complexed with a central metal atom, it is called a metalloporphyrin.

Position Effect A change in the expression of a gene that is brought about by its translocation to a new site in the genome. For example, a previously active gene may become inactive if placed on a new site in the genome.

See also GENOME, TRANSLATION, GENETIC MAP, MAP DISTANCE, PROMOTER

Positional Cloning A technique used by researchers to zero in on the genes responsible for a given trait or disease. A genetic map of the organism's genome is used to make an educated guess as to the precise location of the gene of interest (e.g., near a particular marker, etc.). Then those guessed genes are cloned, inserted into living organisms or cells, and tested to see if the guessed gene causes expression of the protein of interest (e.g., a protein that causes the disease that the researcher is attempting to cure).

See also CLONE (A MOLECULE), GENE, GENE AMPLIFICATION, GENE DELIVERY, DNA PROBE, GENE MACHINE, GENETIC ENGINEERING, GENETIC MAP, GENETIC MARKER, GENOME, MAP DISTANCE, FUNCTIONAL GENOMICS, POSITION EFFECT, EXPRESS

Positive and Negative Selection (PNS) A separation technique; a technique to speed up the task of selecting, from thousands of laboratory specimens, the few cells with precisely the desired genetic changes induced (via genetic engineering). The thousands of genetically altered cells are brought about (produced) by genetic engineering experiments. Many genetic alterations are accomplished by injecting or flooding (specimen) cells with fragments of new genetic material (genes). A few cells are produced that have precisely the desired genetic changes among a large number of cells that do not have the desired changes. This is like a "needle in a haystack." By analogy, the few cells possessing the desired trait represent the needles, whereas the multitude of cells not possessing the trait represent the hay. In order to isolate the few desired cells, the needles must be separated from the hay. PNS gets rid of the nondesired cells and leaves only the cells possessing the desired genetic change. This is accomplished in the following way. The pieces of newly injected genetic material are composed not only of the desired sequence of DNA, but also another piece of DNA (known as a marker) that renders only those cells possessing the desired (genetic) change resistant to certain antibiotic drugs (such as neomycin) and certain antiviral drugs (e.g., Ganciclovir™). When all of the engineered cells are exposed to the drug (which normally kills all of the cells), only those cells possessing the desired genetic change (and the concomitant piece of DNA providing drug resistance) survive, and hence are "selected." The other cells not having the drug resistance are selected against, and die.

See also GENETIC ENGINEERING, GENE, MARKER (GENETIC MARKER), Q-BETA REPLICASE TECHNIQUE, POLYMERASE CHAIN REACTION (PCR) TECHNIQUE

Positive Control Refers to activation (start or increase) of the transcription of a gene owing to the binding (e.g., of a transcription factor, etc.) to a regulatory element.

See also GENE, TRANSCRIPTION, TRANSCRIPTION ACTIVATORS, TRANSCRIPTIONAL ACTIVATOR, REGULATORY ELEMENT, RIBOSWITCHES, METHYLATED

Positive Supercoiling Occurs in double-stranded cyclic DNA molecules having no breaks at all in either strand. If the double helix (of DNA) is wound further in the same direction as the winding of the two strands of the double helix molecule, then the circular duplex itself takes on superhelical turns.

By analogy, supercoiling or superhelicity may be described as follows. A piece of rope can be composed of two or three smaller strands of rope wound around each other to yield the finished rope. This is equivalent to the normal double-stranded DNA. If the ends of the rope are then joined or tied together and the resultant circle of rope is again wound in the same direction as the winding that produced the rope in the first place, supercoils will be formed, and the rope will become a much thicker (supercoiled) but shorter piece.

See also DEOXYRIBONUCLEIC ACID (DNA), DOUBLE HELIX, DNA GYRASE

Postentry Measures Refers to a country's mandatory restrictions on the transport and use of imported agricultural commodities (e.g., to prevent accidental introduction of weed seeds within commodity shipments into that country). Examples of postentry measures include **mandatory covering with tarps** of trucks or railcars transporting the commodity from the port to the processing plant (e.g., flour mill), mandatory frequent mowing of ditches along the roadways between port and processing plant to prevent any (spilled) seeds from growing tall enough to reproduce, etc.

See also INTERNATIONAL PLANT PROTECTION CONVENTION (IPPC), INTRODUCTION, PEST RISK ANALYSIS (PRA), QUARANTINE PEST, TREATMENT SYSTEM

Posttranscriptional Gene Silencing (PTGS)
Refers to an automatic natural response (e.g., in certain plants) to the high buildup (i.e., within such plant cells) of identical mRNA molecules. Because such a high buildup typically occurs as a result of viral infection (of plant), the plant's natural defense system systematically breaks down those mRNA molecules (to fight the viral infection).

This (i.e., triggering the plant to "attack" an unwanted mRNA) can be employed by genetic engineers to "silence" a given gene (i.e., by destruction of **that gene**'s mRNA) via the (cosuppression of) plant's natural PTGS response.

See also GENE TRANSCRIPTION, MESSENGER RNA (mRNA), GENE SILENCING, KNOCKOUT, GENETIC ENGINEERING, VIRUS, COSUPPRESSION, RNA INTERFERENCE (RNAi)

Posttranscriptional Processing (Modification) of RNAs The enzyme-catalyzed processing or structural modifications that RNAs such as mRNAs, rRNAs, and tRNAs must undergo before they are functionally finished products. For example, in eucaryotes, a block of poly A containing at least 200 AMP residues is enzymatically attached to the 3′ end of mRNA in the nucleus of the cell. The mRNAs with the "tail" are then transferred to the cytoplasm and the tail enzymatically removed to form the functional mRNAs. It is believed that the poly A tail aids in the transfer of the complex and targets the complex to the cytoplasm.

See also POSTTRANSLATIONAL MODIFICATION OF PROTEIN, mRNA, rRNA, tRNA

Posttranslational Modification of Protein
Enzymatic processing of a polypeptide chain (i.e., protein) after its translation from its mRNA transcript:

- Glycosylation — addition of carbohydrate moieties to the protein molecule. For example, glycosylation of asparagine, serine, or threonine portions of certain protein molecules is critical for enabling those molecules to function properly, i.e., the cell they are in must be discerned by the body's immune system to be indigenous or foreign.

- Phosphorylation — addition of a phosphate molecular group to the protein molecule. For example, phosphorylation of serine, threonine, or tyrosine portions of a protein molecule is critical for enabling that molecule to be able to function in signaling (e.g., thereby triggering cell growth, cell death, etc.).

- Sulfation — addition of a sulfate molecular group to the protein.

- Acetylation — addition of an acetyl molecular group to the protein.

- Ribosylation — addition of a ribose molecular group to the protein.

- Deamidation — the loss of their side-chain molecular groups by some of the glutamine and asparagine portions of a given protein molecule. For example, such deamidation of some asparagine portions of certain apoptosis-blocking proteins causes loss of that molecule's apoptosis-blocking ability.

- Cleavage — the removal of a portion of the polypeptide chain in order to produce a functional protein in the correct environment.

See also POLYPEPTIDE (PROTEIN), MOIETY, CELL, MESSENGER RNA (mRNA), ENZYME, RIBOSOMES, CARBOHYDRATES, PROTEIN, GLYCOSYLATION, GLYCOPROTEIN, AUTOIMMUNE DISEASE, PHOSPHORYLATION, SIGNALING, APOPTOSIS, RIBOSE, INTEIN, HISTONES

Potato Late Blight A fungal disease of the potato plant (*Solanum tuberosum*) that is caused by the fungus *Phytophthora infestans*. During the 1840s, this plant disease struck the potato crops of Ireland and Europe, leading to the starvation of more than one million people (principally in Ireland, because it was very dependent on potatoes for food).

See also FUNGUS

PPA See PLANT PROTECTION ACT

PPAR Acronym for **peroxisome proliferators activated receptor**. They constitute a "family" of nuclear receptors (i.e., receptor molecules located on cell nucleus) that influence a cell's metabolism of lipids and glucose. PPARs are grouped into two "subfamilies," *PPAR alpha* and *PPAR gamma*. PPAR agonist pharmaceuticals such as GlaxoSmithKline's Avandia™ (resiglitazone) and Takeda Pharmaceuticals' Actos™ (pioglitazone) can help control hyperglycemia and dyslipidemia associated with type II diabetes.

See also CELL, NUCLEUS, RECEPTORS, GENE, EXPRESS, PEROXISOME, METABOLISM, LIPIDS, GLUCOSE (GLc), POLYUNSATURATED FATTY ACIDS (PUFA), AGONISTS, TYPE II DIABETES

PPAR alpha See PPAR

PPAR gamma See PPAR

PPB See ADME TESTS, ADME/Tox

PPFM See PINK-PIGMENTED FACULTATIVE METHYLOTROPH

PPO Acronym for **protoporphyrinogen oxidase**.

See ACURON™ GENE

PR Proteins See PATHOGENESIS-RELATED PROTEINS

Pre-B Cell Colony-Enhancing Factor Abbreviated **PBEF**, it is a hormone (also known as visfatin) that was discovered to act as a growth factor for immature B cells of the immune system in 1994 by B. Samal and colleagues.

See also HORMONE, VISFATIN, B CELLS, GROWTH FACTOR

Prebiotics Chemical compounds or microorganisms (e.g., yeasts), administered alone or in combination (e.g., in the feed rations of animals), generally act to stimulate growth of beneficial types of bacteria in the digestive system of animals (e.g., livestock). These compounds can include some organic acids (e.g., propionic acid, malic acid, etc.).

For example, adding certain strains of yeast (culture) and malate (malic acid) to cattle feed rations has been shown to stimulate *Selenomonas ruminantium* bacteria (growth) in the rumen (i.e., the "first stomach" in cattle). *Selenomonas ruminantium* tend to constitute 22 to 51% of the total bacteria in a typical rumen and are important for optimal digestion (e.g., of the grass eaten by that animal).

Inulin and several fructose oligosaccharides, etc., act as prebiotics in the human digestive system (e.g., by stimulating growth of *Bifidus* species of bacteria in the digestive system).

For animal feed rations, in addition to **fructose** oligosaccharides, transgalacto-oligosaccharides may be added to also act as prebiotics.

See also PROBIOTICS, YEAST, BACTERIA, *BIFIDUS*, INULIN, FRUCTOSE OLIGOSACCHARIDES, TRANSGALACTO-OLIGOSACCHARIDES, STRAIN

Pribnow Box The consensus sequence T-A-T-A-A-T-G centered about ten base pairs before the starting point of bacterial genes. It is a part of the promoter and is especially important in binding RNA polymerase.

See also RNA POLYMERASE, TATA HOMOLOGY, HOMEOBOX, PROMOTER, BASE PAIR (bp)

Primary Structure Refers to the sequence of amino acids in a protein "**molecular**" **chain** or to the linear sequence of nucleotides in a polynucleotide (RNA or DNA) **molecular chain**.

See also POLYPEPTIDE (PROTEIN), AMINO ACID, PROTEIN, STRUCTURAL BIOLOGY, STRUCTURAL GENE, STRUCTURAL GENOMICS, NUCLEOTIDE, PROTEOMICS, DEOXYRIBONUCLEIC ACID (DNA), RIBONUCLEIC ACID (RNA)

Primer (DNA) A short sequence deoxyribonucleic acid (DNA) that is paired with one strand of the template DNA in the polymerase chain reaction (PCR) technique. In PCR testing (e.g., a paternity test), the primer is selected to be complementary to the analytically-relevant sequence of DNA. It is the growing end of the DNA chain and it simply provides a free 3'-OH end at which the enzyme DNA polymerase adds on deoxyribonucleotide units (monomers). Which deoxyribonucleotide is added is dictated by base pairing to the template DNA chain. Without a DNA primer sequence a new DNA chain cannot form, because DNA polymerase is not able to initiate DNA chains.

See also DEOXYRIBONUCLEIC ACID (DNA), SEQUENCE (OF A DNA MOLECULE),

TEMPLATE, COMPLEMENTARY (MOLEC-ULAR GENETICS), DOUBLE HELIX, POLYMERASE, POLYMERASE CHAIN REACTION (PCR), POLYMERASE CHAIN REACTION (PCR) TECHNIQUE, NESTED PCR

Primosome An agglomeration consisting of DNA helicase, primase, etc., that "unwinds" the DNA molecule (within cell) prior to replication. See also DEOXYRIBONUCLEIC ACID (DNA), DNA HELICASE, CELL, UNWIND-ING PROTEIN

Prion Proteinaceous structures (molecules) found in the plasma membrane (surface) of cells, in the brain, and various other tissues of all vertebrates. In addition to a role in signal-ing, one of the functions of (normal) prions [PrP^C] is to help "**capture**" **and deactivate** oxygen free radicals (i.e., oxygen atoms bear-ing an extra electron, which are thus high in energy; e.g., which are sometimes generated in a biological system such as within the body of an organism).

In 1982, Stanley Prusiner discovered that mis-shapen (mutated) versions [PrP^{Sc}] can cause the neurodegenerative disease bovine spongi-form encephalopathy (BSE) in cattle and the neurodegenerative diseases Creutzfeld-Jakob Disease (CJD), kuru, Gerstmann-Straussler-Scheinker syndrome, and fatal familial insom-nia (FFI) in humans. Prusiner named these molecules **prions for "proteinaceous infected particle**," because unlike infectious pathogenic bacteria or viruses, prions do not contain DNA.

When misshapen (isoform of) prions are intro-duced into an animal's central nervous system, they can cause (normal helical shape) prions to adopt the misshaped form (i.e., akin to the pleated folds in an accordion bellows), result-ing in massive neurodegeneration (and death).

The dye named **Congo red** and **IDX** (a deriv-ative of the chemotherapeutic doxorubicin) have shown some ability to slow prion-caused neurodegeneration.

See also PROTEIN, CELL, PLASMA MEM-BRANE, MUTANT, BACTERIA, DEOXYRI-BONUCLEIC ACID (DNA), PROTEIN STRUCTURE, BSE, PROTO-ONCOGENES, STRESS PROTEINS, MONOCLONAL ANTI-BODIES, FREE RADICAL, ANTIOXIDANTS,

HUMAN SUPEROXIDE DISMUTASE (hSOD), SIGNALING, ORGANISM

Proanthocyanidins Refers to phytochemical components (i.e., condensed tannins) within North American cranberries (*Vaccinium mac-rocarpon*), red grapes, and blueberries (genus *Vaccinium*) that impart heath benefits to humans who consume them.

For example, when humans consume these fruits, the proanthocyanidin molecules "tie up" the free radicals that otherwise can cause oxidative stress to the human body.

For example, when humans consume cranberries, these chemical compounds prevent *Escherichia coli* bacteria from adhering to the cells lining the human urinary tract (thereby helping to prevent some urinary tract infections).

See also PHYTOCHEMICALS, FREE RADI-CAL, OXIDATIVE STRESS, ANTIOXI-DANTS, ANTHOCYANIDINS, NUTRA-CEUTICALS, CELL, *ESCHERICHIA COLIFORM (E. COLI)*

Probe A relatively small molecule that can be used to sense the presence and condition of a specific protein, DNA fragment, RNA frag-ment, or nucleic acid by a unique interaction with that macromolecule.

See also DNA PROBE, HYBRIDIZATION (MOLECULAR GENETICS), BACTERIAL ARTIFICIAL CHROMOSOMES (BAC), YEAST ARTIFICIAL CHROMOSOMES (YAC), HUMAN ARTIFICIAL CHROMO-SOMES (HAC), MARKER-ASSISTED SELECTION, SOUTHERN BLOT ANALY-SIS, FLUORESCENCE *IN SITU* HYBRID-IZATION (FISH), BIO–BAR CODES

Probiotics Compounds that (generally) act to stimulate growth of beneficial types of bac-teria within the digestive system of animals (e.g., livestock). For example, organic acids (e.g., propionic acid, acetic acid, lactic acid, citric acid, etc.) act to inhibit the growth/ multiplication of pathogens (i.e., disease-causing microorganisms) in the digestive system of monogastric (i.e., single-stomach) animals such as poultry and swine. Those acids are able to pass through the outer cell membrane (i.e., plasma membrane) of pathogenic bacteria and fungi. Once inside those pathogens' cells, the acids dissociate and acidify the cell interior (which disrupts the cell's protein synthesis, growth, and replication of the pathogen).

See also PREBIOTICS, *BIFIDUS*, CITRIC ACID, FRUCTOSE OLIGOSACCHARIDES, PATHOGEN, MICROORGANISM, BACTERIA, FUNGUS, CELL, ACID, PLASMA MEMBRANE

Procaryotes Simple organisms that lack a distinct nuclear membrane and other organelles. Many structural systems are different between procaryotes and eucaryotes including the DNA arrangement, composition of membranes, the respiratory chain, the photosynthetic apparatus, ribosome size, the presence or lack of cytoplasmic streaming, the cell wall, flagella, the mode of sexual reproduction, and the presence or lack of vacuoles. Some representative procaryotes are the bacteria and blue-green algae.

See also CELL, EUCARYOTE, BACTERIA, NUCLEUS

Process Validation (for production of a pharmaceutical) Defined by U.S. Food and Drug Administration (FDA) as "Establishing documented evidence which provides a high degree of assurance that a specific process will consistently produce a (pharmaceutical) product meeting predetermined specifications and quality characteristics."

See also FOOD AND DRUG ADMINISTRATION (FDA), GOOD MANUFACTURING PRACTICES (GMP), GOOD LABORATORY PRACTICES (GLP), cGMP

Prodrug Therapy Refers to a regime in which pharmaceuticals:

- Are first administered (e.g., injected intravenously) in the form of biologically inactive compounds
- Accumulate in the targeted tissue (e.g., tumor)
- Are then caused to change into biologically active chemicals **at that targeted tissue/location** via a "trigger" (e.g., orally administered nanobody/zymogen)

See also ZYME SYSTEMS, BIOLOGICAL ACTIVITY, ABSORPTION, TUMOR, ORALLY ADMINISTERED, ZYMOGENS, NANOBODIES

Proenzyme See ZYMOGEN

Progesterone A female sex hormone secreted by the ovaries that supports pregnancy and lactation (i.e., milk production).

See also HORMONE, PITUITARY GLAND, ESTROGEN

Programmed Cell Death See p53 GENE, APOPTOSIS, HYPERSENSITIVE RESPONSE

Prokaryotes See PROCARYOTES

Promoter The region on DNA to which RNA polymerase binds and initiates transcription (of RNA). The promoter "promotes" the transcription (expression) of that gene, but the promoter's impact on the timing/degree of gene expression is itself regulated by the molecules that bind to the promoter. For example, the "binding" of RNA polymerase causes transcription of RNA to begin, and the "binding" to promoter of other STATs (i.e., signal transducers and activators of transcription) can regulate the degree to which a given gene is expressed.

A promoter is a region of DNA (deoxyribonucleic acid) that lies "upstream" of the transcriptional initiation site of a gene. The promoter controls where (e.g., which portion of a plant, which organ within an animal, etc.) and when (e.g., which stage in the lifetime of an organism) the gene is expressed. For example, the promoter named "Bce4" is "seed specific" (i.e., it only "promotes" the expression of a given gene's product [e.g., protein, fatty acid, amino acids, etc.] within a plant's seed).

See also POLYMERASE, GENE, EXPRESS, RNA POLYMERASE, CONTROL SEQUENCES, GENE EXPRESSION, BCE4, PLASTID, DEOXYRIBONUCLEIC ACID (DNA), POLYGENIC, TRANSCRIPTION, CAULIFLOWER MOSAIC VIRUS 35S PROMOTER, SIGNAL TRANSDUCERS AND ACTIVATORS OF TRANSCRIPTION (STATs)

Proofreading Any mechanism for correcting errors in nucleic acid synthesis that involves scrutiny of individual (chemical) units after they have been added to the (molecular) chain. This function is carried out by a 3′ to 5′ exonuclease, among others. Proofreading dramatically increases the fidelity of the base-pairing mechanism.

See also SEQUENCING (OF DNA MOLE-
CULES), MISMATCH REPAIR, GENE
REPAIR (NATURAL)

Propionic Acid See PROBIOTICS, *BIFIDUS*

Prostaglandin Endoperoxide Synthase An
enzyme that can exist in several different
forms within the human body to catalyze the
production of prostaglandins.

See also ENZYME, CYCLOOXYGENASE,
ARACHIDONIC ACID, ISOZYMES, PROS-
TAGLANDINS, HIGHLY UNSATURATED
FATTY ACIDS (HUFA)

Prostaglandins A group of cyclic (i.e., circle-
shaped molecule) fatty acids that act as hormones in the body (i.e., promote inflammation
during infections, help promote maintenance
of the tissues of the stomach/kidney/intes-
tines, etc.). Their primary mode of action is
through certain G-protein-coupled receptors.

Originally isolated from sheep and human pros-
tates, prostaglandins are synthesized (i.e.,
"manufactured") by most cells in the body via
chemical reactions catalyzed by the enzymes
cyclooxygenase/prostaglandin endoperoxide
synthase, usually from arachidonic acid (also
docosahexanoic acid).

See also EICOSANOIDS, PROSTAGLANDIN
ENDOPEROXIDE SYNTHASE, CYCLOOX-
YGENASE, ARACHIDONIC ACID, FATTY
ACID, G-PROTEIN-COUPLED RECEP-
TORS, G-PROTEINS, HORMONE,
ENZYME, HIGHLY UNSATURATED FATTY
ACIDS (HUFA), DOCOSAHEXANOIC ACID
(DHA), GLYCYRRHIZIC ACID

Prostate The gland in the body of males that
produces the liquid which carries sperm into
the females (during mating).

In older human males, the prostate will often
become enlarged (e.g., by "antagonism" when
estrogen molecules circulating in the blood
contact its surface). Via the **selective estrogen
effect**, isoflavones (e.g., from soybeans) consumed by such males can displace and replace
those estrogen molecules from the surface of
the prostate (thereby preventing enlargement).

See also ESTROGEN, ISOFLAVONES,
SELECTIVE ESTROGEN EFFECT, RNase 1

Prostate-Specific Antigen (PSA) An antigen
whose concentration increases significantly 5
to 10 yr prior to the (clinical) diagnosis of
prostate cancer. This means that PSA-level

measurements can be utilized in (biomarker)
diagnosis of prostate cancer before symptoms
appear. However, a series of tests is required
in order to accurately gauge the probability of
cancer because PSA levels can also be elevated when a man develops a noncancerous
enlarged prostate.

See also ANTIGEN, TUMOR, TUMOR-
ASSOCIATED ANTIGENS, GENE, CAN-
CER, PROSTATE, RNase 1, RNase 1 GENE,
BIOMARKERS

Prostatitis Refers to noncancerous enlargement of the prostate, which tends to occur in
men as they get older.

See also PROSTATE, PROSTATE-SPECIFIC
ANTIGEN (PSA)

Prosthetic Group A heat-stable metal ion or
an organic group (other than an amino acid)
that is covalently bonded to the apoenzyme
protein. It is required for enzyme function.
The term is now largely obsolete.

See also ION, AMINO ACID, PROTEIN,
ENZYME, APOENZYME, COENZYME

Protease An enzyme that catalyzes the hydrolytic cleavage (breakdown) of proteins. By analogy, the enzyme breaks the link (peptide bond)
holding a chain together. Proteases represent a
whole class of protein-degrading enzymes.

See also HYDROLYTIC CLEAVAGE,
ENZYME, PEPTIDE BOND, TRYPSIN,
CHYMOTRYPSIN, LACTOFERRIN, NEU-
TROPHILS

Protease Nexin I (PN-I) A protein that acts as
an inhibitor of protease.

See also PROTEASE, PROTEIN, PROTEASE
NEXIN II (PN-II)

Protease Nexin II (PN-II) A protein that is
thought to regulate important activities in the
body and brain by inhibiting specific enzymes
and interacting with certain body cells. PN-II
is formed from the metabolic processing of a
precursor molecule known as beta-amyloid.
Recent research indicates that incorrect metabolic processing of beta-amyloid by the body
results in amyloid plaques in the brain. The
amyloid plaques are generally found in victims
of Alzheimer's disease and is directly correlated (in number) with the degree of dementia.

See also PROTEASE NEXIN I (PN-I), REGU-
LATORY ENZYME, PROTEIN, ENZYME,
INHIBITION, METABOLISM

P

Proteasome Inhibitors Refers to any compounds that halt or slow the action of proteasomes in living cells. During 2003, the U.S. Food and Drug Administration (FDA) approved one proteasome-inhibiting pharmaceutical known as Velcade (bortezomib) for the treatment of blood cancer.

See also PROTEASOMES, FOOD AND DRUG ADMINISTRATION (FDA), CANCER

Proteasomes Refers to enzymatic/catalytic bodies that are present within all mammalian cells, which activate certain transcription factors and are involved in causing the cell to "present" antigens (i.e., from pathogens that invaded that cell) on the cell's surface and various other cellular functions. For example, the 26S proteasome degrades (i.e., breaks down) all ubiquinated (i.e., ubiquitin-"tagged") proteins in that cell.

See also ENZYME, PROTEIN, CELL, TRANSCRIPTION FACTORS, ANTIGEN, PATHOGEN, UBIQUITIN

Protein Coined in 1838 by Jons Berzelius. From the Greek word *proteios*, which means "the first" or "the most important" or "of the first rank." Any of a class of high-molecular-weight polymer compounds composed of a variety of α-amino acids joined by peptide linkages. By the synthesis (of this "chain") performed by ribosomes, each protein is the ultimate expression product of a gene. More than one protein can be expressed from a given gene (the particular protein expressed is determined by factors such as the cell's temperature or other environmental variable, presence of STATs, some of which themselves are proteins, presence of certain bacteria, etc.).

During their synthesis (after emerging from cell's ribosome), proteins may also be phosphorylated (i.e., a "phosphate group" is added to the protein molecule), glycosylated (i.e., one or more oligosaccharides is added onto the protein molecule), acetylated (i.e., one or more "acetyl groups" is added to the protein molecule), farnesylated (i.e., a "farnesyl group" is added to the protein molecule), ubiquinated (i.e., a ubiquitin "tag" is added to the protein molecule), sulfated (i.e., a "sulfate group" is added to the protein molecule),

or otherwise chemically modified. Proteins are the "workhorses" of living systems and include enzymes, antibodies, receptors, peptide hormones, etc. Proteins in living organisms respond to changing environmental and other conditions by changing their location within cells, by getting cut into (specific) pieces, by changing which (other) molecules they will bind (adhere) to, etc. All of the amino acids commonly found in (each and every one of the) proteins have an asymmetric carbon atom, except the amino acid glycine. Thus, the protein is potentially chiral in nature.

See also AMINO ACID, GENE, PEPTIDE, ABSOLUTE CONFIGURATION, STEREOISOMERS, CHIRAL COMPOUND, EXPRESS, OLIGOMER, PROTEIN FOLDING, MESSENGER RNA (mRNA), RIBOSOMES, POLYRIBOSOME (POLYSOME), ORGANISM, CELL, SIGNAL TRANSDUCERS AND ACTIVATORS OF TRANSCRIPTION (STATs), CENTRAL DOGMA (NEW), PHOSPHORYLATION, UBIQUITIN, GLYCOSYLATION (TO GLYCOSYLATE), FARNESYL TRANSFERASE

Protein Arrays See PROTEIN MICROARRAYS

Protein Biochips See PROTEIN MICROARRAYS

Protein Bioreceptors See RECEPTORS

Protein C An anticlotting (glyco) protein that prevents postoperative arterial clot formation when administered intravenously. May be synergistic (in its anticlotting effect) with tissue plasminogen activator (tPA).

See also THROMBOMODULIN, TISSUE PLASMINOGEN ACTIVATOR (tPA), PROTEIN, GLYCOPROTEIN

Protein Chips See PROTEIN MICROARRAYS

Protein Engineering The selective, deliberate redesigning and synthesis of proteins. This is done in order to cause the resultant proteins to carry out desired (new) functions. Protein engineering is accomplished by changing or interchanging individual amino acids in a normal protein. This may be done via chemical synthesis or recombinant DNA technology (i.e., genetic engineering). "Protein engineers" (actually genetic engineers) use recombinant

DNA technology to alter a particular nucleoside or triplet (codon) in the DNA (genes) of a cell. In this way, it is hoped that the resulting DNA codes for the different (new) amino acid in the desired location in the protein produced by that cell.

See also PROTEIN, POLYPEPTIDE (PROTEIN), GENE, CODON, GENETIC ENGINEERING, AMINO ACID, ESSENTIAL AMINO ACIDS, SYNTHESIZING (OF PROTEINS)

Protein Expression Consists of (the combination/total of) both translation **and** posttranslational modification of a given protein molecule.

See also PROTEIN, EXPRESS, TRANSLATION, POSTTRANSLATIONAL MODIFICATION OF PROTEIN

Protein Folding The complex interactions of a polypeptide molecular chain with its environment and itself and other protein entities, which cause the polypeptide molecule to fold up into a highly organized, tightly packed, three-dimensional structure. Proved to occur spontaneously for protein molecules outside of living cells by Christian B. Anfinsen during the 1960s.

This ability of polypeptide chains to fold into a great variety of topologies, combined with the large number of sequences (in the molecular chain) that can be derived from the 20 common amino acids in proteins, confers on protein molecules their great powers of recognition and selectivity. How a protein folds up determines its chemical function.

During the 1990s, it was discovered that inside living cells, "chaperone" molecules are needed for proper protein folding to occur. These chaperones are protein molecules (e.g., certain heat-shock proteins) that form a loosely bound complex to suppress incorrect protein folding as the protein molecule is emerging from the cell's ribosome, so protein folding is both complete and correct as soon as the newly formed protein molecule is released from the cell's ribosome. Some diseases (e.g., Alzheimer's disease) can be caused by large amounts of misfolded proteins.

See also AMINO ACID, PROTEIN, POLYPEPTIDE (PROTEIN), RIBOSOMES, CHAPERONES, PRION, ABSOLUTE CONFIGURATION, CONFORMATION, ENZYME, PROTEIN STRUCTURE, ALZHEIMER'S DISEASE, RAPID PROTEIN FOLDING ASSAY

Protein Inclusion Bodies See REFRACTILE BODIES (RB)

Protein Interaction Analysis Refers to a number of different analyses/technologies utilized to determine if a given (e.g., "unknown") protein molecule interacts with a protein molecule whose function is already known (e.g., from previous research, its use as a pharmaceutical, etc.). Through this analysis (e.g., inferring the "new" protein's function by its interactions with the "known" protein), useful information about the "new"/unknown protein can be gathered. Technologies utilized include two-hybrid systems (e.g., yeast two-hybrid system), surface plasmon resonance, nuclear magnetic resonance, mass spectroscopy, tandem affinity purification tagging (TAP), etc.

See also PROTEOMICS, TWO-HYBRID SYSTEMS, PROTEOME CHIP, BIOCHIPS, GENE EXPRESSION ANALYSIS, PROTEIN, GENOMICS, FUNCTIONAL GENOMICS, PROTEIN MICROARRAYS, FLUORESCENCE RESONANCE ENERGY TRANSFER (FRET), SURFACE PLASMON RESONANCE (SPR), NUCLEAR MAGNETIC RESONANCE, MASS SPECTROMETER, TANDEM AFFINITY PURIFICATION TAGGING, QUANTUM DOT

Protein Kinases Enzymes capable of phosphorylating (covalently bonding a phosphate group to) certain amino acid residues in specific proteins. Protein kinases play crucial roles in the regulation of signaling within, and between, cells.

See also KINASES, PHOSPHORYLATION, TYROSINE KINASE, ENZYME, AMINO ACID, PROTEIN, PROTEIN SIGNALING, CELL, TYROSINE KINASE INHIBITORS (TKI)

Protein Microarrays Refers to a piece of glass, plastic, or silicon onto which has been attached a number of **capture agents** (e.g., antibodies, aptamers, enzymes, antigens, receptors, ligands, or other molecules of other chemical compounds that bind or interact with proteins in a specific manner) at specific or known locations on the microarray.

These microarrays (sometimes called "biochips," protein biochips, protein arrays, etc.)

can then be utilized to test (e.g., a single sample) for a wide variety of attributes or effects (on, or by the protein molecules in the sample that is exposed to that microarray).

See also PROTEIN, HIGH-THROUGHPUT SCREENING (HTS), TARGET–LIGAND INTERACTION SCREENING, RECEPTORS, PROTEIN INTERACTION ANALYSIS, PROTEIN STRUCTURE, PROTEOMICS, ANTIBODY, APTAMERS, PROTEOME CHIP, MICROARRAY (TESTING), BIOCHIP, QUANTUM DOT, ENZYMES, CAPTURE AGENT, FUNCTIONAL PROTEIN MICROARRAYS

Protein Quality See AMINO ACID PROFILE, PDCAAS

Protein Sequencer See SEQUENCING (OF PROTEIN MOLECULES), GENE MACHINE, SEQUENCING (OF DNA MOLECULES)

Protein Signaling The "communication" by protein molecules (e.g., to cells) that governs their transport and localization (i.e., their destination in the cell). Discovered and delineated by Guenter Blobel during the 1970s, protein signaling (e.g., via a short sequence of amino acids attached to end of newly synthesized protein molecules) results in proteins traveling to the appropriate cell compartments (e.g., organelles) and/or out of the cell (i.e., secretion).

See also PROTEIN, SIGNALING, SIGNALING MOLECULE, CELL, AMINO ACID, SIGNAL TRANSDUCTION, G-PROTEINS, RIBOSOMES, PROTEIN KINASES

Protein Splicing See SPLICING (OF PROTEIN MOLECULE)

Protein Structure A polypeptide chain may take on a certain structure in and of itself because of the amino acid monomers it contains and their location within the chain. The chain may furthermore interact with other polypeptide chains to form larger proteins known as oligomeric proteins. In what follows, the levels of protein structure normally encountered will be highlighted:

- Primary structure — refers to the backbone of the polypeptide chain and to the sequence of the amino acids it comprises.
- Secondary structure — refers to the shape (recurring arrangement in space in one dimension) of the individual polypeptide chain. In some cases, because of its primary structure, the chain may take on an extended or longitudinally coiled conformation.
- Tertiary structure — refers to how the polypeptide chain (the primary structure) is bent and folded in three-dimensional space to form the normal tightly folded and compact structure.
- Quaternary structure — refers to how, in larger proteins made up of two or more individual polypeptide chains, the individual polypeptide chains are arranged relative to each other. These large multipolypeptide proteins are called oligomeric proteins and the individual chains are called subunits. An example of such a protein is hemoglobin.

See also CONFORMATION, PROTEIN FOLDING, POLYPEPTIDE (PROTEIN), PROTEOMICS, CHAPERONES

Protein Tyrosine Kinase Inhibitor Any compound that inhibits the action of the enzyme **tyrosine kinase**. Examples include genistein and the pharmaceuticals Gleevec™ (imatinib mesylate), Iressa™ (gefinitib), and Tarcera.

See also ENZYME, INHIBITION, TYROSINE KINASE, GENISTEIN (Gen), GLEEVEC™, KINASES

Protein Tyrosine Kinases Refers to a "family" of kinase enzymes in the human body that assist and facilitate the transfer of "phosphoryl groups" from one molecule to another molecule that is "targeted" by that kinase.

Protein tyrosine kinases (PTK) are critical components in the signaling pathways involved in tumorigenesis (tumor creation) and angiogenesis (i.e., creation of new blood vessels to "feed" the growing tumor).

See also TYROSINE KINASE, ENZYME, PHOSPHORYLATION, PROTEIN, KINASES, SIGNALING, SIGNALING MOLECULE, PATHWAY, TUMOR, ANGIOGENESIS, KINOME

Protein-Based Lithography See BIOELECTRONICS, PROTEIN

Protein-Conducting Channel Refers to transmembrane (i.e., through a plasma membrane) holes through which can pass newly synthesized protein molecules, under appropriate conditions. It is also thought that **membrane proteins** (e.g., receptors) enter the relevant membrane (e.g., plasma membrane) via protein-conducting channels (whereupon much of the membrane protein molecule remains embedded in that membrane).

See also PROTEIN, CELL, PLASMA MEMBRANE, RECEPTORS

Protein–Protein Interactions See PROTEIN, PROTEIN INTERACTION ANALYSIS, PROTEIN MICROARRAYS, STRUCTURE–ACTIVITY MODELS, TWO-HYBRID SYSTEMS

Proteolytic Enzymes Enzymes that catalyze the hydrolysis (break down) of proteins or peptides. Proteins (enzymes) that destroy the structure (by peptide bond cleavage) and, hence, the function of other proteins. These other proteins may or may not themselves be enzymes.

See also PROTEASE, UBIQUITIN

Proteome Chip A microarray ("biochip") developed by Michael Snyder et al. during 2001 that has the following properties:

- It has a large number of **known sequence protein molecules** (e.g., all proteins present in a given organism) attached to its surface at known locations (i.e., specific "addresses" on the microarray).
- It utilizes specific **bioactive agents such as certain lipids or biotinylated calmodulin (i.e., calmodulin molecules to which a molecule of biotin is "attached")** in order to determine which of the protein molecules mentioned in the preceding item interacts with relevant bioactive agents. Because calmodulin is a well-known, very well-characterized calcium-binding protein (i.e., bioactive agent) involved in (known) cellular processes, the binding of calmodulin to specific **protein molecules attached to the microarray/biochip** provides critical information about the (cellular, protein–protein, etc.) functions and interactions of those protein molecules **in the organism**.
- It reveals a large amount of data concerning **protein–protein interactions** (e.g., via subsequent application to the microarray of dye-labeled streptavidin to identify the protein molecules VIA THEIR ADDRESSES on the biochip) and **protein–lipid interactions.**

All of the aforementioned are needed in order to determine the organism's proteome.

See also BIOCHIPS, PROTEIN MICROARRAY, PROTEIN INTERACTION ANALYSIS, TARGET–LIGAND INTERACTION SCREENING, MICROARRAY (TESTING), PROTEOME, BIOTIN, ORGANISM, AVIDIN, METABONOMICS

Proteomes See PROTEOMICS

Proteomics The scientific study of an organism's proteins and their role in an organism's structure, growth, health, disease (and/or the organism's resistance to disease, etc.). Those roles are predominantly owing to each protein molecule's tertiary structure or conformation. Some methods utilized to determine which impact results from which protein are:

- Chemical genetics — to compare two same-species organisms (one of which has protein — or a portion of protein — at least partially inactivated by a specific chemical).
- Gene expression analysis — to determine the proteins produced when a given gene is "switched on" by measuring fluorescence of individual messenger RNA (mRNA) molecules (specific to which the particular gene is "switched on" at the time), when that mRNA hybridizes (with DNA pieces corresponding to genes analyzed that were attached to the

P

hybridization surface on the bio-chip).

- Gene expression analysis — to determine the impact when a given gene is "knocked out"/"turned off."
- Protein interaction analysis — to determine if a newly discovered protein molecule interacts with a protein molecule whose function is already known (e.g., from previous research or use as a pharmaceutical). If the newly discovered protein molecule interacts with one whose function is already known, it generally has the same or similar function (in living cells) as the previously known protein molecule. Thus, the function of a newly discovered human protein can sometimes be inferred from a protein molecule discovered earlier in a microorganism (e.g., via expressed sequence tags, model organism, Raman optical activity spectroscopy, etc.).
- *In silico* biology (modeling) — to compare computer-predicted events (e.g., the constituent peptides resulting from protein digestion) with actual or *in vitro* outcomes.

See also PROTEIN, PRIMARY STRUCTURE, CONFORMATION, NATIVE CONFORMATION, TERTIARY STRUCTURE, GENE, GENETIC MAP, GENOMICS, ELECTROPHORESIS, TWO-DIMENSIONAL (2-D) GEL ELECTROPHORESIS, SEQUENCING (OF PROTEIN MOLECULES), GENETIC CODE, CELL, SEQUENCE (OF A PROTEIN MOLECULE), STRUCTURAL GENOMICS, FUNCTIONAL GENOMICS, COMBINATORIAL CHEMISTRY, BIOINFORMATICS, HIGH-THROUGHPUT SCREENING, BIOCHIPS, CHEMICAL GENETICS, GENE EXPRESSION ANALYSIS, FLUORESCENCE, MESSENGER RNA (mRNA), MICROORGANISM, HYBRIDIZATION (MOLECULAR BIOLOGY), HYBRIDIZATION SURFACES, EXPRESS, EXPRESSED SEQUENCE TAGS (EST), ORGANISM, PROTEIN INTERACTION ANALYSIS, *IN SILICO* BIOLOGY, *IN VITRO*, METABONOMICS, PHYLOGENETIC PROFILING, RAMAN OPTICAL ACTIVITY SPECTROSCOPY, KNOCKOUT, KNOCKIN, MODEL ORGANISM

Proto-Oncogenes Cellular genes that can become cancer producing. Proto-oncogenes are activated to oncogenes via different mechanisms, including point mutation, chromosome translocation, insertional mutation, and amplification.

See also ONCOGENES, AMPLIFICATION, MUTATION

Protoplasm Coined by J. E. Parkinje in 1840, it is a general term referring to the entire contents of a living cell; living substance.

See also CELL, NUCLEOPLASM

Protoplast A structure consisting of the cell membrane and all of the intracellular components, but devoid of a cell wall. This (removal of cell's outer wall) can be done to plant cells via treatment with cell-wall-degrading enzymes or electroporation. Under specific conditions (e.g., electroporation), certain DNA sequences (genes) prepared by man can enter protoplasts. The cell then incorporates some or all of that DNA into its genetic complement (genome) and produces whatever product the newly introduced gene codes for. In the case of plant protoplasts, whole plants can be regenerated from the (genetically engineered) protoplasts, resulting in plants that produce whatever products the introduced genes code for.

See also CELL, ENZYME, ELECTROPORATION, GENE, GENETIC ENGINEERING, DEOXYRIBONUCLEIC ACID (DNA), CODING SEQUENCE, PROTEIN, SOYBEAN PLANT, CORN, CANOLA

Protoplast Fusion Refers to the practice of fusing two living cells together by first making each cell into a protoplast, then fusing together the two in order to result in a combined cell that possesses traits from both of the original cells.

See also PROTOPLAST, CELL, TRAIT

Protoxin A chemical compound that only becomes a toxin after it is altered in some way. For example, the B.t. protoxins (e.g., Cry9C, Cry1A (b), Cry1A (c), etc.) only become toxic after they are chemically altered by the alkaline environment inside the gut of certain insects.

See also *BACILLUS THURINGIENSIS (B.t.)*, *B.t. KURSTAKI*, CRY PROTEINS, CRY1A

(b) PROTEIN, CRY1A (c) PROTEIN, CRY9C PROTEIN, *B.T. ISRAELENSIS*, *B.T. TENEBRIONIS*, TARGET (OF A HERBICIDE OR INSECTICIDE)

Protozoa A microscopic, single-celled animal form. A unicellular organism without a true cell wall, which obtains its food phagotropically.
See also PHAGOCYTE

Provitamin A See BETA-CAROTENE, GOLDEN RICE

PrP^C Abbreviation for **prion protein cellular**.
See PRION

PrP^Sc
Abbreviation for **prion protein scrapie**, the misshapen (infectious) form of prion.
See PRION

PRR See PHYTOPHTHORA ROOT ROT

PS See PHOSPHATIDYL SERINE

PSA See PROSTATE-SPECIFIC ANTIGEN (PSA)

Pseudogene A segment of a DNA molecule that acts as a gene (i.e., it codes for a protein molecule product), but its protein product is generally not biologically active.
See also DEOXYRIBONUCLEIC ACID (DNA), GENE, CODING SEQUENCE, PROTEIN, BIOLOGICAL ACTIVITY

Pseudomonas aeruginosa See CITRATE SYNTHASE (CSb) GENE

Pseudomonas fluorescens A normally harmless soil microorganism (bacteria) that colonizes the roots of certain plants. At least one company has incorporated the gene for a protein that is toxic to insects (taken from *Bacillus thuringiensis*) into a *Pseudomonas fluorescens*. This was done in order to confer insect resistance on the plants, the roots of which the genetically engineered *Pseudomonas fluorescens* had colonized.
See also *BACILLUS THURINGIENSIS (B.t.)*, BACTERIA, WHEAT TAKE-ALL DISEASE, GENETIC ENGINEERING, ENDOPHYTE

Psoralen See PSORALENE

Psoralene A toxic chemical (furanocoumarin) to ward off insects, which is naturally produced by (wild-type) plants related to the domesticated celery plant. Also present in small amounts in celery, parsley, parsnips, and dill.
See also TOXIN, PHYTOTOXIN, WILD TYPE, FOOD AND DRUG ADMINISTRATION

(FDA), TRADITIONAL BREEDING METHODS

PST See PORCINE SOMATOTROPIN

Psychrophile An organism that requires a cold environment, such as 0°C (32°F), for growth.
See also MESOPHILE, THERMOPHILE, PSYCHROPHILIC ENZYMES

Psychrophilic Enzymes Enzymes found within certain organisms that are adapted to function in cold environments.
See also PSYCHROPHILE, ENZYME

Pterostilbenes See POLYPHENOLS

PTK Acronym for **protein tyrosine kinase**.
See PROTEIN TYROSINE KINASE

PTM Acronym for **posttranslational modification** (of protein molecules).
See POSTTRANSLATIONAL MODIFICATION OF PROTEIN

PUFA See POLYUNSATURATED FATTY ACIDS (PUFA)

Pure Culture A culture containing only one species of microorganism.
See also CULTURE, CULTURE MEDIUM

Purine A basic nitrogenous heterocyclic compound found in nucleotides and nucleic acids; it contains fused pyrimidine and imidazole rings. Adenine and guanine are examples.

PVP See PLANT VARIETY PROTECTION ACT (PVP)

PVPA See PLANT VARIETY PROTECTION ACT (PVP)

PVR Plant variety rights.
See PLANT VARIETY PROTECTION ACT

PWGF See PLATELET-DERIVED WOUND GROWTH FACTOR, GROWTH FACTOR

Pyralis An insect that is also known as the European corn borer (*Ostrinia nubilalis*).
See also EUROPEAN CORN BORER (ECB)

Pyranose The six-membered ring forms of sugars are called pyranoses. This is because they are derivatives of the heterocyclic compound pyran.
See also SUGAR MOLECULES

Pyrexia Fever; elevation of the body temperature above normal.
See also PYROGEN

Pyrimidine A heterocyclic organic compound containing nitrogen atoms at (molecular ring) positions 1 and 3. Naturally occurring derivatives are components of nucleic acids and coenzymes, uracil, thymine, and cytosine.

P

See also NUCLEIC ACIDS, COENZYMES, URACIL, THYMINE, CYTOSINE, TOXICOGENOMICS

Pyrogen A substance capable of producing pyrexia (i.e., fever).

See also PYREXIA

Pyrophosphate Cleavage The enzymatic removal of two phosphate groups (designated as PP_i) from ATP in one piece, leaving AMP as another product. This cleavage releases more energy, which can be used in certain reactions that require more of a "push" to get them going.

See also ATP, ORTHOPHOSPHATE CLEAVAGE

Pyrrolizidine Alkaloids A class of toxic chemical compounds that are produced naturally by certain plants as a defense mechanism (against predators).

One of the pyrrolizidine alkaloids, **monocrotaline** is consumed (preferentially) by the larvae (caterpillars) of the moth *Utetheisa ornatrix*. The moth subsequently utilizes the monocrotaline content of its body as a defense mechanism against spiders that would otherwise eat it.

See also ALKALOIDS, TOXIN

Q

Q-Beta Replicase A viral RNA polymerase secreted by a bacteriophage that infects *Escherichia coli* bacteria. Q-beta replicase can copy a naturally occurring RNA (molecule) sequence (e.g., from bacteria, viruses, fungi, or tumor cells) at a geometric (i.e., very fast) rate.

See also POLYMERASE, BACTERIOPHAGE, RIBONUCLEIC ACID (RNA), Q-BETA REPLICASE TECHNIQUE

Q-Beta Replicase Technique An RNA assay (test) that "amplifies RNA probes" a researcher is seeking. For instance, by using the Q-beta replicase technique to assay for the presence of RNA that is specific to the AIDS virus, it is possible to detect an AIDS infection in a patient's blood sample long before the infection has progressed to the point where antibodies would appear in the blood.

See also Q-BETA REPLICASE, RNA PROBES, RIBONUCLEIC ACID (RNA), POSITIVE AND NEGATIVE SELECTION (PNS), ASSAY, IMMUNOASSAY, ANTIBODY, POLYMERASE CHAIN REACTION (PCR) TECHNIQUE, COCLONING, WESTERN BLOT TEST

QCM Acronym for **quartz crystal microbalances**.

See QUARTZ CRYSTAL MICROBALANCES

QD Acronym for **quantum dot**.

See QUANTUM DOT

QPCR Acronym for **quantitative polymerase chain reaction**.

Uses include **gene expression analysis** (i.e., quantitatively determining the amounts of each protein being expressed by a cell), genotyping, DNA quantification, etc.

See also POLYMERASE CHAIN REACTION (PCR), CELL, GENE EXPRESSION PROFILING, PROTEIN, GENOTYPE, DEOXYRIBONUCLEIC ACID (DNA)

QSAR See QUANTITATIVE STRUCTURE–ACTIVITY RELATIONSHIP (QSAR)

QSPR See QUANTITATIVE STRUCTURE–PROPERTY RELATIONSHIP (QSPR)

QTL See QUANTITATIVE TRAIT LOCI (QTL)

Quadrupole Ion Trap See ION TRAP

Quantitative Structure–Activity Relationship (QSAR) A computer modeling technique that enables researchers (e.g., drug development chemists) to predict the likely activity (e.g., effect on tissue) of a new compound before that compound is actually created. QSAR is based on data from decades of research investigating the impact on "activity" of the chemical structures of thousands of thoroughly studied molecules.

For example, the biological activity (i.e., bacteria-killing effectiveness) of most antibiotics correlates with their tendency to dimerize (i.e., link two molecules into a single molecular unit).

During the late 1990s, Stephen Fesik and Phil Hajduk created **SAR by NMR,** which is a means for researchers in pharmaceutical companies to utilize NMR (nuclear magnetic resonance) to build the structure–activity model (e.g., of a "candidate pharmaceutical" molecule) for interactions with its **target molecule** (e.g., cell receptors). In SAR by NMR, NMR is utilized to detect even weak binding of **ligands (fragments of the pharmaceutical candidate molecule)** to receptors; then the ligands that successfully bind to target are assembled together into an optimized-to-target pharmaceutical molecule.

See also BIOLOGICAL ACTIVITY, PHARMACOPHORE, ANTIBIOTIC, CELL, RECEPTORS, PHARMACOKINETICS, PHARMACOLOGY, ANALOGUE, RATIONAL DRUG DESIGN, *IN SILICO* SCREENING, POLYMER, STRUCTURE–ACTIVITY MODELS, NUCLEAR MAGNETIC RESONANCE, TARGET (OF A THERAPEUTIC AGENT), LIGAND (IN BIOCHEMISTRY),

TARGET–LIGAND INTERACTION SCREENING

Quantitative Structure–Property Relationship (QSPR) A computer modeling technique that enables scientists to predict the likely properties of a new chemical compound before it is actually created.

See also QUANTITATIVE STRUCTURE–ACTIVITY RELATIONSHIP (QSAR), ANALOGUE, RATIONAL DRUG DESIGN

Quantitative Trait Loci (QTL) Individual-specific DNA sequences that are related to known traits (e.g., litter size in animals, egg production in birds, yield in crop plants.)

See also MARKER (DNA SEQUENCE), TRAIT, LINKAGE, DEOXYRIBONU-CLEIC ACID (DNA), LINKAGE GROUP, LINKAGE MAP, GENE, SEQUENCE (OF A DNA MOLECULE), MARKER-ASSISTED SELECTION, CORN, HIGH-OIL CORN, RESTRICTION FRAGMENT LENGTH POLYMORPHISM (RFLP) TECHNIQUE, RANDOM AMPLIFIED POLYMORPHIC DNA (RAPD) TECHNIQUE, AFLP, SIMPLE SEQUENCE REPEAT (SSR), DNA MARKER TECHNIQUE

Quantum Dot A "molecular structure" that is between 1 and 100 nm in size, so it is midway between molecular and solid states. Quantum dots have been constructed of semiconductor materials (e.g., cadmium selenide), crystallites (grown via molecular beam epitaxy), etc. These semiconductor crystals emit light in the visible, UV, and IR (infrared) wavelengths of the spectrum, depending on their chemical composition and size of the quantum dots, and the specific light source utilized to illuminate them. Quantum dots possessing specific color (emission) combinations can be "attached" to the following:

- Receptors or other proteins via **molecular bridges**
- Specific types of cells (e.g., cancerous cells) via coating them with peptides or other relevant molecules.

These are achieved, for example, by encapsulating clusters of selected quantum dots within polymer beads, which are subsequently attached to a molecular functional group (ligand) that preferentially attaches to **specific types** of cells (e.g., the cancer cells desired to be "color tagged"). When later the tissue is illuminated by light of relevant wavelength, the "tagged" cells glow with the selected colors.

Quantum dots can be utilized to illuminate with different colors the different living tissues (or different structures within a given cell) inside an organism. The color emitted is impacted by the specific tissue each quantum dot is within. Quantum dots could conceivably be constructed to act as receptors (e.g., on "biochips") for specific ligands (e.g., a blood component that is only present in a diseased patient), in a way that would signal the presence of disease when (blood) sample was passed over the quantum dot. That signal might be electronic, emission of light of a specific wavelength, etc.

See also NANOMETERS (nm), NANOTECHNOLOGY, RECEPTORS, MEMS (NANOTECHNOLOGY), BIOCHIP, BIOELECTRONICS, MICROARRAY (TESTING), MOLECULAR BRIDGE, LIGAND (IN BIOCHEMISTRY), CELL, PROTEIN, RECEPTORS, LABEL (FLUORESCENT), PROTEIN INTERACTION ANALYSIS, NANOPARTICLES, PEPTIDE

Quantum Tags See QUANTUM DOT

Quantum Wire A strip or "wire" of (electricity-) conducting material that is 10 nm or less in its thickness or width. Indications from some research show that some forms of DNA molecules might be used as "quantum wires."

See also NANOMETERS (nm), NANOTECHNOLOGY, DEOXYRIBONUCLEIC ACID (DNA), MEMS (NANOTECHNOLOGY), BIOELECTRONICS

Quarantine Pest A pest (e.g., weed, insect, disease, etc.) of potential economic importance to the area (e.g., "pest-free area"), which is thereby endangered (e.g., a weed that would harm local crops, etc.) and is **not yet present in that area**, or is not widely distributed, and is being **officially controlled**.

See also INTERNATIONAL PLANT PROTECTION CONVENTION (IPPC), PEST RISK ANALYSIS (PRA)

Quartz Crystal Microbalances Abbreviated as **QCM**. Refer to biosensors consisting of small quartz crystals (to which is attached a source of appropriate electric current) with sensitive measurement devices utilized to detect when the "attachment" of **specific molecules (e.g., viruses, DNA sequences, and antigens)** to the quartz (or to layers of certain materials previously deposited on the quartz surface) causes the **specific oscillation frequency** of that quartz crystal to change in a way that enables (electronic) identification of the specific molecules attached to the QCM.

See also BIOSENSORS (ELECTRONIC), VIRUS, SEQUENCE (OF A DNA MOLECULE), ANTIGEN

Quaternary Structure The three-dimensional structure of an oligomeric protein, particularly, the manner in which the subunit chains fit together.

See also PROTEIN, OLIGOMER, CONFIGURATION, NATIVE CONFORMATION

Quelling Refers to the impact (on gene expression) of RNA interference.

See also RNA INTERFERENCE (RNAi), EXPRESS, EXPRESSIVITY, GENE

Quencher Dye See MOLECULAR BEACON

Quercetin A "family" of phytochemicals (flavonoids) that is naturally produced in apple, pear, raspberry, red grape, cherry, citrus fruit, tomato, onion, etc. Quercetin is an antioxidant. Research indicates that human consumption of quercetin helps prevent prostate cancer and some other cancers.

Research indicates that human consumption of quercetin leads to suppression of the body's tendency to release histamine.

See also FLAVONOIDS, CHALCONE ISOMERASE, PHYTOCHEMICALS, NUTRACEUTICALS, CANCER, BIOLOGICAL ACTIVITY, HISTAMINE

Quick-Stop The term used to describe how DNA mutants of *Escherichia coli* cease replication immediately when the temperature is increased to 42°C (108°F).

See also *ESCHERICHIA COLIFORM (E. COLI)*

Quorum Sensing Refers to the signaling mechanism utilized by certain microorganisms (e.g., in a biofilm, a population of enteric pathogens within the digestive system of an animal, etc.) in which those microorganisms emit or receive chemical signals until they collectively determine that "enough" of them are present to initiate a **collective** action. Such collective actions can include:

- "Turning on" one or more pathways for production of specific products from certain substrates. For example, certain pathogenic bacteria (e.g., *Vibrio cholerae*) will often live benignly within the digestive system of an animal until "enough" of them are present, as determined via quorum sensing (e.g., utilizing an acyl homoserine lactone signaling molecule). At that point in time, those bacteria collectively turn on a pathway for production of their particular enterotoxin.
- Differentiating into specialized subtypes of cells, which perform different needed functions (for the biofilm or colony to survive).
- Infecting another (host) organism, if the bacteria are pathogenic.
- Sporulating (creation of spores for survival and reproduction).
- Bioluminescing (creation of light).

See also SIGNALING, MICROORGANISM, BACTERIA, PATHOGEN, BIOFILM, SIGNALING MOLECULE, ENTEROTOXIN, DIFFERENTIATION, PATHWAY, SUBSTRATE (CHEMICAL), CHOLERA TOXIN, BIOLUMINESCENCE, GRAM POSITIVE (G+)

R

R Genes Refers to genes within some plants that confer resistance (to certain plant diseases) through **common signaling pathways involved in ("surveillance" and activation of) natural plant defense responses** (e.g., SAR). For example, the gene that codes for (i.e., causes the "manufacture" of) harpin protein is only present in a few bacteria (e.g., *Erwinia amylovora*), but **R genes** (i.e., those responsible for "surveillance" and activation of plant defense responses) **that respond to the presence of harpin** are present within the genomes of numerous species of plants. Thus, the spraying of synthetic harpin protein onto any of those numerous species of (crop) plants causes those particular plants to initiate a protective or defensive response (cascade) against pathogenic bacteria, viruses, fungi, and even some insects.

See also GENE, SIGNALING, PATHWAY, PROTEIN, HARPIN, SPECIES, SYSTEMIC ACQUIRED RESISTANCE (SAR), PATHOGENIC, PATHOGENESIS-RELATED PROTEINS, STRESS PROTEINS, CASCADE, BACTERIA, VIRUS, FUNGUS

RAC See RECOMBINANT DNA ADVISORY COMMITTEE (RAC)

Racemate An equimolar (i.e., equal number of molecules) mixture of the D and L stereoisomers of an optically active compound. A solution of dextrorotary (D) isomer (enantiomer) will rotate the plane in which the light was polarized by a specific number of degrees to the right (dextro), whereas a solution containing the same number of levorotary (L) isomer molecules will rotate the plane in which the light was polarized by the same number of degrees (as in the D isomer case) to the left (levo). The difference between D and L enantiomers is that the rotations of the plane of plane-polarized light are equal in magnitude but opposite in sign. Hence, a 50:50 mixture of both enantiomers (known as a racemic mixture) shows no optical activity. That is, a solution containing a 50:50 mixture of enantiomers will not rotate the plane of plane-polarized light when it is passed through the solution.

See also ENANTIOMERS, STEREOISOMERS, LEVOROTARY (L) ISOMER, DEXTROROTARY (D) ISOMER

Racemic (mixture) See RACEMATE

Radioactive Isotope An isotope with an unstable (atomic) nucleus that spontaneously emits radiation. The radiation emitted includes alpha particles, nucleons, electrons, and gamma rays.

See also ISOTOPE

Radioimmunoassay Invented by Rosalyn Yarlow and Solomon Berson in 1959, it is a very sensitive method of quantitating a specific antigen, using a specific radiolabeled antibody. Functionally, the antibody is made radioactive by the covalent incorporation of radioactive iodine. The radioimmuno probe thus prepared is exposed to its antigen (which may be a protein, a receptor, etc.) in excess (the exact amount will have to be determined). The radiolabeled probe then binds to the antigen, and the unbound, free probe is washed away. The radioactivity is then determined (counted), and by comparison to a standard plot, which has been constructed previously, the amount of antigen (binding) is determined.

See also ANTIBODY, ASSAY, HORMONE, RADIOIMMUNOTECHNIQUE

Radioimmunotechnique A method of using a radiolabeled antibody to quantitate a known antigen.

See also RADIOIMMUNOASSAY, ANTIGEN, ANTIBODY

Radiolabeled From the Latin word *radiare,* meaning "to emit beams."

See LABEL (RADIOACTIVE)

Rafts Term used to refer to **lipid rafts**.

See LIPID RAFTS, PLASMA MEMBRANE

Raman Optical Activity Spectroscopy A chiral-optical spectroscopy tool that is used to

R

investigate the molecular behavior in solution of certain biomolecules such as viruses, nucleic acids, proteins, and carbohydrates.

In ROA spectroscopy, selected-wavelength light is shined onto the biomolecules of interest. Those biomolecules absorb some of the light's energy and become "excited" (i.e., their molecular vibrations increase); then they emit (reflected or scattered) light. That light can be analyzed in order to determine detailed information about the structure and behavior of the biomolecules being analyzed.

For example, an ROA spectrum (i.e., plot of the difference in intensities vs. wavelengths reflected from the biomolecules) also provides information about the conformations and tertiary structures of biomolecules. ROA spectroscopy can also be utilized for structural classification of biomolecules (e.g., in the field of proteomics).

See also PROTEIN, VIRUS, NUCLEIC ACIDS, CARBOHYDRATES, CONFORMATION, NATIVE CONFORMATION, TERTIARY STRUCTURE, PROTEOMICS

Random Amplified Polymorphic DNA (RAPD) Technique A genetic mapping methodology that utilizes as its basis the fact that specific DNA sequences (polymorphic DNA) are "repeated" (i.e., appear in sequence) with gene of interest. Thus, the polymorphic DNA sequences are linked to that specific gene. Their linked presence serves to facilitate genetic mapping (i.e., "location" of specific genes in an organism's genome).

See also GENETIC MAP, SEQUENCE (OF A DNA MOLECULE), RESTRICTION FRAGMENT LENGTH POLYMORPHISM (RFLP) TECHNIQUE, LINKAGE, DEOXYRIBONUCLEIC ACID (DNA), PHYSICAL MAP (OF GENOME), LINKAGE GROUP, MARKER (GENETIC MARKER), LINKAGE MAP, TRAIT, GENOME, GENE, QUANTITATIVE TRAIT LOCI (QTL)

RAPD See RANDOM AMPLIFIED POLYMORPHIC DNA (RAPD) TECHNIQUE

Rapid Microbial Detection (RMD) A broad term used to describe the various testing products or technologies that can be utilized to quickly detect the presence of microorganisms (e.g., pathogenic bacteria in a food processing plant). These testing products are based on immunoassay, DNA probe, electrical conductance or impedance, bioluminescence, and enzyme-induced reactions (e.g., those that produce fluorescence or a color change to indicate the presence of specific microorganism).

See also BIOLUMINESCENCE, MICROBE, BACTERIA, PATHOGEN, IMMUNOASSAY, ENZYME, PROBE, DNA PROBE, ELECTROPHORESIS, HAZARD ANALYSIS AND CRITICAL POINTS (HACCP)

Rapid Protein Folding Assay Refers to an assay or methodology developed by Geoff Waldo in 2001, which initially utilized a fusion protein (made via fusing a gene that codes for green fluorescent protein (GFP) to a gene that codes for the protein being analyzed) in order to indicate when proper or correct folding of that particular protein had occurred (within a cell). Proper or correct folding of the (fusion) protein resulted in green fluorescence. Because of limitations inherent in the initial version of the rapid protein folding assay (RFPA) such as the quite large GFP portion hindering the movement of fusion protein within the cell, during 2005 Geoff Waldo developed a new version of RFPA. That new RFPA incorporates only a **portion** of GFP within the fusion protein (thereby making the resultant fusion protein small enough to both move around the cell and fold without hindrance).

See also ASSAY, CELL, PROTEIN, FUSION PROTEIN, GENE, GENE FUSION, DEOXYRIBONUCLEIC ACID (DNA), CODING SEQUENCE, FLUORESCENCE, LABEL (FLUORESCENT), GREEN FLUORESCENT PROTEIN, CONFORMATION, PROTEIN FOLDING

ras **Gene** Discovered in 1978 by Edward Scolnick, who named it *ras* for "rat sarcoma" (i.e., the particular diseased tissue in which he found it). The *ras* gene is also present in the human genome, and it is an oncogene that (when mutated) is believed to be responsible for up to 90% of all human pancreatic cancers, 50% of human colon cancers, 30% of lung cancers, and 30% of leukemias. The *ras* gene codes for the production (i.e., "manufacture") of *ras* **proteins**, which help to signal each cell to divide and grow at appropriate times; e.g., when free EGF "attaches" to relevant cell receptor on plasma membrane. When the *ras* gene has been damaged or mutated (e.g., via exposure to cigarette smoke or ultraviolet light, etc.), it codes for (i.e., causes to be manufactured in the cell's ribosome) a mutated version of the *ras* protein that can cause the cell to become cancerous (i.e., divide and grow uncontrollably).

See also GENE, ONCOGENES, MUTATION, p53 GENE, GENETIC CODE, MEIOSIS, DEOXYRIBONUCLEIC ACID (DNA), CARCINOGEN, RIBOSOMES, CANCER, TUMOR, *ras* PROTEIN, FARNESYL TRANSFERASE, PROTO-ONCOGENES, PROTEIN, EPIDERMAL GROWTH FACTOR (EGF), EGF RECEPTOR

ras Protein A transmembrane (i.e., through the cell membrane) protein that is coded for by the *ras* gene. The *ras* protein end that is outside the cell membrane acts as a receptor for applicable growth factors (e.g., fibroblast growth factor), and conveys that signal (i.e., to divide or grow) into the cell when that chemical signal (i.e., the growth factor) touches the "receptor end" of the *ras* protein. When the *ras* gene has been damaged or mutated (e.g., via exposure to cigarette smoke or ultraviolet light), it causes excess *ras* proteins to be manufactured, which causes oversignaling of the cell to divide and grow (i.e., cell becomes cancerous).

See also GENE, TRANSMEMBRANE PROTEINS, *ras* GENE, FIBROBLAST GROWTH FACTOR (FGF), ONCOGENES, GENETIC CODE, PROTEIN, p53 PROTEIN, MEIOSIS, CARCINOGEN, RIBOSOMES, DEOXYRIBONUCLEIC ACID (DNA), CANCER, TUMOR, PROTO-ONCOGENES, RECEPTORS, EGF RECEPTOR, CD4 PROTEIN, SIGNALING, SIGNAL TRANSDUCTION, MITOGEN-ACTIVATED PROTEIN KINASE CASCADE

Rational Drug Design The "engineering" (building) of chemically synthesized drugs based on knowledge of receptor modeling and drug–target interactions with the aid of supercomputers, interactive graphics, etc.); the educated, creative design of the three-dimensional structure of a drug, atom by atom, that is, "from the ground up." This approach represents a

major advance over the prior practice of first synthesizing large numbers of compounds (or finding them in nature), followed by thousands of tedious screenings to test for efficacy against a given disease (target). The approach of rational drug design has, however, not yet been perfected and optimized owing, in part, to gaps in our knowledge of drug–receptor interaction (called "docking") and to gaps in our knowledge in general.

See also RECEPTORS, RECEPTOR MAPPING (RM), ANALOGUE, MOLECULAR DIVERSITY, TARGET (OF A THERAPEUTIC AGENT), *IN SILICO* BIOLOGY, FREE ENERGY, HOMOLOGY MODELING, DOCKING (IN COMPUTATIONAL BIOLOGY), *IN SILICO* SCREENING, X-RAY CRYSTALLOGRAPHY

RB See REFRACTILE BODIES

RBS1 Gene A gene that confers on any soybean plant (possessing that gene in its DNA) resistance to the adverse effects of the soilborne fungus *Phialophora gregata*, which can cause the plant disease **brown stem rot (BSR)** in soybean plants.

See also GENE, DEOXYRIBONUCLEIC ACID (DNA), BROWN STEM ROT (BSR), FUNGUS, PATHOGENIC, SOYBEAN PLANT

RBS3 Gene A gene that confers on any soybean plant (possessing that gene in its DNA) resistance to the adverse effects of the soilborne fungus *Phialophora gregata*, which can cause the plant disease known as brown stem rot (BSR) in soybean plants.

See also GENE, DEOXYRIBONUCLEIC ACID (DNA), BROWN STEM ROT (BSR), FUNGUS, PATHOGENIC, SOYBEAN PLANT

rDNA See RECOMBINANT DNA

Reactive Oxygen Species See FREE RADICAL, OXIDATION, OXIDATIVE STRESS

Reading Frame The particular nucleotide sequence that starts at a specific point and is then partitioned into codons. The reading frame may be shifted by removing or adding nucleotides. This would cause a new sequence of codons to be read. For example, the sequence C-A-T-G-G-T is normally read as two codons: C-A-T and G-G-T. If another adenosine nucleotide (A) were inserted between the initial C and A, producing the sequence C-A-A-T-G-G-T, then the reading frame would have been shifted in such a way that the two new (different) codons would be C-A-A and T-G-G, which would code for something completely different.

Se also CODON, GENETIC CODE, FRAME-SHIFT, DEOXYRIBONUCLEIC ACID (DNA), MUTATION

Real-Time PCR Refers to the use of PCR to attempt quantitative (determination of a given DNA sequence within a sample) via coupling of a "molecular beacon" (with a "quencher molecule" attached to it) to the PCR probe.

Thus, while the PCR reaction (cycling) is producing copies of the relevant DNA sequence, the **molecular beacon** (i.e., fluorescent marker) is "unquenched" at the same time, so it fluoresces in direct proportion to the amount of DNA present (which can theoretically be back-calculated to infer the original amount of that particular DNA present in sample prior to initiation of PCR cycling).

See also POLYMERASE CHAIN REACTION (PCR), PROBE, POLYMERASE CHAIN REACTION (PCR) TECHNIQUE, MOLECU-LAR BEACON, MICROARRAY (TESTING), SEQUENCE (OF A DNA MOLECULE), FLUORESCENCE, DEOXYRIBONUCLEIC ACID (DNA)

Reassociation (of DNA) The pairing of complementary single strands (of the molecule) to form a double helix (structure).

See DOUBLE HELIX

RecA The product of the RecA locus (in a gene of) *Escherichia coli*. It is a protein with dual activities, acting as a protease and also able to exchange single strands of DNA (deoxyribonucleic acid) molecules. The protease activity controls the SOS response. The nucleic-acid-handling facility (i.e., ability to exchange single strands of DNA) is involved in recombination or repair pathways.

See also SOS RESPONSE, LOCUS, PRO-TEIN, RIBOSOMES, *ESCHERICHIA COLIFORM (E. COLI)*

Receptor Fitting (RF) A research method used to determine the macromolecular structure that a chemical compound (e.g., an inhibitor) must have in order to fit (in a lock-and-key fashion) into a receptor. For example, a

pain inhibitor compound blocking a pain receptor on the surface of a cell.

See also CD4 PROTEIN, T CELL RECEPTORS, RECEPTORS, RECEPTOR MAPPING (RM), INTERLEUKIN-1, RECEPTOR ANTAGO-NIST (IL-1ra), RATIONAL DRUG DESIGN

Receptor Mapping (RM) A method used to guess (determine) the three-dimensional structure of a receptor binding site extrapolating from the known structure of the molecule binding to it. This approach can be carried out because of the complementary shape of the receptor and the binding molecule. Functionally, the researcher projects the (guessed) properties of the receptor ligands into a mathematical model in which the profile of the receptor is predicted by complementariness (to known chemical molecular structures). The receptor mapping process requires repetitive refinement of the mathematical model to fit properties continually being discovered via the use or interaction of chemical reagents bearing the known molecular structures.

See also CD4 PROTEIN, T CELL RECEP-TORS, RECEPTORS, RECEPTOR FITTING (RF)

Receptor-Mediated Endocytosis See ENDO-CYTOSIS

Receptor Tyrosine Kinase Refers to a "family" of cell surface receptors that respond (i.e., signal transduction) when epidermal growth factor (EGF) or structurally related ligands dock at those receptors.

In cancerous tissues, some receptor tyrosine kinases (RTKs) help initiate tumor proliferation or spread and the related angiogenesis (i.e., creation of new blood vessels to "feed" the growing tumor). For example, the tyrosine kinase inhibitor pharmaceutical GLEEVEC™ can be utilized to treat gastrointestinal stromal tumors, in which it targets the **receptor tyrosine kinase** known as **KIT**.

See also RECEPTORS, CELL, SIGNAL TRANSDUCTION, EPIDERMAL GROWTH FACTOR (EGF), LIGAND (IN BIOCHEMIS-TRY), ENDOCYTOSIS, CANCER, TUMOR, ANGIOGENESIS, GLEEVEC™, MITO-GEN-ACTIVATED PROTEIN KINASE CASCADE

Receptors Functional proteinaceous structures typically found in the plasma membrane (surface) of cells that tightly bind specific molecules (organic, protein, or virus). Some (relatively rare) receptors are located inside the cell's plasma membrane (e.g., free-floating receptor for Retin-A). Both (membrane and internal) types of receptors are a functional part of information transmission (i.e., signaling) to the cell. A general overview is that once bound, both the receptor and its "bound entity," as a complex, are internalized by the cell via a process called endocytosis, in which the cell membrane in the vicinity of the bound complex invaginates. This process forms a membrane "bubble" on the inside of the cell, which then pinches off to form an endocytic vesicle. The receptor then is released from its bound entity by cleavage in the cell's lysosomes. It is recycled (returned) to the surface of the cell (e.g., low-density lipoprotein receptors). In some cases the receptor, along with its bound molecule may be degraded by the powerful hydrolytic enzymes found in the cell's lysosomes (e.g., insulin receptors, epidermal growth factor receptors, and nerve growth factor receptors). Endocytosis (internalization of receptors and bound ligand such as a hormone) removes hormones from circulation and makes the cell temporarily less responsive to them because of the decrease in the number of receptors on the surface of the cell. Hence, the cell is able to respond (to a new signal). A receptor may be thought of as a butler who allows guests (in this case molecules that bind specifically to the receptor) to enter the house (cell) and accompanies them as they enter. Another mode of "reception" occurs when, following binding, a transmembrane protein (e.g., one of the G-proteins) activates the portion of the transmembrane (i.e., through the cell membrane) protein lying inside the cell. That "activation" causes an effector inside the cell to produce a "signal" chemical inside the cell, which causes the cell's nucleus (via gene expression) to react to the original external chemical signal (that bound itself to the receptor portion of the transmembrane protein).

See also CD4 PROTEIN, T CELL RECEPTORS, RECEPTOR FITTING (RF), RECEPTOR MAPPING (RM), LYSOSOMES, INTERLEUKIN-1 RECEPTOR ANTAGONIST (IL-1ra),

CD95 PROTEIN, TRANSFERRIN, VAGINOSIS, SIGNAL TRANSDUCTION, ENDOCYTOSIS, G-PROTEINS, CELL, SIGNALING, PROTEIN, NUCLEAR RECEPTORS, GENE, GENE EXPRESSION, LIVER X RECEPTORS (LXR), RETINOID X RECEPTORS (RXR), FARNESOID X RECEPTORS (FXR), HUMAN IMMUNODEFICIENCY VIRUS TYPE 1 (HIV-1), HUMAN IMMUNODEFICIENCY VIRUS TYPE 2 (HIV-2)

Recessive (gene) See RECESSIVE ALLELE

Recessive Allele Discovered by Gregor Mendel in the 1860s, this refers to an allelic gene whose existence is obscured in the phenotype of a heterozygote by the dominant allele. In a heterozygote, the recessive allele does not produce a polypeptide; it is "switched off." In this case, the dominant allele is the one producing the polypeptide chain (via the cell's ribosome).

See also GENETICS, ALLELE, DOMINANT ALLELE, HOMOZYGOUS, HETEROZYGOTE, POLYPEPTIDE (PROTEIN), CELL, RIBOSOMES

Recombinant DNA (rDNA) DNA formed by the joining of genes (genetic material) into a new combination.

See also RECOMBINATION, GENETIC ENGINEERING, EDITING

Recombinant DNA Advisory Committee (RAC) The former standing U.S. national committee set up in 1974 by the U.S. National Institutes of Health (NIH) to advise the NIH director on matters regarding policy and safety issues of recombinant DNA research and development. Over time, it had evolved to become part of the U.S. government's regulatory process for recombinant DNA research and product approval. The RAC was terminated by the director of the NIH in 1996 because the "human health and environmental safety concerns expressed at the inception (of genetic engineering or biotechnology) had not materialized."

See also INTERIM OFFICE OF THE GENE TECHNOLOGY REGULATOR (IOGTR), GENE TECHNOLOGY OFFICE, GENETIC ENGINEERING, ZKBS (CENTRAL COMMITTEE ON BIOLOGICAL SAFETY), NATIONAL INSTITUTES OF HEALTH (NIH), RECOMBINANT DNA (rDNA),

R

BIOTECHNOLOGY, RECOMBINATION, INDIAN DEPARTMENT OF BIOTECH-NOLOGY, COMMISSION OF BIOMOLEC-ULAR ENGINEERING, GENE TECHNOL-OGY REGULATOR (GTR), GENETIC MANIPULATION ADVISORY COMMIT-TEE (GMAC)

Recombinase A category of enzymes that acts to "cut open" the strand of DNA within a cell (e.g., to "**splice-out**" or "**splice-in**") a given gene. Recombinases normally circulate throughout the cell containing them and initiate repair of cell's (damaged) DNA under certain circumstances.

During 2000, Nam-Hai Chua and Jian-ru Zuo showed that activation of the **gene for recombinase** (via the b estradiol transcription factor) could be done to cause expression of recombinase in a manner that **spliced out** (removed) **antibiotic-resistant** "**marker genes**" from genetically engineered plants.

See also ENZYME, DEOXYRIBONUCLEIC ACID (DNA), GENE, CELL, GENE SPLIC-ING, HOMOLOGOUS RECOMBINATION, GENETIC ENGINEERING, TRANSCRIP-TION FACTORS, ANTIBIOTIC RESIS-TANCE, MARKER GENES (GENETIC MARKER), DNA GLYCOSYLASE

Recombination The joining of genes, sets of genes, or parts of genes into new combina-tions either biologically or through laboratory manipulation (e.g., genetic engineering).

See also GENETIC ENGINEERING, GENE, RECOMBINANT DNA (rDNA), EDITING

Red Biotechnology Term utilized in some countries to refer to **medical** applications of genetic engineering.

See also GENETIC ENGINEERING

Red Blood Cells See ERYTHROCYTES

Redement Napole (RN) Gene A swine gene that causes animals (possessing at least one negative allele of this gene) to produce meat that is more acidic than the average meat and thus has a lower "water-holding" capacity. The RN gene was first identified in the Hampshire breed of swine in France. The Hampshire breed has been known since the 1960s to produce meat that is more acidic than average.

See also GENE, ALLELE, ACID

Reduced-Allergen Soybeans Refer to a bio-technology-derived soybean variety developed by Eliot Herman and Rick Helm in 2002, in which production of the allergenic P34 storage protein (within the seeds) is prevented via gene silencing.

See also ALLERGIES (FOODBORNE), SOY-BEAN PLANT, BIOTECHNOLOGY, GENE, GENE SILENCING, PROTEIN, STORAGE PROTEINS, P34 PROTEIN, RNA INTER-FERENCE (RNAi)

Reduction (biological) The decomposition of complex compounds and cellular structures by heterotrophic organisms. In a given eco-logical system, this heterotrophic decomposi-tion serves the valuable function of recycling organic materials. This occurs because the heterotrophs absorb some of the decomposi-tion products (for nourishment) and leave the balance of the (decomposed) substances for consumption (recycling) by other organisms. For example, bacteria break down fallen leaves on the floor of a forest, thus releasing some nutrients to be utilized by plants.

See also HETEROTROPH

Reduction (in a chemical reaction) The gain of (negatively charged) electrons by a chem-ical substance. When one substance is reduced by another, the other compound is oxidized (loses electrons) and is called the reducing agent.

See also OXIDATION–REDUCTION REAC-TION, OXIDIZING AGENT, TEMPLATE

Redundancy A term used to describe the fact that some amino acids have more than one codon (that codes for production of that amino acid). There are approximately 64 possible codons available to code for 20 amino acids. Therefore, some amino acids will be specified by more than one codon. These (extra) codons are redundant.

See also CODON, GENETIC CODE, RIBO-SOMES

Refractile Bodies (RB) Dense, insoluble (i.e., not easily dissolved) protein bodies (i.e., clumps) that are produced within the cells of certain microorganisms. The refrac-tile bodies function as a sort of natural stor-age device for the microorganism. They are called refractile bodies because their greater density (than the rest of the microorganism's body mass) causes light to be refracted (bent) when it is passed through them. This bending

of light causes the appearance of very bright and dark areas around the refractile body and makes them visible under a microscope. Relatively rare in natural occurrence, refractile bodies can be induced (i.e., caused to occur) in procaryotes (e.g., bacteria) when the procaryotes are genetically engineered to produce eucaryotic (e.g., mammal) proteins. The proteins are stored in refractile bodies. For example, the bacterium *Escherichia coli* can be genetically engineered to produce bovine somatotropin (BST, a cow hormone), which is stored within refractile bodies in the bacterium. After some time of growth when a significant amount of BST has been synthesized, the *Escherichia coli* cells are disrupted (i.e., broken open) and the refractile bodies are removed by centrifugation and washed. They are then dissolved in appropriate solutions to release the protein molecules. This step denatures (unfolds and inactivates) the BST molecules, and they are refolded to their native conformation (i.e., restored to the natural conformation found within the cow) in order to regain their natural activity. The protein is then formulated in such a way as to be commercially viable as a biopharmaceutical. Refractile bodies are also known as inclusion bodies, protein inclusion bodies, and refractile inclusions. One point of interest is that the prerequisite for the generation of a mammalian protein by (in) a living foreign system such as *E. coli* is that the system used to generate the protein (1) must not have an immune system capable of destroying the foreign protein it is making, or (2) the foreign protein made must be camouflaged or protected from any defense mechanisms possessed by the synthesizing organism.
See also PROTEIN, GENETIC ENGINEERING, GENETIC CODE, PROCARYOTES, EUCARYOTE, *ESCHERICHIA COLIFORM (E. COLI)*, BOVINE SOMATOTROPIN (BST), ULTRACENTRIFUGE, CONFORMATION, NATIVE CONFORMATION, PROTEIN FOLDING

Regional Plant Protection Organization (RPPO) See INTERNATIONAL PLANT PROTECTION CONVENTION (IPPC), SPS, NATIONAL PLANT PROTECTION ORGANIZATION (NPPO)

Regulatory Element See REGULATORY SEQUENCE

Regulatory Enzyme A highly specialized enzyme having a regulatory (controlling) function through its capacity to undergo a change in its catalytic activity. There exist two major types of regulatory enzymes: (1) covalently modulated enzymes and (2) allosteric enzymes. Covalently modulated enzymes are enzymes that can be interconverted between active and inactive (or less active) forms by the covalent attachment (or removal) of a modulating metabolite by other enzymes. Hence, the activity of one enzyme can, under certain conditions, be regulated by other enzymes. Glycogen phosphorylase, an oligomeric protein with four major subunits (tetramer), is a classic example of a covalently modulated enzyme. The enzyme occurs in two forms: (1) phosphorylase a, the more active form and (2) phosphorylase b, the less active form. In order for the enzyme to possess maximal catalytic activity (i.e., be phosphorylase a), certain serine residues on all four subunits must have a phosphate covalently attached. If, because of other regulatory signals it has received, the enzyme phosphorylase phosphatase hydrolytically cleaves and removes the phosphate group from the four subunits, the tetramer dissociates into the inactive (or much less active) dimer phosphorylase b. Another enzyme, phosphorylase kinase, is able to rephosphorylate the four specific serine residues of the four subunits at the expense of ATP, and regenerate the active phosphorylase a tetramer.

Allosteric enzymes are those that possess a special site on their surfaces that is distinct from the enzyme's catalytic site and to which specific metabolites (called effectors or modulators) are reversibly and noncovalently bound. The allosteric binding site is as specific for a particular metabolite as is the catalytic site, but it cannot catalyze a reaction and can only bind the effector. The binding of the effector causes a conformation change in the enzyme such that its catalytic activity is impaired or stopped. Allosteric enzymes are normally the first enzymes in, or are near the beginning of, a multienzyme system. The very last product produced by the multienzyme system (the end product) may act as a specific inhibitor of the allosteric enzyme by binding to that enzyme's allosteric site. The binding consequently causes a conformation change to occur in the enzyme, which inactivates it. A classic example of an allosteric enzyme in a multienzyme sequence is the enzyme L-threonine dehydratase, which is the initial enzyme in the enzyme sequence that catalyzes the conversion of L-threonine to L-isoleucine. This reaction occurs in five enzyme-catalyzed steps. The end product L-isoleucine strongly inhibits L-threonine dehydratase, the first enzyme in the five-enzyme sequence. No other intermediate in the sequence is able to inhibit the enzyme. This kind of repression is called feedback or end-product inhibition. It should be noted that allosteric control may be negative (as in the example cited) or positive. In positive control, the effector binds to an allosteric site and stimulates the activity of the enzyme. Furthermore, some allosteric enzymes respond to two or more specific modulators, each modulator having its own specific binding site on the enzyme. An allosteric enzyme that has only one specific modulator is called monovalent, whereas an enzyme responding to two or more specific modulators is called polyvalent. Combinations of these possibilities could lead to very fine tuning of the enzymes involved in the synthesis or degradation of metabolites. Note that in the two examples cited earlier, the common denominator is the structural change that occurs upon execution of the mechanism.

See also METABOLITE, REPRESSIBLE ENZYME

Regulatory Genes Genes whose primary function is to control the state of synthesis of the products of other genes.

See also GENE, MICRORNAs

Regulatory Sequence A DNA sequence involved in regulating the expression of a gene, e.g., a promoter or operator region (in the DNA molecule).

See also OPERATOR, PROMOTER, DOWN PROMOTER MUTATIONS, DOWNREGULATING, TRANSCRIPTION FACTORS

Remediation The cleanup or containment (if chemicals are moving) of a hazardous-waste disposal site to the satisfaction of the applicable regulatory agency (e.g., the Environmental Protection Agency [EPA]). Such cleanup can sometimes be accomplished via use of microorganisms that have been adapted (naturally or via genetic engineering) to consume those chemical wastes that are present in the disposal site.

See also ACCLIMATIZATION

Renaturation The return to the natural structure of a protein or nucleic acid from a denatured (more random coil) state. For example, a protein may be denatured (lose its native [natural] structure) by exposure to surfactants such as SDS or to changes in the pH of the medium, etc. If the surfactant is slowly removed or the pH is slowly readjusted to the optimum for the protein, it will refold (snap) back into its original (native) form.

See also NATIVE CONFIGURATION, DENATURATION, SDS

Renin A proteolytic enzyme that is secreted by the juxtaglomerular cells of the kidney. Its release is stimulated by decreased arterial pressure and renal blood flow resulting from decreased extracellular fluid volume. It catalyzes the formation of angiotensin I from hypertensinogen. Angiotensin I is then converted to angiotensin II by another enzyme located in the endothelial cells of the lungs. Angiotensin II then causes the increase in the force of the heartbeat and constricts the arterioles. This scenario causes a rise in the blood pressure and is thus a cause of hypertension (high blood pressure).

See also HOMEOSTASIS, RENIN INHIBITORS, ATRIAL PEPTIDES

Renin Inhibitors Those chemicals that act to block the hypertensive (i.e., high-blood-pressure-inducing) effect of the enzyme, renin.

See also HOMEOSTASIS, RENIN, ATRIAL PEPTIDES

Rennin See CHYMOSIN

Reovirus A virus containing double-stranded RNA. It is isolated from the respiratory and intestinal tracts of humans and other mammals. The prefix "reo" is an acronym for **respiratory enteric orphan**.

See also RETROVIRUSES

Reperfusion The restoration of blood flow to an occluded (i.e., blocked) blood vessel. May be done biochemically (e.g., via tissue plasminogen activator) or via surgery.

See also HUMAN SUPEROXIDE DISMU-
TASE (hSOD), LAZAROIDS

Replication (of DNA) Reproduction of a
DNA molecule (inside a cell). This process
can be viewed as occurring in stages, in which
the first stage consists of a helicase enzyme
"unwinding" the double helix of the DNA
molecule at a replication origin, forming a
replication fork. At the replication fork, the
two separated (DNA) strands serve as tem-
plates for new DNA synthesis.

That new DNA synthesis is accomplished on
each strand via enzymes known as DNA polymerase, which travel along each (single)
strand, making a second complementary
strand by catalyzing the addition of DNA
bases (to the new, growing strands).

The end result is two new double helices (DNA
molecules), each of which has one chain from
the original DNA molecule and one chain that
was newly synthesized by the DNA polymerase enzymes.

See also DEOXYRIBONUCLEIC ACID (DNA),
DNA POLYMERASE, HELICASE,
ENZYME, REPLICATION FORK, DUPLEX,
DOUBLE HELIX, BASE PAIR (bp), MIS-
MATCH REPAIR

Replication (of virus) Reproduction of the
original virus. This process can be viewed as
occurring in stages, in which the first stage
consists of the adsorption of the virus to the
host cell, followed by penetration of the virus
(or its nucleic acid) into the cell, the taking over
of the cell's biomachinery and harnessing of it
to replicate viral nucleic acid along with the
synthesis of other virus constituents, the correct
assembly of the nucleic acids and other constituents into a functional virus and, finally,
release of the virus from the confines of the cell.

See also VIRUS, CELL, NUCLEIC ACIDS

Replication Fork The point at which strands
of parental duplex DNA are separated in a Y
shape. This region represents a growing point
in DNA replication.

See also REPLICATION (OF DNA), DEOX-
YRIBONUCLEIC ACID (DNA), DUPLEX

Replicon Refers to the nonreplicating viral
RNA particles (e.g., derived by scientists from
the polio virus) utilized to induce apoptosis (i.e.,
"programmed cell death") in brain tumors. Rep-
licons are able to cross the blood–brain barrier

(BBB); they preferentially infect cancer or
tumor cells and then produce proteins that cause
tumor cells to die via apoptosis.

See also VIRUS, REPLICATION (OF VIRUS),
RIBONUCLEIC ACID (RNA), APOPTOSIS,
CELL, BLOOD–BRAIN BARRIER (BBB),
CANCER, TUMOR

Reporter Gene A specific gene that is inserted
into the DNA of a cell so that the cell will
"report" (to researchers) when the following
have occurred:

- Signal transduction has occurred in
  that cell.
- A (linked) gene was successfully
  expressed.

The gene that codes for production of the
enzyme luciferase (which catalyzes bioluminescence, i.e., light production) is one of the
most commonly used **reporter genes**.

For example, when researchers are testing
numerous candidate drugs for their ability to
stop cells from (over) producing a hormone
or growth factor, the researchers need to
quickly know when one of the candidate drugs
has had the desired effect on the cell of interest. By prior insertion into that cell of a gene
(e.g., that causes bioluminescence or a certain
chemical to be produced by the cell when
signal transduction has taken place), that cell
"reports" (when a candidate drug has had the
desired effect on the cell) by producing the
bioluminescence or chemical (coded for by
the reporter gene), which can be rapidly
detected by the researcher (e.g., via light sensors or biosensors placed adjacent to the cell).

Another example is the use of (inserted) **lux gene**
as a reporter gene. The lux gene, which codes
for the bioluminescent **lux protein** (a luminophore), can be inserted into the DNA of certain
bacterial species that can be genetically engineered to biodegrade diesel fuel spilled in soil.
Then, when those engineered bacteria encounter diesel fuel and begin "eating" it (i.e., breaking it down), those engineered bacteria will
glow (bioluminesce) to "report" that they are
biodegrading the spilled diesel fuel.

Another example is the use of such a fluorescent reporter gene (e.g., for **green fluorescent protein**) in "sentinel bacteria" sprayed

R

onto battlefields after a war has ended. Those engineered bacteria produce fluorescent pigments in the presence of explosive chemicals (e.g., TNT), thereby marking landmines and unexploded ordnance for safe removal.

See also GENE, GENETIC ENGINEERING, GENETIC CODE, CODING SEQUENCE, PROTEIN, CELL, BIOLUMINESCENCE, CELL CULTURE, SIGNAL TRANSDUCTION, LINKAGE, HORMONE, GROWTH FACTOR, GREEN FLUORESCENT PROTEIN, BIOSENSORS (ELECTRONIC), LUMINOPHORE, LUX GENE, LUX PROTEIN, DEOXYRIBONUCLEIC ACID (DNA), GUS GENE, BACTERIA, BIOREMEDIATION, HIGH-THROUGHPUT SCREENING (HTS)

Repressible Enzyme An enzyme whose synthesis (rate of production) is inhibited (repressed) when the product it (or it in a multienzyme sequence) synthesizes is present in high concentrations. It is a way of shutting down the synthesis of an enzyme whose product is not required because so much of it is readily available to the cell. When that enzyme product is no longer available (e.g., because the cell has consumed that product), more of the enzyme is synthesized (to catalyze production of the product).

See also REPRESSION (OF AN ENZYME), REGULATORY ENZYME, ENZYME

Repression (of an enzyme) The prevention of synthesis of certain enzymes when their reaction products are present.

See also REPRESSIBLE ENZYME

Repression (of gene transcription or translation) The inhibition of transcription (or translation) by the binding of a repressor protein to a specific site on the DNA (or RNA) molecule. The repressor molecule is the product of one of the following:

• A repressor gene
• Demethylation of a relevant histone

See also REPRESSOR (PROTEIN), TRANSCRIPTION, TRANSLATION, DEOXYRIBONUCLEIC ACID (DNA), HISTONES, METHYLATED

Repressor (protein) Discovered in 1967 by Walter Gilbert et al., this term refers to the product of a regulatory gene; it is a protein that combines both with an inducer (or corepressor) and with an operator region (e.g., of DNA).

See also INDUCERS, COREPRESSOR, OPERATOR, REPRESSION (OF GENE TRANSCRIPTION OR TRANSLATION)

Research Foundation for Microbiological Diseases (includes Institute of Physical and Chemical Research) Also known as **RIKEN**. A Japanese institution that performs research on infectious diseases, among others.

See also NATIONAL INSTITUTE OF ALLERGY AND INFECTIOUS DISEASES (NIAID), KOSEISHO

Residue (of chemical within a foodstuff) See MAXIMUM RESIDUE LEVEL (MRL)

Residue (portion of a protein molecule) See MINIMIZED PROTEINS

Respiration Oxidative process in living cells in which oxygen or an inorganic compound serves as the terminal (final or ultimate) electron acceptor. Aerobic organisms obtain most of their energy from the oxidation of organic fuels. This process is known as respiration.

See also OXIDATION–REDUCTION REACTION, REDUCTION (IN A CHEMICAL REACTION), OXIDATION, OXIDIZING AGENT

Restriction Endoglycosidases A class of enzymes, each of which cleaves (i.e., cuts) oligosaccharides (e.g., the side chains on glycoprotein molecules) at a specific location within the chain. They are an important tool in carbohydrate engineering, enabling the carbohydrate engineer to sequence (i.e., determine the structure of) existing oligosaccharides, to create different oligosaccharides, and to create different glycoproteins via removal, addition, or change of the oligosaccharide chains on glycoprotein molecules.

See also OLIGOSACCHARIDES, GLYCOPROTEIN, CARBOHYDRATE ENGINEERING, GLYCOSIDASES, ENDOGLYCOSIDASE, EXOGLYCOSIDASE, GLYCOFORM, GLYCOBIOLOGY

Restriction Endonucleases A class of enzymes that cleave (i.e., cut) DNA at a specific and unique internal location along its length. These enzymes are naturally produced by bacteria that use them as a defense mechanism against viral infection. The enzymes chop up the viral nucleic acids, and hence, their function is destroyed.

Discovered in 1970 by Werner Arber, Hamilton Smith, and Daniel Nathans, restriction endonucleases are an important tool in genetic engineering, enabling the biotechnologist to splice new genes into the locations of a molecule of DNA where a restriction endonuclease has created a gap (via cleavage of the DNA).

See also VECTOR, ENZYME, POLYMERASE, GENE, GENETIC ENGINEERING, GENE SPLICING, ELECTROPHORESIS

Restriction Enzymes See RESTRICTION ENDONUCLEASES

Restriction Fragment Length Polymorphism (RFLP) Technique A "genetic-mapping" technique that analyzes the specific sequence of bases (i.e., nucleotides) in a piece of DNA (from an organism). Because the specific sequence of bases in their DNA molecules is different for each species, strain, variety, and individual (due to DNA polymorphism), RFLP can be utilized to "map" those DNA molecules (e.g., for plant-breeding purposes, for criminal investigation purposes, etc.).

See also GENETIC MAP, SEQUENCE (OF A DNA MOLECULE), RANDOM AMPLIFIED POLYMORPHIC DNA (RAPD) TECHNIQUE, DEOXYRIBONUCLEIC ACID (DNA), GENOME, PHYSICAL MAP (OF GENOME), LINKAGE, LINKAGE GROUP, MARKER (GENETIC MARKER), LINKAGE MAP, TRAIT, BASE PAIR (bp), DNA PROFILING, POLYMORPHISM (CHEMICAL), NUCLEIC ACIDS, GENETIC CODE, INFORMATIONAL MOLECULES

Restriction Map A pictorial representation of the specific restriction sites (i.e., nucleotide sequences that are cleaved by given restriction endonucleases) in a DNA molecule (e.g., plasmid or chromosome).

See also RESTRICTION SITE, RESTRICTION ENDONUCLEASES, DNA

Restriction Site A nucleotide sequence (of base pairs) in a DNA molecule that is "recognized" and cleaved by a given restriction endonuclease.

See also NUCLEOTIDE, SEQUENCE (OF A DNA MOLECULE), BASE PAIR (bp), DNA,

RESTRICTION ENDONUCLEASES, RESTRICTION MAP

Resveratrol Also known as 3,5,4 trihydroxy stilbene, it is a naturally occurring (in grapes) antifungal agent (e.g., against grape fungus). Resveratrol is thought to be responsible for the fact that consumption of red wine by humans helps their **blood fat (triglycerides)** levels and blood cholesterol levels to be lowered, thereby reducing risk of cardiovascular disease.

Resveratrol is a phytochemical that is produced by certain plants in response to "wounding" (e.g., by fungal growth on plant) or other stress. Plants that produce resveratrol include red grapes, mulberries, soybeans, and peanuts. Resveratrol inhibits cell mutations, stimulates at least one enzyme that can inactivate certain carcinogens, and (when consumed by humans) lowers blood cholesterol and blood fat levels.

Research indicates that consumption of resveratrol by humans can reduce the risk of blood clots, stroke, and certain cancers.

See also PHYTOCHEMICALS, SOYBEAN PLANT, FUNGUS, CARCINOGEN, CELL, CANCER, MUTATION, TRIGLYCERIDES, CHOLESTEROL, ENZYME, INDUCIBLE ENZYMES, ATHEROSCLEROSIS, CORONARY HEART DISEASE (CHD), SIRTUINS

Retinoid X Receptors (RXR) Refer to one "subfamily" among the so-called **orphan receptors**, which sense (via "docking" at RXRs) the presence of retinoids within the cell and thereby regulate the expression of certain genes (e.g., initiating or controlling certain retinoid-dependent regulatory pathways). For example, the retinoid **9-*cis* retinoic acid** (a derivative of vitamin A) can dock at RXRs to initiate one or more crucial regulatory pathways. RXRs can also be activated via docking by several dietary lipids, including docosohexanoic acid (DHA).

Retinoid X receptors (after docking) function as transcription activators or transcription factors, thus controlling or preventing cellular differentiation and proliferation (i.e., they can act to prevent neoplastic growth or cancer).

See also RECEPTORS, NUCLEAR RECEPTORS, ORPHAN RECEPTORS, RETINOIDS, CELL, NUCLEUS, SIGNALING, PATHWAY, EXPRESS, TRANSCRIPTION,

R

TRANSCRIPTION ACTIVATORS, TRAN-SCRIPTION FACTORS, GENE, DIFFEREN-TIATION, DOCOSAHEXANOIC ACID (DHA), NEOPLASTIC GROWTH, CANCER

Retinoids A group of biologically active compounds that are chemical derivatives of vitamin A. Among other effects on living cells, some of the retinoid compounds act to deprive cancerous cells of their ability to proliferate endlessly, so these (formerly cancerous) cells then progress to a natural death (after exposure to an applicable retinoid).

See also CELL, APOPTOSIS, VITAMIN, BIO-LOGICAL ACTIVITY, CANCER, NEO-PLASTIC GROWTH, RETINOID X RECEP-TORS (RXR)

Retroelements See TRANSPOSON

Retroviral Vectors Certain retroviruses that are used by genetic engineers to carry new genes into cells. These molecules become part of that cell's protoplasm.

See also RETROVIRUSES, GENETIC ENGI-NEERING, VECTOR, GENE, PROTOPLASM

Retroviruses From the Latin word *retrovir*, which means "backward man." Oncogenic (i.e., cancer-producing), single-stranded, diploid RNA (ribonucleic acid) viruses that contain (+) RNA in their virions and propagate through a double-helical DNA intermediate. They are known as retroviruses because their genetic information flows from RNA to DNA (reverse of normal). That is, the viruses contain an enzyme that allows the production of DNA, using RNA as a template. Retroviruses can only infect cells in which DNA is replicating, such as tumor cells (because they are constantly replicating) or cells forming the lining of the stomach (because that lining must replace itself every few days).

See also ONCOGENES, DIPLOID, RIBONU-CLEIC ACID (RNA), REVERSE TRAN-SCRIPTASES, CENTRAL DOGMA

Reverse Micelle (RM) Also known as reversed micelle or inverted micelle. A spheroidal structure formed by the association of a number of amphipathic (i.e., bearing both polar and nonpolar domains) surfactant molecules dissolved in organic, nonpolar solvents such as benzene, hexane, isooctane, and oils such as corn and sesame. The structure of an RM is the reverse of that of a micelle. Reverse micelles may be characterized by a structure in which the polar groups of the surfactant and any water present are centrally located with the surfactant hydrocarbon chains pointing outwards to the surrounding hydrocarbon medium. Reverse micelles may be used to solubilize polar molecules (i.e., water and enzymes) in organic nonpolar solvents and oils.

See also AMPHIPATHIC MOLECULES, MICELLE, SURFACTANT

Reverse Phase Chromatography (RPC) A method of separating a mixture of proteins, nucleic acids, and other molecules by specific interactions of the molecules with a hydrophobic (i.e., "water-hating") immobilized phase (i.e., stationary substrate), which interacts with hydrophobic regions of the protein (or nucleic acid) molecules to achieve (preferential) separation of the mixture.

See also CHROMATOGRAPHY

Reverse Transcriptases Also known as RNA-directed DNA polymerases, reverse transcriptases were discovered by Howard Martin Temin and David Baltimore in 1970. They are a class of enzymes first discovered to be present in the RNA of the tumor virus, which allows the synthesis of DNA (complementary to the RNA) using the RNA present in the virus as a template. This is the reverse of what normally happens and hence the name. Reverse transcriptases closely resemble the DNA-directed DNA polymerases (DNA polymerases) in that they require the same materials and conditions as the DNA polymerases (e.g., for RT-PCR).

See also ENZYME, VIRUS, RIBONUCLEIC ACID (RNA), CENTRAL DOGMA (NEW), POLYMERASE, RT-PCR

Reversed Micelle See REVERSE MICELLE (RM)

RFLP (Restriction Fragment Length Polymorphism) Refers to a DNA-testing technology or methodology that is based on the detection of variation in the **length of restriction fragments** when the sample's DNA is first digested with restriction endonucleases and then separated via Southern blot analysis or via electrophoresis.

See also POLYMORPHISM (CHEMICAL), DEOXYRIBONUCLEIC ACID (DNA), RESTRICTION ENDONUCLEASES, SOUTHERN BLOT ANALYSIS, ELECTRO-

PHORESIS, RESTRICTION FRAGMENT LENGTH POLYMORPHISM (RFLP) TECHNIQUE

rh Used to denote compounds (human molecules) made through the use of recombinant DNA technology. Here, "r" stands for recombinant and "h" for human.

See also rhTNF, RECOMBINANT DNA (rDNA), RECOMBINATION, GENETIC ENGINEERING

Rhizoremediation See PHYTOREMEDIATION, *RHIZOBIUM* (BACTERIA)

Rho Factor A protein involved in (chemically) assisting *Escherichia coli* RNA polymerase in the termination of transcription at certain (rho dependent) sites on the DNA molecule.

See also TRANSCRIPTION, POLYMERASE, *ESCHERICHIA COLIFORM (E. COLI)*

rhTNF Acronym for **recombinant human TNF**.

See also TUMOR NECROSIS FACTOR (TNF)

RIA See RADIOIMMUNOASSAY

Ribonuclease 1 Gene A human gene that plays a major role in the regulation of cell proliferation. Research indicates that a mutation in the RNase 1 gene predisposes certain men to get early-onset prostate cancer.

See also GENE, RNase 1 GENE, RNase 1, CELL, PROSTATE, MUTATION, CANCER

Ribonucleic Acid (RNA) A long-chain, usually single-stranded nucleic acid consisting of repeating nucleotide units containing four kinds of heterocyclic, organic bases: adenine, cytosine, guanine, and uracil. These bases are conjugated to the pentose sugar ribose and held in sequence by phosphodiester (chemical) bonds.

The primary function of RNA is protein synthesis within a cell. However, RNA is involved in various ways in the processes of expression and repression of hereditary information. The three main functionally distinct varieties of RNA molecules are (1) messenger RNA (mRNA), which is involved in the transmission of DNA information; (2) ribosomal RNa (rRNA), which makes up the physical machinery of the synthetic process; and (3) transfer RNA (tRNA), which also constitutes another functional part of the machinery of protein synthesis. Recent research indicates RNA can also sometimes be directly involved in protein

synthesis and in the activity of certain enzymes.

See also HEREDITY, GENETIC CODE, PROTEIN, RIBOSOMES, RIBOSOMAL RNA, INFORMATIONAL MOLECULES, INFORMATION RNA (iRNA), MESSENGER RNA (mRNA), TRANSFER RNA (tRNA), NANOTECHNOLOGY, ENZYME

Ribose D-ribose, a five-carbon-atom monosaccharide (i.e., a sugar). It is important to life because it forms, along with the closely allied compound deoxyribose, a part of the molecules that constitute the backbone of nucleic acids.

See also NUCLEIC ACIDS, MONOSACCHARIDES

Ribosomal Adaptor See TRANSFER RNA (tRNA)

Ribosomal RNA See rRNA (RIBOSOMAL RNA)

Ribosomes The molecular "machines" within cells that coordinate the interplay of tRNAs, mRNA, and proteins in the complex process of protein synthesis (manufacture). RNA constitutes nearly two-thirds of the mass of these large (megadalton) molecular assemblies, which are technically **ribozymes** (i.e., an enzyme in which the catalysis is performed by RNA). The formation of a ribosome (in the endoplasmic reticulum of a cell) from individual RNA and protein molecules is largely a self-assembly process, because all of the information needed for the correct assembly of this structure is contained in the primary structure of its (molecular) components. The assembly process is ordered and proceeds in stages. Many ribosomes (in a given cell) can simultaneously translate an mRNA molecule. The structure, consisting of a group of ribosomes bound to an mRNA molecule that is actively synthesizing protein, is called a polyribosome or a polysome. The ribosomes in this (polysome) unit operate independently of each other, each synthesizing a complete polypeptide (protein) "molecular chain."

See also PROTEIN, POLYPEPTIDE (PROTEIN), PROTEIN SIGNALING, PROTEIN FOLDING, POLYCISTRONIC, PROTEIN STRUCTURE, PRIMARY STRUCTURE, TRANSLATION, TRANSCRIPTION, TRANSCRIPTION UNIT, MESSENGER RNA

R

(mRNA), CELL, ENDOPLASMIC RETICU-LUM (ER), TRANSFER RNA (tRNA), rRNA (RIBOSOMAL RNA), DALTON, SELF-ASSEMBLY (OF A LARGE MOLECULAR STRUCTURE), RIBOZYMES, RIBONU-CLEIC ACID (RNA)

Riboswitches Refer to certain noncoding segments within messenger RNA molecules, which act to regulate gene expression (i.e., can **decrease, stop,** or **increase** it) when specific molecules (e.g., metabolites or ligands such as glycine) bind to those riboswitches. For example, during 2004, Ronald R. Breaker and coworkers discovered one riboswitch, in a bacteria, that activates the genes involved in the glycine cleavage pathway in that bacteria.

Many other riboswitches halt gene expression when the concentration of certain metabolites in the cell increase.

See also CELL, MESSENGER RNA (mRNA), TRANSCRIPTION, CODING SEQUENCE, GENE, GENE EXPRESSION, POSITIVE CONTROL, NEGATIVE CONTROL, DOWN-REGULATING, LIGAND (IN BIOCHEMIS-TRY), GLYCINE (Gly), METABOLITE

Ribozymes Discovered by Thomas Cech and Sidney Altman, they are RNA molecules that act as enzymes; that is, they possess catalytic activity and can specifically cleave (cut) other RNA molecules. The ribozyme (RNA) molecule and the other RNA molecule come together, where-upon the ribozyme molecule cuts the other RNA molecule at a specific defined (three-base) site. Because the ribozyme molecule acts as an enzyme in this reaction, the ribozyme molecule is not consumed or destroyed but goes on to similarly "cut" other RNA molecules.

During 2000, Thomas Steitz, Peter Moore et al. proved that **ribosomes** (i.e., the cell's internal protein synthesis "machinery") **are function-ally ribozymes**. During 2002, Scott Basker-ville and David P. Bartel created a ribozyme, via rational design, that catalyzes the ligation (i.e., joining) of RNA molecules to protein molecules. Such ribozymes could potentially be utilized to thereby attach "affinity tags" to certain protein molecules.

See also RIBONUCLEIC ACID (RNA), CATA-LYTIC RNA, BASE (NUCLEOTIDE), ENZYME, CELL, RIBOSOMES, CATALYST, AFFINITY TAG, RATIONAL DRUG DESIGN

Rice Blast A disease that can afflict the domes-ticated rice (*Oryza sativa*) plant. Caused by the filamentous fungi *Magnaporthe grisea* or *Pyric-ularia grisea*, the disease can result in damage to the plant's leaves, stems, and grain, to the point that the plant **appears** to have been "blasted" with projectiles.

See also FUNGUS

Ricin A lethal-to-cells lectin that is naturally produced in castor beans (seeds of the plant *Ricinus communis*). In 1994, Robert J. Ferl and Paul C. Sehnke genetically engineered a tobacco plant to produce ricin. Attached to a pharmaceutical "guided missile" or "magic bullet" such as a monoclonal antibody or the CD4 protein, ricin is potentially useful for treat-ment against some tumors and has been inves-tigated as a possible treatment against acquired immune deficiency syndrome (AIDS).

See also LECTINS, IMMUNOTOXIN, MON-OCLONAL ANTIBODIES (MAb), CELL, CD4 PROTEIN, GENETIC ENGINEERING, FUSION PROTEIN, FUSION TOXIN, SOL-UBLE CD4, PHYTOCHEMICALS, "MAGIC BULLET"

RIKEN Abbreviation for **Rikagaku Kenky-usho,** Japan's Institute of Physical and Chem-ical Research.

See RESEARCH FOUNDATION FOR MICROBIOLOGICAL DISEASES

RISC Acronym for **RNA-induced silencing complex.**

See RNA INTERFERENCE (RNAi)

Rituximab See B LYMPHOCYTES

RMD See RAPID MICROBIAL DETECTION

RN Gene See REDEMENT NAPOLE (RN) GENE

RNA See RIBONUCLEIC ACID (RNA)

RNA Interference (RNAi) Coined by Andrew Fire and Craig Mello in 1998, this term refers to what happens when short strands of (com-plementary) double-stranded RNA (dsRNA) are introduced into living cells. That interaction is either by physical insertion of the dsRNA or by genetic engineering of the organism, so the organism's cells themselves produce that (new) dsRNA. For example, genetic engineers can utilize **T7 RNA polymerase** to cause the pro-duction of such dsRNA within living cells.

Viral infection (i.e., insertion of viral dsRNA) and also microRNAs can cause RNA interference.

If those dsRNAs are relatively long, they are cleaved (cut) by enzymes known as **dimeric RNase III ribonucleases** (also called **dicer enzymes**) into segments approximately 21 to 25 bp (base pairs) in length, called **siRNAs** (**short interfering RNAs** or **small interfering RNAs**). That siRNA (i.e., specific to a selected gene's mRNA) causes specific cellular "cutting enzymes" in RISC (RNA-induced silencing complex) to adhere to the transcribed-from-gene mRNA that the **dsRNA was chosen to be specific to**. Those "cutting enzymes" cut up and mark for destruction the transcribed-from-gene mRNA, thereby negating the effects of that gene. That effect is known as **gene silencing**, and it persists even in the (first generation) offspring of that affected organism.

Thus, RNAi is one methodology that can be utilized by scientists to cause gene silencing or knockout. During 2002, Thomas A. Rosenquist and Gregory J. Hannon created "knockdown" mice via genetic engineering, so those mice (continually) produced the dsRNA that silenced a selected gene. Later, the first-generation offspring of those **knockdown mice** also "silenced" that selected gene in their bodies.

See also SHORT INTERFERING RNA (siRNA), RIBONUCLEIC ACID (RNA), dsRNA, CELL, MICRO-RNAs, GENE, MESSENGER RNA (mRNA), TRANSCRIPTION, GENE SILENCING, CHROMATIN REMODELING, KNOCKOUT, KNOCKDOWN, ENZYME, BASE PAIR (BP), POST-TRANSCRIPTIONAL GENE SILENCING (PTGS), REDUCED-ALLERGEN SOYBEANS, EPIGENETIC, CELLULAR PATHWAY MAPPING, DNA-DIRECTED RNA INTERFERENCE

RNA Polymerase Discovered by Severo Ochoa in 1955, it is an enzyme that catalyzes the synthesis of a complementary mRNA (messenger RNA) molecule from a DNA (deoxyribonucleic acid) template in the presence of a mixture of the four ribonucleotides (ATP, UTP, GTP, and CTP). Also called transcriptase.

See also TRANSCRIPTION, CENTRAL DOGMA (OLD), POLYMERASE, DNA POLYMERASE, PROMOTER, ALTERNATIVE SPLICING, TEMPLATE

RNA Probes See DNA PROBE

RNA Processing See ALTERNATIVE SPLICING

RNA Transcriptase See RNA POLYMERASE

RNA Vectors An RNA (ribonucleic acid) vehicle for transferring genetic information from one cell to another.

See also VECTOR, RETROVIRAL VECTORS

RNA-Induced Silencing Complex See RNA INTERFERENCE (RNAi)

RNAi Acronym for **RNA interference**.

See RNA INTERFERENCE (RNAi)

RNAP Acronym for **RNA Polymerase**.

See RNA POLYMERASE

RNase A category of enzymes that catalyze the destruction of nucleic acids within cells.

See also ENZYME, BARNASE

RNase 1 An enzyme that is coded for by a **RNase 1 gene** (located in "chromosome 1" of the human genome) that has been shown to be associated with an inherited form of prostate cancer in some human families. The **RNase 1** enzyme protects certain cells from viral infections (by triggering apoptosis — cell death), so absence of RNase 1 (e.g. via mutation of its gene, the inactivation of RNase 1, etc.) tends to predispose such individuals (due to that SNP) to prostate cancer.

See also ENZYME, GENE, CELL, RNase, CODING SEQUENCE, CHROMOSOME, RNase 1 GENE, TRANSCRIPTION, LINKAGE, CANCER, PROSTATE, APOPTOSIS, MUTATION, SINGLE-NUCLEOTIDE POLYMORPHISMS (SNPs)

RNase 1 Gene A human gene that plays a major role in the regulation of cell proliferation. Research indicates that a mutation in the RNase 1 gene predisposes men (possessing that SNP) to early-onset prostate cancer.

See also GENE, RIBONUCLEASE 1 GENE, CELL, PROSTATE, MUTATION, CANCER, RNase 1, SINGLE-NUCLEOTIDE POLYMORPHISMS (SNPs)

Rootworm See CORN ROOTWORM

ROS Acronym for **reactive oxygen species**.

See FREE RADICAL

Rosemarinic Acid A phenolic compound (naturally found in some plants) that acts as an antioxidant in the body's tissues when consumed by humans. For example, rosemarinic acid is naturally produced in rosemary

(*Rosemarinus officinalis*) and also in the edible herbs *Origanum vulgare* and *Salvia officinalis*.

See also PHYTOCHEMICALS, ANTIOXI-DANTS, OXIDATIVE STRESS, NUTRA-CEUTICALS

Roving Gene See JUMPING GENES, TRANSPOSITION, TRANSPOSASE, GENE, GENOME, DEOXYRIBONUCLEIC ACID (DNA)

RPFA Acronym for **rapid protein folding assay**.

See RAPID PROTEIN FOLDING ASSAY

Rps1c Gene A gene that confers on any soybean plant (possessing that gene in its DNA) resistance to several strains or races of phytophthora root rot (PRR) disease.

See also GENE, DEOXYRIBONUCLEIC ACID (DNA), SOYBEAN PLANT, PHYTOPHTHORA ROOT ROT

Rps1k Gene A gene that confers on any soybean plant (possessing that gene in its DNA) resistance to as many as 21 strains or races of phytophthora root rot (PRR) disease.

See also GENE, DEOXYRIBONUCLEIC ACID (DNA), PHYTOPHTHORA ROOT ROT, SOYBEAN PLANT

Rps6 Gene A gene that confers on any soybean plant (possessing that gene in its DNA) resistance to some strains or races of phytophthora root rot (PRR) disease.

See also GENE, DEOXYRIBONUCLEIC ACID (DNA), PHYTOPHTHORA ROOT ROT, SOYBEAN PLANT

Rps8 Gene A gene that confers on any soybean plant (possessing that gene in its DNA) resistance to as many as 50 strains or races of phytophthora root rot (PRR) disease.

See also GENE, DEOXYRIBONUCLEIC ACID (DNA), PHYTOPHTHORA ROOT ROT, SOYBEAN PLANT

rRNA (Ribosomal RNA) The nucleic acid component of ribosomes, making up approximately two-thirds of the mass of the bacteria *Escherichia coli* ribosome and approximately one half of the mass of mammalian ribosomes. Ribosomal RNA accounts for nearly 80% of the RNA content of the bacterial cell.

See also NUCLEIC ACIDS, RIBOSOMES, *ESCHERICHIA COLIFORM (E. COLI)*, RIBONUCLEIC ACID (RNA)

RSS Acronym for **recombination signal sequences**.

See GENE SPLICING

RTK Acronym for **receptor tyrosine kinase.**

See **RECEPTOR TYROSINE KINASE**

RT-PCR Acronym for **reverse transcriptase polymerase chain reaction**, a PCR technique that starts with cellular RNA (transcript) and then utilizes reverse transcriptase to create its counterpart DNA, which is then amplified or copied by the PCR (polymerase chain reaction) technique.

See also RIBONUCLEIC ACID (RNA), TRANSCRIPTION, TRANSCRIPTOME, REVERSE TRANSCRIPTASES, DNA POLYMERASE, POLYMERASE CHAIN REACTION (PCR), POLYMERASE CHAIN REACTION (PCR) TECHNIQUE, CAPILLARY ELECTROPHORESIS, DEOXYRIBONUCLEIC ACID (DNA)

Rubitecan A pharmaceutical that either shrinks or halts the growth of pancreatic cancer tumors in humans. The pharmacophore (i.e., **active portion** of molecule) in rubitecan was derived from a Chinese flowering tree (*Camptotheca acuminata*); thus, that "family" of drugs is known as **camptothecins**. Camptothecins inhibit a critical enzyme that is required for cell division to occur (thus, it inhibits rapidly growing tumors).

See also CANCER, PANCREAS, TUMOR, PHARMACOPHORE, ENZYME

Rumen (of cattle) The "first stomach" of cattle (and other bovines).

See PREBIOTICS, MAILLARD REACTION

Rumenic Acid See CONJUGATED LINOLEIC ACID (CLA)

Rusts Various fungal diseases (*puccinia* spp.) that attack small grains plants such as wheat, corn or maize, sorghum, oats, barley, and rye. Its visual appearance is like that of rust on the surfaces of those plants.

See also FUNGUS, WHEAT, CORN

RXR See RETINOID X RECEPTORS (RXR)

S

S1 Nuclease An enzyme that specifically degrades (destroys) single-stranded sequences of DNA.

See also RESTRICTION ENDONUCLEASES, ENZYME, DEOXYRIBONUCLEIC ACID (DNA)

SAAND Acronym for **selective apoptotic antineoplastic drug**.

See SELECTIVE APOPTOTIC ANTINEOPLASTIC DRUG (SAAND)

SAGB Senior Advisory Group on Biotechnology.

See SENIOR ADVISORY GROUP ON BIOTECHNOLOGY (SAGB)

SAGE Acronym for **serial analysis of gene expression.**

See SERIAL ANALYSIS OF GENE EXPRESSION (SAGE)

Salicylic Acid (SA) SA is a signaling molecule in systemic acquired resistance (SAR) when SAR is triggered in plants (e.g., via spray application of COBRA® herbicide to soybean plants, spray application of harpin protein to various plants, chewing by insects on the leaves of tomato plants, and/or the entry of certain pathogenic bacteria or fungi into the plants, etc.).

See also SYSTEMIC ACQUIRED RESISTANCE (SAR), SIGNALING MOLECULE, SOYBEAN PLANT, HARPIN, FUNGUS, PATHOGEN, PROTEIN, PATHOGENESIS-RELATED PROTEINS, JASMONIC ACID

Salinity Tolerance See SALT TOLERANCE

Salmonella A genus of bacteria consisting of more than 2400 serovars (strains or types) that are classified into two species (*Salmonella enterica* and *Salmonella bongori*). All of these serovars are potentially pathogenic (disease causing) to humans. For example, some variants of *Salmonella typhimurium* can cause typhoid fever. The nontyphoid strains of *Salmonella* generally cause enterocolitis that can lead to more serious systemic infections.

Salmonella enteritidis and *Salmonella typhimurium* are increasingly causing outbreaks of foodborne illnesses (e.g., when foods are not washed or cooked properly prior to consumption by humans).

See also BACTERIA, PATHOGEN, PATHOGENIC, STRAIN, COMMENSAL

Salmonella enterica A pathogenic strain of *Salmonella* bacteria that can cause the disease known as typhoid fever in humans. *Salmonella enterica* can cause human macrophages to undergo apoptosis (programmed cell death), thereby enabling *Salmonella enterica* to resist the human cellular immune response.

See also BACTERIA, PATHOGEN, PATHOGENIC, STRAIN, SALMONELLA, MACROPHAGE, CELL, CELLULAR IMMUNE RESPONSE

Salmonella enteritidis (Se) A pathogenic strain of *Salmonella* bacteria that can cause fatal infections in poultry and humans (e.g., when undercooked eggs are eaten by humans).

See also BACTERIA, PATHOGEN, PATHOGENIC, STRAIN, SALMONELLA

Salmonella typhimurium A pathogenic strain of *Salmonella* bacteria that can cause disease in humans (e.g., when contaminated food is not washed and cooked properly prior to consumption).

See also BACTERIA, PATHOGEN, PATHOGENIC, STRAIN, COMMENSAL

Salt Tolerance Refers to the trait (of a plant) that enables a plant to grow or survive in soil that contains a high level of salt. For example, during 2001, Eduardo Blumwald and Hong-Xia Zhang inserted an *AtNHX1* gene from *Arabidopsis thaliana* into a tomato plant (*Lycopersicon esculentum*), and thereby made that tomato plant resistant to salt concentrations up to 200 m*M* (i.e., far higher than it could previously survive). That (*Arabidopsis* origin) gene enables the tomato plant to extract salt from the soil and then sequester and store the salt in vacuoles (i.e., small compartments) within its leaf cells.

See also *ARABIDOPSIS THALIANA*, VACUOLES, TOMATO, ANTIPORTER

Salting Out A technique used for forcing (dissolved) proteins out of a solution by increasing the concentration of salt in the solution. The Na^+ and Cl^- ions derived from the salt compete for and "tie up" water molecules that are solubilizing the protein molecules, thereby rendering them insoluble or increasing their insolubility.

See also PROTEIN.

SAM See SAM-K GENE

Sam-K Gene A gene that is naturally present within the *E. coli* **bacteriophage T3**. If the **sam-k** gene is inserted via genetic engineering into a (fruit crop) plant's genome, it causes greatly **reduced production** of the chemical compound S-adenosylmethionine (SAM) in that plant's fruit.

Because the SAM is normally converted (chemically) into l-aminocyclopropane-1-carboxylic acid (ACC) in the fruits of traditional varieties of (fruit crop) plants, such **sam-k-gene**-containing plants produce fruits that ripen or soften far **slower** than fruit from traditional varieties of those plants, which can reduce spoilage and loss in the harvest and transport of such fruit. That is because ACC is required for fruits to produce ethylene, the plant hormone that triggers (over) ripening or softening of fruit.

See also GENE, BACTERIOPHAGE, *ESCHERICHIA COLIFORM (E. coli)*, GENETIC ENGINEERING, GENOME, ACC, ACC SYNTHASE

Sanitary And Phytosanitary (SPS) Agreement The agreement to GATT/WTO by which WTO member nations agreed to base their technical barriers (re some imports, designed for the protection of human health or the control of animal and plant pests and diseases) only on an assessment of **actual risks** posed by the particular import in question and to only utilize scientific methods in assessing those risks.

See also SANITARY AND PHYTOSANITARY (SPS) MEASURES, WORLD TRADE ORGANIZATION (WTO), SPS

Sanitary And Phytosanitary (SPS) Measures Technical barriers (i.e., against some imports) that are designed for the protection of human health or the control of animal and plant pests and diseases. In the Sanitary and Phytosanitary (SPS) Agreement to GATT/WTO, the WTO member nations agreed to base their SPS measures only on an assessment of **actual risks** posed by the particular import in question and to only utilize scientific methods in assessing those risks.

See also SANITARY AND PHYTOSANITARY (SPS) AGREEMENT, WORLD TRADE ORGANIZATION (WTO), SPS

Saponification Alkaline hydrolysis of triacyl glycerols to yield fatty acid salts. The molecules thus produced are known as surfactants (surface active agents), commonly called soap. The process of soap making.

See also HYDROLYSIS

Saponins A group of phytochemicals (i.e., sugars linked to a triterpene or a steroid molecular subunit) that are produced by certain plants (e.g., the soybean plant, spinach plant, tomatoes, potatoes, ginseng plant, etc.). Evidence suggests that human consumption of saponins (e.g., produced in soybeans) can help to lower a person's blood content of low-density lipoproteins (LDLP) and can help to prevent certain types of cancer.

See also PHYTOCHEMICALS, SUGAR MOLECULES, SOYBEAN PLANT, LOW-DENSITY LIPOPROTEINS (LDLP), CANCER, STEROID

Saponnins See SAPONINS

SAR Acronym for **systemic acquired resistance**.

See SYSTEMIC ACQUIRED RESISTANCE (SAR)

SAR by NMR See QUANTITATIVE STRUCTURE–ACTIVITY RELATIONSHIP (QSAR)

Satellite DNA Many tandem repeats (identical or related) of a short basic repeating unit (in the DNA molecule).

See also DEOXYRIBONUCLEIC ACID (DNA)

Saturated Fatty Acids (SAFA) Fatty acids containing fully saturated alkyl chains (on their molecules). This means that the carbon atoms comprising the chains are held together by one, and not two or three, carbon-to-carbon bond. High levels of dietary SAFA have been related to increased blood cholesterol levels, which tends to lead to coronary heart disease (CHD) in humans. The sole exception is **stearic acid** (also known as stearate), which research has shown has no impact on the blood cholesterol levels of humans who consume it.

Beef fat typically contains approximately 54% saturated fatty acids; sheep fat, 58%; pork fat, 45%; and chicken fat, 32%. In general, fats possessing the highest levels of saturated fatty acids tend to be solid at room temperature, and those fats possessing the highest levels of unsaturated fatty acids tend to be liquid at room temperature. This rule of thumb was the original "dividing line" between the terms "fats" and "oils."

See also FATTY ACID, DEHYDROGENATION, CHOLESTEROL, MONOUNSATURATED FATS, SAPONIFICATION, LPAAT PROTEIN, UNSATURATED FATTY ACID, POLYUNSATURATED FATTY ACIDS (PUFA), CORONARY HEART DISEASE (CHD), PALMITIC ACID, STEARATE (STEARIC ACID), HIGH-STEARATE SOYBEANS, HIGH-STEARATE CANOLA

Saxitoxins Paralytic poisons that are produced by certain shellfish.

See also RICIN

SBO Abbreviation for **soybean oil.**

Scab The common (colloquial) name for *Fusarium* head blight; a disease of wheat (*Triticum aestivum*) that is caused by *Fusarium graminearum* fungus.

See also *FUSARIUM GRAMINEARUM*

Scale-Up The transition step in moving a (chemical) process from an experimental (e.g., "test tube," small, bench) scale to a larger scale, thus producing much more product than the bench scale (e.g., production of tons per year in a chemical plant). A process may require a number of scale-ups, with each scale-up producing more product than the previous one.

Scanning Tunneling Electron Microscopy
See ELECTRON MICROSCOPY (EM)

scCO2 Abbreviation for **supercritical carbon dioxide.**
See SUPERCRITICAL CARBON DIOXIDE

scFv Acronym for **single-chain variable fraction** (of an antibody).
See ANTIBODY SCP
See SINGLE-CELL PROTEIN (SCP)

sd1 Gene See GIBBERELLINS

SDA Acronym for **stearidonic acid.**
See STEARIDONIC ACID

SDM Acronym for **site-directed mutagenesis.**
See SITE-DIRECTED MUTAGENESIS (SDM)

SDS Sodium dodecyl sulfate. Also known as sodium lauryl sulfate (SLS). A surfactant commonly used in biochemical and biotechnological applications for the solubilization of membrane components and hard-to-solubilize (dissolve) molecules. For example, it is often utilized at high concentration in water solution (e.g., along with potassium acetate) to dissolve plant DNA samples (e.g., when a scientist wants to sequence that sample of plant DNA). The SDS/PA in water solution helps the scientist to separate out contaminants that are commonly present in samples from plant tissues (i.e., polysaccharides, proteins, etc.) because DNA molecules are much more soluble in SDS/PA solution than are those contaminant molecules. Above a critical concentration (CMC), SDS forms micelles in water, which are thought to be responsible for its solubilizing action. SDS is also used in such items as shampoo.

See also CRITICAL MICELLE CONCENTRATION, MICELLE, REVERSE MICELLE (RM), PROTEIN, MEMBRANE (OF A CELL), SURFACTANT, DEOXYRIBONUCLEIC ACID (DNA), POLYSACCHARIDES, SEQUENCING (OF DNA MOLECULES), HEXADECYLTRIMETHYLAMMONIUM BROMIDE (CTAB)

"Seedless" Fruits See TRIPLOID

Seed-Specific Promoter See PROMOTER

Selectable Marker Genes See MARKER (GENETIC MARKER)

Selectins Also called LEC-CAMs (leukocyte cell adhesion molecules). A class of molecular, structurally related lectins that mediate (i.e., control, cause, etc.) the contacts between a variety of cells (e.g., leukocytes and endothelial cells) and function as cellular adhesion receptors.

See also RECEPTORS, LECTINS, ADHESION MOLECULE, LEUKOCYTES, ENDOTHELIAL CELLS, ENDOTHELIUM, SIGNAL TRANSDUCTION

Selective Apoptotic Antineoplastic Drug (SAAND) A category of pharmaceuticals that acts to prevent neoplastic growth (i.e., cancer) by allowing normal cell apoptosis to occur again (e.g., by blocking an enzyme that is

S

hindering normal apoptosis) in abnormal pre-cancerous cells and cancerous cells. Examples of SAANDs include **sulindac**, which blocks phosphodiesterases (enzymes).

See also NEOPLASTIC GROWTH, CANCER, TUMOR, APOPTOSIS, CELL, ENZYME, PHOSPHODIESTERASES

Selective Estrogen Effect A term that is used to describe how certain phytochemicals (e.g., flavones, flavonols, isoflavones, etc.) and pharmaceuticals (e.g., Evista/raloxifene, tamoxifen, etc.) possessing molecular structures that are similar to estrogen (a hormone) impart some **beneficial** effect on the human body when consumed by humans, without any of the **adverse** impacts of estrogen (e.g., promotion of the growth of certain tumors by estrogen).

See also PHYTOCHEMICALS, FLAVONOLS, ISOFLAVONES, FLAVONOIDS, ESTROGEN, PHYTOESTROGENS, PROSTATE, GENISTEIN (Gen)

Selective Estrogen Receptor Modulators Abbreviated **SERM**. This term refers to chemical compounds (e.g., isoflavones, the pharmaceuticals Evista/raloxifene and tamoxifen, etc.) that impart some **beneficial** effect on the human body when consumed by humans, without any of the **adverse** impacts of estrogen (e.g., promotion of the growth of certain tumors by estrogen).

See also SELECTIVE ESTROGEN EFFECT, ESTROGEN, ISOFLAVONES, PHYTOCHEMICALS

Selenocysteine See ARCHAEA

Self-Assembling Molecular Machines Refers to nanometer (nm)-sized devices that can be caused to **self**-assemble (from carefully preplanned synthetic components) via affinity or hybridization to each other of molecular (e.g., thiol-, DNA, etc.) segments (attached to the relevant synthetic components).

See also SELF-ASSEMBLY (OF A LARGE MOLECULAR STRUCTURE), ATOMIC FORCE MICROSCOPY, DIP-PEN NANO-LITHOGRAPHY, NANOTECHNOLOGY, DIRECTED SELF-ASSEMBLY, NANOMETERS (nm), OPTICAL TWEEZER, NANO-ELECTROMECHANICAL SYSTEM (NEMS), BIOMOTORS, DEOXYRIBONU-CLEIC ACID (DNA), HYBRIDIZATION (MOLECULAR GENETICS), THIOL GROUP

Self-Assembly (of a large molecular structure) The essentially automatic ordering and assembly of certain molecules into a large structure. Examples of such large molecular structures (often called supramolecular structures or supramolecular assemblies) include nanofibers, nanowires, micelles, reverse micelles, ribosomes, nanotubes, tobacco mosaic virus (TMV), and peptide hydrogels. The first discovery of a self-assembling active biological structure occurred in 1955, when Heinz Frankel-Conrat and Robley Williams showed that TMV could reassemble into functioning, infectious virus particles (after TMV had been dissociated into its components by immersion in concentrated acetic acid).

During 2000, Samuel Stupp designed two-part molecules known as **peptide amphiphiles** (PA), which **assemble themselves** (e.g., when inserted into the space between broken bones inside humans) **into rigid nanofibers possessing specific peptides on their exteriors, that encourage the growth of hydroxyapatite crystals** (a constituent of bone).

In the future, it is hoped that man will be able to "direct" the self-assembly of molecular structures that will serve as the following:

- "Cages" to carefully protect and deliver sensitive or unstable pharmaceuticals to targeted tissues within the body.
- "Crucibles" (i.e., reaction vessels) for small-scale chemical reactions to occur within.
- Computer logic or memory devices (i.e., bioelectronics), connected to each other by nanowires.
- Antibiotics. For example, during the 1990s, M. Reza Ghadiri created "pepide nanotubes" made via self-assembly of certain peptides into tubes (cylinders) of nanometer dimensions. These peptide nanotubes are "membrane active" (i.e., insert one end of themselves into the outer membrane of a cell) and cause the cell (e.g., pathogenic bacteria) contents to "leak out," thus killing the cell (e.g., bacteria).

See also NANOWIRE, MICELLE, CRITICAL MICELLE CONCENTRATION, REVERSE MICELLE (RM), RIBOSOMES, NANO-TUBE, NANOSHELLS, TOBACCO MOSAIC VIRUS (TMV), NANOCRYSTAL MOLECULES, NANOSCIENCE, NANO-TECHNOLOGY, NANOMETERS (nm), BIOELECTRONICS, ANTIBIOTIC, PATHOGEN, BACTERIA, HAIRPIN LOOP, SELF-ASSEMBLING MOLECULAR MACHINES, PEPTIDE, TISSUE ENGI-NEERING, AMPHIPHILIC MOLECULES, DIP-PEN NANOLITHOGRAPHY, SP-1

Semisynthetic Catalytic Antibody An anti-body that is produced (e.g., via monoclonal antibody techniques) in response to a carefully selected antigen (i.e., one of the molecules involved in the chemical reaction that you are trying to catalyze). Such an antibody is then made to be catalytic by "attaching" a (molec-ular) group that is known to catalyze the desired chemical reaction. This attaching is done either via chemical modification of the antibody or via genetic engineering of the cell (DNA) that produces the antibody.

See also CATALYST, ANTIBODY, CATALYTIC ANTIBODY, SITE-DIRECTED MUTAGENE-SIS (SDM), MONOCLONAL ANTIBODIES (MAb), ANTIGEN, GENETIC ENGINEER-ING, ABZYMES

Senescence Refers to the stage of (an annual) plant's life after its seed or fruit has ripened and before the plant dies. During this time period, the plant is primarily respiring (using oxygen) and some metabolites' content increasing.

See also METABOLISM, METABOLITE, RESPIRATION

Senior Advisory Group on Biotechnology (SAGB) An association of approximately 35 of the largest European companies that are engaged in at least some form of genetic engi-neering research or production. Similar to the U.S. Biotechnology Industry Organization (BIO), SAGB works with governments and the public to promote safe and rational advancement of genetic engineering and bio-technology. It was formed in 1989 and is based in Brussels, Belgium.

See also BIOTECHNOLOGY, GENETIC ENGI-NEERING, RECOMBINANT DNA (rDNA), JAPAN BIOINDUSTRY ASSOCIATION, INTERNATIONAL FOOD BIOTECHNOL-OGY COUNCIL (IFBC), BIOTECHNOLOGY INDUSTRY ORGANIZATION (BIO)

Sense Normal (forward) orientation of DNA sequence (gene) in genome.

See also GENE SILENCING, ANTISENSE (DNA SEQUENCE)

Sepsis Also known as systemic inflammatory response syndrome, this life-threatening con-dition ("septic shock") occurs when the body's immune system overresponds to infec-tion (e.g., by gram-negative bacteria) in which release of bacterial endotoxin (lipopolysac-charide, or LPS) occurs. Those immune sys-tem cells (e.g., macrophages, etc.) overpro-duce numerous inflammatory agents (e.g., cytokines) that induce fever, shock, and, sometimes, organ failure.

See also GRAM-NEGATIVE (G), BACTERIA, CYTOKINES, ENDOTOXIN, MACRO-PHAGE

Septic Shock See SEPSIS

Sequence (of a DNA molecule) The specific nucleic acids (and their order) that comprise a given segment of a DNA molecule.

See also DEOXYRIBONUCLEIC ACID (DNA), GENETIC CODE, GENE, CHRO-MOSOMES, NUCLEIC ACIDS, CONTROL SEQUENCES, SEQUENCING (OF DNA MOLECULES), STRUCTURAL GENOM-ICS, COMPLEMENTARY (MOLECULAR GENETICS)

Sequence (of a protein molecule) The spe-cific amino acids (and the order in which they are coupled together) that comprise a given segment of a protein molecule.

See also PROTEIN, AMINO ACID, STRUC-TURAL GENE, LEADER SEQUENCE (PROTEIN MOLECULE), GENOMICS, STRUCTURAL GENOMICS, CHEMICAL GENETICS, SEQUENCING (OF PROTEIN MOLECULES)

Sequence Map A pictorial representation of the sequence of amino acids in a protein molecule, the sequence of nucleic acids in a DNA molecule, or the sequence of oligosaccharide components in a glycoprotein or carbohydrate molecule.

See also SEQUENCING (OF DNA MOL-ECULES), SEQUENCING (OF PRO-TEIN MOLECULES), SEQUENCING (OF OLIGOSACCHARIDES), SEQUENCE

S

(OF A DNA MOLECULE), SEQUENCE (OF A PROTEIN MOLECULE), RESTRICTION MAP

Sequencing (of DNA molecules) The process used to obtain the sequential arrangement of nucleotides in the DNA backbone. The cleavage into fragments (followed by separation of those fragments, which can then be sequenced individually) of DNA molecules by one of several methods as follows:

1. A chemical cleavage method followed by polyacrylamide gel electrophoresis (PAGE) or capillary electrophoresis.
2. A method consisting of controlled interruption of enzymatic replication methods followed by PAGE.
3. A didexyl method utilizing fluorescent "tag" atoms attached to the DNA fragments, followed by use of spectrophotometry to identify the respective DNA fragments by their differing "tags" (which fluoresce at different wavelengths). This (fluorescent tag) variant of the dideoxy method can be automated to "decipher" large DNA molecules (i.e., genomes). Such automated machines are sometimes called "gene machines."

Sequencing of DNA was first done in the mid-1970s by Frederick Sanger.
See also POLYACRYLAMIDE GEL ELECTROPHORESIS (PAGE), GENE MACHINE, CAPILLARY ELECTROPHORESIS, DEOXYRIBONUCLEIC ACID (DNA), SEQUENCE (OF A DNA MOLECULE), BASE EXCISION SEQUENCE SCANNING (BESS), SHOTGUN SEQUENCING, NANOPORE, NEAR-INFRARED SPECTROSCOPY (NIR), COMPARATIVE SEQUENCING, BIOCHIPS

Sequencing (of oligosaccharides) See RESTRICTION ENDOGLYCOSIDASES, SEQUENCE MAP

Sequencing (of protein molecules) The process used to obtain the sequential arrangement of amino acids in a protein molecule.
See also PROTEIN, AMINO ACID, SEQUENCE (OF A PROTEIN MOLECULE)

Sequon A (potential) site on a protein molecule's "backbone" where a sugar molecule (or a chain of sugar molecules, i.e., an oligosaccharide) may be attached.
See also PROTEIN, SUGAR MOLECULES, GLYCOPROTEIN, GLYCOGEN, GLYCOSYLATION, PROTEIN ENGINEERING, OLIGOSACCHARIDES

Serial Analysis of Gene Expression (SAGE) Refers to a methodology of gene expression analysis that is based on the identification of the amount of mRNA transcribed (from each relevant gene) via a "tag" (i.e., a *specific* short mRNA fragment found in the **3 region** of each mRNA transcript). Developed during the 1990s, SAGE involves the following:

• Collecting a single sample of tissue (e.g., **specific type** of cells from a tumor).
• Separating (digesting) short oligonucleotides from each mRNA (messenger RNA) present in the collected cell or tissue.
• Ligating or sequencing those oligonucleotides, and comparing each (sequence) to **known sequences** garnered from the Human Genome Project. The ratios determined of the expressed proteins thereby identified result in a **quantitative determination of gene expression in that specific population of cells** (e.g., tumor cells in this example).

See also GENE, EXPRESS, GENE EXPRESSION ANALYSIS, MESSENGER RNA (mRNA), OLIGONUCLEOTIDE, TRANSCRIPTION, TRANSCRIPTION UNIT, SEQUENCE (OF A DNA MOLECULE), LIGATION

Serine (Ser) A nonessential amino acid; a biosynthetic precursor of several metabolites, including cysteine, glycine, and choline. In 1999, Solomon H. Snyder, Herman Wolosker, and Seth Blackshaw conducted research that showed the some mammals synthesize ("manufacture") D-serine within their brains, where it functions as a neurotransmitter.
See also ESSENTIAL AMINO ACIDS, METABOLITE, CYSTEINE (Cys), GLYCINE (Gly), CHOLINE, NEUROTRANSMITTER

SERM Acronym for **selective estrogen receptor modulators**.
See SELECTIVE ESTROGEN RECEPTOR MODULATORS

Seroconversion The development of antibodies (specific to that disease-causing microorganism) in response to vaccination or natural exposure to a disease-causing microorganism.
See also SEROLOGY, ANTIBODY, IMMUNOGLOBULIN, HUMORAL IMMUNITY, PATHOGEN, POLYCLONAL ANTIBODIES, PASSIVE IMMUNITY

Serologist See SEROLOGY

Serology A subdiscipline of immunology, it is concerned with the properties and reactions of blood sera. It includes the diverse techniques used for the "test tube" measurement of antibody–antigen reactions, including blood typing (e.g., for transfusions), since 1929.
See also MAJOR HISTOCOMPATIBILITY COMPLEX (MHC), OLIGOSACCHARIDES, SERUM LIFETIME

Seronegative Refers to negative results of a serology test.
See also SEROLOGY, HUMORAL IMMUNITY, ANTIBODY

Serotonin An important neurochemical (5-hydroxytryptamine) whose effects on the human brain include mood elevation. Production of serotonin in the brain is increased by ingestion of the amino acid tryptophan (a chemical precursor to serotonin). Elevation of brain levels of serotonin can also be caused by the consumption of herb known as **St. John's Wort** (*Hypericum perforatum*), a West African plant alkaloid known as ibogaine or by the consumption of certain pharmaceuticals such as the antidepressants Prozac™ (trademarked product of Eli Lilly and Company), Zoloft™ (sertraline, trademarked product of Pfizer, Inc.), or Paxil™ (paroxetine, trademarked product of GlaxoSmithKline PLC). In 1997, Marianne Regard and Theodor Landis discovered that humans afflicted with hemorrhagic lesions in the brain (cause of abnormal serotonin activation or production) often became "passionate culinary aficionados."
See also TRYPTOPHAN (Trp), ESSENTIAL AMINO ACIDS, BLOOD–BRAIN BARRIER (BBB), NEUROTRANSMITTER, ALKALOIDS

Serotypes A variety (substrain) of a microorganism that is distinguished from others in strain via its serological effects (within immune system of the host organism it inhabits).
See also BACTERIA, STRAIN, *E. COLI 0157:H7*, SEROLOGY, HUMAN IMMUNODEFICIENCY VIRUS TYPE 1 (HIV-1), HUMAN IMMUNODEFICIENCY VIRUS TYPE 2 (HIV-2)

Serum Blood plasma that has had its clotting factor removed.
See also FACTOR VIII, FACTOR IX, PLASMA

Serum Half-Life See SERUM LIFETIME

Serum Immune Response See HUMORAL IMMUNITY

Serum Lifetime The average length of time that a molecule circulates in an organism's bloodstream before it is cleared from the bloodstream.
See also IMMUNE RESPONSE, ANTIGEN

Sessile Microorganisms that are attached to a (support) substrate directly by their base and not via an intervening peduncle (i.e., stalk). Can also refer to fruit or leaves that are attached directly to the main stem or branch of a plant.
See also VAGILE

Sex Chromosomes Chromosomes whose content is different in the two sexes of a given species. They are usually labeled X and Y (or W and Z); whereas one sex has XX (or WW), the other sex has XY (or WZ). XX (WW) corresponds to the female and XY (WZ), the male.

Sexual Conjugation An infrequent occurrence in which two adjacent bacteria stretch out portions of their (cell) membranes to touch one another, fuse, and then pass transposons, jumping genes, or plasmids to each other.
See also ASEXUAL, BACTERIA, CELL, CONJUGATION, PLASMID, TRANSPOSON, JUMPING GENES

SFE Acronym for **supercritical fluid extraction**.
See SUPERCRITICAL FLUID

Short Hairpin RNA Refers to specific segments of dsRNA (i.e., that bend into a "hairpin-like" molecular shape after they self-assemble) that can either be chemically synthesized by humans to cause RNA interference, or they are formed inside cells when the applicable

DNA-directed RNA interference methodology is utilized.

See also RIBONUCLEIC ACID (RNA), RNA INTERFERENCE (RNAi), GENE, KNOCK-DOWN, CELL, SHORT INTERFERING RNA (siRNA), DNA-DIRECTED RNA INTERFERENCE, dsRNA

Short Interfering RNA (siRNA) Refers to specific short sequences of double-stranded RNA (dsRNA) of less than 30 base pairs (bp) in length that trigger degradation of messenger RNA (mRNA) possessing the same sequence (as those siRNAs) within a cell, as part of the cellular process known as **RNA Interference (RNAi)**.

Because the degradation of mRNA shuts down (quells) production of the corresponding protein, siRNA (via RNAi) constitutes a pathway that cells utilize to regulate or silence gene expression. Relevant promoters within the DNA are silenced via DNA methylation and/or chromatin remodeling. siRNA can be utilized by humans to cause gene silencing or knockout.

In plants and nematodes, such RNA-interference-induced gene silencing spreads (e.g., from the site of dsRNA entry into organism) throughout the organism, apparently via mediation or transport by the transmembrane (i.e., through the plasma membrane) protein known as SID-1.

In animals, such RNA interference tends to be localized at or near the site of dsRNA entry into organism. For example, relevant siRNA has been utilized to quell the overproduction of vascular endothelial growth factor (VEGF) in laboratory animals, thereby helping prevent some age-related macular degeneration (AMD) damage.

See also RIBONUCLEIC ACID (RNA), CELL, ORGANISM, dsRNA, MESSENGER RNA (mRNA), PROTEIN, TRANSMEMBRANE PROTEINS, PATHWAY, DEOXYRIBONU-CLEIC ACID (DNA), GENE, GENE EXPRESSION, RNA INTERFERENCE (RNAi), GENE SILENCING, CHROMATIN REMODELING, DNA METHYLATION, KNOCKOUT, BASE PAIR (bp), PRO-MOTER, POSTTRANSCRIPTIONAL GENE SILENCING (PTGS), AMD, ANGIOGENE-SIS, NEMATODES, PLASMA MEMBRANE

Shotgun Cloning Method A technique for obtaining the desired gene that involves "chopping up" the entire genetic complement of a cell using restriction enzymes, and then attaching each (resultant) DNA fragment to a vector and transferring it into a bacterium, and finally screening those (engineered) bacteria to locate the bacteria that are producing the desired product (e.g., a protein).

See also GENETIC ENGINEERING, GENOME, RESTRICTION ENDONU-CLEASES, VECTOR

Shotgun Sequencing Sometimes called **whole-genome shotgun sequencing**, it was invented by J. Craig Venter and Hamilton O. Smith during the mid-1990s. Shotgun sequencing is a technology for rapid sequencing of (eucaryotic and procaryotic) DNA, in which an organism's genome (DNA) is first fragmented ("broken up"), and then the randomly selected pieces of the DNA are individually sequenced. Those individual pieces' sequences must subsequently be "bridged" (i.e., "assembled" in an overlapping end-by-end pattern) in order to assemble a complete map (e.g., of an organism's chromosome or genome).

See also SEQUENCING (OF DNA MOLE-CULES), DEOXYRIBONUCLEIC ACID (DNA), SEQUENCE (OF A DNA MOLE-CULE), GENOME, DNA "BRIDGES," CHROMOSOME, GENETIC MAP, CHRO-MOSOME WALKING, EUCARYOTE, PRO-CARYOTES

shRNA Acronym for **short hairpin RNA**.
See SHORT HAIRPIN RNA

Shuttle Vector A vector capable of replicating in two unrelated species.
See also VECTOR, REPLICATION (OF VIRUS)

Sialic Acid A sugar (branched-molecule carbohydrate) that the body attaches to surfaces of glycoprotein and glycolipid molecules which it manufactures, to enable those glycoproteins and glycolipids to thereby evade or avoid "clearance mechanisms" (e.g., parts of body's immune system) and thus circulate (e.g., in bloodstream) longer. In the human body, the *Neu5Gc* gene causes sialic acid molecules to be produced on the outer surface of some types of cells.

See also SUGAR MOLECULES, OLIGOSAC-CHARIDES, CARBOHYDRATES, PROTEIN, GLYCOPROTEIN, ANTIBODY, LIPIDS,

HUMORAL IMMUNITY, CELLULAR IMMUNE RESPONSE, GENE, NEU5GC, DEOXYRIBONUCLEIC ACID (DNA), CELL

SID-1 Protein See SHORT INTERFERING RNA (siRNA)

Signal Transducers and Activators of Transcription (STATs) Molecules that cause **signal transduction** to occur (i.e., when a hormone or other chemical "binds" to it), or molecules that cause **transcription** to occur (i.e., when transcription factors "bind" to it). STATs can be attached to solid surfaces (e.g., in a bioassay or biosensor) for use in such research applications as **high-throughput screening**.

See also SIGNAL TRANSDUCTION, HORMONE, TRANSCRIPTION FACTORS, BIOCHIPS, BIOSENSORS (ELECTRONIC), BIOASSAY, HIGH-THROUGHPUT SCREENING (HTS), MICROARRAY (TESTING), TARGET (OF A HERBICIDE OR INSECTICIDE), CASCADE, ACTIVATOR (OF GENE), TRANSCRIPTION ACTIVATORS

Signal Transduction The "reception" and "conversion" of a "chemical message" (e.g., hormone) by a cell. For example, G-proteins (which are embedded in the surface membrane of certain cells but extend through to outside and inside of the membrane) accomplish signal transduction. When a hormone, drug, neurotransmitter, or other signal chemical binds (i.e., "docks") to the receptor (on the exterior of the cell's plasma membrane), the receptor activates the G-protein, which causes an effector inside cell to produce a "signal" chemical inside cell, which causes the cell to react to the original external chemical signal received.

See also CELL, PLASMA MEMBRANE, TRANSMEMBRANE PROTEINS, RECEPTORS, EGF RECEPTOR, *ras* GENE, NUCLEAR RECEPTORS, SIGNALING, G-PROTEINS, MAST CELLS, CD95 PROTEIN, HORMONE, SUBSTANCE P, LECITHIN, CASCADE, KINASES, LIPIDS

Signaling The "communication" that occurs between and within cells of an organism, e.g., via hormones, nitric acid, etc. Such signaling "tells" certain cells to grow, change, or produce specific proteins at specific times.

See also RECEPTORS, PROTEIN, NUCLEAR RECEPTORS, G-PROTEINS, SIGNAL TRANSDUCTION, TRANSDUCTION (GENE), CD95 PROTEIN, HORMONE, PARKINSON'S DISEASE, HARPIN, SUBSTANCE P, LECITHIN, NITRIC OXIDE, SIGNAL TRANSDUCERS AND ACTIVATORS OF TRANSCRIPTION (STATs), PROTEIN SIGNALING, CASCADE, GENE EXPRESSION ANALYSIS, CHOLINE, KINASES, QUORUM SENSING, CELL MOTILITY

Signaling Molecule A molecule utilized to "**signal**" (**communicate**) with cells or to deliver a **signal** to other organisms (e.g., a signal by the soybean plant to attract the beneficial *Rhizobium* bacteria to colonize their roots). For example, the young offspring of fleas can remain immature (larvae) for up to 2 yr in the absence of a food source, until carbon dioxide molecules and heat from a nearby mammal (potential host or food source) **signal them to mature into adults** in order to prey on the mammal.

For example, the larvae of North American tree frogs (*Rara temporaria*) are **signaled** by chemicals that are released into a pond's water when the first such frog larva is killed by a (predatory) dragonfly nymph (i.e., when those dragonflies first arrive each year at a given pond, to prey on the frog larvae). That chemical "signal" causes all of the North American tree frog larvae in that pond to subsequently grow **tails that are twice as large as were grown by them prior to that chemical signal** in order to facilitate their escape from the dragonfly nymphs.

See also SIGNALING, NITRIC OXIDE, G-PROTEINS, HORMONE, SUBSTANCE P, LEUKOTRIENES, ISOFLAVONES, SOYBEAN PLANT, *RHIZOBIUM* (BACTERIA), HARPIN, OCTADECANOID/JASMONATE SIGNAL COMPLEX, SALICYLIC ACID (SA)

Signaling Protein See SIGNALING MOLECULE

Silencing See GENE SILENCING

Silent Mutation A mutation in a gene that causes no detectable change in the biological characteristics of that gene's product (e.g., a protein).

See also EXPRESS, GENE, PROTEIN

Silk A natural, protein polymer with a predominance of alanine and glycine amino acids. Silk is produced by silkworms that have fed on mulberry tree leaves. The body of a silkworm can retain proteins (i.e., raw material for silk) amounting to as much as 20% of its body weight. It is thought that silk may be altered, via genetic engineering of silkworms, to produce fibers of very high strength.

See also GENETIC ENGINEERING, PROTEIN ENGINEERING, AMINO ACID

Simple Protein A protein that yields only amino acids on hydrolysis (i.e., cleavage of the protein molecule into fragments) and does not have other molecular constituents such as lipids or polysaccharide attachments.

See also PROTEIN, AMINO ACID, GLYCOPROTEIN, LIPIDS, POLYSACCHARIDES

Simple Sequence Repeat (SSR) DNA Marker Technique A "genetic mapping" technique that utilizes the fact that microsatellite sequences "repeat" (i.e., appear repeatedly in sequence within the DNA molecule) in a manner enabling them to be used as "markers."

See also GENETIC MAP, SEQUENCE (OF A DNA MOLECULE), RANDOM AMPLIFIED POLYMORPHIC DNA (RAPD) TECHNIQUE, RESTRICTION FRAGMENT LENGTH POLYMORPHISM (RFLP) TECHNIQUE, DEOXYRIBONUCLEIC ACID (DNA), PHYSICAL MAP (OF GENOME), LINKAGE, LINKAGE GROUP, MARKER (GENETIC MARKER), LINKAGE MAP, TRAIT, MICROSATELLITE DNA, QUANTITATIVE TRAIT LOCI (QTL)

Simple Sequence Repeat (SSR) Genetic Markers See SIMPLE SEQUENCE REPEAT (SSR) DNA MARKER TECHNIQUE

Single-Cell Protein (SCP) A protein that is derived from single-celled organisms with high-protein content. Yeast is an example. Generally used in regard to those organisms that are consumed by domesticated animals, or humans. Single-domain antibodies (dAbs) VH "heavy chains" (portion of antibody molecules) produced by genetically engineered *Escherichia coli* cells that act to bind antigens in a manner similar to antibodies or monoclonal antibodies (MAbs). Similar to MAbs, dAbs can be produced in large quantities, and can be used as human or animal therapeutics (e.g., to combat diseases).

See also ANTIBODY, MONOCLONAL ANTIBODIES (MAb), ANTIGEN, *ESCHERICHIA COLI*

Single-Nucleotide Polymorphisms (SNPs) Variations (in individual nucleotides) that occur within DNA at the rate of approximately 1 in every 1300 base pairs in most organisms (approximately 1 in every 100 base pairs in human DNA). SNPs usually occur in the same genomic location (e.g., on the organism's DNA) in different individuals. These variations account for the following:

• Diversity within a given species (e.g., black cattle and white cattle, different human eye colors, different strains or serotypes within a given bacterial species, etc.).

• Some genetic diseases due to one SNP (e.g., cystic fibrosis, sickle cell anemia, familial dysautonomia, (Duchenne) muscular dystrophy, Huntington's disease, neurofibromatosis, and Tay-Sachs disease).

• The body's response to certain pharmaceuticals and food ingredients. For example, the diuretic drug thiazide works to control hypertension in 60% of U.S. African-Americans, but only 8% of U.S. Caucasian people, due to one SNP. For example, certain pharmaceuticals do not have the desired effect in some groups of humans possessing certain specific "grouped SNPs" known as haplotypes. Because those **groupings of SNPs** are linked (i.e., tend to "travel together" as a group within the genetics of a given population), they can collectively confer a given "multiple-SNP trait" to an identifiable subpopulation of individuals. For example, the pharmaceuticals acetaminophen, aspirin, and Valium remain in the bodies of women (who constitute a haplotype for that pharmacogenomic trait) longer than in men.

Methods utilized to identify SNPs include the following:

- Examination of the DNA of populations of individuals with and without a given (genetically related) disease
- Examination of the DNA of populations of individuals with and without a given trait

Four technologies or methodologies for the detection of SNPs (within a sample of DNA taken from such individuals) are the following:

- Capillary electrophoresis
- Denaturing high-performance liquid chromatography (dHPLC)
- FP-TDI assay (i.e., template-directed dye-terminator incorporation with fluorescence polarization detection), which was developed by Pui-Yan Kwok in 1999
- SNP chip

"SNP mapping" (or haplotype mapping) is a "genetic mapping" technique that utilizes the fact that individual nucleotides (within DNA molecule) can exist in different forms (for a particular "site" or location on that DNA molecule), which enables such SNPs to be utilized as "markers." One example would be to track a given SNP vs. occurrence of genetically related disease in a given human population.
See also POINT MUTATION, DEOXYRIBONUCLEIC ACID (DNA), SEQUENCE (OF A DNA MOLECULE), CAPILLARY ELECTROPHORESIS, NUCLEOTIDE, POLYMORPHISM (GENETIC), GENETICS, GENETIC MAP, PHYSICAL MAP (OF GENOME), GENOME, TRAIT, MARKER (GENETIC MARKER), QUANTITATIVE TRAIT LOCI (QTL), DIVERSITY (WITHIN A SPECIES), BASE PAIR (bp), TRANSVERSION, CYSTIC FIBROSIS TRANSMEMBRANE REGULATOR PROTEIN (CFTR), MUSCULAR DYSTROPHY (MD), HUNTINGTON'S DISEASE, MICROARRAY (TESTING), PHARMACOGENETICS, PHARMACOGENOMICS, HAPLOTYPE, SNP MAP, HAPLOTYPE MAP, TOXICOGENETICS, ORGANISM, HEMOGLOBIN, CHROMATOGRAPHY, ALPHA-SYNUCLEIN, FLUORESCENCE POLARIZATION (FP), SNP CHIP, LEPTIN

Single-Stranded DNA Refers to molecules of "unwound" DNA (i.e., half of the double helix DNA). During 2004, Ming Zheng and coworkers discovered that single-stranded DNA (ssDNA) will under certain circumstances (i.e., sonication in water) "coat" the exteriors of carbon nanotubes, thereby rendering them soluble.
See also DEOXYRIBONUCLEIC ACID (DNA), DOUBLE HELIX, APTAMERS, CARBON NANOTUBES

Single-Walled Carbon Nanotubes See CARBON NANOTUBES

Sir2 Gene See SIRTUINS

siRNA Acronym for **short interfering RNA**. See SHORT INTERFERING RNA (siRNA)

SirT1 Gene See SIRTUINS

Sirtuins Also known by the designation **Sir2**, which stands for **Silent Information Regulator 2**, these are a "family" of proteins (NAD-dependent histone deacetylase enzymes) coded for by the **Sir2** gene (e.g., in *Saccharomyces cerevisiae*) or the SirT1 gene (in mammals). Sirtuins are usually overproduced (i.e., *Sir 2* gene is activated) in *Saccharomyces cerevisiae* yeast by very-low-calorie environment (i.e., near "starvation" of the yeast). During 2003, researchers discovered that the phytochemical resveratrol (3,5,4 trihydroxy stilbene) will also activate sirtuins. When those sirtuins are thus activated (e.g., in *Saccharomyces cerevisiae* yeast), the lifespan of that yeast is greatly extended.
Sir2 proteins deacetylate (i.e., remove **acetyl** molecular groups from) the lysine molecular portions of histones. Because histones are components of chromatin (which makes up chromosomes), the deacetylation causes the chromatin or chromosome structure to become compressed in a manner that silences certain segments of the DNA in the chromosome.
See also PROTEIN, ENZYME, DEOXYRIBONUCLEIC ACID (DNA), CODING SEQUENCE, GENE, TRANSCRIPTIONAL ACTIVATOR, POSITIVE CONTROL, RESVERATROL, NAD (NADH, NADP, NADPH), HISTONES, CHROMATIN, GENE SILENCING, SIR2 GENE, SIRT1 GENE

Site-Directed Mutagenesis (SDM) A technique that can be used to make a protein that

S

differs slightly in its structure from what is normally produced (by an organism or cell). A single mutation (in the cell's DNA) is caused by hybridizing the region in a codon to be mutated with a short, synthetic oligonucleotide. This causes the codon to code for a *different* specific amino acid in the protein gene product.

Site-directed mutagenesis holds the potential to enable man to create modified (engineered) proteins that have desirable properties not currently available in the proteins produced by existing organisms. For example, during the 1990s, Georges Fuller and Charles Gerday utilized SDM (starting with a *Bacillus* bacteria from Antarctica that naturally produces subtilisin) to create an enzyme (for subtilisin production) that possessed 20 times the catalytic activity of other subtilisin-production enzymes.

See also MUTANT, MUTATION, POINT MUTATION, ORGANISM, CELL, PROTEIN, ENZYME, CATALYST, CATALYSIS, GENE, INFORMATIONAL MOLECULES, HEREDITY, GENETIC CODE, GENETIC MAP, AMINO ACID, DEOXYRIBONUCLEIC ACID (DNA), CODON, OLIGONUCLEOTIDE, PROTEIN ENGINEERING, BACTERIA, *BACILLUS*

Sitostanol A chemical (ester) that is derived from sitosterol, which is present in pine trees and fibers (e.g., the hull or seed coat) of corn or maize (*Zea mays*) or soybeans (*Glycine max* (L.)). When sitostanol is consumed by humans in sufficient quantities, it causes their total serum cholesterol and their low-density lipoproteins (LDLP) levels to be lowered by approximately 10%, via inhibition (i.e., the sitostanol is preferentially absorbed by the gastrointestinal system instead of cholesterol). During 2000, the U.S. Food and Drug Administration approved a (label) health claim that associates consumption of sitostanols with reduced blood cholesterol content and with reduced coronary heart disease (CHD).

See also ABSORPTION, DIGESTION (WITHIN ORGANISMS), SOYBEAN PLANT, LOW-DENSITY LIPOPROTEINS (LDLP), SERUM LIFETIME, CHOLESTEROL, STEROLS, PHYTOSTEROLS, SITOSTEROL, CORONARY HEART DISEASE (CHD)

Sitosterol A phytosterol that is naturally produced in fibers within soybean (*Glycine max* (L.)) hulls, pumpkin seeds, pine trees, fibers of corn or maize (*Zea mays*) seed coats, etc. Sitosterol can exist in several different molecular forms (e.g., known as α, β, etc.). A human diet containing large amounts of sitosterol and/or certain other phytosterols (e.g., campesterol, stigmasterol, etc.) has been shown to lower total serum (blood) cholesterol and low-density lipoprotein (LDLP) levels, thereby lowering the risk of coronary heart disease (CHD). Evidence indicates that certain phytosterols (including sitosterol) interfere with absorption of cholesterol by the intestines and decrease the body's recovery and reuse of cholesterol-containing bile salts, which causes more cholesterol to be excreted from the body than previously. During 2000, the U.S. Food and Drug Administration approved a (label) health claim that associates consumption of sitosterols with reduced blood cholesterol content and reduced coronary heart disease (CHD).

See also PHYTOSTEROLS, SOYBEAN PLANT, CORN, STEROLS, SITOSTANOL, CAMPESTEROL, STIGMASTEROL, CORONARY HEART DISEASE (CHD), BETA-SITOSTEROL, CHOLESTEROL

SK See SUBSTANCE K

Slime An extracellular (i.e., outside of the cell) material that is produced by some (micro)organisms, characterized by a slimy consistency. The slime is of varied chemical composition. However, usual components are polysaccharides (polysugars) and specific protein molecules.

See also CELL, BIOFILM, POLYSACCHARIDES, PROTEIN

Small Interfering RNA See SHORT INTERFERING RNA (siRNA)

Small RNA See SHORT INTERFERING RNA (siRNA)

Small Ubiquitin-Related Modifier Abbreviated **SUMO,** it is a "partner protein" that readily fuses with certain other protein molecules, and causes the following:

- Enhanced expression of those other protein molecules
- Enhanced solubility of those other protein molecules
- Correct folding of those other protein molecules

See also PROTEIN, FUSION PROTEIN, EXPRESS, EXPRESSIVITY, PROTEIN FOLDING, PROTEIN STRUCTURE, CONFORMATION, UBIQUITIN

Smoothened One of the proteins within the hedgehog signaling pathway that is required for hedgehog signaling to occur.

See also PROTEIN, HEDGEHOG PROTEINS, HEDGEHOG-SIGNALING PATHWAY

Smut See *TELETHIA CONTROVERSIA KOON* SMUT

SNP See SINGLE-NUCLEOTIDE POLYMORPHISMS (SNPs)

SNP Chip Refers to a piece of glass, plastic, or silicon onto which has been placed a large number of **strands of DNA that are complementary to one or more known SNPs** (single-nucleotide polymorphisms). Such "SNP chips" (sometimes known as microarrays) can then be utilized to test a single biological sample for the presence of given SNPs. For example, human blood samples could potentially be tested for the presence of the SNPs responsible for the following:

- Cystic fibrosis
- Sickle cell anemia
- Muscular dystrophy (Duchenne)
- Tay-Sachs disease

For example, human blood samples could potentially be tested for the presence of the following:

- The body's response **or failure to respond to** certain pharmaceuticals (e.g., the diuretic thiazide)
- The body's response **or lack of response to** certain toxins

See also SINGLE-NUCLEOTIDE POLYMORPHISMS (SNP), POINT MUTATION, DEOXYRIBONUCLEIC ACID (DNA), HYBRIDIZATION (MOLECULAR BIOLOGY), COMPLEMENTARY (MOLECULAR GENETICS), MICROARRAY (TESTING), DNA CHIP, BIOCHIP, CYSTIC FIBROSIS TRANSMEMBRANE REGULATOR PROTEIN (CFTR), MUSCULAR DYSTROPHY (MD), HIGH-THROUGHPUT SCREENING (HTS), PHARMACOGENETICS, PHARMACOGENOMICS, SNP MAP, HAPLOTYPE, HAPLOTYPE MAP, TOXIN, TOXICOGENETICS

SNP Map A group of known or detailed SNPs (single-nucleotide polymorphisms) superimposed onto the genome map of an organism (e.g., to facilitate genetic and population studies, such as of genetically-related disease susceptibility).

See also SINGLE-NUCLEOTIDE POLYMORPHISMS (SNPs), ORGANISM, GENOME, GENOMIC SCIENCES, MAPPING (OF GENOME), MAP DISTANCE, MARKER (DNA SEQUENCE), YSTR DNA

SNP Markers See SINGLE-NUCLEOTIDE POLYMORPHISMS (SNPs)

snRNP Acronym for **small nuclear ribonucleoproteins**.

See ALTERNATIVE SPLICING, INTRON, SPLICEOSOMES

Sodium Dodecyl Sulfate See SDS

Sodium Lauryl Sulfate See SDS

Soft Laser Desorption See ICM

Solanine A glycoside neurotoxin (glycoalkyloid) that is naturally present in low levels in potatoes. As a result of this, solanine is present at detectable levels in the bloodstream of humans that consume potatoes. When consumed by humans, solanine acts as a plasma cholinesterase inhibitor. The U.S. Food and Drug Administration (FDA) prohibits the sale in the U.S. of potatoes that contain more (than the stipulated level of solanine); for example, the natural level of solanine in potatoes can unfortunately increase in harvested potatoes that are exposed to direct sunlight.

See also TOXIN, PHYTOTOXIN, CHACONINE, GLYCOSIDE, WILD TYPE, FOOD AND DRUG ADMINISTRATION (FDA), TRADITIONAL BREEDING METHODS, PLASMA, CHOLINESTERASE, INHIBITION

Solid-Phase Synthesis See SYNTHESIZING (OF PROTEINS), SYNTHESIZING (OF DNA MOLECULES)

Solid Support See SUBSTRATE (STRUCTURAL)

Soluble CD4 A synthetic version of the CD4 protein that (when in solution in the bloodstream) interferes with the ability of adhesion molecules on HIV (i.e., AIDS) viruses to infect the relevant human immune system cells.

See also CD4 PROTEIN, ADHESION MOLECULE, SELECTINS, LECTINS, PROTEIN

Soluble Fiber See WATER-SOLUBLE FIBER

Somaclonal Variation The genetic variation (i.e., new traits) that results from the growing of entire new plants from plant cells or tissues (e.g., maintained in culture). Frequently encountered when plants are regenerated (grown) from cells that have been altered via genetic engineering. However, somaclonal variation (i.e., new genetic traits) can occur even in standard tissue culture when plants are regenerated from cells that were part of the same original plant.

See also CELL CULTURE, SOMATIC VARIANTS, CLONE (AN ORGANISM), *AGROBACTERIUM TUMEFACIENS*, BIOLISTIC® GENE GUN, "EXPLOSION" METHOD, SHOTGUN METHOD

Somatacrin See GROWTH-HORMONE-RELEASING FACTOR (GRF or GHRF)

Somatic Cells All eucaryote body cells except the gametes and the cells from which they develop.

See also GAMETE, OOCYTES

Somatic Variants Regenerated plants (i.e., clones) that were derived (produced) from cells that originally came from the same plant that are not genetically identical. Such plants (clones) are called "sports" or somatic variants because they vary (genetically) from the "parent" plant. Sometimes, such somatic variants are developed by humans to produce a new plant variety (e.g., the nectarine is an example of this).

See also SOMACLONAL VARIATION, CELL CULTURE, CLONE (AN ORGANISM), GENOTYPE

Somatomedins A family of peptides that mediates the action of growth hormone on skeletal tissue and stimulates bone formation.

See also HUMAN GROWTH HORMONE (HGH), PEPTIDE, BONE MORPHOGENETIC PROTEINS (BMP)

Somatostatin A 14-amino-acid peptide that inhibits the release of growth hormone.

See also HUMAN GROWTH HORMONE (HGH), GROWTH-HORMONE-RELEASING FACTOR (GRF or GHRF), PEPTIDE

Somatotropin Category of hormone that is produced naturally in the bodies of all mammals, including humans.

See also HORMONE, GROWTH HORMONE, BOVINE SOMATOTROPIN (BST), PORCINE SOMATOTROPIN (PST)

Sonic Hedgehog Protein (Shh) See HEDGEHOG PROTEINS

SOS Protein See SOS RESPONSE (IN *ESCHERICHIA COLI* BACTERIA)

SOS Repair System First postulated by Miroslav Radman in 1970, it refers to a **secondary or alternative** DNA repair system utilized by living cells to repair the cell's DNA when damaged (e.g., by radiation) and such a damage prevents usage of the cell's primary DNA repair system.

See also CELL, DEOXYRIBONUCLEIC ACID (DNA), DNA REPAIR, SOS RESPONSE (IN *ESCHERICHIA COLI* BACTERIA), GENE REPAIR (NATURAL)

SOS Response (in *Escherichia coli* bacteria) The "switching on" of genetic repair machinery in this bacteria when its DNA has been damaged (e.g., by radiation).

See also DEOXYRIBONUCLEIC ACID (DNA), DNA REPAIR, *ESCHERICHIA COLIFORM (E. coli)*, GENE REPAIR (NATURAL)

SOS1 Gene See ANTIPORTER

Southern Blot Analysis Invented in 1975 by Edwin Mellor Southern, it is a test that is performed on biological samples such as restriction endonuclease-digested (i.e., fragmented) plant DNA (e.g., to ascertain if genetic engineering–"inserted" DNA is present in particular plant cells). Gel electrophoresis is used to separate the DNA fragments according to their size, and then those are transferred to a filter (blot).

Radiolabeled DNA probes or RNA probes are added, and the ones that are complementary to each of the (separated, on blot) fragments will hybridize to those respective DNA fragments. The location (i.e., on the blot) and "radioactive label" of those hybridized probes can then be utilized to determine the nature of the initial DNA that was in those plant cells.

See also DEOXYRIBONUCLEIC ACID (DNA), RIBONUCLEIC ACID (RNA), GENETIC ENGINEERING, RESTRICTION

ENDONUCLEASES, ELECTROPHORE-SIS, TWO-DIMENSIONAL (2-D) GEL ELECTROPHORESIS, POLYACRYAMIDE GEL ELECTROPHORESIS (PAGE), RADI-OLABELED, DNA PROBE, COMPLEMEN-TARY (MOLECULAR GENETICS), HYBRIDIZATION (MOLECULAR GENET-ICS), RADIOIMMUNOASSAY

Southern Corn Rootworm Latin name *Diabrotica undecimpunctata hawardii.*

See CORN ROOTWORM

Southwestern Blot A testing methodology utilized to detect **protein–DNA interactions**. It is based on usage of special "labeled" seg-ments of DNA to test (interactions with) pro-tein molecules that were transferred to mem-brane filters via a blotting procedure.

See also PROTEIN, DEOXYRIBONUCLEIC ACID (DNA)

Soy Protein An edible protein (after heat pro-cessing) that is produced within its beans (seeds) by the soybean plant (botanical name *Glycine max* (L.) Merrill). When removed from soybeans via crushing, extrusion, or other processes involving adequate heat treatment, soy protein is (historical average) composed of 2.5% cys-teine, 3.4% histidine, 5.2% isoleucine, 8.2% leu-cine, 6.8% lysine, 1.1% methionine, 5.6% phe-nylalanine, 4.2% threonine, 1.3% tryptophan, 4.2% tyrosine, 5.4% valine, 4% alanine, 7.7% arginine, 6.9% aspartic acid, 19% glutamic acid, 3.7% glycine, 0.1% 4-hydroxyproline, 5.3% proline, and 5.4% serine.

Soy protein (concentrate) is a complete (i.e., "ideal") protein (i.e., it provides all essential amino acids) for humans. It is a good dietary source of calcium with an absorption rate equivalent to milk.

In its initial form (i.e., following crushing or extrusion from soybeans as described in the preceding text), the soy protein is known as soybean meal and contains a bit less than half of protein by weight. If the soy is washed with water (following crushing or extrusion) to remove soluble polysaccharides (e.g., the carbohydrates known as stachyose, raffinose, etc.), the resultant soy protein is known as soy protein concentrate and contains approximately 60% protein by weight. If the soy is washed with water-and-alkali solution, followed by isoelectric precipita-tion of the soluble protein, the result is "iso-lated soy protein" (ISP); and is often known as soy protein isolate or soy isolate. In 1999, the U.S. FDA approved a (label) health claim that associates consumption of soy protein with reduced blood cholesterol content and with reduced coronary heart disease (CHD) in humans.

Consumption of soy protein has been shown to result in upregulation of a human's P53 gene (i.e., a tumor suppressor gene that helps to prevent tissues from becoming cancerous).

See also SOYBEAN PLANT, TRYPSIN INHIBITORS, PROTEIN, CHOLESTEROL, CORONARY HEART DISEASE (CHD), AMINO ACID, ESSENTIAL AMINO ACIDS, "IDEAL PROTEIN" CONCEPT, PROTEIN-DIGESTIBILITY-CORRECTED AMINO ACID SCORING (PCDAAS), FER-RITIN, STACHYOSE, UBIQUINONE, GENE, UPREGULATION, P53 GENE, TUMOR SUPPRESSOR GENES, ONCO-GENES

Soybean Aphid An aphid (*Aphis glycines*) that is native to China, but was accidentally intro-duced into the U.S. during the 1990s (appar-ently via aphid eggs adhering to an ornamental plant). It feeds on the sap of the soybean plant (*Glycine max* (L.)).

See also SOYBEAN PLANT

Soybean Cyst Nematodes (SCN) Microscopic roundworms (*Heterodera glycines*) living in the soil that feed parasitically on roots of the soybean plant. The nematodes use a spear-like mouthpart, called a stylet, to puncture the plant's root cells in order to eat the cell con-tents. This root damage causes the soybean's growth to be stunted, and the plants turn yel-low because of a reduction in nodule forma-tion by the nitrogen-fixing *Rhizobium* bacteria (which normally colonize roots of soybean plants). SCN can combine with a fungus (*Fusarium solani*) to cause a soybean plant disease known as "sudden death syndrome."

As part of integrated pest management (IPM), farmers can utilize naturally resis-tant soybean varieties (e.g., CystX) and/or the parasitic Pasteuria bacteria to help con-trol the soybean cyst nematodes. The *Pas-teuria* bacteria must attach their spores (for reproduction) to juvenile nematodes so that the *Pasteuria* offspring can consume the SCN when the spores later germinate.

See also SOYBEAN PLANT, NITROGEN FIX-ATION, BACTERIA, *RHIZOBIUM* (BACTE-RIA), FUNGUS, SUDDEN DEATH SYN-DROME, ALLELOPATHY, ISOFLAVONES, NEMATODES, CystX

Soybean Meal See SOYBEAN PLANT, SOY PROTEIN

Soybean Oil An edible oil that is produced within its beans (seeds) by the soybean plant (botanical name is *Glycine max* (L.) Merrill). When removed from soybeans via crushing and refining processes, soybean oil is (historical average) composed of 60.8% polyunsaturated fatty acids (PUFA), 24.5% monounsaturated fatty acids, and 15.1% saturated fatty acids. However, soybean varieties have recently been created that possess as little as 7% saturated fatty acids.

See also POLYUNSATURATED FATTY ACIDS (PUFA), FATTY ACID, ESSENTIAL FATTY ACIDS, LECITHIN, HYDROGENATION, SOYBEAN PLANT, HIGH-OLEIC OIL SOY-BEANS, LOW-LINOLENIC-OIL SOY-BEANS, LINOLENIC ACID, OLEIC ACID, LINOLEIC ACID, MONOUNSATURATED FATTY ACIDS, SATURATED FATTY ACIDS, CONJUGATED LINOLEIC ACID

Soybean Plant Botanical name *Glycine max* (L.) Merrill. A green, bushy legume that is the world's single largest provider of protein and edible oil for mankind's use. In summer, this annual plant varies in height from less than 1 ft (0.3 m) to more than 3 ft (1 m). The seeds (soybeans) are borne in pods, and historically have contained 13 to 26% oil and 38 to 45% protein (on a moisture-free basis). Its leaves contain some carotenoids.

The soybean plant has approximately 80,000 genes. It is a self-pollinating plant (i.e., male and female reproductive structures on the same plant, and so it is monoecious).

Soybean hulls (i.e., outer seed coat) contain a total of 0.03 to 0.06% of the plant sterols (phytosterols) campesterol, stigmasterol, and beta-sitosterol (B-sitosterol). Soybeans contain the highest amount of isoflavones of any plant (seeds), i.e., up to 0.3% of each soybean's dry weight.

The traditional soybean, possessing 20% (average) oil content, contains an average of 3% stachyose within its meal (i.e., the solids remaining after the soybean oil is removed).

See also FATTY ACID, PROTEIN, SOY PRO-TEIN, LECITHIN, NITROGEN FIXATION, NODULATION, SOYBEAN OIL, SOYBEAN CYST NEMATODES (SCN), RESVERA-TROL, BROWN STEM ROT, PHYTOPH-THORA ROOT ROT, PEROXIDASE, ISOFLAVONES, LOW-STACHYOSE SOY-BEANS, GENISTEIN (Gen), LIPOXYGEN-ASE (LOX), SAPONINS, CANOLA, CHLO-ROPLAST TRANSIT PEPTIDE (CTP), HERBICIDE-TOLERANT CROP, LOX NULL, PHYTOCHEMICALS, CORN ROOT-WORM, NITRIC OXIDE (NO), MONOE-CIOUS, ALLELOPATHY, LOW-LINOLENIC-OIL SOYBEANS, HIGH-OLEIC-OIL SOY-BEANS, HIGH-PHYTASE (SOYBEANS), HIGH-ISOFLAVONE SOYBEANS, HIGH-STEARATE SOYBEANS, HIGH-SUCROSE SOYBEANS, REDUCED-ALLERGEN SOY-BEANS, WATER-SOLUBLE FIBER, LOW-PHYTATE SOYBEANS, *PHYTOPHTHORA MEGASPERMA f.* sp. *GLYCINEA*, STACHY-OSE, PHYTOSTEROLS, CAMPESTEROL, STIGMASTEROL, SITOSTEROL, BETA-SITOSTEROL (B-SITOSTEROL), SITO-STANOL, PHOSPHATIDYL SERINE, CORO-NARY HEART DISEASE (CHD), SOYBEAN APHID, CAROTENOIDS, TOCOPHEROLS, *Rhizobium* (BACTERIA), PHARMACOENVI-ROGENETICS, UBIQUINONE, CHOLINE, *BRADYRHIZOBIUM JAPONICUM*, P34 PRO-TEIN, REDUCED-ALLERGEN SOYBEANS, NOD GENES, NARK GENE

SP See SUBSTANCE P

SP-1 A protein naturally produced in poplar trees that helps to ensure that protein molecules (e.g., when emerging from cell's ribosomes) are folded correctly. Under certain conditions, SP-1 will self-assemble its molecules into large molecular structures consisting of 12 repeated molecular units.

See also PROTEIN, PROTEIN FOLDING, CELL, CHAPERONES, RIBOSOMES, CONFORMATION, SELF-ASSEMBLY (OF A LARGE MOLECULAR STRUCTURE)

Species A single type (taxonomic group) or organism as determined by the distinguishing characteristics of the particular group of life forms (e.g., the horse is one species among the mammals).

Whereas the horse is easily distinguished from other **obviously** nonsimilar mammals, such as humans, it is less easy to distinguish a horse from a more closely related animal such as a donkey or a zebra.

The so-called "**boundary between different species**" is determined by human assessment or categorization (e.g., whether **systematics** or **cladistics** are utilized by those doing the species categorization and definitions) and sometimes **changes** when more information becomes known at a later date (e.g., if new two-dimensional electrophoresis tests reveal certain species to be genetically related or not).

See also STRAIN, SYSTEMATICS, CLADISTICS, CONSERVED, DIVERSITY (WITHIN A SPECIES), ELECTROPHORESIS, TWO-DIMENSIONAL (2-D) GEL ELECTROPHORESIS

Species Specific Refers to a compound (e.g., a protein), a disease (e.g., a viral infection), or some other effect that only acts in/on one specific species of organism. For example, the antibiotic penicillin kills bacteria by blocking an enzyme that is critical for growth and repair of the bacterial cell wall (i.e., peptidoglycan layer), but penicillin does not harm other species (e.g., man). For instance, bovine somatotropin is a protein hormone that increases growth rate of young cattle and also increases the efficiency of mature cows in converting their feed into milk. Bovine somatotropin has no effect in humans, and (if eaten) is simply digested like any other food protein. It appears that most growth hormones are species specific.

See also SPECIES, HORMONE, PENICILLIN G (BENZYLPENICILLIN)

Specific Activity An enzyme unit defined as the number of moles of substrate converted per unit time to a product by an enzyme preparation under specified conditions of pH, substrate concentration, temperature, etc. Specific enzyme activity units may be expressed as moles of product produced per minute per mg of protein used (or mole of enzyme used if the preparation is pure).

See also MOLE, ENZYME, SUBSTRATE (CHEMICAL)

Spectrophotometer An instrument that measures the concentration of a compound that has been dissolved in a solvent (such as water, alcohol, etc.). The instrument shines a light through the solution, measures the fraction of the light that is absorbed by the solution, and calculates the concentration from that absorbance value.

See also OPTICAL DENSITY (OD), ABSORBANCE (A)

Spinosad ™ A pesticide that is active against certain insects and mites, whose active ingredients (i.e., spinosyn A and spinosyn D) are naturally produced by the soil bacterium *Saccaropolyspora*.

Research shows that Spinosad ™ is effective in controlling the lesser grain borer and other stored-grain insects. Spinosad ™ and its registered trademark are owned by Dow Chemical Company.

See also SPINOSYNS, BACTERIA, WEEVILS

Spinosyns A "family" of pesticidal compounds, active against certain insects and mites, that are naturally produced by some species of bacteria (e.g., *Saccaropolyspora spinosa*).

See also SPINOSAD, BACTERIA, SPECIES

Splice Forms See SPLICE VARIANTS

Splice Variants Refers to the several different proteins that can be expressed from a single given gene via all possible gene transcripts (i.e., different mRNAs resulting from alternative splicing).

See also GENE, PROTEIN, EXPRESS, EXPRESSION, ALTERNATIVE SPLICING, TRANSCRIPTOME

Spliceosomes The cells' entities that process primary RNA to remove introns and to ligate (i.e., attach together) exons, resulting in the mRNA transcript that the cell uses for translation. Spliceosomes consist of a molecular complex made up of both RNA (ribonucleic acid) and snRNPs (small nuclear ribonucleoproteins).

See also TRANSCRIPTION, TRANSLATION, CELL, INTRON, RIBONUCLEIC ACID (RNA), EXON, LIGATION, TRANSCRIPT, MESSENGER RNA (mRNA), ALTERNATIVE SPLICING, SPLICE VARIANTS, EDITING

Splicing The removal of introns and joining of exons in RNA (e.g., genes). Thus, introns are spliced out, whereas exons are spliced together.

See also EXON, INTRON, GENETIC ENGI-
NEERING, RIBONUCLEIC ACID (RNA),
CENTRAL DOGA (NEW), ALTERNATIVE
SPLICING, DIFFERENTIAL SPLICING

Splicing (of protein molecule) The removal
of an intein (i.e., an intervening protein
domain in "center" of a protein molecule)
either spontaneously or by human manipulation, followed by joining together of the
two exteins (i.e., **end segments** of the protein molecule).

See also PROTEIN, INTEIN, EXTEIN,
DOMAIN, SEQUENCE (OF A PROTEIN
MOLECULE), EXCISION (OF PROTEIN
MOLECULE), DOMAIN (OF A PROTEIN)

Splicing Junctions The sequences (in RNA
molecules) of nucleotides immediately surrounding the exon–intron boundaries.

See also EXON, INTRON, SPLICING, ALTER-
NATIVE SPLICING, DIFFERENTIAL
SPLICING, SPLICE VARIANTS, RIBONU-
CLEIC ACID (RNA), NUCLEOTIDE,
SEQUENCE (OF A DNA MOLECULE)

SPM See ATOMIC FORCE MICROSCOPY

Spontaneous Assembly See SELF-ASSEMBLY

SPR Acronym for **Surface Plasmon Resonance**.

See SURFACE PLASMON RESONANCE
(SPR)

SPS Acronym for the **Sanitary and Phytosanitary Standards Agreement of the World
Trade Organization** (WTO), a multinational
trading agreement that "sets the rules" that
govern international trade. Sanitary (i.e., with
regard to human and animal) and phytosanitary (i.e., with regard to plant) standards are
important in preventing the transfer of diseases from one nation to another via international trade. SPS standards are designed to
protect animal, plant, and human life and
health (within WTO member countries) from:

- Entry of pests (e.g., insects, weeds,
  etc.)
- Entry of disease-carrying organisms
  (e.g., European corn borer)
- Entry of disease-causing organisms
  (e.g., *Aspergillus flavus*)
- Toxins, contaminants, or disease-
  causing organisms in foods, beverages, or feedstuffs

WTO member nations are required to base their
SPS standards as much as possible on **existing**
(e.g., Codex Alimentarius, IPPC, and OIE)
**international sanitary and phytosanitary
standards** and practices.

See also SANITARY AND PHYTOSANITARY
(SPS) AGREEMENT, SANITARY AND PHY-
TOSANITARY (SPS) MEASURES, INTER-
NATIONAL PLANT PROTECTION CON-
VENTION (IPPC), INTERNATIONAL
OFFICE OF EPIZOOTICS (OIE), CODEX
ALIMENTARIUS COMMISSION, MAXI-
MUM RESIDUE LEVEL (MRL), WORLD
TRADE ORGANIZATION (WTO), EURO-
PEAN CORN BORER (ECB), *ASPERGILLUS
FLAVUS*

Squalamine A potent antimicrobial agent (steroid, antibiotic) that was discovered in the
tissues of the dogfish shark in 1992. It has
been found to be active against a broad spectrum of bacteria, protozoa, and fungi.
Squalamine was chemically synthesized in
1993.

See also MAGAININS, STEROID, FUNGUS,
BACTERIA, BACTERIOCINS, PROTO-
ZOA, ANTIBIOTIC

Squalene A sterol that is produced in some
plants.

See STEROLS

SRB (Sulfate-Reducing Bacterium) Any
organism that metabolically reduces sulfate to
H_2S (hydrogen sulfide). This includes a variety of microorganisms.

See also REDUCTION (IN A CHEMICAL
REACTION), METABOLISM, MICROOR-
GANISM, FERROBACTERIA

ssDNA Acronym for **single-stranded DNA**.

See also DEOXYRIBONUCLEIC ACID
(DNA), SINGLE-STRANDED DNA,
APTAMERS

SSR See SIMPLE SEQUENCE REPEAT
(SSR) DNA MARKER TECHNIQUE

ssRNA Acronym for **single-stranded RNA**.

See also RIBONUCLEIC ACID (RNA),
INNATE IMMUNE RESPONSE

Stacchyose See STACHYOSE

Stachyose A carbohydrate (oligosaccharide)
that is naturally produced in soybeans (and
some other plants). Stachyose is relatively
insoluble in water, and much less of it is available for digestion by monogastric animals

(e.g., swine, poultry) than the other carbohydrate components within soybeans.

See also CARBOHYDRATES (SACCHARIDES), LOW-STACHYOSE SOYBEANS, OLIGOSACCHARIDES, SOYBEAN PLANT

"Stacked" Genes Refers to the insertion of two or more (synthetic) genes into the genome of an organism. One example of that would be a plant into which has been inserted a gene from *Bacillus thuringiensis (B.t.)*, and a gene for resistance to a specific herbicide.

See also GENE, BIOTECHNOLOGY, GENETIC ENGINEERING, *BACILLUS THURINGIENSIS (B.t.), B.t. KURSTAKI,* GENETICALLY ENGINEERED MICROBIAL PESTICIDES (GEMP), EPSP SYNTHASE, PAT GENE, BAR GENE

Staggered Cuts Scissions (cuts) made in duplex DNA when the two strands of DNA that make up the duplex DNA are cleaved at different points near each other by restriction endonucleases. What is produced is a single-stranded structure (in which the single strands are a number of nucleotide bases long) with a double-stranded core section. This core section is much longer than the single-stranded region.

See also DEOXYRIBONUCLEIC ACID (DNA), RESTRICTION ENDONUCLEASES, STICKY ENDS

Stanol Ester See SITOSTANOL

Stanol Fatty Acid Esters See SITOSTANOL, FATTY ACID

Starch A polymer of glucose molecules (i.e., a polysaccharide) used by plants to store energy. Plants produce starch in two different molecular forms, amylopectin and amylose. For example, the starch content in traditional corn (maize) kernels averages 72 to 76% amylopectin and 24 to 28% amylose.

Starch is broken down by enzymes (amylases) to yield glucose, which can be used as an energy source. The analogous polymer that is used by mammalian systems is called glycogen or, in old usage, "animal starch."

See also GLUCOSE (GLc), ENZYME, AMYLASE, ALPHA AMYLASE (α-AMYLASE), CORN, AMYLOSE, AMYLOPECTIN

Startpoint Refers to the position on a DNA molecule corresponding to the first base incorporated into mRNA.

See also DEOXYRIBONUCLEIC ACID (DNA), MESSENGER RNA (mRNA), EXON, RIBONUCLEIC ACID (RNA), KOZAK SEQUENCE

Stearate (Stearic Acid) A saturated fatty acid containing 18 carbon atoms in its molecular "backbone," which is essentially neutral in effect on coronary heart disease in humans (i.e., does not appreciably increase low-density lipoproteins in the bloodstream). Because of the heart disease neutrality, stearate-containing oils (e.g., high-stearate soybean oil) are an acceptable cooking oil choice, with the resistance to oxidation or breakdown of a saturated fatty acid but no bloodstream-cholesterol increasing effect. In the mid-1990s, the American Cocoa Research Institute/Chocolate Manufacturers Association filed a petition with U.S. Food and Drug Administration (FDA) to differentiate stearate (on food product labels) from the other saturated long-chain fatty acids used as food ingredients. In order to make milk, dairy cows require more stearic acid than that provided by a conventional digestive system alone from the cow's (mainly carbohydrate) diet. Therefore, cows utilize microorganisms living in their rumen (i.e., a special sort of prestomach) to convert carbohydrate (grass) to stearic acid. Thus, high-performance dairy cows might benefit from a diet that contained high-stearate soybeans, if their milk output is limited by dietary stearate availability.

See also FATTY ACID, LOW-DENSITY LIPOPROTEINS (LDLP), SATURATED FATTY ACIDS, FOOD AND DRUG ADMINISTRATION (FDA), HIGH-STEARATE SOYBEANS, FATS, ENOYL-ACYL PROTEIN REDUCTASE, HIGH-STEARATE CANOLA

Stearic Acid See STEARATE

Stearidonate Another name for stearidonic acid.

See STEARIDONIC ACID

Stearidonic Acid A fatty acid that is naturally produced in the seeds of some plants (e.g., *Nasa carunculata, Nasa hornii, Nasa* cf. *magnifica, Borago officinalis* L., etc.). When consumed by humans, stearidonic acid is readily converted into the n-3 fatty acids **eicosapentanoic acid** and **docosahexanoic acid**.

S

See also FATTY ACID, N-3 FATTY ACIDS, EICOSAPENTANOIC ACID (EPA), DOCOSAHEXAENOIC ACID (DHA)

Stearoyl-ACP Desaturase A "family" of enzymes that is naturally produced in oilseed plants. They play the central role in determining the ratio of saturated to unsaturated fatty acids (in the vegetable oils produced from such plants).

See also FATS, FATTY ACID, ENZYME, GENETIC ENGINEERING, GENETIC CODE, LAURATE, HIGH-STEARATE SOYBEANS, HIGH-STEARATE CANOLA

Stem Cell Growth Factor (SCF) A growth factor (glycoprotein hormone) that acts on certain stem cells in a wide variety of ways to increase growth, proliferation, and maturity (into red blood cells or white blood cells).

See also STEM CELLS, GROWTH FACTOR, HORMONE, GLYCOPROTEIN, DIFFERENTIATION, TOTIPOTENT STEM CELLS, COLONY STIMULATING FACTORS (CSFs), ADULT STEM CELL

Stem Cell One The single stem cell in the bone marrow of a fetus from which every immune system cell in the adult is subsequently derived. The primordial stem cell is stimulated to develop into the mature immune system's differentiated, specialized cells by interleukin-7.

See also STEM CELLS, TOTIPOTENT STEM CELLS, INTERLEUKIN-7 (IL-7), EMBRYONIC STEM CELLS, DIFFERENTIATION

Stem Cells Certain cells — present in the bodies of mammals even prior to birth, **also present in adult mammals** — that can grow or differentiate into different cells and tissues of the (adult organism) body. For example, bone marrow (stem) cells, some of which eventually mature into red blood cells or white blood cells. The stem cells that remain in the bone marrow maintain their own numbers by self-renewal divisions, yielding more (adult stem cell) cells to start the maturation process. This maturation process is stimulated and controlled by stem cell growth factor (SCF), granulocyte colony-stimulating factor (G-CSF), and by granulocyte-macrophage colony-stimulating factor (GM-CSF). During 2000, research by Richard Childs showed that stem cells (i.e., collected from a sibling's bloodstream and) transplanted into a patient suffering from kidney cancer could induce generation of a "**new**" **immune system** that could help stop or reverse the kidney cancer.

During 2003, research led by Songtao Shi showed that living stem cells (can be easily collected) remain in a child's baby teeth (i.e., the temporary teeth that begin to fall out when the child is approximately six years old) after they fall out of the child's mouth.

See also CELL, ADULT STEM CELL, MULTIPOTENT ADULT STEM CELLS, ECTODERMAL ADULT STEM CELLS, ENDODERMAL ADULT STEM CELLS, MESODERMAL ADULT STEM CELLS, HEMATOPOIETIC STEM CELLS, RED BLOOD CELLS, WHITE BLOOD CELLS, BASOPHILS, STEM CELL ONE, STEM CELL GROWTH FACTOR (SCF), TOTIPOTENT STEM CELLS, TOTIPOTENCY, EMBRYONIC STEM CELLS, DIFFERENTIATION, IMMUNE RESPONSE, CANCER, MONOCYTES

Stereoisomers Molecules that have the same structural formula, but different spatial arrangements of dissimilar groups (of atoms) bonded to a common atom (in the molecule). Many of the physical and chemical properties of stereoisomers are the same, but there are differences in the crystal structures, in the direction in which they rotate polarized light (that has been passed through a solution of the stereoisomer), and in their use in an enzyme-catalyzed (biological) reaction.

See also RACEMATE, POLARIMETER, DEXTROROTARY (D) ISOMER, EPIMERS, ISOMER, LEVOROTARY (L) ISOMER, ISOMERASE, DIASTEREOISOMERS, ENANTIOMERS, NANOTUBE

Steric Hindrance This term refers to the compression that a group (chemical entity) suffers by being too close to its nonbonded neighbors. If an enzyme and a substrate try to come together in order to react but the substrate has on it a bulky group that disallows close contact between the two (because the group bumps into the enzyme), then the reaction will not occur because of steric hindrance. Seen in another way, two chemical groups bump into each other and cannot get by each other because they are held in place by the bonds that bind them to other atoms. Hindrance of movement or activity occurs because chemical groups bump into each other and cannot occupy the same space.

See also REPRESSION (OF AN ENZYME), INHIBITION, COREPRESSOR, STRUCTURE–ACTIVITY MODELS

Sterile (environment) One that is free of any living organisms or spores. For example, a hypodermic needle that has been sterilized (e.g., by heating it) and is free of living microorganisms is said to be sterile.

See also MICROORGANISM

Sterile (organism) One that is unable to reproduce. For example, a bull that has been castrated is rendered sterile.

See also TRIPLOID, BARNASE

Sterilization See STERILE (ENVIRONMENT), STERILE (ORGANISM)

Steroid A chemical compound composed of a series of four carbon rings joined together to form a (molecular) structural unit called cyclopentanoperhydrophenanthrene. Any of a group of naturally occurring, fat-soluble substances, essential to life, usually classed as lipids. Steroids of importance to the body are the sterols, which are bile acids (produced by the liver, characterized by the presence of a carboxyl group in the molecule's side chain), and the hormones of the sex glands, and the adrenal cortex. In addition, the plant kingdom possesses a wide variety of steroid glycosides.

See also GLYCOSIDE, LIPIDS, HORMONE, CHOLESTEROL, STEROLS, SAPONINS, CORTISOL

Sterols Solid alcohols consisting of ring-structured molecules (i.e., a "ring" made of atoms). Evidence suggests that human consumption of certain phytosterols (i.e., sterols produced in plant seeds) can help to prevent certain types of cancers and can help lower levels of total blood serum cholesterol and low-density lipoproteins (LDLP), thereby reducing risk of coronary heart disease (CHD).

Evidence indicates that those phytosterols interfere with absorption of cholesterol by the intestines, and they decrease the body's recovery and reuse of cholesterol-containing bile salts, which causes more cholesterol to be excreted from the body. Elevated levels in the body of those phytosterols activate LXRs (Liver X Receptors), which thereby act as **cholesterol sensors,** transactivating a "family" of genes that collectively control the catabolism (i.e., break down to yield energy), transport, and elimination of cholesterol, thereby lowering the body's blood cholesterol levels.

During 2000, researcher Joseph Judd fed phytosterols extracted from soybeans (*Glycine max* (L.)) to human volunteers who were already consuming a "low-fat" diet. Their total blood serum cholesterol and low-density lipoproteins (LDLP) levels decreased by more than 10% in a short time.

During 2001, the U.S. FDA approved a (label) health claim that associates the consumption of plant sterols with reduced blood cholesterol content and reduced coronary heart disease (CHD).

Some of the sterols known to impart health benefits when consumed by humans include β-sitosterol (beta-sitsterol) and squalene.

See also PHYTOSTEROLS, STEROID, CHOLESTEROL, RECEPTORS, LIVER X RECEPTORS (LXR), BILE ACIDS, BILE, SITOSTANOL, SOYBEAN PLANT, CAMPESTEROL, STIGMASTEROL, BETA-SITOSTEROL, CORONARY HEART DISEASE (CHD), LOW-DENSITY LIPOPROTEINS (LDLP), FOOD AND DRUG ADMINISTRATION (FDA), PROTEIN, TRANSACTIVATING PROTEIN, CATABOLISM, TRANSACTIVATION

Sticky Ends Complementary single strands of DNA (deoxyribonucleic acid) that protrude from opposite ends of a DNA duplex or from ends of different DNA duplex molecules. They can be generated by staggered cuts in DNA. They are called "sticky" because the exposed single strands can bind (stick) to complementary single strands on another DNA molecule. A hybrid piece of DNA is hence produced (by that binding).

See also STAGGERED CUTS, HYBRIDIZATION (MOLECULAR GENETICS), DUPLEX, ANNEAL, DEOXYRIBONUCLEIC ACID (DNA), BLUNT-END LIGATION, RESTRICTION ENDONUCLEASES

Stigmasterol A phytosterol that is produced within the seeds of the soybean plant (*Glycine max* (L.)), among others. Evidence indicates that human consumption of stigmasterol helps

S

to reduce levels of total serum cholesterol and low-density lipoproteins (LDLP), thereby lowering risk of coronary heart disease (CHD).

Evidence indicates that certain phytosterols (including stigmasterol) interfere with absorption of cholesterol by the intestines and decrease the body's recovery and reuse of cholesterol-containing bile salts, which causes more cholesterol to be excreted from the body.

See also PHYTOSTEROLS, PHYTOCHEMICALS, STEROLS, SOYBEAN PLANT, CHOLESTEROL, CAMPESTEROL, BETA-SITOSTEROL, CORONARY HEART DISEASE (CHD)

STM Acronym for **scanning tunneling microscope**.

See SCANNING TUNNELING MICROSCOPE

Stomatal Pores See GPA1, ABSCISIC ACID

Storage Proteins Refers to proteins whose molecules are utilized as a "store" (for a time) of amino acids to be consumed later. For example, the storage protein known as casein (i.e., in mammalian mother's milk) is such a "store" source of amino acids for baby mammals.

See also PROTEIN, AMINO ACIDS, P34 PROTEIN

STR Markers See YSTR DNA

Strain Organisms or group of the same species that possesses distinctive genetic characteristics that set it apart from others within the same species, but the differences are not "severe" enough for it to be considered a different breed or variety (of that species). The basic taxonomic unit of microbiology. Can also be used to designate a population of cells derived from a single cell.

See also SPECIES, CELL, CLONE (AN ORGANISM)

Streptavidin A bacterial-origin protein that possesses natural anticancer properties (e.g., it causes human promyelocytic leukemia cells to die when pure streptavidin enters those cells). Streptavidin has a specific and high affinity for biotin (i.e., it "sticks" tightly to the biotin molecule). This can be utilized by researchers to perform the following, among others:

- "Label" certain large molecules of interest, by attaching biotin molecules

to them via a chemical reaction (this is known as **biotinylation**).

- Similarly attach a fluorophore, enzyme, colored bead or quantum dot, etc. to molecules of streptavidin.

- Apply the specific high affinity of streptavidin–biotin for research and diagnostics within microarrays, affinity chromatography, and other separation methodologies.

See also PROTEIN, CELL, CANCER, BIOTIN, MOLECULAR BRIDGE, FLUOROPHORE, ENZYME, QUANTUM DOT, MICROARRAY (TESTING), AFFINITY CHROMATOGRAPHY, CARBON NANOTUBES, BACTERIA

Streptococcus Refers to bacteria of the genus *Streptococcus*. Among the diseases that can be caused by some strains of *Streptococcus* is **necrotizing fasciitis** (so-called "flesh-eating bacteria" disease), which is caused by Group A *Streptococcus*.

See also BACTERIA, GENUS, *STREPTOCOCCUS MUTANS*

Streptococcus mutans The strain of *Streptococcus* bacteria that grows on the surface of teeth and can contribute to causing tooth "decay."

See also STRAIN, BACTERIA, *STREPTOCOCCUS*

Stress Proteins Discovered by Italian biologist Ferruchio Ritossa in the 1960s, these molecules are also called heat-shock proteins. Proteins made by many organisms' (plant, bacteria, and mammal) cells when those cells are stressed by environmental conditions such as certain chemicals, pathogens, or heat. Heat-shock proteins function as molecular chaperones to protect protein molecules from folding prematurely or incorrectly within the cells they are produced in.

When corn or maize (*Zea mays* L.) is stressed during its growing season by high nighttime temperatures, the plant switches from its normal production of ("immune system" defense) chitinase to production of heat-shock (i.e., stress) proteins instead.

Stress proteins are also produced by tuberculosis and leprosy bacteria after these bacteria have invaded (i.e., infected) cells in the human body in an attempt by those bacteria to mimic the stress proteins that (mammal) cells would normally manufacture to repair damage done to the (mammal) cells. This mimicry makes it more difficult for the immune system to recognize and attack those pathogenic bacteria (and/or repair misshaped protein molecules in the body's cells).

Similarly, production of stress proteins helps some types of cancer cells to avoid being attacked by the immune system. Because consumption of genistein by humans causes a reduction in the production of stress proteins, genistein may thereby help the human immune system to destroy cancerous cells. In 1996, Richard I. Morimoto discovered that two stress proteins known as HSP 90 and HSP 70 help to ensure that certain crucial proteins in cells are folded into the configuration or conformation needed by that cell.

See also ANTIGEN, IMMUNE RESPONSE, PATHOGEN, PROTEIN, PROTEIN FOLDING, CONFORMATION, CHAPERONES, PROTEIN STRUCTURE, ABSOLUTE CONFIGURATION, PRION, CHITINASE, AFLATOXIN, GENISTEIN, CANCER, LIPOXYGENASE (LOX), PHYTOALEXINS

Stress Response Proteins See STRESS PROTEINS

Stress Responsive Proteins See STRESS PROTEINS

Stromelysin (MMP-3) A collagenase (enzyme) that "clears a path" through living tissue, ahead of tumor cells, thereby enabling a cancer to spread within the body.

See also COLLAGENASE, ENZYME, CANCER, TUMOR

Structural Biology Refers to the study of **molecular physical structures** and their impact on life processes (e.g., whether or not a given protein molecule can bind to another, how "tightly" an antibody or an enzyme bind to the molecules they each act upon, etc.).

See also NUCLEAR MAGNETIC RESONANCE, GENE, STRUCTURAL GENE, HOMOLOGY MODELING, PROTEIN, ENZYME, ACTIVE SITE, CATALYTIC SITE, ANTIBODY, AVIDITY (OF AN ANTIBODY), PRIMARY STRUCTURE, PROTEIN FOLDING, CONFORMATION,

NATIVE CONFORMATION, TERTIARY STRUCTURE, STERIC HINDRANCE, SUBSTRATE (CHEMICAL), STRUCTURE–ACTIVITY MODELS, CYTOSKELETON, DOMAIN (OF A PROTEIN)

Structural Gene A gene that codes for any RNA (ribonucleic acid) or protein product other than a regulator molecule. It determines the primary sequences (i.e., the amino acid sequences) of a polypeptide (protein).

See also GENE, EXPRESS, POLYPEPTIDE (PROTEIN), AMINO ACID, PRIMARY STRUCTURE, RIBONUCLEIC ACID (RNA)

Structural Genomics Study of, or discovery of, where (gene) sequences are located within the genome and what (DNA) subunits comprise those sequences.

See also GENE, SEQUENCE (OF A DNA MOLECULE), DEOXYRIBONUCLEIC ACID (DNA), SEQUENCING (OF DNA MOLECULES), GENOME, GENOMICS, PRIMARY STRUCTURE, STRUCTURAL BIOLOGY

Structural Proteomics See PROTEOMICS, STRUCTURAL BIOLOGY, STRUCTURE–ACTIVITY MODELS

Structure–Activity Models Refers to models (e.g., of protein molecules) from which their biological activity (e.g., impact on a cell's metabolism, etc.), ligand-binding sites, steric hindrance, avidity, etc. can be calculated or inferred.

See also PROTEIN, CONFORMATION, NATIVE CONFORMATION, TERTIARY STRUCTURE, BIOLOGICAL ACTIVITY, CELL, METABOLISM, PROTEIN FOLDING, DISULFIDE BOND, LIGAND (IN BIOCHEMISTRY), STERIC HINDRANCE, AVIDITY (OF AN ANTIBODY), STRUCTURAL BIOLOGY, QUANTITATIVE STRUCTURE–ACTIVITY RELATIONSHIP (QSAR)

STS Sulfonylurea (Herbicide)-Tolerant Soybeans These are soybeans that have been bred (via insertion of **ALS gene** by traditional breeding methods) to resist the (weed-killing) effects of sulfonylurea-based herbicides. The ALS gene was discovered by Scott Sebastian in 1986.

See also GENE, GENETIC ENGINEERING, HTC, ALS, ALS GENE, BAR GENE, PAT GENE, EPSP SYNTHASE, GLYPHOSATE OXIDASE, HERBICIDE-TOLERANT CROP

Stx Shiga-like toxins.

See also TOXIN, TOXIGENIC *E. COLI*, ENTEROHEMORRHAGIC *E. COLI*, *ESCHERICHIA COLIFORM 0157:H7 (E. COLI 0157:H7)*

Substance K See TACHYKININS

Substance P A neuropeptide (i.e., peptide produced by cells of the nervous system) that is involved in activation of the immune system, pain sensation, and (when in excess) some psychiatric disorders. In the case of chronic, intractable pain (hypersensitivity), approximately 1% of the nerve cells in the human spine process substance P (thereby "transmitting" its pain message via signal transduction). In 1997, Patrick Mantyh showed that killing those (1%) cells relieved chronic pain hypersensitivity without impairing sense of touch or normal (beneficial) pain sensation in humans.

See also TACHYKININS, PROTEIN, POLYPEPTIDE (PROTEIN), SIGNAL TRANSDUCTION, SIGNALING, PEPTIDE, NEUROTRANSMITTER

Substantial Equivalence See CANOLA, ORGANIZATION FOR ECONOMIC COOPERATION AND DEVELOPMENT (OECD)

Substantially Equivalent See SUBSTANTIAL EQUIVALENCE

Substrate (chemical) The substance acted upon, e.g., by an enzyme. For example, the enzyme amylase catalyzes the breakdown of starch molecules into glucose polysaccharide molecules; starch is the substrate (of the enzyme amylase).

See also ENZYME, AMYLASE, CATALYST, SUBSTRATE (STRUCTURAL), LUCIFERIN

Substrate (in chromatography) The (usually solid or gel) substance that attracts and non-covalently binds (interacts) with one or more of the molecules in a solution that is passed over that substrate (e.g., in a chromatography column). This preferential binding (interaction with the substrate) enables one or more of the solution's molecular ingredients to be separated from the others.

See also CHROMATOGRAPHY

Substrate (structural) The substance (support) to which the agent of interest (e.g., a molecule) is attached. For example, some catalyst molecules are chemically attached to nonreactive solids to preserve the catalyst from being flushed away when the chemical substrate (the molecule to be converted by the catalyst) is washed by the catalyst immobilized on the structural substrate.

See also SUBSTRATE (CHEMICAL), CATALYST, HYBRIDIZATION SURFACES, BIOFILM

Sudden Death Syndrome A plant disease caused by the *Fusarium solani* fungus, which sometimes afflicts soybean plants.

See also SOYBEAN PLANT, SOYBEAN CYST NEMATODES (SCN)

Sugar Molecules See OLIGOSACCHARIDES, POLYSACCHARIDES, MONOSACCHARIDES, CARBOHYDRATES, ALDOSE, GLYCOBIOLOGY, PYRANOSE, GLUCOSE (GLc), FURANOSE, GLYCOPROTEIN, SIALIC ACID

Suicide Genes See GENE, P53 GENE, APOPTOSIS

Sulfate-Reducing Bacterium See SRB (SULFATE-REDUCING BACTERIUM)

Sulforaphane A compound that is naturally produced within cruciferous plants such as broccoli, cabbage, and kale. Also within horseradish.

Consumption of sulforaphane results in higher levels of (induced) phase II detoxification enzymes in the digestive system. Research indicates that human consumption of significant amounts of sulforaphane helps to lower the risk of several cancers. Research also has shown that sulforaphane can kill *Helicobacter pylori* bacteria.

See also NUTRACEUTICALS, PHYTOCHEMICALS, CANCER, *H. PYLORI*, ENZYME, INDUCIBLE ENZYMES, PHASE II DETOXIFICATION ENZYMES

Sulfosate An active ingredient in some herbicides, it kills plants (e.g., weeds) by inhibiting the crucial plant enzyme EPSP synthase.

Chemically, sulfosate is a trimethylsulfonium salt of the same organic acid as glyphosate, so sulfosate can be applied over crops (e.g., soybeans) that have been genetically engineered to be tolerant to glyphosate-based herbicides.

See also ENZYME, EPSP SYNTHASE, CP4 EPSPS, GLYPHOSATE, ACID, SOYBEAN PLANT, HERBICIDE-TOLERANT CROP, GENETIC ENGINEERING

SUMO Acronym for **small ubiquitin-related modifier**.

See SMALL UBIQUITIN-RELATED MODI-
FIER

Superantigens Certain types of antigens that
activate a large proportion of an organism's
immune system T cells. These superantigens,
which thus overactivate the organism's
immune system, are thought to be responsible
for some autoimmune diseases (in which T
cells attack and destroy the organism's own
healthy tissues).

See also ANTIGEN, T CELLS, AUTOIM-
MUNE DISEASE

Supercoiling Also known as superhelicity.
The coiling of a closed duplex DNA (deoxyribonucleic acid molecule) in space so that
it crosses over its own axis.

See also DEOXYRIBONUCLEIC ACID
(DNA), HELIX, DUPLEX, DOUBLE
HELIX, POSITIVE SUPERCOILING

Supercritical Carbon Dioxide A   solvent
that, when combined with water and an appropriate surfactant (e.g., fluoroethers), forms a
solvent system that can effectively dissolve
large biological molecules without causing
those molecules to lose biological activity.
Carbon dioxide is a gas at normal (atmospheric) pressure and ambient temperature,
but in its *supercritical state* — temperature
above 31.3°C (88°F) and pressure greater than
72.9 atm — carbon dioxide becomes a dense
(sort of) liquid. Some coffee processors have
used supercritical carbon dioxide as a solvent
to remove caffeine from coffee.

In 1995, Keith Johnston added the surfactant
ammonium carboxylate perfluoropolyether to
a supercritical carbon dioxide system containing water, and proved that the large biological
molecule bovine serum albumin dissolved
inside the micelles that form via water droplet
surrounded by fluoroether molecules. Subsequent to that Eric Beckman proved that the
protease *subtilisin Carlsberg* can be extracted
from crude (impure) cell broth, because that
protease preferentially dissolves in a supercritical carbon dioxide–water system containing fluoroether amphiphiles as surfactants.

See also BIOLOGICAL ACTIVITY, SURFAC-
TANT, MICELLE, REVERSE MICELLE
(RM), BROTH, PROTEASE, SUPERCRITI-
CAL FLUID, ALBUMIN, AMPHIPHILIC
MOLECULES

Supercritical Fluid Refers to a material that
has been heated to a temperature above its
(normal atmospheric pressure) boiling point
but is kept in a state that resembles a liquid
via the application of high pressure. Less commonly, refers to a liquid that has been cooled
to a temperature below its normal freezing
point but is kept in a liquid state by various
means.

For example, water will remain a "liquid" up
to a temperature of 375°C (617°F) if it is
placed under enough pressure. Ammonia
will remain "liquid" up to a temperature of
133°C (271°F) if it is placed under enough
pressure despite the fact that ammonia normally becomes a gas (at standard atmospheric pressure) whenever the temperature
is higher than −33.35°C (−30°F). One predatory mite (*Alaskozetes antarcticus*) living
in Antarctica is able to survive subfreezing
temperatures by preventing ice crystals from
forming (i.e., supercritical water) inside its
body; even when the environmental temperature is below the freezing point (i.e., supercritical). Most supercritical fluids have
unique physical properties (e.g., they are
often better solvents than their true liquid
forms). Some supercritical fluids (e.g.,
supercritical carbon dioxide) can be used to
extract biological molecules (e.g., chlorophyll) from mixtures (e.g., ground up plant
leaves). After the biological molecule has
dissolved out of the mixture, the biological
molecule is recovered by releasing pressure
so that the carbon dioxide returns to gaseous
form and drifts away.

See also SUPERCRITICAL CARBON DIOXIDE

Superoxide Dismutase (SOD) See HUMAN
SUPEROXIDE DISMUTASE (hSOD)

Superparamagnetic Nanoparticles See NANO-
PARTICLES

Suppressor Gene A gene that can reverse the
effect of a specific type of mutation in other
genes, such as a premature termination
sequence.

See also GENE, TRANSWITCH®

Suppressor Mutation A mutation that totally
or partially restores a function that was lost
by a primary mutation. It is located at a site
in the gene different from the site of the primary mutation.

See also GENE

Suppressor T Cells Those T cells (thymus-derived lymphocytes) that are triggered (after other types of T cells and other immune system cells have successfully fought off an infection) to gradually slow down and halt the body's immune response (to the now-conquered pathogen). Discovered by Tomio Tada in 1971, suppressor T cells suppress B cell activity. Failure to halt the immune response in time could lead to harm to the body by its own immune system. The B and T lymphocytes are indistinguishable in size and general morphology. Only the existence or nonexistence of certain proteins on their cell surfaces distinguishes the two classes of lymphocytes. See also CELLULAR IMMUNE RESPONSE, PATHOGEN, B LYMPHOCYTES, T CELLS, AUTOIMMUNE DISEASE

Supramolecular Assembly Phrase utilized to refer to a very large molecular structure. See SELF-ASSEMBLY (OF A LARGE MOLECULAR STRUCTURE), OPTICAL TWEEZER, NANOWIRE

Surface Plasmon Resonance (SPR) A testing technology that enables real-time detection of interactions (e.g., "binding"/ligand, etc.) between protein molecules (attached to a gold surface on a sensitive glass "sensor chip") and other molecules (e.g., pharmaceutical candidate compounds, toxins, etc.) passed over those attached protein molecules. When certain metal surfaces (e.g., gold, silver, etc.) are struck by light of relevant wavelength, **electromagnetic charge oscillations known as surface plasmons** are generated. By shining a highly focused beam of light (e.g., laser, polarized light, etc.) on the bottom of the gold surface (i.e., through the transparent glass "chip") and measuring changes in refractive index of the chip/gold/reflected light, the **mass change** (e.g., caused by pharmaceutical molecule binding to an attached protein such as an antibody or receptor-target) **can be determined** from the SPR it induces on gold surface. See also SURFACE PLASMONS, PROTEIN, LIGAND (IN BIOCHEMISTRY), ANTIBODY, RECEPTORS, PROTEIN INTERACTION ANALYSIS, TARGET–LIGAND INTERACTION SCREENING

Surface Plasmons Refers to a sort of nanometer-scale "shock wave" (electromagnetic excitation) that occurs when light of applicable wavelength is shined on certain metal surfaces (i.e., the plasmons are caused by the light waves striking the "free" electrons at the surface of those metal atoms).

When such light is shined through tiny holes in those metals, such as through a nanometer-scale metal mesh, [more light emerges from the far side of the nanomesh than would be predicted via classical optics]. That is because — in addition to the light that actually **passes through** the mesh openings — some of the light that strikes the "edge of the openings" undergoes the following:

- Light is converted to surface plasmons.
- Light transits the thickness of the metal mesh in the form of surface plasmons, **traveling through the free electrons that rim each mesh opening** while also creating large electric fields around the openings.
- Then, these surface plasmas are reconverted into light on the far side of the metal mesh.

See also NANOMETERS (nm), NANOSCIENCE, NANOTECHNOLOGY, SURFACE PLASMON RESONANCE (SPR)

Surfactant Acronym for **surface active agent.** Amphipathic molecules (i.e., molecules that contain both a polar and nonpolar domain), which, due to their unique properties, position themselves at interfacial regions (surfaces) such as an oil–water interface. When surfactants are dissolved above a certain critical concentration in either water or nonpolar solvents, they may form micelles or reverse micelles, respectively. Surfactants are commonly used to solubilize cell membrane components and other hard to solubilize molecules. See also AMPHIPATHIC MOLECULES, AMPHIPHILIC MOLECULES, MICELLE, REVERSE MICELLE (RM), SDS, ADJUVANT (TO A HERBICIDE)

Sustainable Development Defined in the 1987, United Nations report Our Common Future to be development (e.g., economic development) that meets the needs of the present, without compromising the ability of future generations to meet their own needs.

See also CONSERVATION TILLAGE, GLO-MALIN, NO-TILLAGE CROP PRODUCTION, LOW-TILLAGE CROP PRODUCTION, EARTHWORMS

Switch Proteins Refers to certain protein molecules that signal a plant when environmental conditions are so dry (or cold, etc.) that the plant needs to protect itself (via extreme measures) to survive.

See also TREHALOSE, PROTEIN, SIGNALING, TRANSCRIPTION FACTORS, CBF1, SEQUENCE (OF A DNA MOLECULE), REGULATORY SEQUENCE

Switching (e.g., on/off) of Genes See GENE, GENETIC CODE, CODING SEQUENCE, DEOXYRIBONUCLEIC ACID (DNA), SEQUENCE (OF A DNA MOLECULE), REGULATORY SEQUENCE, TRANSCRIPTION FACTORS, CBF1, COLD HARDENING, CESSATION CASSETTE

SWNT Acronym for **single-walled carbon nanotube**.

See CARBON NANOTUBES

Syk Protein See MAST CELLS

Symbiotic Refers to the mutually beneficial living together of organisms in an intimate association or union. For example, **lichen** are a life form consisting of algae and a fungus growing together as a unit on a solid surface (e.g., a tree trunk or a rock). Each helps the other to survive and grow.

Mycorrhizae consist of plant roots and a fungus growing together as a unit within soil. Each helps the other to survive and grow.

See also ALGAE, FUNGUS, *RHIZOBIUM (BACTERIA)*, MYCORRHIZAE, PHARMACOENVIROGENETICS, ANTIBIOSIS

Synapse From Greek, meaning *"point of contact."* See DENDRITES

Synthase See ACC SYNTHASE, EPSP SYNTHASE, ENZYME, CP4 EPSPS, CITRATE SYNTHASE (CSb) GENE, GLUTAMINE SYNTHETASE, ALS GENE, LOW-PHYTATE SOYBEANS

Synthesizing (of DNA molecules) The building (i.e., polymerization manufacture) of a known sequence of nucleotides into a chain called an oligonucleotide (of which genes are made) or DNA (deoxyribonucleic acid). Invented by Har Gobind Khorana and his colleagues at the University of Wisconsin–Madison in 1968, this process enables scientists to create genes or gene fragments for use in research.

In 1973, Robert Bruce Merrifield developed a means to partially automate the oligonucleotide assembly process. This led to automated machines that can now rapidly manufacture a gene fragment, gene, or DNA probe.

See also GENE MACHINE, NUCLEOTIDE, OLIGOMER, OLIGONUCLEOTIDE, SYNTHESIZING (OF PROTEINS), DEOXYRIBONUCLEIC ACID (DNA), DNA PROBE, SYNTHESIZING (OF OLIGOSACCHARIDES)

Synthesizing (of oligosaccharides) Chemical synthesis (i.e., manufacture) of a known oligosaccharide (structure). For example, a synthesis of a defined-sequence oligosaccharide (molecular) "branch" at a specific site on a glycoprotein in order to "cover up" an antigenic site on that glycoprotein molecule (e.g., so the glycoprotein can be used as a pharmaceutical).

See also OLIGOSACCHARIDES, GLYCOPROTEIN, ANTIGEN, ANTIGENIC DETERMINANT, RESTRICTION ENDOGLYCOSIDASES

Synthesizing (of proteins) Chemical synthesis (manufacture) of a known protein molecule. Devised based upon the solid-phase synthesis methodology developed by Robert Bruce Merrifield in 1963, the desired proteins are assembled by repetitive coupling of the constituent amino acids to a growing polypeptide backbone that itself is attached to a polymeric support (substrate). This procedure has been automated, so it is now possible to make proteins via automated synthesizers.

See also PROTEIN, POLYPEPTIDE (PROTEIN), AMINO ACID, SUBSTRATE (STRUCTURAL), COMBINATORIAL CHEMISTRY, SYNTHESIZING (OF DNA MOLECULES)

Synthetase See SYNTHASE

Synthetic Biology Refers to the study of biology/life by creating synthetic versions of "parts" of it and observing how those parts "work." For example, during 2003, Hamilton O. Smith and J. Craig Venter (re)created the phiX174 bacteriophage by synthesizing its

5386 base pairs from original chemicals. They discovered that it functioned just like other phiX174 bacteriophages. During 1990, Peter G. Schultz had developed cells whose DNA coded for amino acids in **addition to** the 20 naturally occurring amino acids. During the late 1990s, Drew Endy developed numerous distinct segments of DNA that **both** code for specific desired proteins **and also work well together** (when both of those segments are inserted into a given cell to each do a specific task). And such "parts" working together in living systems have been extensively modeled *in silico*.

See also BIOLOGY, BACTERIOPHAGE, SYNTHESIZING (OF DNA MOLECULES), BASE PAIR (bp), CELL, DEOXYRIBONU-CLEIC ACID (DNA), SEQUENCE (OF A DNA MOLECULE), CODING SEQUENCE, AMINO ACID, *IN SILICO* BIOLOGY

Systematic Activated Resistance See SYS-TEMIC ACQUIRED RESISTANCE (SAR)

Systematics An extension of taxonomy, it is the scientific classification of living organisms.

Systemic Acquired Resistance (SAR) Discovered in 1992 (applicable to harpin-induced SAR) and in 1996 by J.A. Ryals, U.H. Neuenschwander, M.G. Willits, A. Molina, H.-Y. Steiner, and M.D. Hunt, SAR is a sort of "immune (cascade) response" by a plant to an infection (e.g., by bacteria, fungus, etc.). One example of this is the production of stress proteins or pathogenesis-related proteins when certain plants are attacked by certain pathogens. Via such SAR response triggered by low-level fungal or viral infection, many plants successfully resist fungal, bacterial, or viral attacks.

In 1998, the U.S. Environmental Protection Agency (EPA) approved one herbicide (COBRA™ owned by Valent Corp.), whose active ingredient is the chemical LACTOFIN, to be applied to soybean plants "at or near bloom stage" in order to trigger SAR against **white mold disease**. In 2000, the U.S. EPA approved a harpin protein to be applied to some crops in order to trigger SAR against certain plant diseases.

See also PATHOGENESIS-RELATED PRO-TEINS, PHYTOALEXINS, R GENES, ISOFLAVONES, SOYBEAN PLANT, FUN-GUS, IMMUNE RESPONSE, VIRUS, PATHOGEN, STRESS PROTEINS, SALI-CYLIC ACID (SA), JASMONIC ACID, HARPIN, CASCADE, WHITE MOLD DIS-EASE

Systemic Inflammatory Response Syndrome See SEPSIS

Systeomics A term coined during 2002 by the California Separation Science Society. Defined as the integration of genomics, proteomics, and metabonomics.

See also GENOMICS, PROTEOMICS, META-BONOMICS

T

T Cell Growth Factor (TCGF) Also known as interleukin-2.

See INTERLEUKIN-2 (IL-2)

T Cell Modulating Peptide (TCMP) A short protein chain that is thought to restrain certain types of T cells from attacking an arthritis-afflicted patient's tissues (mainly cartilage). Arthritis is caused by the arthritis sufferer's own immune system attacking the body's cartilage tissues.

See also CYTOTOXIC T CELLS, HELPER T CELLS (T4 CELLS), LYMPHOCYTE, SUPPRESSOR T CELLS, T CELL RECEPTORS, AUTOIMMUNE DISEASE, TUMOR NECROSIS FACTOR (TNF)

T Cell Receptors Antibody-like transmembrane (i.e., across the cell's surface membrane) proteins located on the surface of T cells. These trigger the (cellular) immune response that is mounted by T cells when these receptors bind to antigens (foreign pieces of antigenic protein) that have been "presented" to these receptors by an MHC protein which itself is located on the surface of phagocytic (i.e., scavenging, pathogen-ingesting) B lymphocyte. Antibodies in the blood recognize native antigen macromolecules (i.e., large molecules), whereas T cell receptors recognize fragments derived from those antigen macromolecules (upon presentation at the surface of B lymphocytes following ingestion and digestion by the B lymphocytes).

See also ANTIBODY, ANTIGEN, MAJOR HISTOCOMPATIBILITY COMPLEX (MHC), PROTEIN, T CELLS, CELLULAR IMMUNE RESPONSE, PHAGOCYTE, B LYMPHOCYTES, CYTOTOXIC T CELLS, HELPER T CELLS, SUPPRESSOR T CELLS

T Cells A class of thymus-derived lymphocytes that include helper T cells (also known as T helper cells or T_H cells), suppressor T cells, and cytotoxic T cells (also known as killer cells or CTL for cytotoxic T lymphocyte). These cells mediate (i.e., control/direct) the cellular response of the human immune system in very complex ways (e.g., synthesis of leukotrienes). T cells are involved in the activation of B cells.

See also CELLULAR IMMUNE RESPONSE, CYTOTOXIC T CELLS, HELPER T CELLS (T4 CELLS), LYMPHOCYTE, SUPPRESSOR T CELLS, T CELL RECEPTORS, T CELL MODULATING PEPTIDE (TCMP), ALLERGIES (FOODBORNE), DENDRITIC CELLS, LEUKOTRIENES

T Lymphocytes See T CELLS, LYMPHOCYTE, LYMPHOKINES, THYMUS

T-DNA See Ti PLASMID

t-IND Treatment Investigational New Drug Application to the U.S. Food and Drug Administration (FDA).

See "TREATMENT" IND REGULATIONS

T3 See SAM-K GENE

T4 Cells See HELPER T CELLS (T4 CELLS)

Tachykinins A class of neuropeptides (i.e., peptides produced by cells of the nervous system; neurons) that includes neurokinin A, neurokinin B, eledoisin, physalaemin, kassinin, substance P, and substance K. Some of these neuropeptides (e.g., Substance P) are picked up by mast cells, lymphocytes, and monocytes and cause those three types of immune system cells to release certain lymphokines (e.g., tumor necrosis factor, interleukin-1 etc.), thus activating the immune system.

See also MAST CELLS, LYMPHOCYTE, MONOCYTES, TUMOR NECROSIS FACTOR (TNF), INTERLEUKIN-1 (IL-1)

TAG See TRIACYLGLYCEROLS

Tagged (molecules or cells) Also sometimes referred to as **labeling (molecules or cells)**.

See AFFINITY TAG, AFFINITY, AFFINITY CHROMATOGRAPHY, EXPRESSED SEQUENCE TAGS (EST), BACTERIAL EXPRESSED SEQUENCE TAGS (BEST), LABEL (FLUORESCENT), LABEL

(RADIOACTIVE), MOLECULAR BEACON, QUANTUM DOT, CELL SURFACE ENGINEERING, MICROARRAY (TESTING), DNA MICROARRAY, BIO–BAR CODES, NANOPARTICLES

Tandem Affinity Purification Tagging Abbreviated "TAP tagging," it refers to one particular method of **protein interaction analysis**. In TAP tagging, the scientist first creates a **fusion protein** by fusing a TAP tag (short segment of known amino acids) onto the thoroughly known target protein. Next, the scientist introduces that fusion protein into living cells in which **the proteins that will hopefully interact with the target protein** are present. When the TAP-tagged fusion protein is recovered after some time, the **cell proteins that ligand-interacted with that fusion protein** are determined by utilizing the following:

- An **antibody that is specific to the TAP tag** to capture the tagged fusion protein along with the ligands that are bound to that fusion protein.
- A protease buffer to cleave off those bound ligands
- A calcium-containing solution with calmodulin-coated beads to remove any remaining protease and impurities
- Mass spectrometry or two-dimensional gel electrophoresis to determine precisely **what those ligands** (to the known fusion protein) **are**.

See also PROTEIN INTERACTION ANALYSIS, PROTEIN, AMINO ACID, CELL, POLYPEPTIDE (PROTEIN), FUSION PROTEIN, LIGAND (IN BIOCHEMISTRY), PROTEASE, MASS SPECTROMETER, TWO-DIMENSIONAL (2-D) GEL ELECTROPHORESIS, ANTIBODY, AFFINITY CHROMATOGRAPHY

Tannins Refers to a large category of chemical compounds that are produced in many plant species. Some of the tannins are beneficial to health when consumed by humans (e.g., the proanthocyanidins within cranberries, cocoa, chocolate, etc.).
See also PROANTHOCYANIDINS

TAP Tagging See TANDEM AFFINITY PURIFICATION TAGGING

Taq **DNA Polymerase** A 94-kDa DNA polymerase that was originally isolated from the thermophilic archaean *Thermus aquaticus*. Commonly utilized to catalyze PCR reactions due to its heat resistance (needed for thermal cycles utilized in the PCR technique).
See also DNA POLYMERASE, POLYMERASE, KILODALTON (kDa), DEOXYRIBONUCLEIC ACID (DNA), BACTERIA, THERMOPHILIC BACTERIA, PCR, POLYMERASE CHAIN REACTION (PCR) TECHNIQUE, *ARCHAEA*

Target (of a herbicide or insecticide) The molecule (e.g., receptor, enzyme, etc.) within a weed plant or within a pest (insect) that a given herbicide or insecticide is aimed at (e.g., when scientists are conducting research aimed at creating that herbicide or insecticide). For example, glyphosate-containing herbicides act on the (target) crucial plant enzyme EPSP synthase. For example, insect-resistant transgenic plants containing "**B.t. genes**" act on (target) receptors inside the digestive system of specific insect species via the **B.t. protoxin**.
See also RECEPTORS, ENZYME, GLYPHOSATE, EPSP SYNTHASE, TRANSGENIC (ORGANISM), PROTOXIN, HERBICIDE-TOLERANT CROP, PAT GENE, GLUTAMINE, GLUTAMINE SYNTHETASE, CORN, BIOLOGICAL ACTIVITY, TARGET–LIGAND INTERACTION SCREENING

Target (of a therapeutic agent) The molecule (e.g., receptor) or moiety that a given drug or therapeutic regimen (e.g., gene delivery) is aimed at (i.e., when scientists are working to create/discover that drug or regimen).
Targets can be normally occurring constituents of the body (e.g., receptors, enzymes, factors, hormones, ion channels, nuclear receptors, DNA, etc.) or nonnormal constituents of the body (e.g., tumors, antigens on tumor surfaces, etc.), or (external, invading) pathogenic agents (e.g., microorganisms, viruses, parasites, etc.).
See also ENZYME, FACTOR, HORMONE, ION CHANNELS, NUCLEAR RECEPTORS, DEOXYRIBONUCLEIC ACID (DNA), TUMOR, MICROORGANISM,

BIOLOGICAL ACTIVITY, PATHOGEN, PATHOGENIC, VIRUS, PHARMACO-PHORE, GENE DELIVERY, RECEPTORS, MOIETY, COMBINATORIAL CHEMIS-TRY, COMBINATORIAL BIOLOGY, SIG-NALING, SIGNAL TRANSDUCTION, G-PROTEINS, TUMOR NECROSIS FACTOR (TNF), HIGH-THROUGHPUT SCREEN-ING (HTS), MULTIPLEXED ASSAY, TAR-GET–LIGAND INTERACTION SCREEN-ING, FLUORESCENCE MAPPING, LABEL (RADIOACTIVE), VALIDATION (OF TAR-GET), BIOCHIPS, QUANTITATIVE STRUCTURE–ACTIVITY RELATIONSHIP (QSAR), WHOLE-CELL PATCH-CLAMP RECORDING

Target Validation See VALIDATION (OF TARGET)

Target-Ligand Interaction Screening A methodology of high-throughput screening (HTS) that is utilized to screen a large number of candidates (e.g., compounds) based upon their interaction (e.g., chemical binding) to a preselected target (e.g., receptor molecule present within a cell membrane, molecule placed on a biochip or other bioassay to facilitate HTS, molecule present on the surface of a nematode utilized in HTS, etc.).

See also HIGH-THROUGHPUT SCREENING (HTS), TARGET (OF A THERAPEUTIC AGENT), TARGET (OF A HERBICIDE OR INSECTICIDE), COMBINATORIAL CHEMISTRY, COMBINATORIAL BIOL-OGY, LIGAND (IN BIOCHEMISTRY), RECEPTORS, SIGNAL TRANSDUCTION, NUCLEAR RECEPTORS, BIOCHIP, SIG-NAL TRANSDUCERS AND ACTIVATORS OF TRANSCRIPTION (STATs), *CAE-NORHABDITIS ELEGANS (C. ELEGANS)*, SURFACE PLASMON RESONANCE (SPR), TWO-HYBRID SYSTEMS, QUAN-TITATIVE STRUCTURE–ACTIVITY RELATIONSHIP (QSAR)

TAT The name of a protein that helps the HIV ("AIDS virus") to cross the human cell plasma membrane, thereby enabling infection of those cells by HIV (human immunodeficiency virus).

TAT is the main activator of HIV gene expression in cells. It is a protein that complexes with TAR (a 60-nucleotide sequence found in all viral messenger ribonucleic acid) to mediate

synthesis of proteins (in an infected cell) necessary for HIV to reproduce.

See also TATA HOMOLOGY, HUMAN IMMUNODEFICIENCY VIRUS TYPE 1 (HIV-1), HUMAN IMMUNODEFICIENCY VIRUS TYPE 2 (HIV-2), GENE, EXPRESS, NUCLEOTIDE, MESSENGER RNA (mRNA), VIRUS, PROTEIN, PLASMA MEMBRANE, CELL

TATA Homology An adenine-thymidine-rich (gene) sequence present 20 to 30 nucleotides "upstream" of the transcription start site on most eucaryotic protein-coding genes; it is required for correct expression. Recent research indicates that blocking this portion of the (gene) sequence may inhibit ability of the AIDS virus to reproduce.

See also GENE, GENETIC CODE, NUCLE-OTIDE, ADENINE, SEQUENCE (OF A DNA MOLECULE), TAT, TRANSCRIP-TION, STARTPOINT, EUCARYOTE, COD-ING SEQUENCE, HOMOLOGY, PRIB-NOW BOX, PROMOTER, SEQUENCE (OF A PROTEIN MOLECULE)

Taxol A phytochemical that is naturally produced in some plants and protects them from the plant pathogen known as **water mold**. Coined during the 1960s by Monroe E. Wall when it was originally isolated from the Pacific yew tree (genus *Taxus*), this word is now a trademark of the Bristol-Myers Squibb Co. Taxol now refers to the antitumor pharmaceutical sold by this company. The active compound from the Pacific yew tree is now known as paclitaxel.

Both Taxol and paclitaxel act by binding and stabilizing microtubules in cells (thereby halting or preventing the uncontrolled cell growth/proliferation that is cancer).

See also CHEMOTHERAPY, PACLITAXEL, CANCER, CELL, MICROTUBULES, TUBULIN

TBT Acronym for the **Technical Barriers to Trade (TBT) Agreement** to WTO.

See also TECHNICAL BARRIERS TO TRADE (TBT) AGREEMENT, WORLD TRADE ORGANIZATION (WTO)

TCGF See T CELL GROWTH FACTOR (TCGF)

TCK Smut See *TELETHIA CONTROVERSIA KOON* SMUT

T

Technical Barriers to Trade (TBT) Agreement The agreement to GATT/WTO according to which WTO member nations agreed to base their import (restrictive) regulations and standards (e.g., mandatory packaging, package marking, testing, certification, labeling requirements, etc.) — known as TBT measures — only on scientific assessments of actual risks (i.e., for those TBT measures intended to protect human health, animal and plant health, or the environment) and to require **only** those TBT measures that do not create unnecessary obstacles to international trade.

See also WORLD TRADE ORGANIZATION (WTO), SPS, SANITARY AND PHYTOSANITARY (SPS) AGREEMENT, SANITARY AND PHYTOSANITARY (SPS) MEASURES, TECHNICAL BARRIERS TO TRADE (TBT MEASURES)

Technical Barriers to Trade (TBT) Measures These are (restrictive) import regulations, standards (e.g., mandatory packaging, package marking, testing, certification and labeling requirements, etc.). Some of them are designed to protect human health, animal and plant health, and the environment. In the Technical Barriers to Trade (TBT) Agreement to GATT/WTO, the WTO member nations agreed to base their TBT measures **only** on requirements that do not create unnecessary obstacles to international trade.

See also TECHNICAL BARRIERS TO TRADE (TBT) AGREEMENT, SPS, WORLD TRADE ORGANIZATION (WTO)

Technology Protection System See CESSATION CASSETTE

Telethia Controversia Koon **Smut** A fungal disease that sometimes afflicts wheat (*Triticum aestivum*) plants.

See also FUNGUS, WHEAT

Telomerase An enzyme that enables the repair of telomeres (thereby stabilizing their length, and preventing shortening of the telomeres). The telomerase enzyme is only present in cancerous cells (thereby enabling the "immortality" of cancerous cells). Human telomerase contains an RNA component and a catalytic-protein component (i.e., a member of the reverse transcriptase "family" of enzymes).

See also REVERSE TRANSCRIPTASES, CANCER, NEOPLASTIC GROWTH, ZYGOTE, TELOMERES, ENZYME, ONCOGENES, HYBRIDOMA, MONOCLONAL ANTIBODIES (MAb), AGING

Telomeres Assemblies consisting of protein and DNA sequences (that do not code for proteins), which are located at the (end) tips of chromosomes.

Telomeres protect the ends of chromosomes, prevent chromosomes from fusing to each other, and serve to limit the maximum number of times that a given cell divides (in the cell's "lifetime"). Telomeres' DNA consists of the sequence GGGGTT repeated many times.

With the exception of certain types of cells (e.g., zygotes, cancerous cells, "immortal" hybridoma cells), portions of each telomere break off each time that the cell containing that chromosome divides. This shortening process serves to limit the lifetime (i.e., number of replications) of those (noncancerous, nonzygote, nonhybridoma, etc.) cells.

See also DEOXYRIBONUCLEIC ACID (DNA), CODING SEQUENCE, PROTEIN, CHROMOSOMES, SEQUENCE (OF A DNA MOLECULE), TELOMERASE, MITOSIS, MITOGEN, CANCER, GAMETE, CELL, AGING, RETINOIDS, HYBRIDOMA

Template In general terms, it is a mold or pattern that can be copied or its shape reproduced. When used with reference to molecular dimensions, it is a macromolecular mold or pattern for the synthesis of another macromolecule.

For example, during 2003 Angela Belcher, Daniel Solis, and Chuanbin Mao genetically engineered a pencil-shaped bacteriophage known as **M13** so that it expressed and incorporated into its capsid a **peptide that causes and controls nucleation/condensation** onto it of specific nanometer-size (conductor) particles. After those nanoparticles thereby become **deposited in a very specific order** onto the bacteriophage's pencil-shaped template, exposure to very high temperature removes the bacteriophage, leaving a solid NANOWIRE. For example, during 2003, Susan Lindquist did the following:

- Triggered the self-assembly of *Saccharomyces cerevisiae* (yeast) amyloid protein to thereby create 10-nm-wide fibers

- Placed those fibers onto specially designed electrodes and then reacted colloidal gold particles with cysteine molecular groups protruding from those fibers
- Filled in the spaces between the gold particles bound to fiber via a reductive deposition procedure that deposited both gold and silver atoms

This resulted in a NANOWIRE possessing an average diameter of 100 nm. Also, during 2002, William A. Drucker and Chang-Hyun Jang were able to utilize the enzyme acetylcholinesterase as a template to create a precisely structured strip 70-nm wide deposited onto a prepared gold surface. After first coating the gold surface with a carboxylic acid (film), they were able to adhere onto it a film of acetylcholinesterase; then by scratching away a strip via utilization of an atomic force microscope tip (stylus), they were able to to lay down a 70-nm wide strip (onto the gold) of thiocholine cleaved from acetylcholine-containing solution.

See also MACROMOLECULES, ENZYME, NANOMETERS (nm), NANOWIRE, BACTERIOPHAGE, GENETIC ENGINEERING, PEPTIDE, ACETYLCHOLINESTERASE, ACETYLCHOLINE, DEOXYRIBONUCLEIC ACID (DNA), RNA POLYMERASE, STRUCTURAL GENE, INFORMATIONAL MOLECULES, HEREDITY, GENE, GENETIC CODE, GENETIC MAP, BIOSENSORS (CHEMICAL), GENOSENSORS, RIBONUCLEIC ACID (RNA), GENE REPAIR (DONE BY HUMANS), CODON, EXON, CHIMERAPLASTY, NANOTECHNOLOGY, NANOPARTICLES, BIOELECTRONICS, PRIMER (DNA), ATOMIC FORCE MICROSCOPE, YEAST, SELF-ASSEMBLY (OF A LARGE MOLECULAR STRUCTURE), CYSTEINE (Cys), REDUCTION (IN A CHEMICAL REACTION)

Teosinte Refers to a "family" of specific wild plants (*Zea diploperennis*) native to southern Mexico, Guatemala, Honduras, and Nicaragua, which are related to domesticated corn/maize (*Zea mays* L.).
See also CORN, WILD TYPE

Termination Codon Also known as **terminator sequence**. One of three triplet sequences

(U-A-G, U-A-A, or U-G-A) found in DNA molecules (genes) that cause termination of protein synthesis; they are also called nonsense codons. The sequences cause the termination of the peptide chain and its release in free form.
See also CODING SEQUENCE, CODON, DEOXYRIBONUCLEIC ACID (DNA), GENETIC CODE, NONSENSE CODON, SEQUENCING (OF DNA MOLECULES), CONTROL SEQUENCES

Terminator See TERMINATION CODON

Terminator Cassette See CESSATION CASSETTE

Terminator Sequence See TERMINATION CODON

Terpenes A category of chemical compounds (cyclic hydrocarbon molecules) that are produced by plants, especially conifers, oranges, and certain blue-green algae (e.g., *Oscillatoria perornata*).
For example, the drug Taxol (paclitaxel) is a diterpene (i.e., molecule consisting of two terpene units) extracted from the Pacific yew tree (genus *Taxus*).
Also, the blue-green algae *Oscillatoria perornata* produce the terpene **2-methyl-isoborneol**. When catfish (*Ictalurus furcatus*) consume such algae, it accumulates in their bodies and imparts an undesirable (musty) flavor to their meat.
See also TAXOL, PACLITAXEL, SAPONINS

Terpenoids See TERPENES

Tertiary Structure The three-dimensional folding of the polypeptide (i.e., protein) molecular chains that characterizes a protein molecule in its native state.
See also PROTEIN STRUCTURE, PROTEIN, POLYPEPTIDE (PROTEIN), CONFORMATION, PROTEIN FOLDING, NATIVE CONFORMATION, PROTEOMICS, TRANSCRIPTOME

Testosterone An androgen (steroid hormone) that is biochemically synthesized (made) from androstenedione, which is itself synthesized from progesterone. Testosterone is responsible for the development of male secondary sex characteristics in humans such as greater strength, larger body size, facial hair and a deeper voice, etc.
See also STEROID, ESTROGEN

T

Tetrahydrofolic Acid The reduced, active coenzyme form of the vitamin folic acid; involved in C_1 transfers. Tetrahydrofolate (also known as FH_4) serves as an intermediate carrier (molecule) of methyl, hydroxy-methyl, or formyl groups (all containing one carbon atom) in a relatively large number of enzymatic reactions in which such one-carbon groups are transferred from one metabolite to another.

See also COENZYME

Tetraploid Refers to organisms that possess four sets of chromosomes instead of the normal two sets of chromosomes. Conversion of a diploid (i.e., two sets of chromosomes) organism to tetraploid can be done by humans. For example, by soaking seeds in certain chemicals such as colchicine, scientists can cause the resultant (plant) to become tetraploid. This is utilized to create mutated plant varieties with new traits.

See also CHROMOSOMES, COLCHICINE, DIPLOID, MUTATION BREEDING

TG See TRIGLYCERIDES

TGA The government regulatory agency charged with approving all pharmaceutical products sold within Australia.

See also FOOD AND DRUG ADMINISTRATION (FDA), KOSEISHO, COMMITTEE FOR PROPRIETARY MEDICINAL PRODUCTS (CPMP), EUROPEAN MEDICINES EVALUATION AGENCY (EMEA), MEDICINES CONTROL AGENCY (MCA), COMMITTEE ON SAFETY IN MEDICINES, BUNDESGESUNDHEITSAMT (BGA), GENE TECHNOLOGY OFFICE

TGF See TRANSFORMING GROWTH FACTOR-ALPHA (TGF-ALPHA), TRANSFORMING GROWTH FACTOR-BETA (TGF-BETA)

Thale Cress Common name for *Arabidopsis thaliana*.

See *ARABIDOPSIS THALIANA*

Thermal Hysteresis Proteins Also referred to as "antifreeze proteins" or AFPs, these are a class of proteins/glycoproteins (possessed by some organisms) that inhibit the formation of ice crystals inside the cells of that organism when those cells are exposed to temperatures colder than 32°F (0°C).

See also PROTEIN, ORGANISM, CELL, GLYCOPROTEIN

Thermoduric An organism that can survive high temperatures but does not necessarily grow at such temperatures.

See also THERMOPHILE, MESOPHILE, EXTREMOPHILIC BACTERIA, PSYCHROPHILE, ENDOPHYTE

Thermophile An organism whose optimum temperature for growth is close to, or exceeds, the boiling point of water (100°C, 212°F).

See also EXTREMOPHILIC BACTERIA, THERMOPHILIC BACTERIA, THERMODURIC, MESOPHILE, PSYCHROPHILE, EUCARYOTE

Thermophilic Bacteria Literally "heat-loving" bacteria. They are a category of thermophiles generally found near geothermal vents beneath bodies of water.

See also THERMOPHILE, THERMODURIC, EXTREMOPHILIC BACTERIA, MESOPHILE, PSYCHROPHILE

Thioesterase A "family" of enzymes that is naturally produced within some plants, such as the California bay tree (*Umbellularia californica*). Thioesterase catalyzes those plants' production of the fatty acid **laurate**.

See also FATS, FATTY ACID, LAUROYL-ACP THIOESTERASE, ENZYME, LAURATE, CANOLA, HIGH-LAURATE CANOLA

Thiol Group Refers to a specific chemical entity (on a molecule).

See CYSTEINE (Cys), CYSTINE

Thioredoxin See ALLERGIES (FOOD-BORNE)

Threonine (Thr) A crystalline, α-amino acid considered essential for normal growth of animals. It is biosynthesized (i.e., made) from aspartic acid and is a precursor of isoleucine in microorganisms.

See also ESSENTIAL AMINO ACIDS

Thrombin The key to thrombus (blood clot) formation. Thrombin is a proteolytic enzyme that cleaves fibrinogen into (molecular) pieces, which then spontaneously assemble themselves into fibrin, which forms a clot.

See also THROMBUS, THROMBOSIS, THROMBOMODULIN, THROMBOLYTIC AGENTS, FIBRIN, FIBRINOLYTIC AGENTS, CASCADE

Thrombolytic Agents Bloodborne compounds (such as tissue plasminogen activator) that work to disintegrate (break up or lyse) blood clots.

See also FIBRIN, FIBRINOLYTIC AGENTS, TISSUE PLASMINOGEN ACTIVATOR (tPA)

Thrombomodulin A cell surface protein found on endothelial cells that plays a key role in modulating the final step in the coagulation process. After thrombin binds to thrombomodulin, thrombin loses its ability to cleave fibrinogen to form fibrin. In addition, once thrombin binds to thrombomodulin, thrombin's activation of protein C is increased 200-fold and this activated protein C then degrades factors Va and VIIIa, which are both required for the production of thrombin from prothrombin. Hence, thrombomodulin modulates the activity of the enzyme thrombin, causing a cessation of full-blown clotting activity.

See also THROMBIN, PROTEIN, PROTEIN C, THROMBOSIS, PATHWAY, PATHWAY FEEDBACK MECHANISMS

Thrombosis The intravascular (i.e., inside of blood vessel) formation of a blood clot.

See also THROMBIN, THROMBUS, THROMBOLYTIC AGENTS, TRIGLYCERIDES, FIBRIN, FIBRINOLYTIC AGENTS, TISSUE PLASMINOGEN ACTIVATOR (tPA), PLAQUE

Thrombus The blood clot itself. The mass of blood coagulated *in situ* in the heart or other blood vessel. For example, such a clot causes a heart attack when the coagulation occurs in the vessels feeding the heart.

See also THROMBIN, THROMBOSIS, THROMBOLYTIC AGENTS, FIBRIN, TRIGLYCERIDES, FIBRINOLYTIC AGENTS

Thymine (Thy) A pyrimidine component of nucleic acid first isolated from the thymus. Its hydrogen-bonding counterpart in RNA is uracil.

See also NUCLEIC ACIDS, PYRIMIDINE, BASE (NUCLEOTIDE), THYMUS, RIBONUCLEIC ACID (RNA)

Thymoleptics A class of drugs that primarily exerts their effect on the brain, influencing "feeling" and behavior.

Thymus A gland that enables cells of the immune system of mammals to mature. In humans, it lies behind the breast bone and extends upward as far as the thyroid gland. The thymus is the place in the body where T lymphocytes are "taught" to distinguish foreign (e.g., pathogen's) antigens from "self" cell antigens, to avoid immune responses in which the body's immune system attacks organs and other cells within the body (resulting in autoimmune disease). Any T lymphocytes that remain "autoreactive" (i.e., would tend to attack "self" cells, such as organs in the body) are destroyed by the thymus via a cytotoxic mechanism.

An example of an autoimmune disease is multiple sclerosis (MS), in which the body's acetylcholine receptors are attacked by the body's immune system. Because cetylcholine is crucial in the transmission of nerve impulses to the body's muscles, such destruction of acetylcholine receptors results in loss of control of the body's muscles.

See also T LYMPHOCYTES, CYTOTOXIC, RECEPTORS, T CELLS, IMMUNE RESPONSE, PATHOGEN, ANTIGEN, NEUROTRANSMITTER, ACETYLCHOLINE, AUTOIMMUNE DISEASE

Thyroid Gland A gland that is found on both sides of the trachea ("windpipe") in humans. This gland secretes the hormone thyroxine, which increases the rate of metabolism.

See also THYROID-STIMULATING HORMONE (TSH), GRAVE'S DISEASE

Thyroid-Stimulating Hormone (TSH) A hormone that causes the thyroid gland to secrete additional amounts of thyroxine.

See also THYROID GLAND, GRAVE'S DISEASE

Ti Plasmid Abbreviation for **tumor-inducing plasmid** or **tumor induction plasmid**. It is the plasmid of *Agrobacterium tumefaciens* bacteria that naturally has a part of its DNA (T DNA) transferred to a plant when *Agrobacterium tumefaciens* infects that plant (e.g., via a wound in the plant).

After it has been transferred into the plant, that Ti plasmid DNA segment (now known as T-DNA or **transferred DNA**) inserts itself into the plant's DNA, where it causes cells to grow into tumor-like structures known as galls. The **Ti plasmid** can be modified so that it can be utilized (by genetic engineers) to insert genes from other organisms into plants.

See also PLASMID, BACTERIA, *AGROBACTERIUM TUMEFACIENS*, CELL,

DEOXYRIBONUCLEIC ACID (DNA), GENE, GENETIC ENGINEERING

TIRF Microscopy Refers to microscopy systems/microscopes that utilize **total internal reflection fluorescence** to help visualize (e.g., thin layers of biological tissue). For example, instead of using chemical stains to try to "color" various tissues/cells differently to make them easier to see/differentiate under a conventional light microscope, scientists can instead do the following:

- Utilize **fluorescent proteins** such as green fluorescent protein or Kusabira Orange (which will differentially adhere to different tissues/cells)
- Genetically engineer (e.g., living cells) to express one or more of the fluorescent proteins in one or more cellular structures (or within tissues)

With the cell/tissue sample thus **fluorescently labeled**, the scientist can then utilize one of the fluorescent microscopes available (e.g., confocal microscope equipped with a relevant laser source to "light up" the fluorescent proteins) to view the fluorescence-illuminated/colored cell/tissue in three dimensions.
See also FLUORESCENCE, CELL, PROTEIN, GREEN FLUORESCENT PROTEIN, KUSABIRA ORANGE, GENETIC ENGINEERING, TRANSFECTION, EXPRESS, GRAM STAIN, CONFOCAL MICROSCOPY

Tissue Array See LIVE CELL ARRAY

Tissue Culture The growth and maintenance (by researchers) of cells from higher organisms *in vitro*, that is, in a sterile test tube or petri dish environment that contains the nutrients necessary for cell growth. One use of tissue culture is to produce **disease-free** offspring from certain (valuable, high-quality) crop plants.
Another use of tissue culture methods is for "embryo rescue" to enable "wide crosses" between two different species of plants. In this procedure, pollen from one plant species (e.g., a wild plant possessing disease resistance) is induced to fertilize a plant from another species (e.g., a domesticated crop). The resultant fertilized plant embryo, which would not grow on its own, is "rescued" via tissue culture methods. Following maturation, that wide cross (i.e., a hybrid plant from two species that normally would not cross) produces fertile seeds on its own without any need for further intervention by man.
See also CELL, ORGANISM, CULTURE MEDIUM, SPECIES, HYBRIDIZATION (PLANT GENETICS)

Tissue Engineering Refers to the technologies utilized to induce the following:

- Injected liver, cartilage, etc., cells to grow within the recipient organism's body and form entire (integral) tissues.
- Extant cells within the body to grow and form desired (integral) tissues via precise injection of relevant compounds (e.g., certain growth factors, growth hormones, etc.).

During the 1980s, Robert S. Langer invented degradable "scaffolds" made of lactic acid-glycolic acid copolymer fibers. When these "scaffolds" are "seeded" with cells (e.g., propagated in vats or transplanted from another organism), the cells grow together to form tissue. This scaffold technology can also be utilized to grow skin tissue, blood vessels, corneas, nerves, etc.
During 2000, Samuel Stupp created two-part molecules known as **peptide amphiphiles** (PA), which self-assemble into nanofibers which encourage bone growth (e.g., when inserted into the space between human broken bone fragments).
See also TISSUE CULTURE, CELL, ORGANISM, GROWTH FACTOR, GROWTH HORMONE (GH), SELF-ASSEMBLY (OF A LARGE MOLECULAR STRUCTURE)

Tissue Plasminogen Activator (tPA) A glycoprotein that possesses thrombolytic (i.e., blood-clot-dissolving) activity. It is used as a drug to dissolve clots and acts by first binding to fibrin (clots). It then activates (i.e., proteolytically cleaves) plasminogen (molecules) to yield plasmin, a bloodborne enzyme that itself cleaves molecular bonds in the fibrin clot. The plasmin molecules diffuse through the fibrin clot and cause the clot to dissolve

rapidly. With the dissolution of the clot, blood flow to the formerly blocked blood vessel (e.g., the heart) is restored.
See also THROMBUS, THROMBIN, THROMBOLYTIC AGENTS, GLYCOPROTEIN, FIBRIN, FIBRINOLYTIC AGENTS

TKI See TYROSINE KINASE INHIBITORS

TLR Acronym for **toll-like receptors**.
See INNATE IMMUNE RESPONSE

TME (N) Abbreviation for "true metabolizable energy (corrected for nitrogen)"; a measure of the amount of energy that a given animal (e.g., chicken) can extract from a given feed ration.
See also METABOLISM, CHEMOMETRICS, CALORIE

TMEn See TME (N)

Tobacco Budworm See *HELIOTHIS VIRESCENS (H. VIRESCENS)*

Tobacco Hornworm Caterpillars (pupae) of the Lepidopteran insect *Manduca sexta.*
Tobacco hornworm is susceptible to Cry1A (b) protein (e.g., they are killed if they eat plants genetically engineered to contain Cry1A (b) protein).
See also CRY1A (b) PROTEIN

Tobacco Mosaic Virus (TMV) One the of smallest viruses, consisting of some 2200 chains of identical polypeptides and a molecule of RNA. All of the genetic/heredity information of the tobacco mosaic virus is contained in its RNA.
The first discovery of a self-assembling, active biological structure occurred in 1955 when Heinz Frankel-Conrat and Robley Williams showed that TMV will reassemble into functioning, infectious virus particles after the TMV has been dissociated into its components via immersion in concentrated acetic acid. The TMV virus infects the leaves of tomato and tobacco plants, causing disease. Tobacco plants can be genetically engineered to resist TMV infection. A tomato plant genetically engineered to resist TMV infection has been commercially available since 1992.
See also GENETIC ENGINEERING, CAPSID, VIRUS, RNA, POLYPEPTIDE (PROTEIN), GENE, INFORMATIONAL MOLECULES, HEREDITY, SELF-ASSEMBLY (OF A LARGE MOLECULAR STRUCTURE)

Tocopherols A "family" of different molecular forms of vitamin E, each of which has a saturated phytyl "tail" attached to the "backbone" of the molecule. Commercial tocopherols are extracted from soybeans, although some are also naturally present in canola and sunflower.
See also VITAMIN, SOYBEAN PLANT, VITAMIN E

Tocotrienols A "family" of different molecular forms of vitamin E, each of which has an unsaturated isoprenoid side chain attached to the "backbone" of the molecule.
Tocotrienols are naturally present in oil palm (*Elaeis guineensis*) and in cereal grains (e.g., oats, barley, rye, and rice bran).
See also VITAMIN, ISOPRENE, VITAMIN E

Toll-Like Receptors See INNATE IMMUNE RESPONSE

Tomato A green bushy plant, botanical name *Lycopersicon esculentum*. The wild type is native to South America, but the domesticated tomato is grown worldwide today. Its fruit, known as tomatoes, are a natural source of the antioxidant carotenoid **lycopene**, a phytochemical whose consumption has been linked to a reduction in coronary heart disease and some cancers (e.g., prostate cancer).
See also LYCOPENE, PHYTOCHEMICALS, ANTIOXIDANTS, CANCER, CAROTENOIDS, CORONARY HEART DISEASE (CHD), WILD TYPE

Tomato Fruitworm See *HELICOVERPA ZEA (H. ZEA)*

Topotaxis See TROPISM

TOS See TRANSGALACTO-OLIGOSACCHARIDES

Total Internal Reflecton Fluorescence See TIRF MICROSCOPY

Totipotency The ability to grow/differentiate into all of the types of cells/tissues constituting an (adult) organism's body.
See also STEM CELL ONE, CELL, ZYGOTE, CELL DIFFERENTIATION, CELL DIFFERENTIATION PROTEINS, TOTIPOTENT STEM CELLS

Totipotent Stem Cells Bone marrow cells that (when signaled) mature into both red blood cells and white blood cells. Receptors on the surface of totipotent stem cells "grasp" passing blood cell growth factors (e.g., interleukin- 7,

T

stem cell growth factor, etc.), bringing them inside these stem cells and thus causing the maturation and differentiation into red and white blood cells. These receptors are called FLK-Z receptors.

See also STEM CELL ONE, STEM CELLS, WHITE BLOOD CELLS, GROWTH FACTOR, RECEPTORS, CELL DIFFERENTIATION PROTEINS, CELL DIFFERENTIATION, CELL

Toxic Substances Control Act (TSCA) A 1976 American federal law under which the U.S. Environmental Protection Agency (EPA) has regulated the release of genetically engineered organisms (e.g., bacteria or plants) that produce natural insecticides. This is based on legal analogy to synthetic chemical insecticides, which are clearly regulated under TSCA.

See also OAB (OFFICE OF AGRICULTURAL BIOTECHNOLOGY), FEDERAL INSECTICIDE FUNGICIDE AND RODENTICIDE ACT (FIFRA), GENETICALLY ENGINEERED MICROBIAL PESTICIDES (GEMP), WHEAT TAKE-ALL DISEASE, *BACILLUS THURINGIENSIS (B.t.)*

Toxicogenomics A branch of toxicology that deals with the reactions between toxins and the **specific differences in response** of different organisms **owing to their different genomes/DNA** (of the different individuals that consume the same toxin). For example, some rare humans can tolerate eating certain poisonous mushrooms (which sicken or kill all other humans that consume those particular mushroom species).

Some humans can tolerate intimate exposure to urushiol oil toxin in poison oak (*Rhus diversiloba*), which harms other humans (e.g., causes oozing, itching rash, etc.).

During 2001, scientists identified a human genetic variation that makes some cancer patients approximately seven times more likely to have a toxic reaction to the common chemotherapy drug **irinotecan** used to treat colorectal cancer. Some rare humans are unable to degrade (break down) pyrimidine-containing pharmaceuticals, owing to those humans' lack of a gene coding for production in their body of a specific pyrimidine-degrading enzyme (abbreviated DHPDH). The goal of toxicogenomics in that case is to **avoid**

administering pyrimidine-containing pharmaceuticals (e.g., the anticancer drug **5-fluorouracil**) to those humans. One way to accomplish that goal would be via genetic testing, to determine which individuals lack the gene for DHPDH before any pyrimidine-containing pharmaceuticals are administered.

During 2001, Fred Gould, David Heckel, and Linda Gahan showed that a rare, recessive gene (allele) known as **BtR-4** could confer (on tobacco budworms possessing two copies of that particular gene) resistance to at least some of the "Cry" proteins (which kill all other tobacco budworms that consume those proteins).

The subgroup of **all those individuals whose DNA (genome) causes their bodies to resist the effects of a given toxin**, or be unable to degrade other toxins, is known as a haplotype. A haplotype could (theoretically) be as small as one individual, because the particular resistance-to-toxin could result from one single-nucleotide polymorphism (SNP).

See also GENE, GENOMICS, PHARMACOGENOMICS, TOXIN, MUTAGEN, PHARMACOGENETICS, GENOME, DEOXYRIBONUCLEIC ACID (DNA), HAPLOTYPE, SINGLE-NUCLEOTIDE POLYMORPHISMS (SNPs), RECESSIVE ALLELE, CRY PROTEINS, CELL ARRAY, TOBACCO BUDWORM, LIVE CELL ARRAY, ENZYME, CHEMOTHERAPY, ADME/Tox, CELLULAR PATHWAY MAPPING

Toxigenic E. coli See ENTEROHEMORRHAGIC *E. COLI*, *ESCHERICHIA COLIFORM 0157:H7 (E. COLI 0157:H7)*

Toxin A substance (e.g., produced in some cases by fungi, weeds, ants, or disease-causing microorganisms) that is poisonous to certain other living organisms.

See also ANTITOXIN, ABRIN, RICIN, COLICINS, BACTERIOCINS, *ESCHERICHIA COLIFORM 0157:H7 (E. coli 0157:H7)*, ENTEROHEMORRHAGIC *E. COLI*, *PFIESTERIA PISCICIDA*, PHYTOTOXIN, *PHOTORHABDUS LUMINESCENS*, ENTEROTOXIN, GLUCOSINOLATES, ALKALOIDS, AFLATOXIN, MYCOTOXINS, FUNGUS

TPS See TECHNOLOGY PROTECTION SYSTEM

Tracer (Radioactive Isotopic Method) A metabolite that is labeled by incorporation of an isotopic atom into its structure. The metabolic fate of the labeled metabolite can then be traced in intact organisms. That is, one is able to ascertain where (in what kind of structure) the metabolite ends up as well as the transformation products (intermediate molecules) that were involved in its formation. Certain atoms of a given metabolite are labeled. This is done by substituting radioactive isotopes for the atom in question. Because an atom is replaced by an isotope, the metabolite as a whole is chemically and biologically indistinguishable from its normal analogue. The presence of the isotope allows the metabolite and its transformation products to be detected and measured. Without this technique, many aspects of metabolism could not have been studied. These include the process of photosynthesis, metabolic turnover rates, and the biosynthesis of proteins and nucleic acids.

See also REASSOCIATION (OF DNA), RADIOACTIVE ISOTOPE, RADIOIMMUNOASSAY

Traditional Breeding Methods A phrase utilized by some people to refer to some or most techniques/technologies utilized by crop plant breeders prior to some arbitrarily chosen date (after which some people feel that "genetic engineering" arrived abruptly). For example, in 1992 Tim Croughan discovered a single rice (*Oryza sativa*) plant that had survived what should have been a lethal dose of an imidazolinone-based herbicide owing to a (mutated) gene in its DNA that made it resistant to imidazolinones. That plant was then propagated via straightforward breeding to yield seeds still sown today.

Many years ago, some other crops similarly were given new traits (e.g., herbicide tolerance, compositional improvements, etc.) via mutation breeding (i.e., soaking seeds or pollen in mutation-causing chemicals such as colchicine, or bombardment of seeds by ionizing radiation to cause random genetic mutations, followed by grow-out and selection of the particular mutation desired such as herbicide tolerance — as described in the preceding text).

Other crops were given new traits by crossing them with related wild plants. This occasionally resulted in extremely high levels of natural toxicants in those plants/seeds (e.g., solanine, psoralene, etc.).

Still others were given new traits by wide-crossing them with other domesticated species (e.g., the tangelo is a hybrid of the grapefruit and the tangerine). The U.S. Food and Drug Administration (FDA) regulates all new crop plants similarly (e.g., also requires testing of plants produced via "traditional breeding methods" for the potential presence of introduced or increased natural toxicants).

See also GENETIC ENGINEERING, HERBICIDE-TOLERANT CROP, GENETICS, MUTATION, MUTATION BREEDING, HIGH-OLEIC SUNFLOWERS, TRAIT, CANOLA, SOYBEAN PLANT, CORN, SOLANINE, PSORALENE, FOOD AND DRUG ADMINISTRATION (FDA), BARLEY, HYBRIDIZATION (PLANT GENETICS), MARKER (DNA SEQUENCE), MARKER-ASSISTED SELECTION, POINT MUTATION, SOMACLONAL VARIATION, SOMATIC VARIANTS, WIDE CROSS, EMBRYO RESCUE, TISSUE CULTURE, COLCHICINE

Traditional Breeding Techniques See TRADITIONAL BREEDING METHODS

Trait A characteristic of an organism, which manifests itself in the phenotype (physically). Many traits are the result of the expression of a single gene, but some are polygenic (result from simultaneous expression of more than one gene). For example, the level of protein content in soybeans is controlled by five genes.

See also PHENOTYPE, GENOTYPE, EXPRESS, GENE, POLYGENIC, PROTEIN, CALLIPYGE

***trans*-Acting Protein** A *trans*-acting protein has the exceptional property of acting (having an effect) only on the molecule of DNA (deoxyribonucleic acid) from which it was expressed.

See also EXPRESS, *cis*-ACTING PROTEIN

Transactivating Protein Refers to a specific protein that "switches on" a cascade of genes/gene regulation.

See also PROTEIN, TRANSACTIVATION, GENE, CASCADE, GENE EXPRESSION CASCADE, STEROLS, TRANSCRIPTION

ACTIVATORS, VIRAL TRANSACTIVATING PROTEIN, LIVER X RECEPTORS (LXR)

Transactivation Refers to the activation (i.e., start/increase) of transcription via the "binding" of a transcription factor to a given DNA regulatory sequence.

See also TRANSCRIPTION, TRANSCRIPTION FACTORS, REGULATORY SEQUENCE, STEROLS, LIVER X RECEPTORS (LXR)

Transaminase A large group of enzymes that catalyze the transfer of the amino group from any one of at least 12 amino acids to a keto acid to form another amino acid. Also known as aminotransferases.

See also ENZYME, AMINO ACID

Transamination The reaction of the enzymatic removal and transfer of an amino group from one specific compound to another.

See also TRANSAMINASE, AMINO ACID

Transcript Term used to refer to the various segments of messenger RNA (mRNA) that result from transcription of a gene.

See also GENE, TRANSCRIPTION, MESSENGER RNA (mRNA), TRANSCRIPTOME, CENTRAL DOGMA (NEW)

Transcriptase See RNA POLYMERASE

Transcription The enzyme-catalyzed process whereby the genetic information contained in one strand of DNA (deoxyribonucleic acid) is used as a template to specify and produce a complementary mRNA strand. Transcription may be thought of as a rewriting of the information contained in DNA into RNA. The language, however, is the same — both are nucleic acid based. This is in contrast to translation, in which the information is translated from one language (RNA, nucleic acid based) into another language (protein, amino acid based).

See also GENE EXPRESSION, TRANSLATION, MESSENGER RNA (mRNA), GENETIC CODE, DEOXYRIBONUCLEIC ACID (DNA), TRANSCRIPTION FACTORS, TRANSCRIPTION UNIT, ANTICODING STRAND, ACTIVATOR (OF GENE), EDITING

Transcription Activators Refers to transcription factors (proteins and other molecules) that interact with regulatory sequences within DNA (in cell). By binding directly to those regulatory sequences (usually at multiple sites on the sequence), and "recruiting" modifying molecules (chromatin remodeling elements) to also come to the sites on the DNA, transcription activators cause transcription (of a given gene) to begin or to increase.

Classes of transcription activators include:

- **Nuclear Receptors**: These receptors (in the cell's outer membrane) convey a "signal" from outside the cell all the way into the DNA within the cell's nucleus. For example, when the steroid hormone cortisol (i.e., a chemical "signal") binds to the glucocortiod receptor (GR) in cells, the GR (protein molecule) enters the cell's nucleus and binds to the **glucocorticoid response element** (i.e., a specific regulatory sequence) in that cell's DNA. This then causes a **second** GR molecule to bind to that same glucocorticoid response element. The binding of the two (i.e., a GR dimer) to the glucocorticoid response element "activates" (i.e., starts) transcription of the gene (in the DNA molecule) immediately adjacent to the glucocorticoid response element.

- **Catabolite Activator Proteins (CAP)**: CAPs activate transcription by binding to the DNA — near Class I or Class II CAP promoter sites on the DNA molecule — and RNA polymerase (RNAP), which results in an amalgamated molecular structure known as **RNAP promoter complex**.

See also PROTEIN, GENETIC CODE, CODING SEQUENCE, CELL, NUCLEUS, REGULATORY SEQUENCE, TRANSCRIPTION, TRANSCRIPTION FACTORS, DEOXYRIBONUCLEIC ACID (DNA), GENE, ACTIVATOR (OF GENE), SIGNAL TRANSDUCERS AND ACTIVATORS OF TRANSCRIPTION (STATs), NUCLEAR RECEPTORS, CAP, RNA POLYMERASE, SIGNALING, G-PROTEINS, CD4 PROTEIN, HORMONE, RETINOID X RECEPTORS, CORTISOL, POSITIVE CONTROL

Transcription Factor Binding Site Refers to a sequence (segment) of DNA within an organism's genome (DNA) that is "recognized" and bound (i.e., "adhered to") by a transcription factor, thereby activating (or repressing, for **repressor**) transcription.
See also SEQUENCE (OF A DNA MOLECULE), ORGANISM, DEOXYRIBONUCLEIC ACID (DNA), TRANSCRIPTION FACTORS, TRANSCRIPTION

Transcription Factors Proteins and other chemical compounds that interact with each other and with regulatory sequences within DNA (when immediately adjacent to the DNA in a cell), to either facilitate (i.e., "turn on") or inhibit (i.e., "turn off") the activity (i.e., coding for proteins) of that DNA's genes. Transcription factors have the following potential benefits:

- Cure diseases (e.g., by blocking the deleterious effects of certain disease-causing genes).
- Assist farmers in crop protection (e.g., by **switching on** the genes that cause crop plants to initiate "cold hardening," or certain types of insect resistance mechanisms).
- Improve human health (e.g., PUFA modulation of genes, modulation of genes by some vitamins, etc.).

Some transcription factors are an integral component in certain **gene expression cascades**. For example, a gene expression cascade is initiated by the first gene causing expression of a transcription factor, which then **itself** interacts with the cell's DNA to either cause or speed up yet **another** gene expression. The protein resulting from that second gene expression is yet **another** transcription factor which triggers another (i.e., third) gene expression, and so on.
See also PROTEIN, GENETIC CODE, CODING SEQUENCE, DEOXYRIBONUCLEIC ACID (DNA), CELL, INHIBITION, GENE, P53 GENE, TRANSCRIPTION, P53 PROTEIN, CBF1, COLD HARDENING, REGULATORY SEQUENCE, EXPRESS, GENE EXPRESSION, GENE EXPRESSION CASCADE, DOWNREGULATING, VITAMIN, POLYUNSATURATED FATTY ACIDS (PUFA), RECOMBINASE, ACTIVATOR (OF GENE), ZINC FINGER PROTEINS, TRANSCRIPTION ACTIVATORS, TRANSCRIPTION FACTOR BINDING SITE, OLEIC ACID, FATTY ACID BINDING PROTEINS

Transcription Unit A group of genes that code for functionally related RNA molecules or protein molecules. This group of genes is expressed (transcribed) together (i.e., as a unit, thus the name).
See also EXPRESS, GENE, TRANSCRIPTION, TRANSLATION, GENETIC CODE, CODING SEQUENCE, DEOXYRIBONUCLEIC ACID (DNA), RIBONUCLEIC ACID (RNA), RIBOSOMES

Transcriptional Activator A regulatory sequence that binds (i.e., adheres to) a DNA transcription control sequence, and thereby activates (i.e., begins or increases) the transcription of a gene.
See also REGULATORY SEQUENCE, GENE, DEOXYRIBONUCLEIC ACID (DNA), TRANSCRIPTION, TRANSCRIPTION FACTOR, CONTROL SEQUENCE, GENE EXPRESSION, TRANSACTIVATION

Transcriptional Profiling See TRANSCRIPTION, GENE EXPRESSION PROFILING, METABOLITE PROFILING, GENE EXPRESSION ANALYSIS

Transcriptional Repressor A regulatory sequence (segment of DNA) that "binds" (i.e., adheres to) a **DNA transcription control sequence**, and thereby represses (decreases or halts) the transcription of a gene.
See also REGULATORY SEQUENCE, GENE, DEOXYRIBONUCLEIC ACID (DNA), TRANSCRIPTION, TRANSCRIPTION FACTOR, CONTROL SEQUENCE, GENE EXPRESSION, POSITIVE CONTROL, DOWNREGULATING, TRANSACTIVATION

Transcriptome Refers to the entire (complete, possible) set of all gene **transcripts** (i.e., mRNA segments resulting from gene transcription process) in a given organism and also to knowledge of their roles in that organism's structure, growth, health, disease (and that organism's resistance to disease), etc. These roles are predominantly owing to the impact of each protein

T

molecule (i.e., resulting from the mRNA segments being **translated** in cells' ribosomes), which is itself because of the protein molecule's composition **and its tertiary conformation** (which determines the protein's impact in the organism's tissues, metabolism, etc.).

More than one protein can result from each gene in an organism's genome, due to:

- Interactions **between** genes
- Interactions between genes and their (protein) products
- Interactions between genes and some environmental factors

Mechanistically, this results in different proteins being produced during the translation process via:

- **Alternative splicing** of the mRNA transcript. For example, a single intronic base substitution that is present within the IKAP gene, i.e., the allele responsible for the disease known as **Familial Dysautonomia** affects the splicing of the IKAP transcript (i.e., the mRNA segment that determines which specific protein is subsequently "manufactured" by the ribosomes). Up to eight different proteins can be produced from each human gene via alternative splicing.
- Varying translation start or stop site (on the gene).
- **Frameshifting** (i.e., different set of triplet codons in the mRNA/transcript is translated by the ribosome).

See also GENE, TRANSCRIPT, MESSENGER RNA (mRNA), CODING SEQUENCE, TRANSLATION, CODON, PROTEIN, GENOME, GENETIC CODE, CENTRAL DOGMA (NEW), ORGANISM, CONFORMATION, METABOLISM, TERTIARY STRUCTURE, INTRON, BASE, ALTERNATIVE SPLICING, FRAMESHIFT, SPLICE VARIANTS, SPLICEOSOMES

Transduction (gene) The transfer of bacterial genes (DNA) from one bacterium to another by means of a (temperature or defective) bacterial virus (bacteriophage). There exist two kinds of transduction: specialized and general.

In the case of **specialized transduction**, a restricted group of host genes become integrated into the virus genome. These "guest" genes usually replace some of the viral genes and are subsequently transferred to a second bacterium. In the case of **generalized transduction, host genes become a part of the mature virus particle in place of, or in addition to, the virus DNA.** However, in this case the genes can come from virtually any portion of the host genome and this material does not become directly integrated into the virus genome. In the case of plants, the vector can be *Agrobacterium tumefaciens*.

See also BACTERIOPHAGE, VECTOR, GENETIC CODE, *AGROBACTERIUM TUMEFACIENS*, RETROVIRAL VECTORS, GENE DELIVERY, TRANSFECTION

Transduction (signal) See SIGNAL TRANSDUCTION

***trans* Fatty Acids** One of the two isomeric forms that fatty acids can exist in. *Trans* fatty acids are naturally present in some meat and dairy products (which constitute approximately 5% of the average American diet).

See also FATTY ACID, ISOMER, STEREOISOMERS, HYDROGENATION

Transfection This term has several different meanings, depending on the context in which it is used:

- A word utilized most generally to refer to insertion of DNA segments (genes) into cells (e.g., via electroporation, endocytosis, etc.). For example, insertion of a gene that codes for green fluorescent protein (GFP) into a cell in such a manner that it causes the cell (or **class of cells**) to fluoresce under certain conditions/illumination.
- A word utilized since 1998 to refer to insertion of certain double-stranded RNA (dsRNA) segments into cells (via electroporation, certain RNA polymerases, certain viral infections, etc.); to cause RNA interference (RNAi)/knockout/silencing.
- A word utilized to refer to insertion of (**complementary-to-constitutive**

mRNA) antisense oligonucleotides, to cause cosuppression/knockdown.

- A word utilized to refer to insertion of a **DNA biologically active protein** (e.g., transcription factors, STATs, etc.) or other DNA/RNA biologically active small molecule.

- A special case of transformation in which an appropriate recipient strain of bacteria is exposed to (free) DNA isolated from a transducing phage with the "take-up" of that DNA by some of the bacteria and consequent production and release of complete virus particles. The process involves the direct transfer of genetic material from donor to recipient.

See also MARKER (GENETIC MARKER), TRANSFORMATION, ELECTROPORATION, GENE, VIRUS, CELL, BACTERIA, DEOXYRIBONUCLEIC ACID (DNA), TRANSDUCTION (GENE), GREEN FLUORESCENT PROTEIN (GFP), CODING SEQUENCE, FLUORESCENCE, PROTEIN, RIBONUCLEIC ACID (RNA), RNA INTERFERENCE (RNAi), dsRNA, MESSENGER RNA (mRNA), KNOCKOUT, GENE SILENCING, ANTISENSE (DNA SEQUENCE), KNOCKDOWN, DOWNREGULATING, COMPLEMENTARY (MOLECULAR GENETICS), TRANSCRIPTION FACTORS, SIGNAL TRANSDUCERS AND ACTIVATORS OF TRANSCRIPTION (STATs), BIOLOGICAL ACTIVITY, REPORTER GENE

Transfer RNA (tRNA) Discovered in 1957 by Mahlon Bush Hoagland, they are a class of relatively small RNA (ribonucleic acid) molecules of molecular weight 23,000 to about 30,000. tRNA molecules act as carriers of specific amino acids during the process of protein synthesis. Each of the 20 amino acids found in proteins has at least one specific corresponding tRNA. Attachment of an amino acid to a tRNA molecule forms an active (amino-acyl) tRNA, which then functions as a **ribosomal adaptor** (tRNA adaptor). The tRNA binds covalently with "its" specific amino acid and "leads" it to the ribosome for incorporation into the growing peptide chain.

See also RIBONUCLEIC ACID (RNA), MOLECULAR WEIGHT, AMINO ACID, MESSENGER RNA (mRNA)

Transferases Enzymes that catalyze the transfer of functional groups to molecules (from other molecules).

See also TRANSAMINASE, ENZYME, HEDGEHOG PROTEINS, GLYCOSYL-TRANSFERASES

Transferred DNA See Ti PLASMID

Transferrin The protein molecule that is responsible for transporting iron (molecules) to tissues throughout the body, via the circulatory system.

See also PROTEIN, TRANSFERRIN RECEPTOR, HEME, BLOOD–BRAIN BARRIER (BBB)

Transferrin Receptor The receptor molecule (located on the surface of cells throughout the body) that is responsible for binding to transferrin molecules, then bringing those iron-rich transferrin molecules into the cell where the iron is released to be used by the cell.

See also TRANSFERRIN, RECEPTORS, HEME, BLOOD–BRAIN BARRIER (BBB)

Transformation The process in which free DNA is transferred directly into a competent recipient cell. The direct transfer of genetic material from donor to recipient. The acquisition (e.g., by bacteria cells) of new genetic markers (new traits coded for by the new DNA) via the process of transformation.

See also DEOXYRIBONUCLEIC ACID (DNA), TRANSFECTION, MARKER (GENETIC MARKER)

Transforming Growth Factor-Alpha (TGF-Alpha) An angiogenic growth factor produced by tumor cells. It is able to induce specific malignant characteristics in normal cells (such as fibroblasts), thereby "transforming" them. TGF-alpha appears to possess a variety of potentially useful pharmaceutical properties, such as powerful stimulation of scar tissue formation following wounding of a tissue, as indicated by preliminary research.

See also TRANSFORMING GROWTH FACTOR-BETA (TGF-BETA), GROWTH FACTOR, NERVE GROWTH FACTOR (NGF), TUMOR, FIBROBLASTS, ANGIOGENIC GROWTH FACTORS

T

Transforming Growth Factor-Beta (TGF-Beta) An angiogenic growth factor produced by tumor cells, it is able to induce specific malignant characteristics in normal cells (such as fibroblasts), thereby "transforming" those cells from epithelial phenotype to mesenchymal phenotype (thereby enabling cell motility). TGF-beta stimulates blood vessel growth, even though it inhibits the division of endothelial cells. TGF-beta is a strong "attracting agent" for macrophages (i.e., TGF-beta is chemotactic), and appears to be responsible for the high concentrations of macrophages that are often found in tumors. TGF-beta has shown immunosuppressive activity (i.e., it suppresses the immune system). For example, TGF-beta works together with osteoinductive factor (OIF) to promote bone formation by first causing connective tissue cells to grow together to form a matrix of cartilage (e.g., across a bone break), after which bone cells slowly replace that cartilage.

See also TRANSFORMING GROWTH FACTOR-ALPHA (TGF-ALPHA), GROWTH FACTOR, OSTEOINDUCTIVE FACTOR (OIF), EPITHELIUM, IMMUNOSUPPRESSIVE, NERVE GROWTH FACTOR (NGF), TUMOR, FIBROBLASTS, ANGIOGENIC GROWTH FACTORS, MITOGEN, ENDOTHELIAL CELLS, CHEMOTAXIS, MACROPHAGE, CELL MOTILITY

Transgalacto-oligosaccharides A "family" of oligosaccharides (produced via enzymatic conversion of lactose, using β-glucosidase enzyme), some of which help to foster the growth of beneficial **bifidobacteria** in the lower colon of monogastric animals (e.g., humans, swine, etc.).

See also OLIGOSACCHARIDES, PREBIOTICS, BACTERIA, BIFIDOBACTERIA, *BIFIDUS*, ENZYME

Transgene A "package" of genetic material (i.e., DNA) that is inserted into the genome of a cell via gene splicing techniques. May include promoters, leader sequence, termination codon, etc.

See also DEOXYRIBONUCLEIC ACID (DNA), GENE SPLICING, GENOME, LEADER SEQUENCE, PROMOTER, GENETIC CODE, TERMINATION CODON (SEQUENCE), GENETIC ENGINEERING, CASSETTE

Transgenic An organism whose gamete cells (sperm/egg) contain genetic material originally derived from an organism **other** than the parents, or in addition to the parental genetic material.

See also GENETIC ENGINEERING, GAMETE, NUCLEAR TRANSFER

Transgressive Segregants Refers to offspring (e.g., created within a formal crop seed company breeding program) that possess significantly **different** traits/phenotypes than their parents. It results when allele pairs get separated from each other during meiosis (and subsequently sorted into different cells).

See also GENE, ALLELE, TRAIT, PHENOTYPE, CELL, MEIOSIS, EPISTASIS

Transgressive Segregation A plant-breeding (propagation) technique, in which *genetically very different* members of the *same species* are mated with each other. The offspring of that mating can be more healthy, productive (e.g., fast growing), and uniform than their parents, a phenomenon known as "hybrid vigor."

See also GENETICS, SPECIES, F1 HYBRIDS, HYBRIDIZATION (PLANT GENETICS)

Transit Peptide A peptide that when fused to a protein acts to transport that protein between compartments within eucaryotic cells. Once inside the "destination compartment," the transit peptide is cleaved off the protein and that protein is then free (to do its designed task).

See also PEPTIDE, PROTEIN, EUCARYOTE, CELL, FUSION PROTEIN, GATED TRANSPORT, VESICULAR TRANSPORT, CHLOROPLAST TRANSIT PEPTIDE (CTP)

Transition Refers to the replacement (i.e., in DNA or RNA molecule) of one purine by another purine; or one pyrimidine by another pyrimidine.

See also PURINE, PYRIMIDINE, DEOXYRIBONUNCLEIC ACID (DNA), RIBONUCLEIC ACID (RNA), BASE SUBSTITUTION

Transition State (in a chemical reaction) That point in the chemical reaction at which the reactants (i.e., chemical entities about to react with each other) have been "brought to the brink." It is a point in the chemical reaction process in which an "activated condition" is reached. From this point the probability of the reaction going to completion and yielding a product is very high. The transition state separates (energetically) products from reactants. It is viewed as being at the top of the energy barrier separating reactants and products. The reacting species in the transition state can, because of their location at the "top" of the energy barrier, "fall" to either products or reactants.

See also CATALYST, ENDERGONIC REACTION, ACTIVATION ENERGY, FREE ENERGY, CATALYTIC ANTIBODY, SEMI-SYNTHETIC CATALYTIC ANTIBODY, EXERGONIC REACTION

Translation The process by which protein molecules are synthesized (made) whereby the genetic information present in an mRNA molecule directs the order of incorporation of specific amino acids and, hence, the growth of the polypeptide chain during protein synthesis. One can think of translation as the process of translating one language into another. In this particular case the nucleic-acid-based language represented by mRNA is translated into the amino-acid-based language of proteins.

See also CODING SEQUENCE, CODON, RIBOSOMES, MESSENGER RNA (mRNA), AMINO ACID, RIBOSOMES, SPLICEO-SOMES, PROTEIN, GENE, GENETIC CODE, ALTERNATIVE SPLICING

Translational Repression See MICRO-RNAs

Translocation Genetic mutation in which a section of a chromosome breaks off and moves to a new (abnormal) position in that (or a different) chromosome.

See also GENE, CHROMOSOMES, GENETIC CODE, CODING SEQUENCE, TRANSPOSITION, DEOXYRIBONU-CLEIC ACID (DNA), MUTATION, INTRO-GRESSION, JUMPING GENES, HOT SPOTS

Translocation (of protein molecules) The movement of a protein molecule:

- From one location/compartment within a cell to another location.
- Across a cellular membrane (e.g., a plasma membrane).

See also PROTEIN, CELL, MEMBRANES (OF A CELL), MEMBRANE TRANSPORT, MEMBRANE TRANSPORTER PROTEIN, LEADER SEQUENCE (PROTEIN MOLE-CULE), GATED TRANSPORT, CHAPER-ONES, PLASMA MEMBRANE

Transmembrane Proteins Refers to those protein molecules that extend from one side of a cell membrane to the other side of that membrane.

For example, G-proteins are transmembrane proteins that act to accomplish signal transduction (i.e., convey "signal" from outside the cell to one or more internal cell parts). EGF receptors bind to EGF molecules (e.g., passing by in the blood), then both enter the cell (through the cell membrane) together, where the EGF stimulates growth/division of that cell.

See also PROTEIN, CELL, PLASMA MEM-BRANE, RECEPTORS, MEMBRANE (OF A CELL), MEMBRANE TRANSPORT, ABC TRANSPORTERS, EGF RECEPTOR, G-PROTEINS, CECROPHINS (LYTIC PRO-TEINS), MAGAININS, SIGNAL TRANS-DUCTION, SIGNALING, EPIDERMAL GROWTH FACTOR (EGF), GATED TRANS-PORT, PORIN, SID-1 PROTEIN

Transport Proteins Refers to protein molecules that are utilized to carry (i.e. transport) compounds within the body of an organism. For example, the transport protein known as hemo-globin is used by the human body to transport oxygen from the lungs to all of the cells of the body. For example, fatty acid binding proteins (FABP) are used by cells to transport specific fatty acids from the cell's plasma membrane to the needed destination within the cell's interior.

See also PROTEIN, ORGANISM, CELL, HEMOGLOBIN, FATTY ACID, FATTY ACID BINDING PROTEINS, PLASMA MEMBRANE

Transposable Element See TRANSPOSON

Transposase An enzyme that is required for transposition to occur (i.e., assists movement of a transposon from one location to another within a cell's DNA). It is coded for by the transposon known as the P element.

See also TRANSPOSITION, TRANSPOSON, ENZYME, GENETIC CODE, CODING SEQUENCE, DEOXYRIBONUCLEIC ACID (DNA)

Transposition Movement of a gene or set of genes from one site in the genome to another without a reciprocal exchange (of DNA).

See also GENE, JUMPING GENES, GENOME, TRANSPOSON, TRANSPOSASE, HOT SPOTS, DEOXYRIBONUCLEIC ACID (DNA)

Transposon A DNA (deoxyribonucleic acid) sequence (segment of molecule) able to replicate and insert one copy (of itself) at a new location in the genome (i.e., a transposition of location). Discovered in 1950 by geneticist Barbara McClintock in corn (maize) plants (*Zea mays* L.) and in bacteria a decade later by Joshua Lederberg, transposons can either carry genes along one organism's genome, or even into another organism's genome (e.g., via sexual conjugation, in bacteria). By such sexual conjugation, transposons can carry genes that confer new phenotypic properties (e.g., resistance to certain antibiotics, for a given bacterial cell).

See also DEOXYRIBONUCLEIC ACID (DNA), REPLICATION (OF VIRUS), GENOME, TRANSPOSITION, TRANSPOSASE, SEQUENCE (OF A DNA MOLECULE), CORN, JUMPING GENES, GENE, SEXUAL CONJUGATION, PHENOTYPE, CONJUGATION

Transversion The substitution of a purine for a pyramidine, or of a pyramidine for a purine (at a specific site, within a given nucleotide in a molecule of DNA). That substitution generally results from a mutation in an organism's DNA.

See also NUCLEOTIDE, DEOXYRIBONUCLEIC ACID (DNA), SINGLE-NUCLEOTIDE POLYMORPHISMS (SNPs), MUTATION, BASE SUBSTITUTION

TRANSWITCH® A "sense" technology used to "turn off" (suppress) a gene (e.g., the one that causes tomato to ripen) that causes an unwanted effect (e.g., premature softening of tomato). TRANSWITCH® and its registered trademark are owned by DNA Plant Technology Corp.

See also GENE SILENCING, SUPPRESSOR GENE, SENSE

Trastuzumab A ("humanized") monoclonal antibody-against-HER-2-gene that was approved by the U.S. Food and Drug Administration (FDA) during 2002 for use as a pharmaceutical in conjunction with chemotherapy against metastatic breast cancer.

See also MONOCLONAL ANTIBODIES (MAb), CANCER, METASTASIS, FLUORESCENCE *IN SITU* HYBRIDIZATION (FISH), FOOD AND DRUG ADMINISTRATION (FDA), HUMANIZED ANTIBODY, GENE, HER-2 GENE

"Treatment" IND Regulations Food and Drug Administration (FDA) regulations promulgated in 1987 to provide a more rapid formal pharmaceutical approval mechanism than the usual IND (Investigational New Drug) regulatory approval process. Its purpose is to enable drug developers to provide promising experimental drugs to patients suffering from immediately life-threatening diseases or certain serious conditions (e.g., acquired immune deficiency syndrome, or AIDS) before complete data on that drug's efficacy or toxicity are available.

See also IND, FOOD AND DRUG ADMINISTRATION (FDA), DELANEY CLAUSE, KOSEISHO, COMMITTEE FOR PROPRIETARY MEDICINAL PRODUCTS (CPMP)

Treatment Investigational New Drug See "TREATMENT" IND REGULATIONS

Treatment System Also sometimes called **Treatment Process**. Refers to the measures utilized (e.g., by an agricultural-commodity-importing country) to prevent the **introduction** of a **"quarantine pest"** into a **"pest-free area."**

For example, some countries that are free of relevant insect pests, may require that certain agricultural commodities (i.e., containing that live pest) be fumigated with specific pesticides before those commodity shipments are allowed to enter that country.

See also INTERNATIONAL PLANT PROTECTION CONVENTION (IPPC), QUARANTINE PEST, INTRODUCTION

Trehalose A disaccharide (simple sugar) that is naturally synthesized (i.e., "manufactured") by many plants and animals in response to the stresses of freezing, heating, or drying. That is because trehalose protects certain proteins (needed for life) and prevents loss of crucial volatile (i.e., easily evaporated) compounds from organisms during those stressful (e.g., dry, frozen, or hot) conditions. Trehalose also provides a source of quick energy after the stressful conditions have passed. That is why dried baker's yeast (which contains up to 20% trehalose by weight) can be stored in its dry state for many years, yet quickly leavens bread dough within minutes of being rehydrated (i.e., rewetted).

Trehalose accomplishes this protection by forming a nonhygroscopic "glass" on the surfaces of cells and large molecules. It immobilizes and stabilizes large molecules (e.g., proteins), but still allows water to diffuse out so that complete drying can occur. Thus, trehalose has potential as a food additive to keep proteins (e.g., eggs) fresh in the dried form. In 1991, the U.K. approved trehalose for use in food. Trehalose hydrolyzes (e.g., during digestion) into two molecules of glucose.

Owing to its trehalose content, the Resurrection Plant (also known as **Rose of Jericho**) can be "resurrected" (after years in a state of total desiccation) by rehydrating it.

See also DISACCHARIDES, PROTEIN, GLUCOSE (GLc), HYDROLYSIS, CONFORMATION, "SWITCH" PROTEINS, TERTIARY STRUCTURE, PROTEIN FOLDING

Tremorgenic Indole Alkaloids A "family" of toxic alkaloids (chemical compounds) that are naturally produced (e.g., within some plants) by certain fungi (i.e., which sometimes grow in those plants).

For example, the alkaloid known as **Penitrem D** is produced by certain fungi that grow in some grass species. It causes tremors, weakness, lack of coordination, and convulsions in animals that consume those fungus-infested grasses.

See also ALKALOIDS, TOXIN, FUNGUS, ENDOPHYTE

Triacyglycerides See TRIGLYCERIDES

Triacylglycerols See TRIGLYCERIDES

Trichoderma harzianum A microorganism that possesses (natural) fungicide activity.

See also *BACILLUS THURINGIENSIS (B.t.)*, WHEAT TAKE-ALL DISEASE, FUNGUS, FUNGICIDE

Trichosanthin An enzyme extracted from a specific Chinese plant. It has been discovered to cut apart the ribosomes in some cells that are infected with the HIV (i.e., AIDS) virus, thus potentially stopping the virus and preventing infection of additional cells.

See also RIBOSOMES, ACQUIRED IMMUNE DEFICIENCY SYNDROME (AIDS), ENZYME, PROTEIN, HUMAN IMMUNODEFICIENCY VIRUS TYPE 1 (HIV-1), HUMAN IMMUNODEFICIENCY VIRUS TYPE 2 (HIV-2)

Triglycerides The primary constituent of fats or oils, triglycerides are molecules that consist of three fatty acids attached to a glycerol "molecular backbone." More accurately called **triacylglycerols**, although long-term historical usage of "triglycerides" has made the latter term more common (though not totally accurate).

Similarly, the term "**diglyceride**" is often used to refer to those molecules that consist of two fatty acids attached to a glycerol "molecular backbone." "Diglycerides" (more accurately called **diacylglycerols**) can result from the splitting off (i.e., hydrolysis) of one fatty acid from a triacylglycerol ("triglyceride") molecule (e.g., during fat breakdown/oxidation), or from the combination of two fatty acids with glycerol (e.g., during synthesis of fats).

The "**triglyceride level**" in human bloodstream refers to the blood's content of noncholesterol total fats. Research during the 1990s provided evidence that high blood levels of triglycerides in humans (e.g., immediately after meals) can contribute to thrombosis.

See also FATS, THROMBOSIS, FATTY ACID, SATURATED FATTY ACIDS (SAFA), LPAAT PROTEIN, UNSATURATED FATTY ACID, HYDROLYSIS, OXIDATION (OF FATS, OILS, OR LIPIDS), ADIPOCYTES, FRUCTOSE OLIGOSACCHARIDES, BIFIDUS, POLYUNSATURATED FATTY ACIDS (PUFA), DIACYLGLYCEROLS, MEDIUM-CHAIN TRIACYLGLYCERIDES

Triploid Refers to organisms that possess three sets of chromosomes instead of the normal two sets. Conversion of a diploid (i.e., two sets of chromosomes) organism to triploid can be done by man (e.g., certain fish, "seedless" grapes, etc.). For example, fish are ordinarily diploid. By exposing fish eggs to certain specific combinations of temperature and pressure immediately after fertilization of those eggs, scientists can cause the resultant fish to become triploid. Triploid fish are unable to reproduce. This sterility is desired by man, in order to prevent certain fish (e.g., those that have been genetically engineered) from mating with wild fish.

Such induced (triploid) sterility also prevents the (genetically engineered) fish from wasting energy on the act of reproduction, so they grow faster and larger. That transfer (of energy use from reproduction to growth) also holds true for "seedless" grapes, watermelons, etc.
See also DIPLOID, CHROMOSOMES, WHEAT

tRNA Abbreviation for **transfer RNA**.
See TRANSFER RNA (tRNA)

Tropism Orientation movement of a sessile organism in response to a stimulus. Movement of curvature due to an external stimulus that determines the direction of movement. Also known as topotaxis.
See also SESSILE, CHEMOTAXIS

Trypsin A proteolytic (protein **molecular chain**-cutting) enzyme that is produced by the pancreas, to facilitate digestion within certain animals.

Trypsin cleaves polypeptide (protein) molecular chains on the carboxyl (group) side of arginine and lysine units (residues), and it is often utilized by man to break apart protein molecules (e.g., to enable scientists to study its constituent peptides).
See also ARGININE (Arg), LYSINE (Lys), PROTEIN, PEPTIDE, POLYPEPTIDE (PROTEIN), PROTEOLYTIC ENZYMES, PROTEASES, CHYMOTRYPSIN, TRYPSIN INHIBITORS, DIGESTION (WITHIN ORGANISMS), COWPEA TRYPSIN INHIBITOR (CpTI)

Trypsin Inhibitors Compounds present in certain plants (e.g., squash, soybeans, etc.) that inhibit the activity (i.e., protein cleavage, which aids digestion) of proteases (i.e., protein-cleaving enzymes such as trypsin or chymotrypsin) in the digestive systems of monogastric (i.e., single-stomach) animals (which include swine, poultry, and humans). Trypsin inhibitors present in some varieties of squash include the **Ecballium elaterium trypsin inhibitor (EETI)**. Trypsin inhibitors present in traditional varieties of soybeans (botanical name *Glycine max* (L.) Merrill) include:

- The Kunitz trypsin inhibitor (TI), which was first isolated and crystallized by M. Kunitz in 1945. It combines tightly with molecules of trypsin on a 1:1 basis, and thereby reduces the rate of protein cleavage effected by the trypsin enzyme, which inhibits the animal's digestion of proteins.

- The Bowman-Birk trypsin inhibitor (BB T.I.), which was first described by D. E. Bowman in 1944. It combines with molecules of trypsin and chymotripsin, and thereby reduces the rate of protein cleavage effected by the trypsin and chymotrypsin enzymes; which inhibits the animal's digestion of proteins.
  NOTE: During 2000, research by Frank Meyskins and William Armstrong indicated that consumption of BB T.I. in a manner that "bathes" mouth tissues (for extended periods of time) inhibits the development of the precancerous mouth lesions that can become oral cancer.

- Certain free fatty acids and their acyl-CoA esters, which reduce the rate of protein cleavage effected by the trypsin enzyme, which inhibits the animal's digestion of proteins.

Heating of soybeans to a temperature of 212° (100°C) for 15 min causes these trypsin inhibitors to be rendered inactive in soybeans, so the animal's digestion is unimpeded when it is fed soy that has been thus heated.
See also TRYPSIN, CHYMOTRYPSIN, SOYBEAN PLANT, PROTEIN, PROTEASES, ENZYME, PROTEOLYTIC ENZYMES, DIGESTION (WITHIN ORGANISMS), POLYPEPTIDE (PROTEIN), BIOLOGICAL ACTIVITY, ACYL-CoA, COWPEA TRYPSIN INHIBITOR (CpTI), EETI, ORAL CANCER

Tryptophan (Trp) Discovered in 1900 by Frederick Hopkins, tryptophan is an essential amino acid. It is a precursor of the important biochemical molecules: indoleacetic acid, serotonin, and nicotinic acid. L-Tryptophan is used as a common feed additive for livestock to ensure that their diet includes an adequate amount of this essential amino acid.
See also ESSENTIAL AMINO ACIDS, STEREOISOMERS, SEROTONIN, AMINO ACID

TSH See THYROID-STIMULATING HORMONE (TSH)

Tuberculosis See *MYCOBACTERIUM TUBERCULOSIS*

Tubulin A cell protein that comprises microtubules in eucaryotic cells. Such microtubules fulfill a number of cellular functions, and are required for cell mitosis (i.e., the **cell reproduction process** in which a cell divides into two identical cells).

When the drugs **paclitaxel** or Taxol™ are administered to body (e.g., in chemotherapy), they bind tubulin, which halts cell division and causes apoptosis in the affected cells (e.g., tumor cells) by binding **Bc1-2** (a protein that prevents apoptosis in cells).

Tubulin analogues present in bacterial cells include **FtsZ**, which is the principal cytoskeleton component of the **Z-ring** that first constricts, then divides the cells into two different cells during mitosis.

See also CELL, PROTEIN, EUCARYOTE, MICROTUBULES, MITOSIS, PACLITAXEL, TAXOL, CANCER, CHEMOTHERAPY, APOPTOSIS, ANALOGUE, CYTOSKELETON, MOTOR PROTEINS

Tumor A mass of abnormal tissue that resembles normal tissues in structure, but which fulfills no useful function (to the organism) and grows at the expense of the body. Tumors may be malignant or benign. Malignant tumors (which infiltrate adjacent healthy tissues) can result from oncogenes or carcinogens. They can eventually kill their host if unchecked.

Epidermal growth factor encourages rapid cell growth in more than 50% of human tumors.

See also CANCER, ANGIOGENESIS, ONCOGENES, PROTO-ONCOGENES, CELL, CARCINOGEN, TYROSINE KINASE, TYROSINE KINASE INHIBITORS (TKI), ATP SYNTHASE, EPIDERMAL GROWTH FACTOR (EGF)

Tumor-Associated Antigens Discovered by Thierry Boon in 1991, these are distinctive protein molecules that are produced in the surface membrane of tumor cells. These protein molecules are used by the body's cytotoxic T cells to recognize (and destroy) tumor cells, so such proteins hold promise for use in vaccines.

See also MAJOR HISTOCOMPATIBILITY COMPLEX (MHC), MACROPHAGE, TUMOR, T CELL RECEPTORS, ANTIGEN, T CELLS, PROTEIN, CELL, CYTOTOXIC T CELLS, HUMAN LEUKOCYTE ANTIGENS (HLA)

Tumor-Infiltrating Lymphocytes (TIL cells) The white blood cells of a cancer patient that have been:

1. Taken from that patient's tumor (where those white blood cells had been attempting to combat the cancer, albeit unsuccessfully)
2. Stimulated with doses of interleukin-2 (to make the lymphocytes more effective against the cancer)
3. Multiplied *in vitro* (i.e., outside of the patient's body) to make them more numerous (and thus more likely to successfully combat the cancer)

When these "souped-up" lymphocytes (white blood cells) are reintroduced into the patient's body, the lymphocytes (now called TIL cells because they have been souped up) attack the cancer tumor (malignant growth) more vigorously than before.

See also TUMOR, WHITE BLOOD CELLS, LYMPHOCYTE, LYMPHOKINES, T CELLS, CYTOTOXIC T CELLS

Tumor Necrosis Factor (TNF) Literally, *tumor death factor.* More precisely called **tumor necrosis factor-α**, it is an adipokine (i.e., protein synthesized by adipose cells, which helps regulate the immune system) that has shown potential to combat (kill) malignant (cancer) tumors.

Tumor necrosis factor was discovered to be 10,000 times more toxic in humans than in rodents, where it had been tested for toxicity prior to human clinical tests. This example illustrates one potential pitfall of nontarget animal testing in that sometimes animal testing does not accurately reflect or foretell what will happen in humans.

Another drawback of using TNF-α as a drug to combat human tumors is the fact that it is one of the substances released by the body in excess (in the disease rheumatoid arthritis) that destroys tissue in the joints (TNF causes both inflammation and joint damage).

When released as part of the AIDS (disease), TNF causes cachexia, which is a wasting away of the

T

body due to the body's reduced ability to process nutrients received via digestion. The pharmaceuticals known as Remicade™ (infliximab), and Humira ™ (adalimumab) are monoclonal antibodies approved by the U.S. Food and Drug Administration (FDA) as treatments to inhibit the structural damage (to body joints) of the autoimmune disease rheumatoid arthritis.

The pharmaceutical known as Enbrel™ (etanercept) is a fusion protein approved by the U.S. Food and Drug Administration (FDA) as a treatment to inhibit the structural damage (to body joints) of the autoimmune disease rheumatoid arthritis.

Each of these three pharmaceuticals specifically block tumor necrosis factor-α.

See also ADIPOKINES, ADIPOSE, LYMPHOKINES, NECROSIS, TUMOR, TUMOR-INFILTRATING LYMPHOCYTES (TIL CELLS), PROTEIN, AUTOIMMUNE DISEASE, T-CELL-MODULATING PEPTIDE (TCMP), DIGESTION (WITHIN ORGANISMS), TOXICOGENOMICS, RHEUMATOID ARTHRITIS, MONOCLONAL ANTIBODIES (MAb), ADALIMUMAB, FUSION PROTEIN, FOOD AND DRUG ADMINISTRATION (FDA)

Tumor Necrosis Factor-α See TUMOR NECROSIS FACTOR (TNF)

Tumor Suppressor Genes Also called anticancer genes. Genes within a cell's DNA that code for (i.e., cause to be manufactured in cell's ribosomes) proteins that hold the cell's growth in check. If these genes are damaged (e.g., by radiation, by a carcinogen, or by chance accident in normal cell division), they no longer hold cell growth in check, and the cell becomes malignant (if the cell's DNA also contains a gene called an *oncogene*). Oncogenes must be present for the cell to become malignant, but oncogenes cannot cause a cell to become malignant until a tumor suppressor gene is damaged. As with all genes, tumor suppressor genes are inherited in two copies (alleles, one from each parent) and either copy can code for the proteins necessary for cell growth control. However, an organism that is born with one defective copy of a tumor suppressor gene (or in whom one copy is damaged early in life) is especially prone to cancer (malignancy).

See also GENE, p53 GENE, GENETIC CODE, MEIOSIS, DEOXYRIBONUCLEIC ACID (DNA), CARCINOGEN, RIBOSOMES, ONCOGENES, CANCER, TUMOR, PROTO-ONCOGENES, PROTEIN

Tumor Suppressor Proteins Proteins that are coded for (i.e., caused to be manufactured in the cell's ribosomes) by tumor suppressor genes (e.g., the p53 gene). Such proteins (e.g., the p53 protein) then act on the cell's DNA in order to prevent uncontrolled cell growth and division (i.e., cancer).

See also TUMOR SUPPRESSOR GENES, GENE, p53 GENE, PROTEIN, GENETIC CODE, MEIOSIS, DEOXYRIBONUCLEIC ACID (DNA), RIBOSOMES, ONCOGENES, CANCER, TUMOR, CELL, PROTO-ONCOGENES

Turnover Number The number of molecules of a product produced per minute by a single-enzyme molecule when that enzyme is working at its maximum rate. That is, the number of substrate molecules converted into a product by one enzyme molecule per minute when that enzyme is "going (catalyzing) as fast as it can."

See also ENZYME, TRANSFERASES, PROTEASE, PROTEIN KINASES, PROTEOLYTIC ENZYMES, TRANSAMINASE

Two-Dimensional (2-D) Gel Electrophoresis
A technology/methodology discovered by Patrick O'Farrell in 1975 to separate the various proteins within a given biological sample prior to their analysis. The proteins are moved by applying an electrical field in two distinct directions.

The sample is moved through two different gels (i.e., two different dimensions). The initial gel has a pH gradient that separates the different proteins based on their respective isoelectric points (i.e., separated on the basis of the protein molecule's charge).

The second gel (dimension) the sample is moved through is a gel that separates the protein molecules based on their individual molecular weights. That gel acts as a "molecular sieve" (i.e., smaller proteins move faster — and farther — than larger proteins through this gel in a fixed amount of time).

A fixed-time gel run (i.e., with appropriate gel and the appropriate electrical fields applied to the gel) leaves a scientist with as many as 1,000 "spots" (of individual protein molecules) on the gel. Each spot is a collection of the molecules of one protein from the original sample (mixture). To identify the proteins in the spots, the scientist can do the following:

- Stain them (e.g., with ethidium bromide, etc.), then illuminate them with a special (UV) light and assesses the entire gel with an electronic image scanner (or assess it visually).
- Cut out each spot from the gel and analyze it (e.g., via use of MALDI-TOF mass spectrometer) to determine the identity of the protein in the spot.

From the pattern (coupled with intensity) of the spots, two such gels could be utilized to do the following:

- Confirm if two sample organisms were the same species/strain/variety.
- Determine the differences (in gene expression) between samples of diseased vs. healthy tissues.

See also PROTEIN, GEL, ELECTROPHORESIS, AGAROSE, POLYACRYLAMIDE GEL ELECTROPHORESIS (PAGE), PAGE, ISOELECTRIC POINT, GENE EXPRESSION ANALYSIS, PROTEOMICS, MOLECULAR WEIGHT, SPECIES, MALDI-TOF-MS, ISOELECTRIC FOCUSING (IEF)

Two-Hybrid Systems Refers to yeast or bacterial "systems" (test systems built by scientists) that are utilized to detect specific protein–protein interactions (e.g., identification of the gene that codes for the **protein which is found to specifically interact with a known protein** when the latter is exposed to a sample containing numerous "unknown" proteins). Two-hybrid systems take advantage of the fact that certain transcriptional factors possess **two** distinctly separate functional domains. One of those two domains must interact with a second domain (e.g., in a fusion protein containing a portion of a known protein) in order to cause transcription (e.g., of

the *GAL4* gene in the yeast two-hybrid system).

The oldest two-hybrid system is that utilizing the *GAL4* transcriptional activation system of *Saccharomyces cerevisiae* yeast. *GAL4* is required to initiate expression of proteins that are central to galactose metabolism in that yeast.

See also PROTEIN, FUSION PROTEIN, GENE, CODING SEQUENCE, DOMAIN (OF A PROTEIN), GENE EXPRESSION, TARGET–LIGAND INTERACTION SCREENING, LIGAND (IN BIOCHEMISTRY), PROTEIN MICROARRAYS, TRANSCRIPTION, TRANSCRIPTIONAL ACTIVATOR, YEAST TWO-HYBRID SYSTEM

Type I Diabetes The form of diabetes disease that usually strikes young people (thus, it was formerly known as juvenile or insulin-dependent diabetes). It is characterized by the body's immune system (antibodies) destroying the insulin-producing cells (Beta cells) of the pancreas. If not treated in time (i.e., via insulin injections), the person can die suddenly. Even when treated, the person is at increased risk of blindness, atherosclerosis, coronary heart disease, heart attack, stroke, and kidney disease.

See also DIABETES, BETA CELLS, PANCREAS, INSULIN, INSULIN-DEPENDENT DIABETES MELLITIS (IDDM), CALPAIN-10, ATHEROSCLEROSIS, CORONARY HEART DISEASE (CHD), TYPE II DIABETES, ANTIBODY

Type II Diabetes The form of diabetes disease that usually strikes people who are older than 40 years old. Also known as adult-onset diabetes or non-insulin-dependent diabetes, it is characterized by the body's tissues becoming insensitive to insulin. Effects on the body include increased likelihood of blindness, atherosclerosis, coronary heart disease, heart attack, stroke, and kidney disease.

See also DIABETES, INOSITOL, INSULIN-DEPENDENT DIABETES MELLITIS (IDDM), INSULIN, CALPAIN-10, ATHEROSCLEROSIS, CORONARY HEART DISEASE (CHD), TYPE I DIABETES, PPAR

Type Specimen The actual physical specimen (e.g., a stuffed lizard or a dried insect) that a scientist (who describes and names a previously unknown species) must place in a museum (or other recognized repository) in order to have the right to name that newly discovered species. This "officially deposited specimen" is required so that:

1. Comparisons can later be made if there is ever a doubt whether another "new" species is simply a member of this same species (and thus already named).
2. Taxonomists (who determine and keep the official scientific names by which scientists must refer to each of the world's organisms) can name each of the newly discovered species in accordance with the complex rules of the International Codes for Nomenclature. Examples of such names in this glossary are *Arabidopsis thaliana, Escherichia coli,* and *Agrobacterium tumefaciens.*
3. Patent claims for genetically engineered organisms can later be enforced.

See also SPECIES, STRAIN, CLADISTICS, CHAKRABARTY DECISION, AMERICAN TYPE CULTURE COLLECTION (ATCC), CONSULTATIVE GROUP ON INTERNATIONAL AGRICULTURAL RESEARCH (CGIAR)

Tyrosine (Tyr) A phenolic α-amino acid. It is a precursor of the hormones epinephrine, norepinephrine, thyroxine, and triiodothyronine. It is also a precursor of the molecule known as melanin (which is the pigment of a suntan).

See also AMINO ACID, HORMONE

Tyrosine Kinase Inhibitors (TKI) Refers to various chemical compounds that inhibit the activity of tyrosine kinase enzyme (inside the body). Examples of TKI include genistein and the pharmaceuticals Iressa™ (gefinitib), Gleevec (imatinib mesylate), and Tarcera™.

Because the activity of tyrosine kinase helps cancerous (tumor) cells to metastasize (spread/grow), consumption by humans of relevant TKI acts to help prevent spreading of certain cancers.

See also ENZYME, KINASES, TYROSINE KINASE, PROTEIN TYROSINE KINASE INHIBITOR, BIOLOGICAL ACTIVITY, CANCER, CELL, TUMOR, GENISTEIN, ISOFLAVONES, GLEEVEC™

T

U

Ubiquinone Also called **coenzyme Q**, ubiquinone is present in all cells of eucaryotic organisms. Ubiquinone "escorts" nutrients across cell walls, where it plays an assisting role in the formation of adenosine triphosphate (ATP) in the cell's mitochondria. Significant dietary sources of ubiquinone include soybeans, fish, meat, nuts, etc.

See also ENZYME, COENZYME, EUCARYOTE, ORGANISM, ADENOSINE TRIPHOSPHATE (ATP), MITOCHONDRIA, SOYBEAN PLANT, SOY PROTEIN

Ubiquitin A small protein present in all eucaryotic cells (i.e., it is ubiquitous), which plays an important role in "tagging" other protein molecules (e.g., old ones that are degraded, misfolded, or no longer needed) so that they are destined (marked) for destruction (via proteolytic cleavage). Such proteins are then broken down in cell's proteasomes and their constituents recycled because they are damaged or no longer needed by the body. The ubiquitin molecules are then available for reuse.

Tagging or marking for destruction occurs via fusion of the ubiquitin to the relevant protein molecules, and the "tagged" protein molecules are said to have been **ubiquitinated**. The overall ubiquitination process was discovered and delineated during the 1970s and 1980s by Irwin Rose, Aaron Ciechanover, and Avram Hershko. Ubiquitination is also critical in cell division processes, DNA repair processes, apoptosis, transport of certain proteins from a cell's surface to the interior of cell, and protein synthesis processes. In some specific instances, the fusion of ubiquitin to certain protein molecules in cells causes that "partner protein" to be expressed in amounts larger than previously expressed.

See also EUCARYOTE, PROTEIN, PROTEIN FOLDING, CONFORMATION, PROTEOLYTIC ENZYMES, PROTEASOMES, DENATURATION, CELL, GENE, EXPRESS, RIBOSOMES, APOPTOSIS

Ubiquitin–Proteasome Pathway See UBIQUITIN

Ubiquitinated See UBIQUITIN

Ultracentrifuge A high-speed centrifuge that can attain revolving speeds up to 85,000 rpm and centrifugal fields to 500,000 times gravity. The machine is used to sediment (i.e., cause to settle out) and, hence, separate macromolecules (i.e., large molecules) and macromolecular structures in a mixture or solution. In general, a centrifuge is a machine that whirls test tubes around rapidly, like a merry-go-round, to force the heavier suspended materials (in the solutions in the test tubes) to move to the bottoms of the test tubes before the lighter material.

Ultrafiltration A (mixture) separation methodology that uses the ability of synthetic semipermeable membranes (possessing appropriate physical and chemical natures) to discriminate between molecules in the mixture primarily on the basis of the molecules' size or shape.

Invented and developed by Dr. Roy J. Taylor in the 1950s and 1960s, ultrafiltration is typically utilized for the separation of relatively high-molecular-weight solutes (e.g., proteins, gums, polymers, and other complex organic molecules) and colloidally dispersed substances (e.g., minerals, microorganisms, etc.) from their solvents (e.g., water).

See also DIALYSIS, MEMBRANE TRANSPORT, MICROORGANISM, MOLECULAR WEIGHT, PROTEIN, POLYMER, HOLLOW FIBER SEPARATION

Union for Protection of New Varieties of Plants (UPOV) A group of the world's countries that have jointly agreed to mutually protect the intellectual property (of owners, breeders) that is inherent in new plant varieties developed by man. These **intellectual property protections** are often collectively referred to as "**Breeder's Rights**." Established in 1961, the secretariat for this union (UPOV) is in Geneva, Switzerland.

See also PLANT VARIETY PROTECTION ACT (PVP), U.S. PATENT AND TRADEMARK OFFICE (USPTO), PLANT'S NOVEL TRAIT (PNT), PLANT BREEDER'S RIGHTS (PBR), EUROPEAN PATENT CONVENTION, EUROPEAN PATENT OFFICE (EPO), MUTUAL RECOGNITION AGREEMENTS (MRAs), COMMUNITY PLANT VARIETY OFFICE

Units (U) A measure (quantitation) of biological activity of a substance as defined by various standardized assays (tests).
See also ASSAY, BIOASSAY

Unsaturated Fatty Acid A fatty acid containing one or more double bonds (between individual atoms of the molecule).
See also FATTY ACID, DESATURASE, MONOUNSATURATED FATS, POLYUNSATURATED FATTY ACIDS (PUFA)

Unwinding Protein A protein that binds (i.e., adheres to) single-stranded DNA, and thereby aids or stabilizes the unwinding of the DNA molecule's normal (helical or wound-up) structure.
See also PROTEIN, DOUBLE HELIX, DEOXYRIBONUCLEIC ACID (DNA), PLECTONEMIC COILING, HELICASE, GENE REPAIR (NATURAL), MISMATCH REPAIR, PRIMOSOME

UPOV See UNION FOR PROTECTION OF NEW VARIETIES OF PLANTS (UPOV)

Upregulating See TRANSCRIPTIONAL ACTIVATOR, POSITIVE CONTROL

Upregulation See POSITIVE CONTROL, TRANSCRIPTIONAL ACTIVATOR

Uracil A pyrimidine base, important as a component of ribonucleic acid (RNA). Its hydrogen-bonding counterpart in DNA is thymine.
See also PYRIMIDINE, RIBONUCLEIC ACID (RNA), BASE (NUCLEOTIDE), DEOXYRIBONUCLEIC ACID (DNA)

Uridine A nucleoside form of uracil.
See also URACIL, NUCLEOSIDE

Urokinase A thrombolytic (i.e., clot-dissolving) enzyme used as a biopharmaceutical.
See also THROMBOLYTIC AGENTS, TISSUE PLASMINOGEN ACTIVATOR (tPA), FIBRINOLYTIC AGENTS

U.S. Patent and Trademark Office (USPTO) A U.S. government agency based in Washington, D.C., that is responsible for common patent protection matters for all of the 50 U.S. states and its territorial possessions. The USPTO allows the patenting of new and unique microbes, plants, and animals, as well as the new and unique methods to produce such biotechnology advances.
See also EUROPEAN PATENT OFFICE (EPO), CHAKRABARTY DECISION, MICROBE, GENETIC ENGINEERING, PLANT'S NOVEL TRAIT (PNT), PLANT BREEDER'S RIGHTS (PBR), BIOTECHNOLOGY, AMERICAN TYPE CULTURE COLLECTION (ATCC)

USPTO See U.S. PATENT AND TRADEMARK OFFICE (USPTO)

V

Vaccine Any substance, bearing antigens on its surface, that causes activation of an animal's immune system without causing the actual disease. The animals' immune system components (e.g., antibodies) are then prepared to quickly vanquish those particular pathogens when they later enter the body.

See also DNA VACCINES, "NAKED" GENE, EDIBLE VACCINES, PEYER'S PATCHES, ANTIGEN, CELLULAR IMMUNE RESPONSE, HUMORAL IMMUNITY, CARRIER PROTEIN, CELL SURFACE ENGINEERING

Vaccinia A nonpathogenic virus that is believed to be a (modified) form of the virus that causes cowpox. *Vaccinia* readily accepts genes (inserted into its genome via genetic engineering) from pathogenic viruses so it can be used to make vaccines that do not possess the risk inherent in attenuated-virus vaccines (i.e., that the attenuated virus "revives" and causes disease). Such genetically engineered *Vaccinia* codes for (presents) the proteins of the pathogenic virus on its surface, which activates the immune system (e.g., of vaccinated animal) to produce antibodies against that pathogenic virus.

See also VACCINE, PATHOGENIC, VIRUS, GENE, GENE DELIVERY, GENETIC ENGINEERING, ATTENUATED (PATHOGENS), ANTIBODY, MACROPHAGE, COMPLEMENT CASCADE, CELLULAR IMMUNE RESPONSE, PHAGOCYTE

Vacuoles A membrane-bound sac within a cell, within which water, food, waste, or salt, etc., are temporarily stored. Also, refers to pigments in certain plant cells.

See also PLASMA MEMBRANE, CELL, ANTHOCYANIDINS

VAD Acronym for **Vitamin A Deficiency**.

See also GOLDEN RICE, VITAMIN, BETA-CAROTENE, CAROTENOIDS

Vagile Wandering or roaming (e.g., a microorganism that is not attached to a solid support tends to "wander" through its environment as it gets pushed about by currents of air or liquid).

See also SESSILE, VAGILITY

Vagility The ability of organisms to disseminate (e.g., spread throughout a given habitat).

See also VAGILE

Vaginosis The process whereby a cell internalizes an entity (such as a virus or a protein) that has bound to the cell's outer membrane. Once that "bound entity" is inside the cell, the cell membrane fuses together again.

See also NUCLEAR RECEPTORS, RECEPTORS, ENDOCYTOSIS, TRANSFERRIN, VIRUS, BLOOD–BRAIN BARRIER (BBB)

Validation See VALIDATION (OF TARGET), PROCESS VALIDATION

Validation (of target) The process of verifying that a selected "**target**" (e.g., receptor, ion channel, DNA segment, etc.) **of pharmaceuticals** functions as expected in a given disease process.

For protein "targets" (e.g., receptors), validation is done by cloning and expressing the gene that codes for that protein target (to evaluate its **biological impact** on the disease, **which cells** it is expressed in, etc.). Another tool utilized is short interfering RNA (siRNA).

Validation of a target often involves linking together the results of several different studies (e.g., clinical studies with patients who are suffering from a specific disease but were treated with different agents, etc.).

See also TARGET (OF A THERAPEUTIC AGENT), BIOMARKERS, RECEPTORS, NUCLEAR RECEPTORS, ION CHANNELS, DEOXYRIBONUCLEIC ACID (DNA), CODING SEQUENCE, HIGH-THROUGHPUT SCREENING (HTS), TARGET–LIGAND INTERACTION SCREENING, SHORT INTERFERING RNA (siRNA)

Valine (Val) An amino acid considered essential for normal growth of animals. It is biosynthesized (made) from pyruvic acid.

See also AMINO ACID, ESSENTIAL AMINO ACIDS, ALS GENE

Value-Added Grains See VALUE-ENHANCED GRAINS

Value-Enhanced Grains Grains that possess novel traits that are economically valuable (e.g., higher-than-normal protein content, better **quality** protein, higher-than-normal oil content, etc.). For example, high-oil corn (maize) possesses a kernel oil content of 5.8% or greater vs. oil content of 3.5% or less for traditional No. 2 yellow corn.

Glutamate dehydrogenase (GDH) corn (maize) possesses a kernel protein content that tends to be approximately 10% greater than the protein content of traditional corn (maize) varieties.

High-amylose corn possesses a kernel amylose content of 50% or more of the total kernel starch, etc.

See also HIGH-OIL CORN, PROTEIN, AMY-LOSE, HIGH-AMYLOSE CORN, OPAGUE-2, FLOURY-2, GENETIC ENGINEERING, LOW-PHYTATE CORN, LOW-PHYTATE SOYBEANS, TRAIT, HIGH-LYSINE CORN, HIGH-METHIONINE CORN, HIGH-PHYTASE CORN AND SOYBEANS, HIGH-OLEIC-OIL SOYBEANS, HIGH-STEARATE SOYBEANS, GLUTAMATE DEHYDROGENASE, HIGH-SUCROSE SOYBEANS, HIGH-LAURATE CANOLA, HIGH-LACTOFERRIN RICE

van der Waals Forces The relatively weak forces of attraction between molecules that contribute to intermolecular bonding (i.e., binding together two or more adjacent molecules). Historically, it was thought that van der Waals forces were always weaker than the hydrogen bond forces responsible for intramolecular bonding. However, in 1995, Dr. Alfred French discovered that van der Waals forces are primarily responsible for holding together a mass of cellulose molecules, with hydrogen bonding playing a lesser role. During 2000, Kellar Autumn discovered that van der Waals forces (acting between **foot skin hairs** of a gecko and the surface on which the foot is placed) are responsible for enabling the Tokay gecko (*Gecko gecko*) to climb vertical surfaces and also to hang upside-down. These forces work (to "adhere" a gecko's foot) even underwater or in a vacuum.

See also CELLULOSE, CELLULASE, MOLECULAR WEIGHT, WEAK INTER-ACTIONS, IMMOBILIZATION

Vascular Endothelial Growth Factor (VEGF) A human growth factor (GF) that causes angiogenesis (i.e., growth or proliferation of blood vessels or endothelium and also endothelial cells). Discovered in 1989 by Napoleone Ferrara.

See also GROWTH FACTOR, ENDOTHE-LIUM, ENDOTHELIAL CELLS, ANGIO-GENESIS, APTAMERS

Vector The agent used (by researchers) to carry new genes into cells. Plasmids currently are the biological vectors of choice, although viruses and other biological vectors such as *Agrobacterium tumefaciens* bacteria or BACs are increasingly being used for this purpose. Nonbiological vectors include the metal microparticles (coated with genes), which are "shot" into cells by the Biolistic® gene gun.

See also PLASMID, GENE, CELL, RETRO-VIRAL VECTORS, PROTOPLASM, *AGRO-BACTERIUM TUMEFACIENS*, BACTERIA, BIOLISTIC® GENE GUN, MICROPARTI-CLES, BACULOVIRUS EXPRESSION VECTORS (BEVs), BAC

VEGF Acronym for **vascular endothelial growth factor.**

See VASCULAR ENDOTHELIAL GROWTH FACTOR (VEGF)

Vernalization Refers to the process by which plants "sense" the cold of winter and activate the plant's innate defense response to cold stress, thereby they await spring to begin their flowering.

For example, in the wheat plant (*Triticum aestivum*), a gene known as **VRN2** represses flowering. However, exposure of that plant to prolonged cold will downregulate that gene (thereby enabling flowering to begin when spring's warm weather arrives).

During 2003, Kan Wang and coworkers were able to initiate earlier vernalization in soybean, corn (maize), and rice plants via insertion of a **VRN2 analogous** tobacco plant gene. One result of that was to confer greater resistance to cold temperatures.

See also WHEAT, GENE, DOWNREGU-LATING

Vertical Gene Transfer See OUTCROS-SING

V

Very-Low-Density Lipoproteins (VLDL)
VLDLs and LDLPs are the specific lipoproteins that are most likely to **deposit cholesterol** on artery walls inside the human body, which increases risk of coronary heart disease (CHD).
See also LOW-DENSITY LIPOPROTEINS (LDLP), LIPOPROTEIN, APOLIPOPROTEINS, CHOLESTEROL

Vesicle A small vacuole.
See VESICULAR TRANSPORT, VACUOLES

Vesicular Transport (of a protein) One of three means for a protein molecule to pass between compartments within eucaryotic cells. The compartment "wall" (membrane) possesses a "sensor" (receptor) that detects the presence of correct protein (e.g., after that protein has been synthesized in the cell's ribosomes), and then bulges outward along with that protein molecule. The membrane bulge containing the protein then "breaks off" and carries (transports) the protein to its destination in another compartment in the cell.
See also PROTEIN, EUCARYOTE, CELL, RIBOSOMES, MICROTUBULES, SIGNALLING, VAGINOSIS, ENDOCYTOSIS, GATED TRANSPORT

VFP Acronym for **visible fluorescent proteins**.
See VISIBLE FLUORESCENT PROTEINS

Viral Transactivating Protein The specific protein used by a lytic virus to "switch on" the cascade of gene regulation by which that virus "takes over" a healthy cell and subverts its molecular processes (machinery) to produce virus components. This (transactivating) protein is key to the whole lytic cycle of the virus and, therefore, a potential target for therapeutic intervention.
See also LYTIC INFECTION, TRANSACTIVATING PROTEIN, VIRUS, PROTEIN, CELL, GENE CASCADE, TRANSACTIVATING PROTEIN

Virion An intact virus particle (e.g., prior to it entering a cell to "infect" the cell). A virion consists of a protein coat (known as a **capsid**) around a central core composed of genetic material (DNA or RNA).
See also VIRUS, CELL, CAPSID, PROTEIN, RIBONUCLEIC ACID (RNA), DEOXYRIBONUCLEIC ACID (DNA)

Viroid Refers to certain plant pathogens (i.e., plant-disease-causing virus-like entities) capable of reproducing on their own (unlike a true virus).
See also PATHOGEN, VIRUS

Virotherapy Refers to the use of viruses (i.e., modified to prevent any harm to patent) in the treatment of a disease (e.g., cancer).
Examples include:

- During the 1950s, researchers showed that an adenovirus was able to attack and kill cervical cancer cells.
- During 2005, Stephen Russell and Irvin S. Y. Chen were able to "infect" cancer cells in mice with modified viruses, which killed the cancer cells but did not harm the adjacent healthy tissues.

See also MAGIC BULLET, VIRUS, CANCER, ADENOVIRUS

Virtual HTS See *IN SILICO* SCREENING, HIGH-THROUGHPUT SCREENING (HTS)

Virus A simple, noncellular particle (entity) that can reproduce only inside living cells (of other organisms), which was first proved to exist in 1892 by Dimitry Ivanovsky. The simple structure of viruses is their most important characteristic. Most viruses consist only of a genetic material — either DNA (deoxyribonucleic acid) or RNA (ribonucleic acid) — and a protein coating. This (combination) material is categorized as a nucleoprotein. Some viruses also have membranous envelopes (coatings). They are able to "inject" their genetic material into (host) cells because the internal pressure inside viruses is greater than inside the host cells.

Viruses are "alive" in that they can reproduce — although only by taking over a cell's "synthetic genetic machinery" — but they have none of the other characteristics of living organisms. Viruses cause a large variety of significant diseases in plants and animals, as well as humans. Viruses can (e.g., as one part of the disease) cause **gene silencing**.

In 1970, it was discovered that some RNA viruses (known as retroviruses) are able to utilize viral reverse transcriptase to cause (infected) cells to make DNA copies of those particular viruses. That "viral DNA" is then able to incorporate itself into the (infected) cell in a manner that transforms that cell into a cancer cell. For example, infections by hepatitis B virus, hepatitis C virus, and some human papilloma viruses can lead to cancer. Viruses present a philosophical problem to those who speak of living and nonliving systems because in and of itself a virus is not "alive" as we understand life, but rather represents "life potential" or "symbiotic life."

See also VACCINIA, NUCLEOPROTEINS, RETROVIRUSES, TOBACCO MOSAIC VIRUS (TMV), VIRAL TRANSACTIVATING PROTEIN, GENE DELIVERY, ADENOVIRUS, REPLICON, NFκB, CANCER, REVERSE TRANSCRIPTASES, NEOANTIGEN, KINESIN

Viscosity A measure of a liquid's resistance to flow, as expressed in units called poise (P; gm per cm per sec). The degree of "thickness" or "syrupiness" of a liquid.

Visfatin A protein discovered during 2004 by Iichiro Shimomura, which is secreted by visceral adipose cells (i.e., **vis**ceral **fat** tissue surrounding the body's organs). In some aspects, visfatin has some of the same effects as insulin (e.g., stimulate glucose uptake by the body, which lowers blood sugar levels). Visfatin binds to insulin receptors in the body without interfering with the same binding by insulin. Visfatin is sometimes called **PBEF.**

See also PROTEIN, ADIPOKINES, ADIPOSE, GLUCOSE (GLc), INSULIN, RECEPTORS, PBEF

Visible Fluorescent Proteins Refers to a number of proteins, many of them naturally present in some species of organisms, which visibly fluoresce when illuminated with light of relevant wavelength. Examples include green fluorescent protein (GFP), cyan fluorescent protein (CFP), yellow fluorescent protein (YFP), kusabira orange, etc.

See also GREEN FLUORESCENT PROTEIN, KUSABIRA ORANGE

Vitafoods See NUTRACEUTICALS

Vitamers See VITAMIN

Vitamin The modern term that is based on the original phrase "**vital amine**" (or "**vitamine**"), which was coined by Casimir Funk in the early 1900s. Most vitamins are actually "families" of chemically related isomers (i.e., vitamers) that cause the same or similar metabolic impact (benefit) in most animals (including humans) that consume those vitamins. Some compounds are vitamins for certain species of animals but are not for certain other species. In general, a vitamin is an organic compound required in tiny amounts (for optimal growth, proper biological functioning, and maintenance of health of an organism). Vitamins are commonly classified into two categories — fat soluble and water soluble. Vitamins A, D, E, and K are fat soluble, whereas vitamin C (ascorbic acid) and members of the vitamin B complex group are water soluble.

In general, the vitamins play catalytic and regulatory roles in the body's metabolism. Among the water-soluble vitamins, the B vitamins apparently function as coenzymes (nonprotein parts of enzymes). Vitamin C's coenzyme role, if any, has not been established. Part of the importance of vitamin C to the body may arise from its strong antioxidant action. The functions of the fat-soluble vitamins are less well understood. Some of them, too, may contribute to enzyme activity; others are essential to the functioning of cellular membranes (on the surface of cells).

Some vitamins act as transcription factors. Vitamin A is able to regulate the expression of certain genes in the embryos of mammals via one of its metabolites, retinoic acid. Those embryo cells contain nuclear receptors (which bring the retinoic acid "signal" from outside into the cell's nucleus) on their cell membrane surface. Retinoic acid then (via the nuclear receptors) regulates the expression of the genes that cause embryonic cell differentiation into complex body structures, such as legs and arms, of the growing embryo.

See also ENZYME, CATALYST, COENZYME, METABOLISM, METABOLITE, GENE, EXPRESS, BETA-CAROTENE, EMBRYOLOGY, RETINOIDS, PROTEIN, CELL, RECEPTORS, SIGNALING, CHOLINE, SIGNALING MOLECULES, SIGNAL TRANSDUCTION, NUCLEAR HORMONE RECEPTORS, LYCOPENE, LUTEIN, FATS, TRANSCRIPTION FACTORS, SPECIES, AVIDIN, VITAMIN E, BIOTIN, TOCOPHEROLS, TOCOTRIENOLS, ANTIOXIDANTS, INOSITOL

V

Vitamin E Refers to a group of related, naturally occurring compounds consisting of tocopherol and tocotrienol "families." It is a fat-soluble vitamin with antioxidant properties (i.e., helps prevent lipids in the body from breaking down). Vitamin E is especially effective in preventing oxidation of low-density lipoproteins (so-called "bad cholesterol"), whose oxidation products (e.g., beta hydroxycholesterol) can be deposited onto the interior walls of blood vessels (e.g., arteries) in the form of **plaque** (which can result in the disease atherosclerosis) and/or adversely increasing blood platelet aggregation (e.g., clotting).

Vitamin E occurs naturally in soybeans, cereal grains, etc., so it can be considered a phytochemical. In 2000, the Institute of Medicine of the U.S. National Academy of Sciences issued a report that called for an increase in the amount of vitamin E consumed each day, to improve citizens' health.

See also VITAMIN, OXIDATIVE STRESS, ANTIOXIDANTS, PHYTOCHEMICALS, OXIDATION, LIPIDS, CHOLESTEROL, LOW-DENSITY LIPOPROTEINS (LDLP), ATHEROSCLEROSIS, PLAQUE, PLATELETS, PHYTOCHEMICALS, NATIONAL ACADEMY OF SCIENCES (NAS), TOCOPHEROLS, TOCOTRIENOLS, SOYBEAN PLANT

Volicitin A chemical compound produced by beet armyworm caterpillars (*Spodoptera exigua*) after they have consumed some linoleic acid (in plants they chew on, such as corn or maize). The body cells of beet armyworm caterpillars conjugate (i.e., chemically join) the linoleic acid molecules on to glutamine molecules. The conjugated molecule, consisting of one linoleic acid (molecule) joined to one glutamine (molecule), is known as volicitin.

When beet armyworm caterpillars subsequently chew on corn or maize plants, some volicitin is inadvertently inserted by those caterpillars into the tissue of the corn (maize). That volicitin causes the corn (maize) plant to emit certain compounds known as **green leafy volatiles** that have the following functions:

- Attract the types of wasps that are natural enemies of the beet armyworm, leading those wasps to attack the beet armyworm caterpillars that are feeding on the maize or corn.
- Activate natural innate chemical defense systems within nearby corn (maize) plants.

See also LINOLEIC ACID, CORN, GLUTAMINE, CELL, OCTADECANOID–JASMONATE SIGNAL COMPLEX

Voltage-Gated Ion Channel A transmembrane (i.e., extending from one side of a cell membrane to the other side) ion channel. Passage (e.g., of ions or atoms) through a voltage-gated ion channel is controlled (i.e., this channel is opened or closed) by a membrane potential (i.e., **electrical charge difference** between one side of the cell membrane and the other).

See also ION CHANNELS, ION, CELL, MEMBRANES (OF A CELL), PLASMA MEMBRANE

Volume Rendering Refers to technologies utilized (e.g., in confocal microscopes, ultrasound imaging machines, data mining, etc.) to convert numerous "slices" (two-dimensional) of a given three-dimensional volume (e.g., the inside of a living cell, a living organ within a body, etc.) into a compiled-together three-dimensional image.

See also DATA MINING, CONFOCAL MICROSCOPY, CELL

Vomitoxin See *FUSARIUM*, MYCOTOXINS

VRN2 Gene See VERNALIZATION

W

Water Activity (A$_w$) A measure of the amount of "free" **unbound** water (e.g., in a processed food product) that is available to sustain the growth of microorganisms (spoilage) and to sustain undesired chemical reactions (e.g., "staling" of baked food products). Most bacteria are unable to grow in foods possessing a water activity below 0.90. Most yeasts and molds that cause spoilage cannot grow in foods possessing a water activity below 0.80. Sugars can be added to certain foods in order to increase A$_w$, because they "bind up" the (formerly) free water present.

See also MICROORGANISM, HYDRO-PHILIC, BACTERIA, YEAST, *PENICIL-LIUM*

Water-Soluble Fiber Food fiber (e.g., oat fiber, barley fiber, carob fiber, soybean fiber, guar gum fiber) that dissolves in water. Water-soluble fiber apparently absorbs low-density lipoproteins (LDLP) in the intestine before the fiber passes from the body; also these fibers inhibit absorption of LDLP by the body's intestinal walls by increasing the viscosity of the intestinal contents. These two effects thus lower the amount of "bad" cholesterol (i.e., LDLP can lead to hardening or blockage of arteries) in the body and thereby lower the risk of coronary heart disease (CHD). Additional to those two effects, water-soluble fiber also absorbs or binds bile acid and causes it to be excreted with the fiber. This helps to lower cholesterol levels in the body (bloodstream) because the liver synthesizes ("manufactures") more bile acids (to replace those absorbed and removed by the fiber) from cholesterol.

Water-soluble fiber from oat bran is a polysac-charide in a form known as beta-glucan (β) and is composed entirely of glucose (molecular) units. U.S. FDA regulations also include gums, pectins, mucilages, and certain hemi-celluloses in the category of water-soluble fiber. Soybean flour or meal is also a source of water-soluble fiber.

In 1997, the U.S. FDA approved a (label) health claim that associates consumption of beta-glu-can oat fiber with reduced blood cholesterol content and with reduced coronary heart disease (CHD). In 1998, the U.S. FDA approved a (label) health claim that associates soluble fiber from psyllium husks with reduced risk of coronary heart disease (CHD).

See also HIGH-DENSITY LIPOPROTEINS (HDLPs), LOW-DENSITY LIPOPROTEINS (LDLP), POLYSACCHARIDES, GLUCOSE (GLc), FOOD AND DRUG ADMINISTRA-TION (FDA). ATHEROSCLEROSIS, CORO-NARY HEART DISEASE (CHD), SOYBEAN MEAL, SOYBEAN PLANT, HIGH-MAN-NOGALACTAN SOYBEANS, CHOLES-TEROL, PLAQUE

Waxy Corn Refers to corn (maize) hybrids that produce kernels in which the starch con-tained is at least 99% amylopectin as against the average of 72 to 76% amylopectin in tra-ditional cornstarch.

See also CORN, STARCH, AMYLOPECTIN

Waxy Wheat Refers to varieties of wheat (*Triticum aestivum*) that produce a higher amylopectin content and, thus, a lower amy-lose content in the starch within their seeds than traditional varieties of wheat. For example, bread flour made from **waxy wheat** would contain 0 to 3% amylose vs. 24 to 27% amylose in bread flour made from traditional varieties of wheat. Because bread made from such waxy (i.e., lower amylose) wheat becomes firm at a much slower rate than bread made from traditional wheat vari-eties, these breads would probably require less shortening (added to the flour) to keep it soft.

See also WHEAT, STARCH, AMYLOSE, AMYLOPECTIN

Weak Interactions The forces between atoms that are less strong than the forces involved in a covalent (chemical) bond (between two atoms). Weak interactions include ionic (chemical) bonds, hydrogen bonds, and van der Waals forces.

See also VAN DER WAALS FORCES

Weevils A term that refers to a number of insects that consume grains (i.e., grown and used by man). Many of the weevils consume and proliferate in stored grains (e.g., the Indian meal moth *Plodia interpunctella*) and stored grain products (e.g., flour, etc.).

One example of a weevil is the insect known as the pea weevil, which lay their eggs on pea pods or dried peas. When the larvae hatch, they burrow into the pod and eat the peas.

The insect *Theocolax elegans* attacks the larvae of maize weevils (*Sitophilus granarius* and *Triboleum castaneum*), rice weevils (*Sitophilus oryzae*), and the lesser grain borer. Thus, it could potentially be added to grain storage bins (silos) as part of an integrated pest management (IPM) program. Research indicates that the "green" pesticide Spinosad is effective in controlling the lesser grain borer and other weevils. Spinosad and its registered trademark are owned by Dow Chemical Company.

See also INTEGRATED PEST MANAGE-MENT (IPM), BIOTIN, AVIDIN, ALPHA AMYLASE INHIBITOR-1, SPINOSAD, SPINOSYNS

Western Blot Test A test that is performed on biological samples such as blood (after centrifugation to remove red blood cells from the blood) to **detect proteins** (e.g., AIDS-related antibodies) individually. Gel electrophoresis is used to separate the AIDS antigen proteins of killed (known) AIDS viruses. Next, the protein bands (resulting from the gel electrophoresis) are exposed to the blood being tested and (AIDS) antibodies stick to specific individual antigens (bands), which are then identified (as being present in the tested blood) using dyes.

See also ACQUIRED IMMUNE DEFICIENCY SYNDROME (AIDS), ANTIBODY, ANTI-GEN, ELECTROPHORESIS, POLYACRYLA-MIDE GEL ELECTROPHORESIS (PAGE), BASOPHILIC, BUFFY COAT (CELLS)

Western Corn Rootworm Latin name *Diabrotica virgifera virgifera* LeConte.

See CORN ROOTWORM

WGSS Acronym for **whole-genome shotgun sequencing.**

See SHOTGUN SEQUENCING

Wheat Refers to a family of related small grains that descended from the natural crossing of three Middle East grasses (*Triticum monococcum*, *Aegilops speltoids*, and *Triticum tauscii*) centuries ago. As a result, wheat's genome is triploid (i.e., it incorporates three complete sets of deoxyribonucleic acid [DNA]), and contains approximately 17 billion base pairs (bp).

Wheat is historically an annual plant that can attain a height of 4 ft (1.2 m), although variations (e.g., shorter) have been bred. The Latin name for traditional (bread) wheat is *Triticum aestivum* and that for durum (pasta) wheat is *Triticum durum desf.* Historically, wheat kernels have contained 15% or less protein. Most of the rest of the kernel is composed of starch (amylose and amylopectin).

See also GENOME, DEOXYRIBONUCLEIC ACID (DNA), BASE PAIR (bp), HYBRID-IZATION (PLANT GENETICS), TRIPLOID, WHEAT TAKE-ALL DISEASE, WHEAT SCAB, KARNAL BUNT, WHEAT HEAD BLIGHT, GLUTEN, GLUTENIN, PRO-TEIN, STARCH, AMYLOSE, AMYLOPEC-TIN, *TELETHIA CONTROVERSIA KOON* SMUT, OXALATE OXIDASE

Wheat Head Blight See *FUSARIUM*

Wheat Scab See *FUSARIUM*

Wheat Take-All Disease A fungal disease that attacks wheat (*Triticum aestivum*) plant roots and causes dry rot and premature death of the plant.

Certain strains of *Brassica* plants and *Pseudomonas* bacteria produce compounds that can act as natural antifungal agents against the wheat take-all fungus.

See also FUNGUS, BACTERIA, GENETI-CALLY ENGINEERED MICROBIAL PESTI-CIDES (GEMP), *BRASSICA*, ALLELOPATHY

Whiskers™ A trademarked method for inserting DNA (genes) into plant cells so that those plant cells will then incorporate that new DNA and express the proteins coded for by that DNA.

Developed by ICI Seeds Inc. (Garst Seed Company) in 1993, Whiskers™ is an alternative method of inserting DNA into plant cells (e.g., the Biolistic® gene gun, *Agrobacterium tumefaciens*, the "shotgun" method, etc.); it consists of needle-like crystals ("whiskers") of silicon carbide.

The crystals are placed in a container along with the plant cells and then mixed at high speed, which causes the crystals to pierce the plant cell walls with microscopic "holes" (passages). Then, the new DNA (gene) is added, which flows into the plant cells. The plant cells then incorporate the new genes, and thus they have been genetically engineered.

See also BIOLISTIC® GENE GUN, *AGROBACTERIUM TUMEFACIENS*, "SHOTGUN" METHOD, GENETIC ENGINEERING, GENE, BIOSEEDS, CODING SEQUENCE, PROTEIN, CELL, DEOXYRIBONUCLEIC ACID (DNA)

White Biotechnology Term utilized in some countries to refer to **industrial** applications of genetic engineering. One example would be production of laccase in genetically engineered organisms.

See also GENETIC ENGINEERING, LACCASE

White Blood Cells See LEUKOCYTES

White Corpuscles See LEUKOCYTES

White Mold Disease The common name that is used to refer to a plant disease caused under certain conditions (e.g., moist, humid, etc.) by the *Sclerotinia sclerotiorum* fungus.

In 1998, the U.S. Environmental Protection Agency (EPA) approved one herbicide (COBRA™ owned by Valent Corporation), whose active ingredient is the chemical LACTOFIN, to be applied to soybean plants "at or near bloom stage" in order to trigger **systemic acquired resistance (SAR,** a sort of "immune response") in those soybean plants against white mold disease. Use of no-tillage crop production (methodology) for some crops helps to reduce the incidence of white mold disease.

See also FUNGUS, SYSTEMIC ACQUIRED RESISTANCE (SAR), NO-TILLAGE CROP PRODUCTION, SOYBEAN PLANT

Whole-Cell Patch-Clamp Recording Developed by Bert Sakmann and Erwin Neher in 1976, this is a method for measuring the current or potential of a single ion channel.

Although the initial 1976 technique was slow and laborious (i.e., "hook up" the cell to electrodes to measure electrical potential),

several companies have since developed easier and faster methodologies to measure the electrical potential across a cell's ion channels as that cell is exposed to one or more pharmaceutical candidate compounds.

See also CELL, MEMBRANE, ION, ION CHANNELS, TARGET (OF A THERAPEUTIC AGENT), HIGH-THROUGHPUT SCREENING (HTS)

Whole-Genome Shotgun Sequencing See SHOTGUN SEQUENCING

Wide Cross Refers to the plant-breeding technologies or techniques that are utilized to cross two plant species that would not normally cross in nature.

See also TRADITIONAL BREEDING METHODS, TISSUE CULTURE, SPECIES

Wide Spectrum See GRAM STAIN

Wild Type The traditional or historical form of an organism as ordinarily encountered in nature, in contrast to domesticated strains, natural mutant, or laboratory mutant individuals (organisms). One example of a measurable difference between the two types is that the wild strains of animals respond to the presence of EMF fields (e.g., weak magnetic fields such as those generated near power transmission cables), but laboratory strains of the same animals do not.

See also STRAIN, MUTANT, PHENOTYPE, GENOTYPE, PSORALENE, SOLANINE

Wobble The ability of the third base in a tRNA (transfer RNA) anticodon to form a hydrogen bond with any of two or three bases at the 3′ end of a codon. This wobble (nonspecificity) allows a single tRNA species to recognize several different codons.

See also TRANSFER RNA (tRNA), CODON, BASE PAIR (bp), REDUNDANCY

World Trade Organization (WTO) The international organization consisting of more than 100 nations that signed the General Agreement on Tariffs and Trade (GATT), which contained 38 Articles that lay out the rules and procedures that signatory countries must observe in their conduct of international trade and trade policy.

GATT was WTO's predecessor body. The WTO permits signatory countries to ban specific imports from other countries in order to protect the health of humans, animals, or plants. Such import bans are allowed based on the (GATT/WTO) Agreement on Sanitary and Phytosanitary Measures, or the Agreement on Technical Barriers to Trade, which were approved in 1994 by GATT. WTO was established on January 1, 1995.

The WTO's Agreement on Sanitary and Phytosanitary (SPS) Measures requires that such import bans must be based on sound, internationally agreed science. WTO recognizes only the following three international science organizations in order to resolve SPS disputes between member nations:

- Codex Alimentarius Commission — for foods and food ingredients
- International Plant Protection Convention (IPPC) — for plants
- International Office of Epizootics (OIE) — for animal diseases

See also SPS, CODEX ALIMENTARIUS COMMISSION, INTERNATIONAL PLANT PROTECTION CONVENTION (IPPC), INTERNATIONAL OFFICE OF EPIZOOTICS (OIE)

WP 900 See Z-DNA

WTO See WORLD TRADE ORGANIZATION (WTO)

X

X Chromosome A sex chromosome that usually occurs paired in each female cell, and single (i.e., unpaired) in each male cell in those species in which the male typically has two unlike sex chromosomes (e.g., humans).
See also CHROMOSOMES, IMPRINTING

X Receptors See LIVER X RECEPTORS (LXR), FARNESOID X RECEPTORS (FXR), RETINOID X RECEPTORS (RXR)

X-Ray Crystallography The use of diffraction patterns produced by x-ray scattering from crystals (of a given material's molecules) to determine the three-dimensional structure of the molecules. First done in 1958 by Max Perutz and John Cowdery Kendrew (to determine a myoglobin molecule structure), x-ray crystallography data is also utilized today for efforts such as rational drug design.
See also PROTEIN, CONFIGURATION, CONFORMATION, TERTIARY STRUCTURE, PROTEIN FOLDING, RATIONAL DRUG DESIGN

Xanthine Oxidase An enzyme responsible for production of free radicals in the body. See also ENZYME, HUMAN SUPEROXIDE DISMUTASE (hSOD)

Xanthophylls A "family" of carotenoids (i.e., plant-produced pigments that act as protective antioxidants in photosynthetic plants and in the bodies of animals that consume those carotenoids). Xanthophylls are produced by yellow carrots and other plants.
Consumption of xanthophylls by humans and animals assists development of healthy eye tissue.
Research indicates that consumption of xanthophylls by humans helps prevent lung cancer and some other cancers.
See also CAROTENOIDS, ANTIOXIDANTS, OXIDATIVE STRESS, CANCER

Xenobiotic Compounds Compounds (e.g., veterinary drugs, agrochemical herbicides, etc.) that are designed to be used in an ecosystem comprising more than one species. For example, herbicides intended to kill weeds but leave commercial crops undamaged, or veterinary drugs intended to kill parasitic worms but leave the host livestock unharmed.

Xenogeneic Organs From the Greek word *xenos*, meaning "stranger." Xenogeneic literally means "strange genes." Refers to genetically engineered (e.g., "humanized") organs that have been grown within an animal of another species. For example, several companies are working to engineer and grow — inside swine — a number of organs to be transplanted into humans that need those organs (e.g., due to loss of their own organs via disease or accident). If successful, this would free human organ transplant recipients from having to continually use immunosuppressive drugs in order to keep their body from "rejecting" the new organ.
See also IMMUNOSUPPRESSIVE, GRAFT-VERSUS-HOST DISEASE (GVHD), CYCLOSPORIN, MAJOR HISTOCOMPATIBILITY COMPLEX (MHC), GENETIC ENGINEERING

Xenogenesis The (theoretical) production of offspring that are genetically different from and genotypically unrelated to either of the parents.
See also GENOTYPE, TRANSGENIC, HEREDITY, GENETICS, MEIOSIS, GENETIC CODE

Xenogenetic Organs See XENOGENEIC ORGANS

Xenogenic Organs See XENOGENEIC ORGANS

Xenograft See XENOTRANSPLANT

Xenotransplant From the Greek word *xenos,* meaning "stranger." Xenotransplant is the implantation of an organ or limb from one species to another organism in a different species. When performed in animals, "rejection" of the transplant by the recipient's immune system is a common response.

See also GRAFT-VERSUS-HOST DISEASE (GVHD), XENOGENEIC ORGANS

Xenotropic Virus A virus that can grow or reproduce within one or more species **other** than its normal host species.

See also VIRUS, ZOONOSES, SPECIES

X

Y

Y Chromosome A sex chromosome that is characteristic of male zygotes (and cells) in species in which the male typically has two unlike sex chromosomes.

See also CHROMOSOMES

YAC See YEAST ARTIFICIAL CHROMOSOMES (YAC)

Yeast A fungus of the family *Saccharomycetaceae*, which is used especially in the making of alcoholic liquors and as a leavening agent in bread making.

Some strains of yeast cells are also commonly used in bioprocesses because they are relatively simple to genetically engineer (via recombinant DNA) and relatively easy to propagate (via fermentation) to yield desired products (e.g., proteins).

See also FUNGUS, STRAIN, PREBIOTICS, FERMENTATION, GENETIC ENGINEERING, YEAST ARTIFICIAL CHROMOSOMES (YAC), RECOMBINANT DNA (rDNA)

Yeast Artificial Chromosomes (YAC) Pieces of DNA (usually human DNA) that have been cloned (made) inside living yeast cells. Whereas most bacterial vectors cannot carry DNA pieces that are larger than 50 base pairs, YACs can typically carry DNA pieces that are as large as several hundred base pairs.

See also YEAST, CHROMOSOMES, HUMAN ARTIFICIAL CHROMOSOMES (HAC), BACTERIAL ARTIFICIAL CHROMOSOMES (BAC), *ARABIDOPSIS THALIANA*, DEOXYRIBONUCLEIC ACID (DNA), CLONE (A MOLECULE), VECTOR, BASE PAIR (bp), MEGA-YEAST ARTIFICIAL CHROMOSOMES (MEGA YAC)

Yeast Episomal Plasmid (YEP) A cloning vehicle used for introduction of constructions (i.e., genes and pieces of genetic material) into certain yeast strains at high copy number. YEP can replicate in both *Escherichia coli* and certain yeast strains.

See also PLASMID, CASSETTE, CLONE (AN ORGANISM), GENE, GENETIC ENGI-NEERING, *ESCHERICHIA COLIFORM (E. COLI)*, COPY NUMBER

Yeast Two-Hybrid System The oldest of the two-hybrid systems, utilized to analyze protein–protein interactions.

Discovered in 1989 by Stanley Fields, it utilizes the fact that the **gene activation system** for *Saccharomyces cerevisiae* yeast's *GAL4* gene is activated by a transcriptional factor possessing **two** distinctly separate functional domains. One of those two domains must interact with a second domain (i.e., in a genetically engineered yeast-created fusion protein containing a portion of the "known" protein) in order to cause transcription of the *GAL4* gene. *GAL4* is required to initiate expression of proteins that are central to galactose metabolism in that yeast.

See also TWO-HYBRID SYSTEMS, PROTEIN, PROTEIN INTERACTION ANALYSIS, GENE, GENE EXPRESSION, GENETIC ENGINEERING, TRANSCRIPTION, TRANSCRIPTIONAL ACTIVATOR, CODING SEQUENCE, DOMAIN (OF A PROTEIN), FUSION PROTEIN, GALACTOSE (Gal), METABOLISM

YFP Acronym for **Yellow Fluorescent Protein**. See VISIBLE FLUORESCENT PROTEINS.

YSTR DNA Refers to **Y chromosome Short Tandem Repeat** DNA, which is DNA found only in men (because only men have the Y chromosome).

Utilizing certain specific **STR markers** (i.e., based on detectable repeated DNA sequences in Y chromosome), YSTR DNA can be utilized for some genetic studies (e.g., to track parentage) and for some forensic efforts (e.g., crime evidence determination). SNPs within such YSTR DNA can be utilized to increase the "completeness" of some SNP maps.

See also DEOXYRIBONUCLEIC ACID (DNA), Y CHROMOSOME, SEQUENCE (OF A DNA MOLECULE), MARKER (DNA SEQUENCE), SINGLE-NUCLEOTIDE POLYMORPHISMS (SNPs), SNP MAP

Y

Z

Z-DNA A left-handed helix (molecular structure) of DNA, in contrast to A-DNA and B-DNA which are right-handed helix structures. The difference is in the direction of the double-helix twist. Z-DNA has the most base pairs per turn (in the helix), and so has the least twisted structure; it is very "skinny" and its name is taken from the zigzag path that the sugar-phosphate "backbone" follows along the helix. This is quite different from the smoothly curving path of the backbone of **B-DNA**. The Z-form of DNA has been found in polymers that have an alternating purine-pyrimidine sequence.

One possible biological importance of Z-DNA is that it is much more stable at lower salt concentrations, and there is a possibility that the Z-DNA form (of DNA within cells) is the cause of certain diseases (e.g., certain cancers).

During 2000, Jonathan Chaires/Waldernar Priebe/John Trent showed that WP 900 (i.e., the enantiomer of daunorubicin, a natural chemical compound which inhibits cancer) binds tightly (and selectively) to a Z-DNA polymer.

See also CELL, DEOXYRIBONUCLEIC ACID (DNA), B-DNA, HELIX, DOUBLE HELIX, A-DNA, PURINE, BASE PAIR (bp), PYRIMIDINE, ENANTIOMERS, CANCER

Z-ring See TUBULIN

Zearalenone One of the mycotoxins (i.e., toxins produced by a fungus), it causes reproductive difficulties in swine (e.g., reduced sperm production, halting of estrus, etc.) when consumed by animals (e.g., in contaminated grain such as corn/maize). It causes a variety of adverse health impacts when consumed by some other species of animals. Zearalenone is produced by certain strains of *Fusarium* fungi (e.g., *Fusarium culmorum, Fusarium graminearum, Fusarium crookweliense, Fusarium oxysporum*, etc.) when climate (e.g., moisture and temperature) conditions during the grain growing season, combined with entry points (e.g., holes chewed into the grain plants by insects) facilitate growth of those *Fusarium* strains in grain.

See also TOXIN, MYCOTOXINS, FUNGUS, STRAIN, *FUSARIUM*, LACTONASE, *FUSARIUM GRAMINEARUM*

Zeaxanthin A carotenoid (i.e., "light harvesting" compound utilized in photosyntheis) that is naturally produced in Brussels sprouts, summer squash, maize, avocado, green beans, and dark green leafy vegetables. Zeaxanthin is also naturally present within the retina of the human eye.

Zeaxanthin is a phytochemical/nutraceutical whose consumption by humans has been shown to reduce risk of the disease age-related macular degeneration, a leading cause of blindness of older people.

See also CAROTENOIDS, PHOTOSYNTHESIS, PHYTOCHEMICALS, NUTRACEUTICALS

Zebra Fish The fish *Danio rerio*.

See also MODEL ORGANISM

ZFP Acronym for **zinc finger protein**.

See ZINC FINGER PROTEINS.

Zinc Finger Proteins Protein molecules (transcription factors) bearing at least one **"finger shaped"** molecular appurtenance which acts to either repress, or to activate transcription (i.e., of the gene the "finger" touches within the DNA molecule). For example, nuclear receptors contain two zinc fingers which target those receptors to **hormone response elements** (i.e., specific DNA sequences that initiate the activation of applicable gene(s) for that receptor).

Thus, zinc finger proteins could potentially be utilized in FUNCTIONAL GENOMICS (i.e., to study the specific function of a given gene).

Zinc finger DNA-binding proteins possess two domains:

- A "DNA recognition domain" which locates and binds itself to a specific DNA sequence
- A "functional domain" which initiates (or inhibits) transcription

Zinc finger proteins are also sometimes involved in DNA repair.

See also NUCLEAR RECEPTORS, PROTEIN, GENE, TRANSCRIPTION, REPRESSION (of gene transcripton), PROMOTER, DEOXYRIBOUCLEIC ACID (DNA), FUNCTIONAL GENOMICS, DOMAIN (OF A PROTEIN), SEQUENCE (OF A DNA MOLECULE), INITIATION FACTORS, INHIBITION, TRANSCRIPTION FACTORS, EDITING, DNA REPAIR

ZKBS (Central Committee on Biological Safety) The advisory body on safety in gene-splicing labs and plants for the German Government's Ministry of Health. It is the German counterpart of the American Government's Recombinant DNA Advisory Committee (RAC), Australia's Genetic Manipulation Advisory Committee (GMAC), Brazil's National Biosafety Commission (CTNBio), and the Kenya Biosafety Council.

The ZKBS is composed of 10 experts from the biology and ecology sectors, trade union representatives, plus representatives from the industrial sector and environmental pressure groups. The ZKBS advises the Ministry of Health and the individual German States (Länder), which regulate all recombinant DNA (i.e., gene-splicing) activities in Germany.

See also GENETIC MANIPULATION ADVISORY COMMITTEE (GMAC), CTNBio, KENYA BIOSAFETY CONCIL, GENE TECHNOLOGY OFFICE, RECOMBINANT DNA ADVISORY COMMITTEE (RAC), GENETIC ENGINEERING, RECOMBINANT DNA (rDNA), RECOMBINATION, BIOTECHNOLOGY, INDIAN DEPARTMENT OF BIOTECHNOLOGY, COMMISSION OF BIOMOLECULAR ENGINEERING

Zoonoses Diseases that are communicable from animals to humans.

Examples would include the diseases anthrax (caused by *Bacillus anthracis*), tularemia (caused by *Francisella tularensis*), etc.

Zoonotic See ZOONOSES

Zygote A fertilized egg formed as a result of the union of the male (sperm) and female (egg) sex cells. The zygote gives rise to the placenta (lining of the uterus) in addition to growing into (adult organism) body.

See also X CHROMOSOME, Y CHROMOSOME, TELOMERES, GAMETE, ORGANISM, CELL, CELL DIFFERENTIATION

Zyme Systems Chemical reactions characterized by the presence of an inactive precursor of an enzyme. The enzyme is activated via another enzyme that normally removes an extra piece of peptide chain at a physiologically appropriate time and place.

See also ZYMOGENS, FIBRIN, PRO-DRUG THERAPY, DIGESTION (WITHIN ORGANISMS), NANOBODIES

Zymogens The enzymatically inactive precursors of certain proteolytic enzymes. The enzymes are inactive because they contain an extra piece of peptide. When this peptide is hydrolyzed (clipped away) by another proteolytic enzyme the zymogen is converted into the normal, active enzyme. Zymogens are sometimes referred to as **proenzymes**. The reason for the existence of zymogens may be to protect the cell, its machinery, and/or the place of manufacture within the cell from the potentially harmful or lethal effects of an active, proteolytic enzyme. In other words, the strategy is to activate the enzyme only when and especially where it is needed.

See also ENZYME, PROTEOLYTIC ENZYMES, FIBRIN, ZYME SYSTEMS, LIPOPROTEIN-ASSOCIATED COAGULATION (CLOT) INHIBITOR (LACI), PRO-DRUG THERAPY, NANOBODIES

Z